Ferret Medicine and Surgery

Ferret Medicine and Surgery

CATHY A. JOHNSON-DELANEY, DVM

Kirkland, Washington, USA

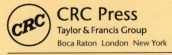

CRC Press
Taylor & Francis Group
Boca Raton London New York

CRC Press is an imprint of the
Taylor & Francis Group, an **informa** business

CRC Press
Taylor & Francis Group
6000 Broken Sound Parkway NW, Suite 300
Boca Raton, FL 33487-2742

First issued in paperback 2018

ISBN-13: 978-1-4987-0787-9 (hbk)
ISBN-13: 978-0-367-11245-5 (pbk)

Cover image of Zeus, courtesy of Vondelle McLaughlin.

DEDICATION

*I would like to dedicate this book to my husband Michael; Williard 'Skip' Nelson DVM; the staff
and ferrets of the Washington Ferret Rescue & Shelter; and all of my beloved ferrets over the years:
Simon, Robbie, Buddy, Tichuk, Cinnamon, Cyrano, Jack, Surfer, John, D'Argo, Stark, Chiana, Aeryn,
Moya, Annabelle the one-kidney wonder, Mittens, Gandolf, Pete, Claudia, Myka, Lena and Jinks.*

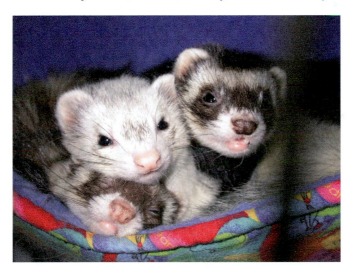

(Aeryn, Moya, Chiana)

CONTENTS

CHAPTER **11**   **EMERGENCY CARE**   **113**
John R. Chitty and Cathy A. Johnson-Delaney

CHAPTER 15   **DISORDERS OF THE EARS AND EYES**   **219**
Cathy A. Johnson-Delaney

CHAPTER 16   **DISORDERS OF THE HAEMIC, IMMUNOLOGICAL AND LYMPHATIC SYSTEMS**   **237**
Samantha Swisher and Angela M. Lennox

INTRODUCTION

In this book I have attempted to cover veterinary aspects of an incredible little creature – our domestic ferret (*Mustela putorius furo*). The book is designed to provide quick, concise information of immediate use to the practitioner.

Each chapter of disorders is designed to be inclusive although there are cross references to other chapters throughout, and there may be some highlights of anatomy and physiology included with each as a review.

It is not intended to be a complete textbook on ferrets but a working book to provide ready information. For more details, the reader is referred to Fox JG, Marini RP (eds). *Biology and Diseases of the Ferret, 3rd Edition* (2014), Wiley Blackwell; and Lewington JH (ed). *Ferret Husbandry, Medicine and Surgery, 2nd Edition* (2007), John H. Saunders Elsevier Ltd.

Much of the information is from experience, with references listed for further reading. The information is biased to that of the EU, UK, and US sources and conditions encountered.

I hope that the book provides a useful source and summary for the inexperienced and experienced veterinary practitioner, nurse/technician and veterinary student working with ferrets.

I want to thank all the contributors for the wealth of ferret medical knowledge they brought to the book. I could not have done it without you!

I would appreciate feedback and experiences that can add to future information resources.

Cathy A. Johnson-Delaney

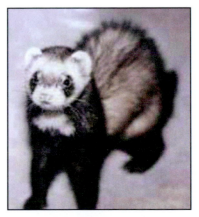

Fig. 1 Robbie McFerret Delaney, the first ferret to receive Lupron™ for adrenal disease.

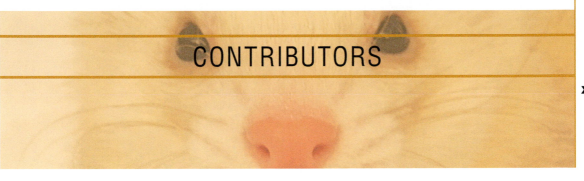

CONTRIBUTORS

John R. Chitty BVetMed CertZooMed CBiol
MSB MRCVS
Anton Vets
Andover, Hampshire, UK

Cathy A. Johnson-Delaney DVM
Washington Ferret Rescue and Shelter
Kirkland, Washington, USA

Angela M. Lennox DVM Dipl. ABVP (Avian) Exotic
Companion Mammal DECZM (Small Mammal)
Avian and Exotic Animal Clinic of Indianapolis
Indianapolis, Indiana, USA

Anna Meredith MA VetMB PhD CertLAS
DZooMed Dipl. ECZM MRCVS
Professor
Personal Chair of Zoological and Conservation
Medicine
Head of Exotic Animal and Wildlife Service
Hospital for Small Animals
Royal (Dick) School of Veterinary Studies
University of Edinburgh
Easter Bush Veterinary Centre
Roslin, Midlothian, Scotland

Susan E. Orosz PhD DVM Dipl. ABVP (Avian)
Dipl. ECZM (Avian)
Bird and Exotic Pet Wellness Center
Toledo, Ohio, USA

David Perpiñán DVM MSc Dipl. ECZM
(Herpetology) MRCVS
Lecturer in Exotic Animal and Wildlife Medicine
Hospital for Small Animals
Royal (Dick) School of Veterinary Studies
University of Edinburgh
Easter Bush Veterinary Centre
Roslin, Midlothian, Scotland

Jenna Richardson BVM&S, MRCVS
Hospital for Small Animals
Royal (Dick) School of Veterinary Studies
University of Edinburgh
Easter Bush Veterinary Centre
Roslin, Midlothian, Scotland

Nico J. Schoemaker DVM PhD Dipl. ECZM
(Small Mammal & Avian) Dipl. ABVP (Avian)
Division of Zoological Medicine
Department of Clinical Sciences of Companion
Animals
Faculty of Veterinary Medicine
Utrecht University
Utrecht, Netherlands

Samantha Swisher DVM
Avian and Exotic Animal Clinic of Indianapolis
Indianapolis, Indiana, USA

Yvonne R.A. van Zeeland DVM MVR PhD Dipl.
ECZM (Avian & Small Mammal)
Division of Zoological Medicine
Department of Clinical Sciences of Companion
Animals
Faculty of Veterinary Medicine, Utrecht
University
Utrecht, Netherlands

The following contributed images to this book:

Natalie Antinoff DVM DABVP (Avian)
Gulf Coast Veterinary Specialists
Houston, Texas, USA

Ferran Bargalló LV
Zoològic Badalona Veterinària
Badalona (Barcelona), Spain

Timothy Baszler DVM PhD Dipl. ACVP
Director and Pathologist
Washington Animal Disease Diagnostic
   Laboratory
Washington State University
Pullman, Washington, USA

Donald Brown DVM PhD
Vermont Veterinary Cardiology Services
Peak Veterinary Referral Center
Williston, Vermont, USA

Vittorio Capello DVM Dipl. ECZM
   (Small Mammal) Dipl. ABVP (Exotic Companion
   Mammals) European Veterinary Specialist in
   Zoological Medicine (Small Mammal)
Specialista in Malattie dei Piccoli Animali
   Clinica Veterinaria
S. SiroClinica Veterinaria Gran Sasso
Milano, Italy

Kevin Farlee BS
President
Washington Ferret Rescue & Shelter
Kirkland, Washington, USA

Michael Garner DVM DACVP
NW Zoopath
Monroe, Washington, USA

Jordi Jiménez LV
Clínica Veterinària Els Altres
Barcelona, Spain

Vondelle McLaughlin
Shelter Director
Washington Ferret Rescue & Shelter
Kirkland, Washington, USA

Drury Reavill DVM DABVP (Avian and Reptile
   & Amphibian Practice) DACVP
Zoo/Exotic Pathology Service
Carmichael, California, USA

Robert A. Wagner VMD Dipl. ABVP
   (Exotic Companion Mammals)
Chief of Surgical Veterinary Services
Associate Professor Medicine
Division of Laboratory Animal Resources
University of Pittsburgh
Pittsburgh, Pennsylvania, USA

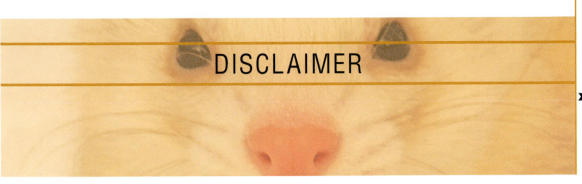

DISCLAIMER

THE dosages in this text are derived from published literature. Many dosages are empirical or based on clinical experience. Caution should be used because most uses and dosages listed are extra label. The authors have made every attempt to verify all dosages and references. Despite this, errors in the original sources or in the preparation of this book may have occurred. Users of this text should evaluate all dosages prior to use to determine that they are reasonable. The authors and publisher cannot be held responsible for misuse or misapplication of the material in this book.

5-HT	5-hydroxytryptamine	CT	computed tomography
ACD	adrenal cortical disease	cTnI	serum cardiac troponin I
ACE	angiotensin-converting enzyme	cTnT	serum cardiac troponin T
ACTH	adrenocorticotropic hormone	CVC	cranial vena cava
ADV	Aleutian disease virus	CVM	Center for Veterinary Medicine
AF	atrial fibrillation	DAP	diastolic arterial pressure
AFA	American Ferret Association	DCM	dilated cardiomyopathy
AGD	adrenal gland disease	DEW	dark-eyed white
AGID	agar gel immunodiffusion	DIC	disseminated intravascular
AHI	Animal Health Institute		coagulation
ALT	alanine aminotransferase	DIM	disseminated idiopathic
AMDUCA	Animal Medicinal Drug Use		myofasciitis
	Clarification Act	DM	diabetes mellitus
Ao	aorta	DV	dorsoventral
AV	atrioventricular	ECE	epizootic catarrhal enteritis
AVD	acquired valvular disease	ECG	electrocardiogram/graphy
AVMA	American Veterinary Medical	EDTA	ethylenediamine tetraacetic acid
	Association	EIA	enzyme immunoassay
BAL	bronchoalveolar lavage	ELDU	extra-label drug use
BALT	bronchiole-associated lymphoid	ELISA	enzyme-linked immunosorbent
	tissue		assay
BEW	black-eyed white	EM	erythema multiforme
BID	bis in die (Latin), twice a day	EMH	extramedullary haematopoiesis
BNP	b-type natriuretic peptide	EPSS	E-point to septal separation
bpm	beats per minute	ET	endotracheal tube
BUN	blood urea nitrogen	EU	European Union
CAV	chicken anaemia virus	FCoV	feline coronavirus
CBC	complete blood count	FDA	Food and Drug Administration
CD(V)	canine distemper (virus)	FFDCA	Federal Food, Drug and
CEP	counterimmunoelectrophoresis		Cosmetic Act
CHF	congestive heart failure	FIP	feline infectious peritonitis
CN	cranial nerve	FNA	fine needle aspirate
CNS	central nervous system	FRECV	ferret enteric coronavirus
CP	crude protein	FRSCV	ferret systemic coronavirus
CRI	constant rate infusion	FS	fractional shortening
CRT	capillary refill time	FSH	follicle-stimulating hormone
CSD	congenital sensorineural deafness	GALT	gastric mucosa-associated
CSF	cerebrospinal fluid		lymphoid tissue

GDV	gastric dilatation volvulus	prn	*pro re nata* (when necessary)
GGT	gamma-glutamyl transferase	PT	prothrombin time
GI	gastrointestinal	PTH	parathyroid hormone
GMS	Grocott's methenamine silver stain	PTT	partial thromboplastin time
GnRH	gonadotropin-releasing hormone	PU	polyuria
GyV	gyrovirus	PUFA	polyunsaturated fatty acid
H&E	haematoxylin and eosin (stain)	PZ-CCK	pancreozymin–cholecystokinin
hCG	human chorionic gonadotrophin	RAAS	renin–angiotensin–aldosterone
HCM	hypertrophic cardiomyopathy		system
HEV	hepatitis E virus	RBC	red blood cell
HIV	human immunodeficiency virus	RNA	ribonucleic acid
HSD	hydroxysteroid dehydrogenase	RT-PCR	reverse transcriptase PCR
IBD	inflammatory bowel disease	SA	sinoatrial
IM	intramuscular	SAP	systolic arterial pressure
IO	intraosseus	SARS	severe acute respiratory disorder
IP	intraperitoneal	SARS CoV	SARS coronavirus
IT	intratracheal	SC	subcutaneous
IV	intravenous	SD	standard deviation
IVC	intravenous circulation	SE	standard error
IVS	interventricular septum thickness	SID	once a day
LAAD	left atrium appendage diameter	SSI	surgical site infection
LES	lower oesophageal sphincter	SVT	supraventricular tachycardia
LH	luteinising hormone	TB	tuberculosis
LMN	lower motor neuron	TEM	transmission electron microscopy
LN	lymph node	THC	tetrahydrocannabinol
LVID	left ventricular internal diameter	TS	total solids
LVW	left ventricular wall thickness	TSH	thyroid-stimulating hormone
MAP	mean arterial pressure	UCCR	urinary corticoid:creatinine ratio
ME	metabolisable energy	UMN	upper motor neuron
MEA	mean electrical axis	UV	ultraviolet
MEN	multiple endocrine neoplasia	VC	vena cava
MRI	magnetic resonance imaging	VCPR	veterinarian–client–patient
MSH	melanocyte stimulating hormone		relationship
NAPQI	N-acetyl-p-benzoquinoneimine	VD	ventrodorsal
NFE	nitrogen-free extract	V-hob	vasectomised hob
NSAID	non-steroidal anti-inflammatory	VIP	vasoactive intestinal peptide
	drug	VP	vena porta
PAS	periodic acid-Schiff stain	VPC	ventricular premature complex
PBGM	portable blood glucose meter	WBC	white blood cell
PCR	polymerase chain reaction	WFRS	Washington Ferret Rescue &
PCV	packed cell volume		Shelter
PD	polydipsia	WHO	World Health Organisation
PDAB	preoperative donated autologous	WHO-REAL	WHO Revised European–
	blood		American Lymphoma
PNS	peripheral nervous system	ZN	Ziehl–Neelsen stain
PO	per os (Latin), by mouth		

CHAPTER 1

GENERAL INFORMATION

Cathy A. Johnson-Delaney

1

The domestic ferret, *Mustela putorius furo* (also known as *Mustela furo*) was derived from the European polecat, *Mustela putorius*. There is some debate whether there may also be Asiatic, Siberian or Ethiopian polecat in the lineage. Genome work so far points to just the European polecat. Its Latin name is descriptive, translating as 'smelly little thief'. The domestic ferret is also known as the fitch ferret. It is considered to have been domesticated around 2000 years ago. It was introduced into the United States (USA) in the late 19th century. It is the only domesticated member of the Mustelidae. Domestication has led to very few significant changes in appearance or anatomy from the polecat, with coat colour, patterns, length and eye colour being the most significant source of human-influenced variation. Ferrets are all one blood type. An intact female ferret is termed a 'jill', while an ovariectomised female is a 'sprite'. An intact male ferret is termed a 'hob', while an orchiectomised male is a 'gib'.

The ferret is used for hunting, for fur, as a laboratory animal and as a pet. It is only in the past 30–40 years that the ferret has really gained popularity as a pet. In the USA it is ranked third most popular after cats and dogs (**Fig. 1.1**). It is still used for hunting rabbits and rats in many parts of the world. It has a long history of skill in flushing rabbits. The ferret can turn in the diameter of its body so is ideal for getting into animal tunnels (**Fig. 1.2**). It was also used on ships to control vermin. Because it is a successful hunter, several states in the USA (California, Hawaii) have made owning the ferret illegal. However, no feral colonies exist in the USA and the likelihood of ferrets hunting native prey species in California is remote. In the USA, there are urban and suburban predators such as hawks, coyotes, and even raccoons that may kill the lost ferret. There are pet ferrets in California despite the illegality. Several municipalities including New York City have made ferrets illegal, citing

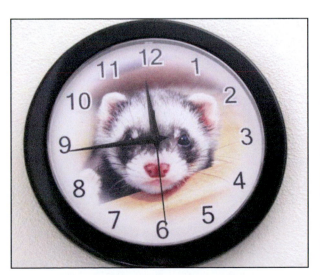

Fig. 1.1 **Time for ferrets. Popularity of ferrets and ferret-related products.**

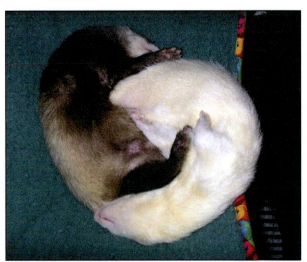

Fig. 1.2 **Ferrets can turn in the diameter of their bodies. They often sleep contorted.**

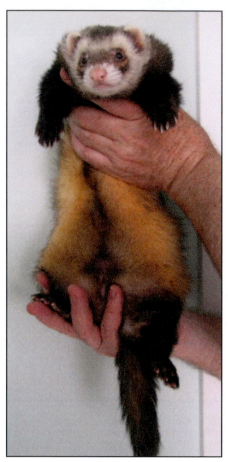

Fig. 1.3 **Sable male 'fitch' ferret, pink nose.**

public health reasons (bite wounds). Ferrets are regulated in some states and they require a permit to own them (Georgia).

The use of ferrets for the fur trade has largely fallen out of favour. The fur was referred to as 'fitch'. Fur of the ferret was also used in the manufacture of paint brushes, labeled 'sable' (**Fig. 1.3**).

LABORATORY ANIMAL

The ferret is a vital part of influenza research as it contracts human influenza. Recently it has been determined that it lacks sialic acid, as humans do, which makes it susceptible to the virus. Ferrets are being used as a smaller alternative to cats and dogs and are currently omitted from the United States Animal Welfare Regulations (United States Department of Agriculture).

Research uses for the ferret include:

- Canine distemper.
- Cardiology.
- Cystic fibrosis (genetic knock-out model).
- Emesis: used to screen compounds for emesis potential.
- *Helicobacter pylori* (*Helicobacter mustelae*: gastritis, ulcers, gastric neoplasia, inflammatory bowel disease, ulcerative colitis).
- Influenza (human, swine H1N1, avian H5N1).
- Intubation practice (oropharyngeal anatomy is similar to a human infant's).
- Neuroanatomy.
- Neuroendocrinology.
- Pulmonary.
- Reproductive physiology.
- SARS (severe acute respiratory syndrome – SARS coronavirus, SARS-CoV).
- Toxicology.
- Vesicular stomatitis.
- Virus-induced neoplasms.

CHAPTER 2

NORMATIVE DATA INCLUDING COAT COLOURS

Cathy A. Johnson-Delaney

NORMATIVE DATA

Because the ferret is used in research, biological data have been established (*Table 2.1*).

CLASSIFICATIONS

Ferrets can be classified by the coat colour coupled with the coat pattern, eye colour, mask type and

Table 2.1 **Selected normative data**

PARAMETER	VALUE
Lifespan (average)	5–8 years
Body temperature	38.8°C (37.8–40°C)
Chromosome number (diploid)	40
Dental formula	2(I3/3, C1/1, P4/3, M1/2)
Vertebral formula	C7, T14–15, L5–7, S3–4, C14–18
Age of sexual maturity	4–12 months
Adult bodyweight	Female 700–1200 g; male 1000–2000 g
Water intake	75–100 mL/24 h
Urine volume	26–28 mL/24 h
Blood pressure:	
Non-sedated	140–164 mmHg systolic
	110–125 mmHg diastolic
Sedated (butorphanol, midazolam at 0.2 mg/kg each)	95–155 mmHg systolic
	51–89 mmHg diastolic
Arterial blood pressure:	
Mean systolic	Female 133 mmHg; male 161 mmHg (conscious)
Mean diastolic	110–125 mmHg (anaesthetised)
Heart rate	200–400 beats/min
Cardiac output	139 mL/min
Circulation time	4.5–6.8 s
Blood volume	75 mL/kg
Respiration rate	33–36/min
Gastrointestinal transit time	3–4 hours

Cerebral spinal fluid values are in Appendix 1.
Coagulation parameters are in Appendix 2.
Haematology and serum chemistry values are in Appendix 3.
Hormone values are in Appendix 4.
Urine values are in Appendix 5.

nose pattern. Currently there is a range of at least 30 coat colour variations recognised at ferret shows by the American Ferret Association and various ferret societies. Detailed genetics of coat colour can be found in Lewington (2007). An Angora ferret has long hair and can be any coat colour or pattern. Recently a blue-eyed ferret mutation has been seen.

Nose patterns (Figs 2.1–2.7)

Nose patterns can be black, outlined, speckled, spots, 'T' or pink.

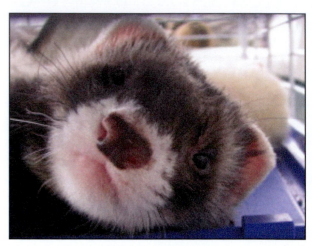

Fig. 2.1 **Black nose (dark sable).**

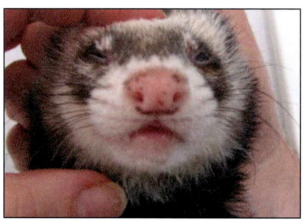

Fig. 2.2 **Outlined or ringed nose (dark sable).**

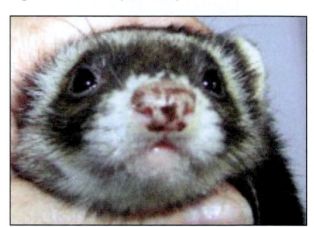

Fig. 2.3 **Speckled or freckled nose (sable).**

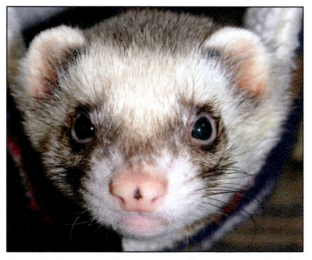

Fig. 2.4 **Spot nose (brown eyes, silver). (Courtesy of Vondelle McLaughlin.)**

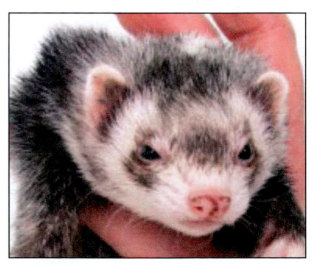

Fig. 2.5 **T nose (silver mitt).**

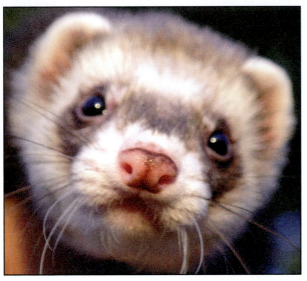

Fig. 2.6 T nose (chocolate). (Courtesy of Vondelle McLaughlin.)

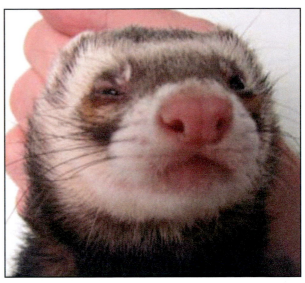

Fig. 2.7 Pink nose (sable).

Eye colours (Figs 2.8–2.11, *Table 2.2*)

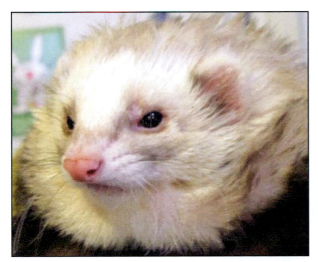

Fig. 2.8 Black eyes of a hob, partly angora coat, hood pattern.

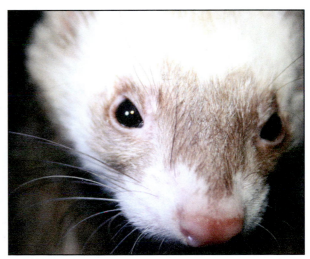

Fig. 2.9 Brown eye. (Courtesy of Vondelle McLaughlin.)

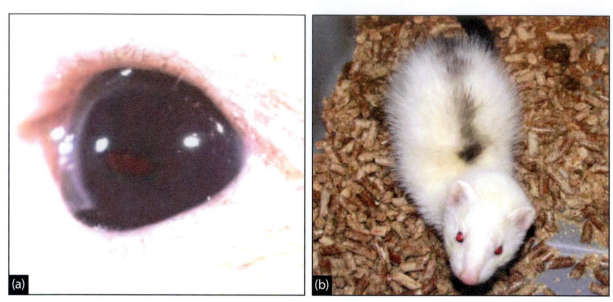

Fig. 2.10 (a) Ruby/burgundy eye; note red tapetum (Courtesy of Kevin Farlee); (b) 8 weeks old with marked pattern and ruby eyes.

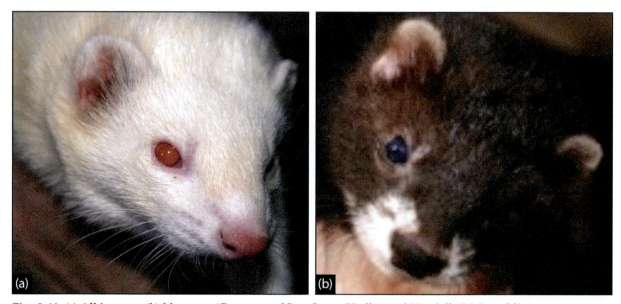

Fig. 2.11 (a) Albino eye; (b) blue eye. (Courtesy of Sara Jayne Hadley and Vondelle McLaughlin.)

Table 2.2 **Eye colour combinations**		
EYE COLOUR	**IRIS**	**TAPETUM**
Black	Black	Pigmented
Brown	Brown	Pigmented
Ruby (burgundy)	Light brown	Non-pigmented
Pink (albino)	Non-pigmented	Non-pigmented
Blue	Not described	Not described

Coat colours (Figs 2.12–2.36, *Table 2.3*)

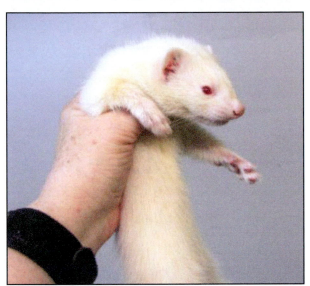

Fig. 2.12 Albino.

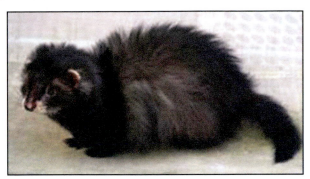

Fig. 2.13 Black, angora coat. (Courtesy of Angel Ferret.)

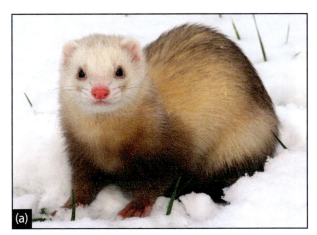

(a)

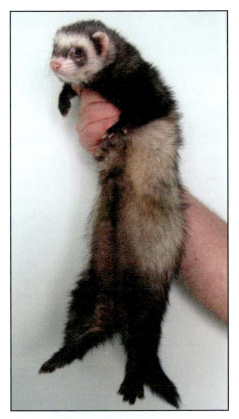

Fig. 2.14 Black (dark) sable.

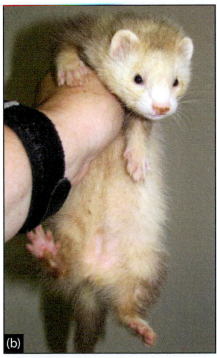

(b)

Fig. 2.15 (a) Champagne (Courtesy of Vondelle McLaughlin); (b) champagne, 8 weeks old.

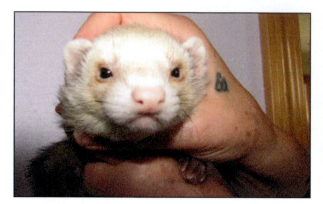

Fig. 2.16 Champagne face.

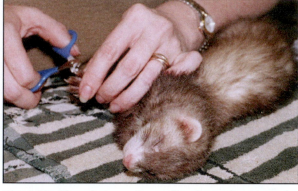

Fig. 2.18 Chocolate getting nails trimmed.

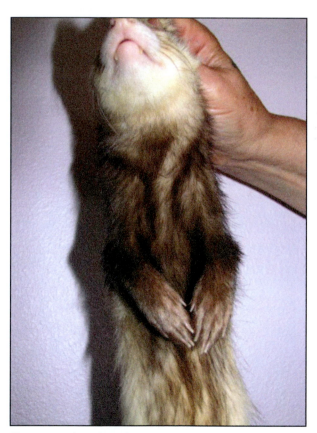

Fig. 2.17 Chocolate (brown).

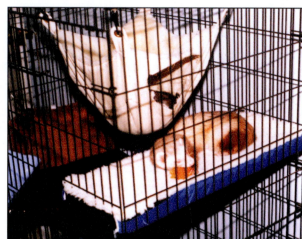

Fig. 2.19 Cinnamon coat colour, with ferret chewing on a commercial treat.

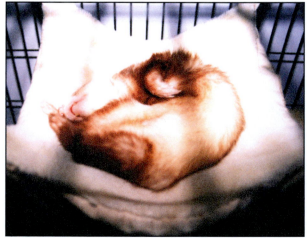

Fig. 2.20 Cinnamon coat colour.

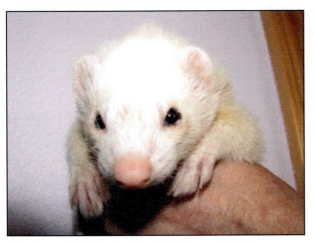

Fig. 2.21 Dark-eyed white (black-eyed white), DEW or BEW.

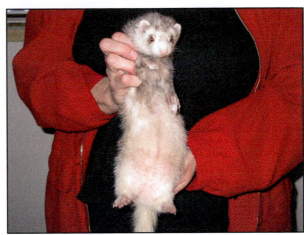

Fig. 2.22 Silver.

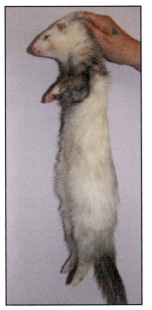

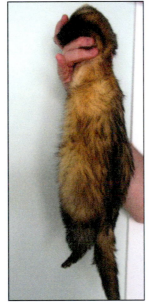

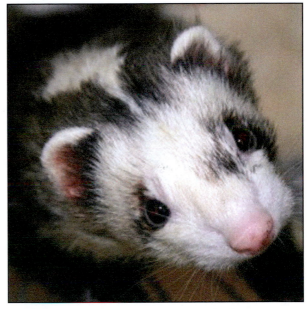

Fig. 2.23 Light silver.

Fig. 2.24 Sable (fitch).

Fig. 2.25 Blaze pattern (note: all are deaf). (Courtesy of Vondelle McLaughlin.)

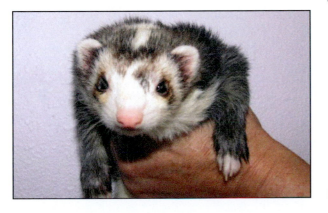

Fig. 2.26 Blaze pattern, silver coat.

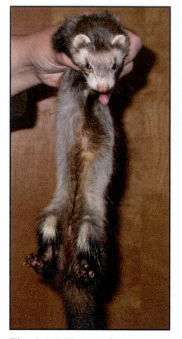
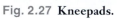

Fig. 2.27 **Kneepads.**

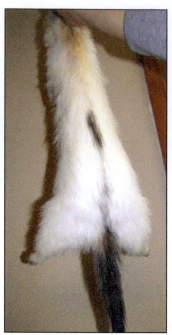

Fig. 2.28 **Marked (spotted).**

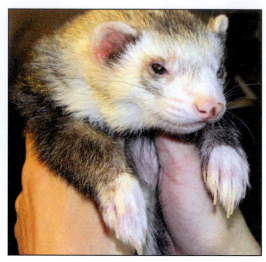

Fig. 2.29 **Mitt.**

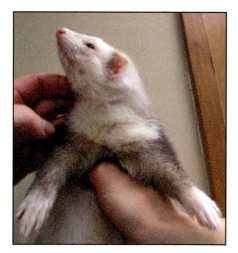

Fig. 2.30 **American Panda (silver with mitts).**

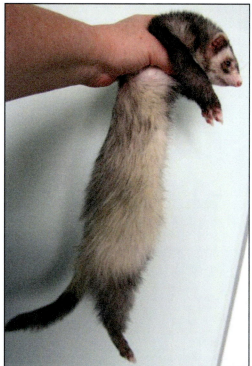

Fig. 2.31 **Point.**

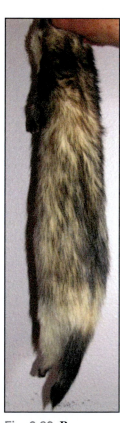

Fig. 2.32 **Roan.**

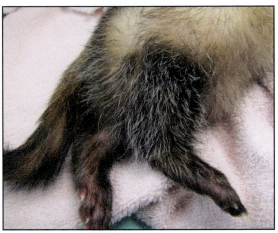

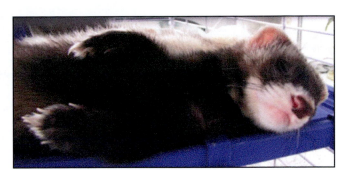

Fig. 2.34 Solid except for white tips of toes.

Fig. 2.33 Roan legs.

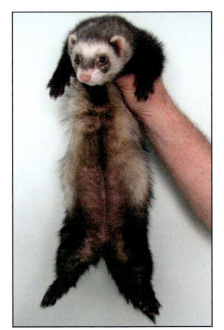

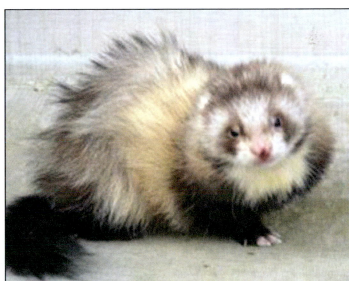

Fig. 2.36 Angora. (Courtesy of Angel Ferret.)

Fig. 2.35 Standard.

Table 2.3 Coat colours

COLOUR	COAT GUARD HAIRS	EYES	NOSE
Albino	White	Pink	Pink
Black	Solid colour black	Black	Black
Black sable (dark sable)	Black prominent	Black/brown	Black, speckled, spots, outlined, T
Champagne	Light brown	Brown	Pink, speckled, spots, outlined, T but with light brown colouring not black
Chocolate (Siamese)	Brown	Black/brown	Pink, brown, speckled, spots, outlined, T
Cinnamon	Red	Brown	Pink, speckled, spots, outlined, T but with light brown to red colouring not black
Dark-eyed white DEW (Black-eyed white BEW)	White	Black/brown	Pink
Silver (light, dark)	Sparse black guard hairs. Get whiter with age	Black/brown/ruby (burgundy)	Pink, black, speckled, spots, outlined, T
Sable (fitch)	Black, under fur is white to yellowish	Black/brown	Pink, black, speckled, spots, outlined, T

Key: BEW, black-eyed white; DEW, dark-eyed white.

Patterns (*Table 2.4*)

Table 2.4 Pattern types

PATTERN	DESCRIPTION	MASK
Blaze (note: these are deaf)	Wide white stripe from forehead to shoulder, white mitts or toe tips, white knee patches, may be speckled	Colour rings around eyes or colour smudges below eyes
Hood	White head, rest of body normal coat colour	No mask – face is white
Kneepads	White fur over knees	Normal mask for coat colour
Marked (spotted)	White with black spots along spine and tail	No mask – face is white
Mitt	White feet or toes	Normal mask for the coat colour
Panda (note: these are deaf)	Full white head, including neck and throat. American Panda may also have speckled belly, white knee patches, mitts, and toe tips	May have colour rings around eyes, otherwise no mask
Point	Distinct difference in colour concentration between the body colour and the colour points (legs, tail)	V-shaped
Roan	50% colour guard hairs (any colour, usually black) and 50% white guard hairs	V-shaped usually dark marked
Solid	No colour contrasts between points (legs and tail) and the body. Solid colour from mask to tail tip	T-bar mask
Standard	Moderate colour contrasts between points (legs and tail) and the body	Full mask
Angora coat	Long hair. Can be any colour or pattern	Mask appropriate with colour, pattern

CHAPTER 3

APPLIED CLINICAL ANATOMY AND PHYSIOLOGY

Cathy A. Johnson-Delaney

INTRODUCTION

The ferret is similar in many ways to other carnivores (**Fig. 3.1**); however, the differences will be highlighted. The ferret has a rapid metabolism, as do other members of the Mustelidae. The average body temperature is 38.8°C (range 37.8–40°C).

ADRENAL GLANDS

The left adrenal gland lies at the cranial pole of the left kidney and adjacent to the caudal vena cava. Its blood supply comes from short vessels arising from the abdominal aorta and caudal vena cava. It is also drained by the adrenal lumbar vein. All three of these need to be ligated during adrenalectomy. There are also numerous small vessels in the fat surrounding the gland. It measures approximately 6–8 mm in length.

The right adrenal gland lies at the cranial pole of the right kidney and lies on the dorsal surface of the caudal vena cava. Its vasculature arises from the abdominal aorta and usually drains through a short vein or directly into the caudal vena cava. It measures approximately 8–11 mm (**Figs 3.2–3.4**).

Adrenal glands function as with other mammals, although they are also the source of sex steroids when they become stimulated by luteinising hormone (LH) (see Chapter 14).

BRAIN

The ferret brain has been used in developmental and system neuroscience studies. The gross anatomy and gyral/sulcal cortical folding pattern and functionality are similar to those in other carnivores, but especially in cats. (There is a detailed chapter on this: 'Neuroanatomy of the ferret brain' by Lawes

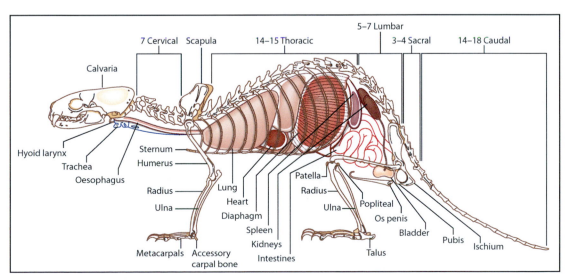

Fig. 3.1 Overall anatomy diagram.

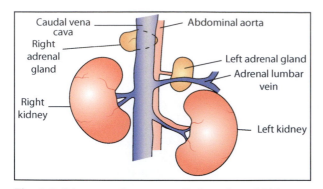

Fig. 3.2 **Diagram of anatomy of adrenals and kidneys.**

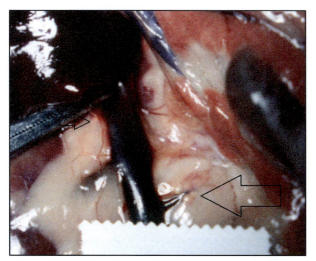

Fig. 3.3 *In situ* adrenal location. Large arrow: left adrenal; small arrow: part of right adrenal gland.

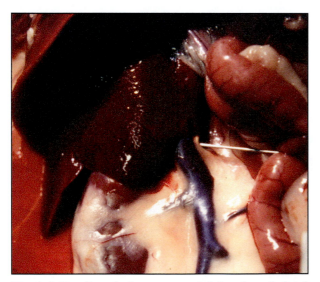

Fig. 3.4 **Needle pointing at part of right adrenal gland overlapping the dorsal surface of the caudal vena cava.**

and Andrews in Fox JG, *Biology and Diseases of the Ferret, 2nd edition*, 1998, pp. 71–102.) The brain is approximately 36 mm long and 24 mm wide. From a dorsal view, the forebrain appears nearly triangular and overlaps the cerebellum (**Fig. 3.5**). Part of the medulla is visible caudal to the cerebellum. Visible on the ventral surface are the forebrain, midbrain, hindbrain and lateral aspects of the cerebellum (**Fig. 3.6**). The forebrain is composed of the telencephalon (olfactory bulbs, cerebrum) and diencephalon (optic chiasma, pituitary, mammillary bodies). The midbrain contains the crus cerebri, mammillary peduncle and tectum. The hindbrain is composed of the pons and medulla. A lateral view of these structures is shown in **Fig. 3.7**.

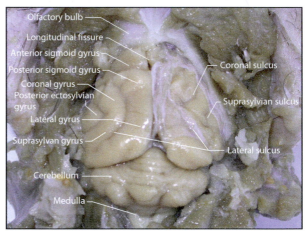

Fig. 3.5 **Brain, dorsal view.**

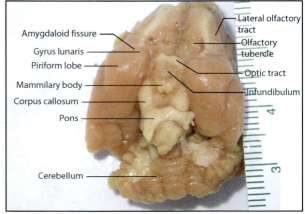

Fig. 3.6 **Brain, ventral view.**

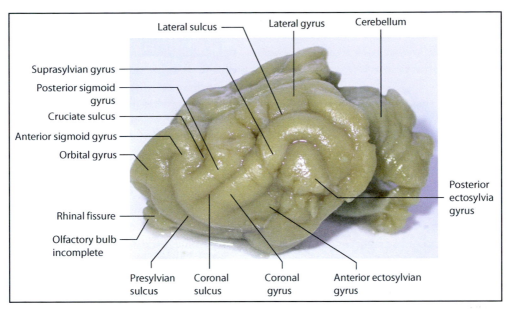

Lateral sulcus — Lateral gyrus — Cerebellum

Suprasylvian gyrus

Posterior sigmoid gyrus

Cruciate sulcus

Anterior sigmoid gyrus

Orbital gyrus

Posterior ectosylvia gyrus

Rhinal fissure

Olfactory bulb incomplete

Presylvian sulcus   Coronal sulcus   Coronal gyrus   Anterior ectosylvian gyrus

Fig. 3.7 **Brain, lateral view.**

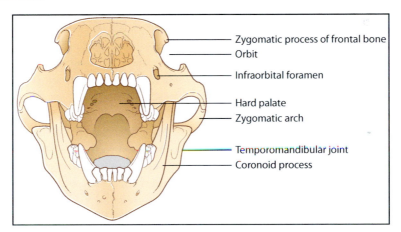

Zygomatic process of frontal bone
Orbit

Infraorbital foramen

Hard palate
Zygomatic arch

Temporomandibular joint
Coronoid process

Fig. 3.8 **Diagram of the skull.**

DENTAL ANATOMY AND PHYSIOLOGY (SEE CHAPTER 19)

The ferret is a strict carnivore and has a teeth and jaw structure to accommodate such a diet (**Fig. 3.8**). The jaws are short with the articular condyle of the mandible fitting into a transverse articular fossa. This has a postarticular process preventing dislocation upon wide opening, for a strong bite. The muscles of mastication include a well-developed masseter muscle that originates at the zygomatic arch and inserts on the masseteric fossa, condyloid crest and mandibular angular process. The digastric

muscle originates on the jugular process and tympanic bulla and passes to the ventral border of the caudal portion of the mandible. It has the action of opening the jaw. The major adductor muscle of the lower jaw is the temporalis. This is well developed in the hob (male). The deep pterygoid muscles, lateral and medial, assist the masseter and temporalis muscles in the crushing and chewing motion of closing the jaws.

The tooth-bearing arcades of the jaws are approximately equal in length, but the lower arcade is narrower and fits medially to the upper arcade. This allows for the shearing motion during chewing. The six upper incisors are slightly longer than the six lower incisors. The second incisors of the mandible are set back from the others. The mandibular canines close in front of the maxillary canines.

While usually there are four premolars in Carnivora, only three are present in the ferret (**Fig. 3.9**). The first premolar has been lost in development. The last maxillary carnassial tooth (third cheek tooth) is the fourth premolar. It has three roots. There is a single molar in the maxillary arcade that has three roots. It is wider in the buccolingual breadth compared to the mesiodistal length, making it appear to be rooted at right angles to the rest of the teeth. It has a narrow depressed waist that separates its lingual side from the buccal side of the crown. There are two small cusps on the buccal part and a single cusp on the lingual part. This tooth may be overlooking in an awake ferret examination due to its location. The large mandibular carnassial tooth (fourth cheek tooth) is the first molar. All living mustelids only have the first molar in the maxilla and both the first and second molars in the mandible. The first mandibular molar has a crown with three distinct cusps. Two form the blades of the carnassial and the smaller, lower cusp, in conjunction with the second molar, interlocks with the cusps of the maxillary molar (**Fig. 3.10**). The first mandibular molar has two roots, although sometimes there is an accessory slender central root present. The second mandibular molar is a small tooth with a single root

and a simple crown with a minor ridge and cusplets. It does not occlude with any maxillary teeth, but helps with the crushing function for the caudal cusp of the first mandibular molar. Congenitally this tooth may be missing in many pet ferrets. There is speculation that it is in the evolutionary process of becoming lost or vestigial as has happened in other carnivores.

Mustelids crush their food using the postcarnassial molars. Another adaptation is the overlapping and interdigitation of the mandibular arcade by the motions necessary to process plant materials and abrasive food, but this does allow the dorsoventral movement necessary for the cheek teeth and carnassials to shear tissue-based foods. The temporomandibular joint effectively locks the mandible into the skull, preventing the loss of bite force during predation. The maxillary canines and cheek teeth are aligned into what effectively become arches; this is a common adaptation of carnivores that strengthens the skull without adding bone mass. The canine teeth form a tight interlock when the mouth is closed. The biomechanics of these adaptations are markedly different from those of herbivores.

It is likely that the shift from a whole-prey diet to one of dry kibbles may have deleterious impacts on the function of the ferret's specific dental adaptations, although this has yet to be the focus of a published research study. Kibble is crunchy and abrasive, a selling point to reduce dental

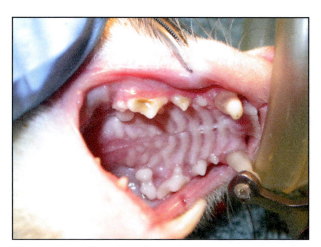

Fig. 3.9 **Maxillary dental arcade.**

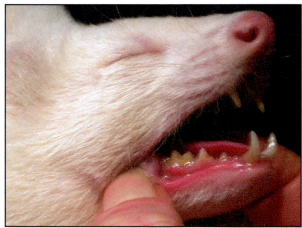

Fig. 3.10 **Mandibular dental arcade.**

calculus, but chewing kibble may cause structural changes to the tooth and underlying bony support. This ultimately causes excessive wear of the tooth and may result in fractures or loss of the tooth. In short, the ferret's dentition is not well suited to having to grind kibble.

The domestic ferret has 28–30 deciduous teeth (di3–4/3: dc1/1: dm3/3). The permanent dental formula is I3/3: C1/1: PM3/3: M1/2 = 34 (note: if M2 is missing, then M1/1 = 32).

Ferrets have a relatively large oral cavity. The labial commissures extend further caudally than the carnassial teeth. The orbicularis oris muscle is moderately well developed. The lower lip is closely attached to the mandibular gingiva, with little flexibility.

GASTROINTESTINAL ANATOMY AND PHYSIOLOGY (SEE CHAPTER 13)

General physiology
The ferret has a short intestinal transit time of 148–219 minutes when fed a meat-based diet. Kits may have a more rapid transit time; as little as 1 hour. This rapid transit time contributes to the inefficiency of absorption. The small intestine is approximately 5 times longer than the ferret's body. In comparison, a cat's small intestine is 8–10 times the length of the body. Concentrations of at least some intestinal brush border enzymes (e.g. lactase) are lower in ferrets than in other species. Weaning-age kits have less lactase per gram of jejunal mucosa than mature rats. This results in soft stool appearance within an hour when an adult ferret drinks an ounce (28 g) of milk. The digestive system is under vagal and sacral innervation. The tract is spontaneously active even under anaesthesia. Motility can be moderated with atropine. The stomach spontaneously produces acids and proteolytic enzymes. Histamine and vagal stimulation provoke more secretions.

Gut closure for antibody absorption occurs in kits between 28 and 42 days of age. Ferrets can absorb beta carotene and convert it to retinoic acid. Carbohydrases and proteolytic activity take place distally in the jejunum rather than more proximally in the duodenum.

Gut content is reduced within 4–6 hours in the ferret to the same extent as an overnight fast in a dog or cat. Because of this rapid intestinal transit time and small meals eaten, ferrets should not be fasted more than 3 hours prior to surgery. Growing kits or juveniles become irritable and may be likely to bite after a long fast. Ferrets with insulinomas may become severely hypoglycaemic if fasted for more than 1–2 hours. If it is necessary to empty the gastrointestinal (GI) tract in a ferret with insulinoma, it is acceptable to continue to feed the ferret concentrated, low-volume supplements such as Nutri-Cal®(Vetoquinol USA, Inc., Ft Worth, TX) until 1–2 hours before surgery.

Tongue
The tongue is fairly long and freely movable. It can be pulled forwards to expose the tracheal entrance as in other mammals. The tonsil crypts are visible on either side of the oral cavity. The lingual frenulum can be the site of grass awn penetrations in working ferrets in the summer. The tongue possesses von Ebner's glands in the crypts of the taste buds that synthesise neutral secretory glycoproteins and peroxidase. It has four types of papillae. Filiform and fungiform (fewer) papilla lie on the rostral three-quarters. Vallate papillae lie in a V shape at the base of the tongue. In the fold just rostral to the tonsillar fossa are the folate papilli.

Salivary glands
There are five pairs of salivary glands: the parotid (seromucous), mandibular (mucous), sublingual (mucous), molar and zygomatic. The molar and zygomatic glands secrete mainly mucous but partly serous. The opening of the parotid duct is at the level of the maxillary carnassial tooth. The mandibular gland opens on a sublingual papilla and joins with several small ducts from the sublingual gland. The molar or buccal gland's duct opens into the oral cavity just opposite the mandibular molars. The zygomatic gland has several ducts opening opposite the upper cheek teeth. Duct openings should be examined routinely during any oral examination or procedure. Damage to the glands can result in mucoceles that may need surgical repair.

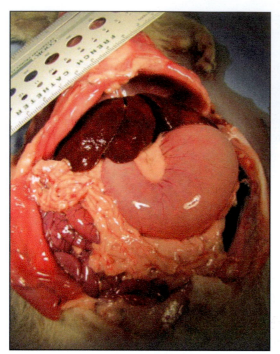

Fig. 3.11 **Stomach with normal anatomic positioning with the liver, intestines and spleen.**

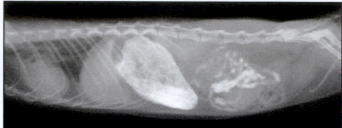

Fig. 3.12 **Lateral radiograph with contrast showing stomach and small intestines.**

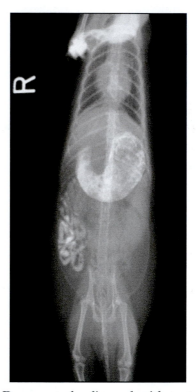

Fig. 3.13 **Dorsoventral radiograph with contrast showing the positions of the stomach and small intestines.**

Oesophagus

This is long (17–19 cm in a ferret of 1 kg) reaching nearly to mid-body. It is composed of striated muscle. The mucous membranes lie in longitudinal folds except when dilated. The three points of constriction are at the origin, the point where the left bronchus crosses it, and just cranial to the diaphragm at the oesophageal hiatus. It initially lies dorsal to the trachea, but changes to the left of the trachea from the thoracic inlet caudally. It enters the abdomen between the liver lobes.

Stomach

The ferret has a simple stomach, similar in shape to that of the dog (**Figs 3.11–3.13**). There is prominent vasculature of the stomach as well as a prominent lymph node lying in the lesser curvature. It is innervated by parasympathetic fibres from the vagus nerve and sympathetic fibres via the coeliacomesenteric plexus. The stomach has considerable storage capacity (100 mL of milk in 10 minutes in an adult). Eighty per cent of a meal is stored in the proximal stomach.

The lower oesophageal sphincter (LES) and the mechanisms of gastro-oesophageal reflux in the ferret are being used as an animal model. Transient LES relaxation is the mechanism and is unassociated with swallowing in the ferret, just as in the human. Gastric infusions of glucose, lipid and gas are all effective in provoking gastro-oesophageal reflux in the ferret. Lipid and glucose stimulate acid secretion.

The fundus of the stomach and the LES are co-innervated by vagal preganglionic motor neurons as these sections work in tandem: the LES must relax to accommodate food during ingestion or preceding emesis. The antrum of the stomach provides mixing and propulsion of contents for gastric emptying and is innervated by neurons responding to differing neurotransmitters.

Ferrets are spontaneous secretors of hydrochloric acid. It is natural for them to cache food and eat small amounts frequently, rather than gorging every day or two like most carnivores. Because of the gastric physiology and strong emetic responses, they are used as animal models of emesis. Serotonin at 10 mg/kg successfully blocks cisplatin-induced emesis. An antiemetic pursued in the ferret model has been delta-9-tetrahydrocannabinol (Δ9-THC), the cannabinoid that is antiemetic in humans. Ferrets have the cannabinoid-1 receptor in the dorsal motor vagal nucleus, with cell bodies in the area postrema, nucleus tractus solitarius and nodose ganglion. This receptor mediates the antiemetic action of cannabinoids. Δ9-THC was found to cause gastro-oesophageal reflux due to the relaxation of the LES. This effect may have implications in the treatment of gastro-oesophageal reflux and other upper GI disorders.

The ferret stomach also secretes acid in response to histamine, pentagastrin and calcium. There is a low concentration of free histamine in the stomach. The ferret lacks the histamine-forming enzyme (L-histidine decarboxylase) in the stomach, although histamine-destroying activity is present. Histamine also stimulates secretion of proteolytic enzymes. Histamine H2 receptor antagonists abolish the acid secretion response to exogenous histamine or exogenous stimulation with pentagastrin. Atropine only reduces acid secretion by 30%. Gastrin is secreted in the gastric antrum and duodenum. Hypoglycaemia induced by insulin produces a sustained stimulation of acid secretion. This is particularly relevant to ferrets with insulinomas; therapy needs to include medications that decrease acid secretion.

Intestine

The ferret intestine consists of 3 sections: the duodenum, the jejunoileum, and the colon (**Fig. 3.14**). The small intestine is short, about 190 cm (5 times

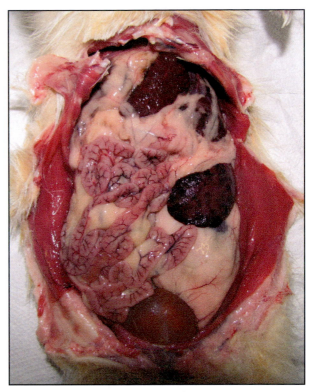

Fig. 3.14 *In situ* positioning of the intestines, omentum reflected cranially and showing moderately enlarged spleen and left renal cyst.

body length). There is no distinct junction between the jejunoileum and the colon. There is no caecum. Villi and goblet cells are present in all sections. It has an unsophisticated gut flora. The usual anaerobic flora abundant in most mammals are scanty in the ferret, probably in part because of the abbreviated large intestine. The large intestine is only approximately 10 cm long in an adult male. Ferrets raised in an isolator after caesarean derivation had no intestinal problems that are common to other germ-free animals; however, they did require vitamin K supplementation, suggesting that gut flora do play an essential part in some of the digestive processes. Ferrets that are treated for weeks or months with broad-spectrum antibiotics do not seem to experience GI upsets such as diarrhoea.

The duodenum is the proximal segment. The duodenum is innervated by vagal preganglionic parasympathetic neurons originating in the dorsal motor nucleus of the vagal nerve in the brainstem. The major duodenal papilla contains the common opening for the bile and pancreatic ducts. This is located about 3 cm from the pylorus. The minor papilla may be absent. Brunner's glands are present in the submucosa of the duodenum proximal to the bile duct. The glands produce only neutral mucosubstances as in humans.

The jejunal and ileal segments cannot be distinguished and may be referred to as the jejunoileum that ends at the ascending colon. The small intestine is innervated by the vagus nerve and the sympathetic trunks arise from the coeliac and cranial mesenteric plexus.

Motility is affected by the hormones secretin, PZ-CCK (pancreozymin-cholecystokinin), an unidentified vasoconstrictor, vasoactive intestinal peptide (VIP), and substance P. VIP inhibits jejunal motor activity due to vagal simulation while substance P excites activity. Both increase water secretion by jejunal epithelium. The muscular layer has a higher concentration of these hormones than the epithelium. Jejunal motility mediated by hormones is not blocked by atropine. 5-hydroxytryptamine 3 receptor agonist (5-HT$_3$) as well as synthetic serotonin receptor agonists induce large contraction and defaecation. The basal colonic motility pattern is not changed, and the large contractions can be blocked with a receptor antagonist. The implications of this model are for testing pharmaceuticals for constipation without undesired changes in gut motility patterns. Cervical (mechanical) vagus stimulation will affect motility. This has significant implications for the clinician who during intubation may manipulate the neck and thorax and inadvertently stimulate the vagus nerve and intestinal motility at the beginning of surgery.

The large intestine is composed of the colon and rectum. There is no caecum and no ileocolic junction. The junction is inferred by the presence of the anastomoses of the jejunal artery with the ileocolic artery. This is adjacent to the mesenteric lymph node. The colon consists of the ascending, transverse, and descending colon, with the largest being the descending. The colon is only about 10 cm long and ends at the anus, which is closed by an internal sphincter of smooth muscle and an external sphincter of striated muscle. The external sphincter encloses the openings from the anal sacs. The colon is innervated by autonomic fibres from the vagus, cranial and caudal mesenteric plexus.

There are tubular glands and goblet cells in the colon. These secrete sulphated mucosubstances. The motility of the colon resembles that of a dog ileum. Motility is vagus-dependent and mediated by cholinergic and non-cholinergic fibres. Sacral innervation is excitatory. Retroperistalsis begins in the colon which may be the genesis of vomiting in the ferret.

LIVER AND GALLBLADDER

The liver fits into the mould of the diaphragm (**Fig. 3.15**). It is relatively large compared to the average ferret bodyweight. An 800–1150 g animal could have a liver of 35–59 g. The liver has right lateral, right medial, left medial and left lateral lobes. The gallbladder is found between the quadrate and right medial lobes. It is large and can contain 0.5–1.0 mL of bile (**Fig. 3.16**). The caudate lobe must be reflected to observe the right adrenal gland. There is often a tissue attachment of the caudate lobe to the caudal vena cava. The bile duct opens into the duodenal papillae along with the pancreatic ducts.

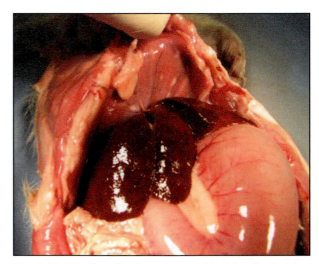

Fig. 3.15 The liver fits into the mould of the diaphragm.

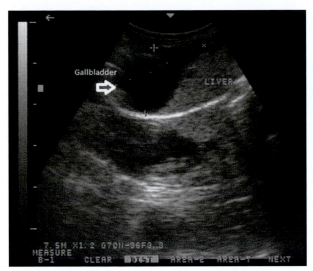

Fig. 3.16 Ultrasonogram showing the gallbladder and liver.

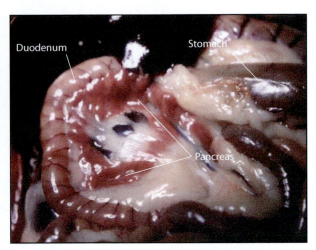

Fig. 3.17 The pancreas is a C-shaped structure between the stomach and duodenum. In this picture there are two small pieces of splenic tissue.

The gallbladder contracts in response to cholecystokinin. Cholecystokinin is found throughout the GI tract. This contraction inhibits gastric emptying and stimulates small intestine and colonic motility. The contractile response directly affects smooth muscles and/or neurons, which furthers intestinal motility.

EXOCRINE PANCREAS AND BILIARY SYSTEM

The pancreas is an elongate, lobulated, C-shaped organ (**Fig. 3.17**). It lies attached between the stomach and duodenum. The cranial portion extends along the stomach and spleen. The caudal portion extends along the descending duodenum and curves into fat lying between the duodenum and stomach. The ducts from the cranial portion and caudal portion join and empty in the duodenal papillae along with the common bile duct.

The exocrine pancreas and biliary system are also under vagal stimulation. There is a trophic relationship with capillary connections between the islets and the exocrine pancreatic tissue. A bile salt-dependent lipase is produced. The adult jill (female) mammary tissue is high in this enzyme. Ferret milk has activity 10–20 times higher than human milk. If lipase elevations are present in the blood, consider pancreatic inflammation or disease.

HEART AND CARDIOVASCULAR (SEE CHAPTER 12)

The heart is cone shaped and is similar to that of other carnivores. It usually lies between the sixth and eighth ribs (**Figs 3.18, 3.19**). The apex is to the left of midline. It is 4-chambered, consisting of left and right auricles and left and right ventricles. For auscultation purposes it lies more caudal in the chest than is usual for other carnivores. The heart ligament joins it to the sternum and contains fat. On radiology the heart appears to be slightly elevated from the sternum. If there is cardiac disease some of the fat may be lost and the heart appears to rest on the sternum.

There are unpaired innominate (brachiocephalic) arteries at the base of the neck. There are two common carotid arteries in the neck. Other vascular structures are similar to other mammals.

The heart rate is between 200 and 400 beats per minute. Cardiovascular parameters are listed in *Table 3.1*.

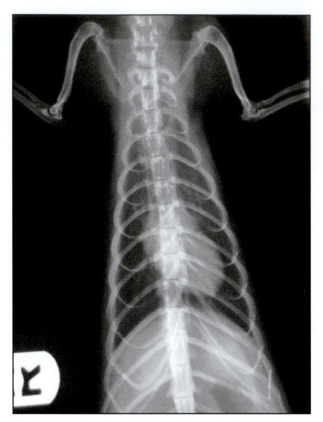

Fig. 3.18 Ventrodorsal (VD) radiograph of normal heart laying approximately between the sixth and eighth ribs.

Table 3.1 Basic cardiac parameters

PARAMETER	VALUES
Blood pressure: 　Non-sedated 　Sedated (butorphanol, 　midazolam at 0.2 mg/kg 　each)	140–164 mmHg systolic 95–155 mmHg systolic
Mean diastolic blood pressure	110–125 mmHg (anaesthetised)
Heart rate	200–400 beats/min
Cardiac output	139 mL/min
Circulation time	4.5–6.8 seconds
Blood volume	Jill: 40 mL; hob: 60 mL (5–7% of bodyweight)

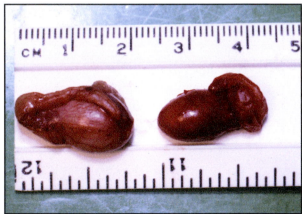

Fig. 3.20 Anal glands.

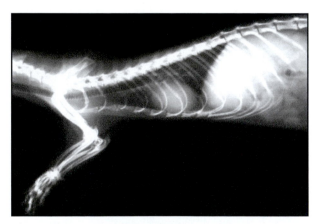

Fig. 3.19 Lateral radiograph of normal heart and thorax.

INTEGUMENT (SEE CHAPTER 21)

The skin has numerous sebaceous glands that give the animal its musky smell. The well-developed anal glands have a different musk odour (**Fig. 3.20**).

Intact hobs and oestrous jills may have a distinctive musky odour even after removal of the anal glands. This is because of normal sebaceous secretions. There are no skin sweat glands. Ferrets are vulnerable to heat stress when ambient temperature reaches 32°C. The ferret coat goes through seasonal moults. Starting in spring the ferret will lose the undercoat that is present in the winter, and coat colour tends to darken with the guard hairs being prominent. White ferrets tend to become yellowish with age. The coat colours are illustrated in Chapter 2. The skin of the dorsal neck is thickened allowing for protection from bites, and also provides the 'scruff' for restraint.

MUSCULOSKELETAL (SEE CHAPTER 17)

The vertebral formula is C7, T14-15, L5-7, S3-4, with varying coccygeal number (usually >15). There may be 14 or 15 ribs with 14 on one side and 15 on the other (**Figs 3.21–3.24**). The first 11 ribs on each side articulate between vertebrae. The remainder each articulate with a single vertebra. The first 10 pairs of ribs attach to the sternum. The last 5 ribs make up the costal arch. The first ribs are relatively small as are the last 2, which makes the thoracic inlet narrow in contrast to other animals for the passage of the trachea, oesophagus and large blood vessels. This can be significant when there is chest pathology. The remaining ribs are unattached and end in the flank musculature. The chest is large compared to body size.

The spine is flexible. The ribcage can be compressed around the heart. The ferret can compress

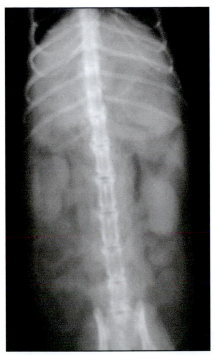

Fig. 3.21 **VD radiograph showing transitional rib right side, with 5 lumbar vertebrae.**

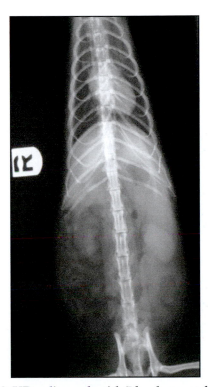

Fig. 3.22 **VD radiograph with 7 lumbar vertebrae.**

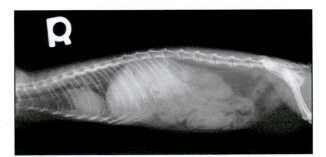

Fig. 3.23 **Lateral view, T14, L6.**

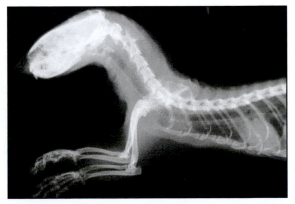

Fig. 3.24 **Lateral view, normal skeleton.**

itself and turn in the diameter of its body. There are 5 digits on each foot with strong non-retractable toenails that are very useful for digging and climbing. These usually require routine clipping in pet ferrets.

The appendicular skeleton is naturally fine with light bones. The long bones are of matchstick diameter. The femur is used for intraosseous blood transfusion.

SKULL

The skull shows characteristics of all carnivores (**Fig. 3.25**). It has unclosed zygomatic bones to the eye orbit like the dog, in contrast to the cat. One-third of the skull represents the short facial region. The brain case is relatively large.

REPRODUCTIVE TRACT

Males have paired testes in an external scrotum (**Fig. 3.26**). This becomes prominent in breeding season when the testicles enlarge (**Fig. 3.27**). The os penis is J-shaped (**Fig. 3.28**). The females have paired ovaries that lie just caudal to the kidneys (**Fig. 3.29**). The broad and suspensory ligaments attach the ovaries to the wall of the abdominal cavity. The uterus is bicornate with a short body and single cervix. The vagina is short and dilatable. The vulva is made up of the vestibule, well-developed clitoris and labia. During the breeding season the vulva is enlarged.

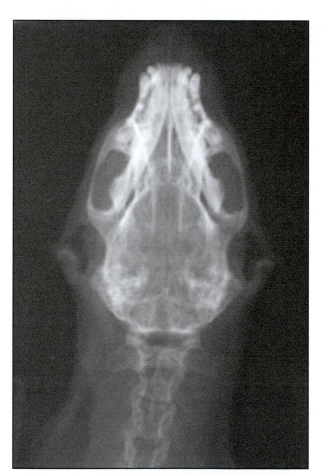

Fig. 3.25 **VD radiograph, normal skull.**

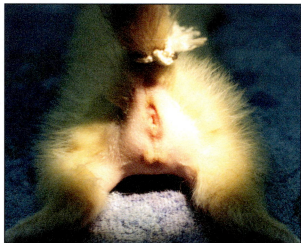

Fig. 3.26 **Intact male showing scrotum. The patient is positioned for neutering.**

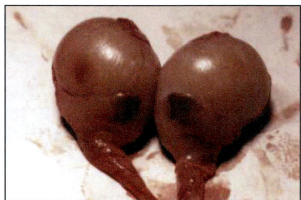

Fig. 3.27 **Testicles in season.**

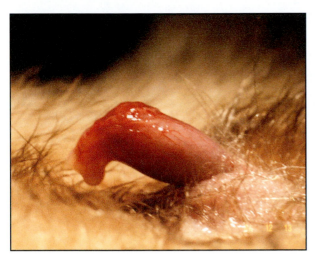

Fig. 3.28 **J-shaped os penis.**

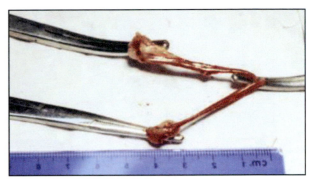

Fig. 3.29 **Normal uterus and ovaries.**

RESPIRATORY TRACT

Upper respiratory tract

The nasal cavity separates into left and right by the nasal septum. Both are connected via the nasopharyngeal opening to the pharynx. The middle ear is joined to the pharynx by the Eustacean tubes that have slit-like openings. The larynx contains the thyroid, epiglottic, cricoid, and arytenoid cartilages (**Fig. 3.30**). The sesamoid and interarytenoid cartilage lie within the interarytenoid muscles. The thyroid cartilage articulates with the thyrohyoid bone, which articulates with the median unpaired basihyoid bone. The vocal folds attach to the arytenoid and cricoid cartilages. The muscles that close the glottis also attach to these two cartilages.

Lungs

There are two left lobes (apical and diaphragmatic) and 4 lobes to the right lung (apical, middle, diaphragmatic and accessory) (**Figs 3.31, 3.32**). The apical and middle lobes form a cardiac notch. The left lung is found from the first to the tenth intercostal space, with the caudal surfaces in contact with the dome-shaped diaphragm. The two left lobes are separated at the sixth or seventh intercostal space by an oblique fissure. The lungs occupy from the first to the tenth or eleventh intercostal space in the thorax. Microscopic structure of the lungs is similar to other carnivores although they

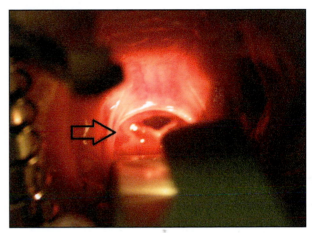

Fig. 3.30 **Normal epiglottis. Arrow is pointing to an ulcer on pharyngeal mucosa.**

contain excess submucosal glands in the bronchial wall and extra terminal bronchioles. This is similar to humans and makes them a good model for pulmonary research studies.

The lungs have a large volume in relation to bodyweight. Total lung capacity is nearly 3 times that which would be predicted based on body size, as compared with other mammals, hence ferrets' value as experimental animals for research into human conditions such as cystic fibrosis and influenza.

Trachea

In a 1 kg ferret the trachea is approximately 9 cm long to the tracheal bifurcation that lies at the fifth intercostal space. The trachea has 60–70 C-shaped rings of cartilage along its length. The thoracic inlet is narrow compared to other carnivores. It contains

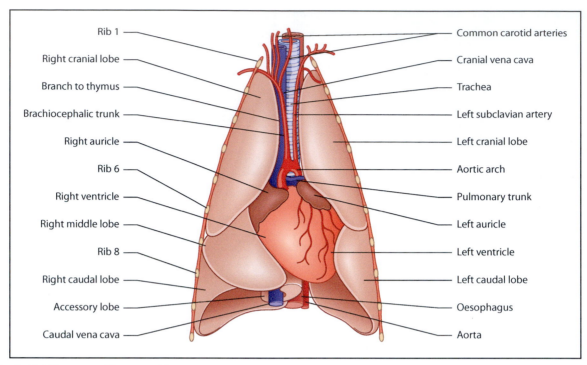

Fig. 3.31 **Diagram of lungs and heart.**

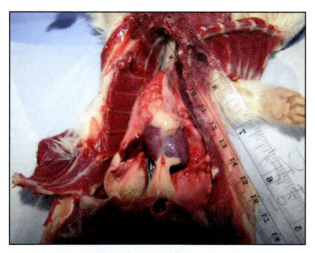

Fig. 3.32 **Necropsy, abnormal lungs but illustrating lobes and position.**

anterior mediastinal lymph nodes and the trachea, oesophagus and major blood vessels. Any enlargement of any of these structures can interfere with chest function.

Respiration rate is 33–36 per minute.

SPECIAL SENSES

Ear and hearing

The external ear consists of the pinna and an external ear canal. The pinna is set close to the head and is half-moon shaped. It is approximately 2 cm wide in adult hobs and points forwards. Some ferrets have a flatter, wider pinna that is larger compared to the head size; this is probably a genetic defect.

Adult ferrets' hearing range is 4–15 kHz. Kits aged 32 days respond to 1–6 kHz but at a higher threshold. Adult frequency response patterns have been recorded at 39–42 days. Neonates put out distress cries of 100 kHz, and jills with litters respond to calls above 16 kHz.

Deafness in ferrets is linked with coat colour (Chapter 15) (**Fig. 3.33**). This is Waardenburg syndrome, which is a dominant genetic fault. Hearing at 32 days of age can be checked with a loud clap.

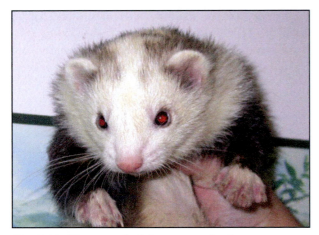

Fig. 3.33 Blaze-marked ferrets are deaf.

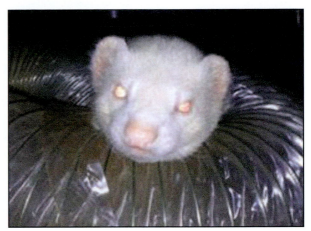

Fig. 3.34 Albino ferret showing eye shine from a non-pigmented tapetum.

Eye and vision

Ferret kits are born with their eyes closed and the eyelids do not open until 28–34 days postnatally. The ferret globe is small at 7.0 ± 0.24 mm with a relatively large lens at 3.4 ± 0.15 mm. It has a wide cornea for optimal light gathering in low light conditions. The ferret eye is optimised for function in dim and dark environments. This is an adaptation for hunting prey at dawn and dusk. The ferret's eyes are widely spaced laterally giving a field of view around 270 degrees but a relatively poor degree of binocularity of only about 40 degrees frontally. The pupil is ovoid allowing the eye a greater range of variation to admit light with a mydriatic pupil. The ferret has a horizontally orientated long axis, presumably optimised to scan the horizon for prey on the ground.

Pigmented individuals include the natural sable with brown to black iris and pigmented tapetum, and the dark-eyed whites (black-eyed whites) have a brown iris and pigmented tapetum, whereas the albino ferret has no pigment (**Fig. 3.34**) (see Chapter 2). There is also a 'ruby' eye that has a pigmented iris and non-pigmented tapetum. This colouration frequently shows with the silver coat that turns to white as the ferret ages. Ferrets have a holangiotic fundus with retinal blood vessels radiating from the optic disc. The vessels appear magnified due to the effect of their unusually large lens. Pigmented ferrets have the green-blue reflective eye shine from the tapetum lucidum. Albinos lack this reflectivity but histologically have a tapetum similar to the pigmented one.

The ferret retina has been well studied. It is considered that ferret vision has less acuity than the cat's. The ferret's visual resolution according to Snellen acuity is 20/170 in bright light and 20/350 in dim light. The threshold of light needed for vision in the ferret is considered to be 5–7 times lower than that of man. The ferret retina has a high proportion of rods in the photoreceptor layer. The rods predominate to the cones in the ratio 50–60:1. There are twelve cortical visual areas. Ferrets can detect red colour only. There are defects in the optokinetic reflex in albino ferrets. This is associated with defective neurogenesis and abnormal neurogenesis in the visual cortex. Thus albino ferrets have problems with motion detection, which is shown behaviourally. Albino ferrets do not appear to have poorer ability in visual discrimination when compared to their pigmented counterparts. There does appear to be lower visual acuity although it is not statistically significant.

The nictitating membrane is well developed. It has lymphoid tissue that can be a site of lymphoma.

Nasal structure and olfaction

The ferret nasal cavity is similar to that of long-nosed dogs. It is formed by the maxilla and nasal bones dorsally and laterally. The maxillary and palatine bones supply the cavity floor. The bony nasal aperture is divided into two symmetrical halves. The ethmoid bone complex is located between the brain case and the facial part of the skull and consists of the ethmoid labyrinth, cribriform plate and median bone plate of the nasal septum. The labyrinth is composed of many delicate scrolls that attach to the cribriform plate and occupy the fundus of the nasal cavity. The conchae, which are shaped as bony scrolls, project into each nasal fossa. The mucosa within acts as a baffle to warm and clean inspired air. The conchae are divided as in the dog, into small dorsal and large ventral portions. The olfactory mucosa that lines the conchae contains olfactory nerve cells. The ethmoid plate does not completely pass ventral to the cartilage of the nasal septum to divide the nasal fossa as it does in the dog. This makes it more difficult to pass a nasal tube.

SPLEEN

The ferret spleen lies from the upper left to lower right abdominal cavity (**Fig. 3.35**). It is attached to the liver and stomach by the gastrosplenic ligament. It is crescent shaped and purplish brown. Its size in a 1 kg ferret is approximately 5 × 2 × 0.8 cm. With anaesthesia it can greatly enlarge, with blood storage estimated at between 15–30% of its size. For this reason, its size should be estimated on palpation prior to any sedation or anaesthesia for radiography or ultrasonography. It also tends to enlarge with age

and also disease conditions. It becomes a primary site of extramedullary hematopoiesis surplanting the bone marrow. For this reason, a bone marrow biopsy should always be done prior to splenectomy. It can be a site of lymphoma.

THYMUS

The thymus lies in the cranial mediastinum in the thoracic inlet. It is large in young ferrets but may be replaced by fat in adults.

THYROID AND PARATHYROID GLANDS

The bilobed thyroid glands are elongate and flattened structures, reddish-brown in colour lying just caudal to the larynx alongside the trachea. They are approximately 1 cm in length. The thyroid glands are joined ventrally with a thin isthmus that lies across the trachea. The parathyroid glands appear as tiny white masses at the cranioventral area of the thyroids. These glands function as in other carnivores (**Fig. 3.36**).

URINARY TRACT (SEE CHAPTER 22)

The kidneys palpate movably in the abdomen (**Fig. 3.2**). The left kidney lies further caudal than

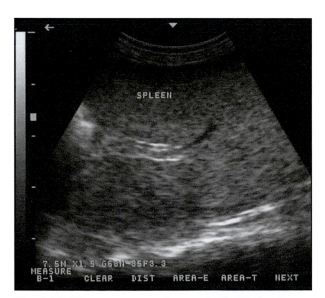

Fig. 3.35 Ultrasonogram of normal splenic tissue.

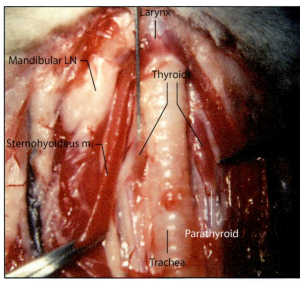

Fig. 3.36 Normal thyroids and parathyroid. LN, lymph node.

the right kidney. The cranial pole of the right kidney is covered by the caudate lobe of the liver. The left kidney is covered by the spleen. Vasculature for each is supplied by their respective artery and vein. A study was done to measure normal kidneys (Appendix 9). The mean size of the right kidney is 30.13 × 14.83 mm. The mean size of the left kidney is 29.33 × 14.63 mm. This equates to just a little over the length of two vertebrae. Both kidneys drain via their respective ureters to the bladder. Kidney structure and function is similar to other carnivores.

The bladder is small and usually may only hold up to 10 mL with low pressure. The urine is voided through the urethra. In the males, the prostate glandular tissue surrounds the urethra as it exits the bladder for approximately 1 cm just at the entrance to the pelvic canal. In the female, the urethra opens at the vaginovestibular junction. In the males, the urethra after exiting the pelvic canal proceeds cranially to open at the prepuce mid ventral abdomen. This is similar to the anatomy of the dog. The os penis is J-shaped (**Fig. 3.28**).

CHAPTER 4

FERRET BEHAVIOUR, HOUSING AND HUSBANDRY

Anna Meredith

INTRODUCTION

Ferrets make endearing, entertaining, easily trained and highly rewarding pets and are popular in many countries around the world. To work effectively with ferrets in a clinical setting, to get the best out of ferret ownership and to ensure ferret welfare in both the home and veterinary environment, it is important to have a good understanding of the fundamental needs and natural behaviour of the species (**Fig. 4.1**).

Domestication of the ferret has led to very few significant changes in appearance or anatomy from its wild counterpart, the European polecat, with coat colour being the most significant source of human-influenced variation. The ferret has also retained the majority of its natural behavioural repertoire. Ferrets can manage in the wild and might survive as feral animals if there is a food source and no predators such as hawks. Wild polecats and feral ferrets are essentially solitary nocturnal predators, but one significant feature of domestication is that domestic ferrets are much more sociable, due to retention of juvenile behavioural characteristics, as in domestic cats and dogs. This feature may also be attributable in part to neutering. Another difference is that domestic ferrets are intrinsically less frightened of people and novel environments or objects than the wild polecat (Poole, 1972). Although naturally most active at dawn and dusk and overnight to coincide with wild prey activity, pet ferrets adapt easily to their owners' routines and can be habituated to be more active during the day and sleep at night by feeding and encouraging activity during these times (**Fig. 4.2**).

BEHAVIOUR

Normal ferret behaviour can be described as 'all or nothing'. Reflecting their role as an intelligent carnivorous predator, a healthy ferret is either asleep or 'full on', i.e. highly alert, constantly active and investigative, and will not spend time awake doing nothing or

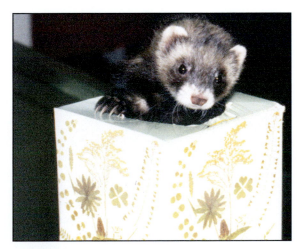

Fig. 4.1 **Ferret playing in a tissue box.**

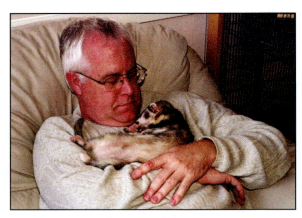

Fig. 4.2 **Ferret in the arms of the owner.**

spend any significant time resting, other than briefly 'slumping' (see below) between bouts of activity or play. Normal ferret behaviour is frequently perceived as exuberant and joyful, and it is easy to imagine that ferrets have a sense of fun and humour (See the Ferret Ten Commandments, *Box 4.1*). Lethargy, reduced levels of alertness or reluctance to be active or interactive indicate that a ferret is unwell.

Locomotion

Ferrets are constantly in motion when awake. Their elongated thin body shape with long back and short legs gives them a typical sinuous or 'slinky' appearance when moving, and they can turn and change direction in a very restricted space. This trait has led to the popular pastime of ferret racing, where bets are placed on ferrets entered singly at the same time into one end of a line-up of long opaque tubes to see which one emerges first from the other end, in the hope that they do not turn and come back out of the entrance (**Fig. 4.11**).

Locomotory behaviours seen in ferrets include:

- Walking – with a typical ambling gait, head held close to the ground and the body stretched out.
- Running – generally a scampering motion involving repeated arching of the back.
- Running backwards, and a 'back up then charge' manoeuvre (**Fig. 4.12**).
- Slither/slink/belly crawl – may be seen when playing (see below) or as part of scent-marking behaviour.

Box 4.1 The Ferret Ten Commandments (courtesy C. Johnson-Delaney)

1. Thou shalt poo in corners (**Fig. 4.3**).
2. Thou shalt bite thy brethren and lick thy humans (**Fig. 4.4**).
3. Thou shalt revere milk and dairy products above all things except Ferretone® & Nutri-Cal®.
4. Thou shalt despise anything labelled 'For ferrets'.
5. Thou shalt climb everything in sight and take the good stuff (**Fig. 4.5**).
6. When placed in a cage or locked room, thou shalt beat loudly upon the door in protest (**Fig. 4.6**)!
7. Thou shalt lurk and seek opportunities (**Fig. 4.7**).
8. Thou shalt love, honour and steal shoes and socks (**Fig. 4.8**).
9. Thou shalt expose the roots of all plants (**Fig. 4.9**).
10. Thou shalt hide those things that should not see the light of day (**Fig. 4.10**).

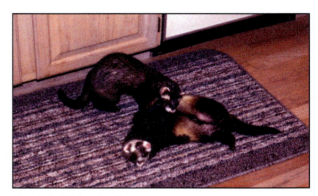

Fig. 4.4 **Biting in play.**

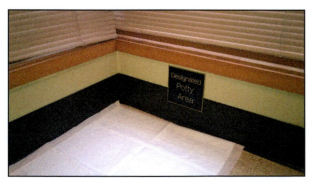

Fig. 4.3 **Designated toilet area in a veterinary examination room. (Courtesy of Kevin Farlee.)**

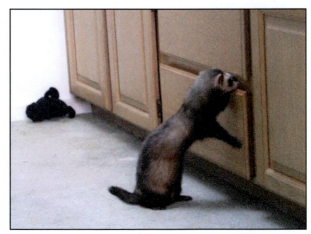

Fig. 4.5 **Beginning the climb up the cabinets.**

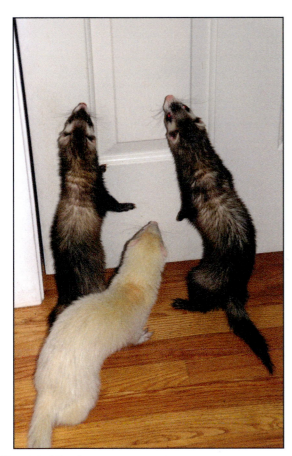

Fig. 4.6 **Wanting to get out.**

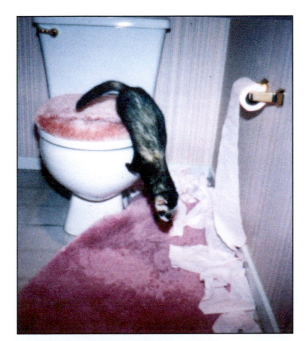

Fig. 4.7 **Attacking the toilet paper roll.**

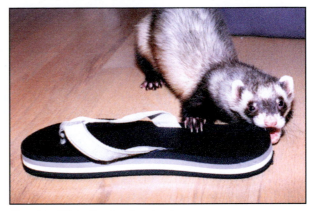

Fig. 4.8 **This flip flop is mine!**

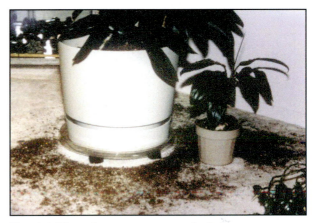

Fig. 4.9 **Plant damage courtesy of a ferret.**

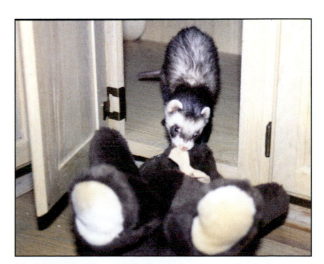

Fig. 4.10 **Pulling stuffed toy into the cupboard.**

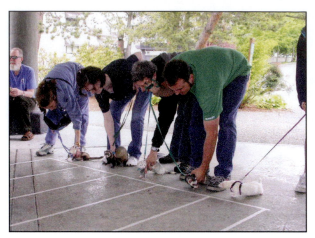

Fig. 4.11 Ferret race held at a 'Frolics' event.

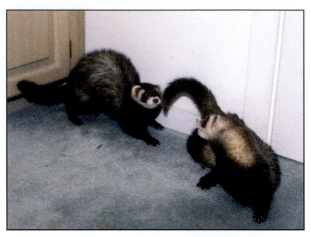

Fig. 4.12 Ferrets backing up in play behaviour.

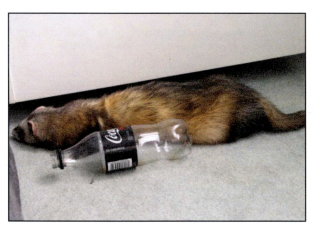

Fig. 4.13 Ferret slumping during playtime.

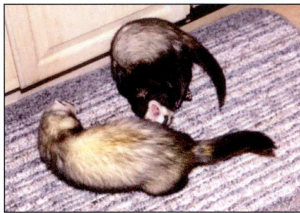

Fig. 4.14 Flipping during play.

- Slumping – a sudden slump to the floor with body flattened to the ground, eyes open and back legs splayed for a few minutes; seen between bouts of intense play/activity. This is often called 'pelting' or 'speedbump. (**Fig. 4.13**).
- Hopping – play (see below), excitement.
- Galloping.
- Digging – natural tunnelling/exploratory behaviour.
- Spinning/pivoting – usually during play (**Fig. 4.14**).
- Jumping.
- Climbing.
- Dancing – the ferret springs into the air with back arched and sways from side to side, often with the mouth wide open and making a hissing sound, dancing forwards or backwards or in

place. Much enjoyed by owners, this is referred to variously as the 'weasel war dance', the 'dance of joy', or the 'happy dance', among other terms. Although it may appear alarming if unused to ferret behaviour, this dance behaviour is a sign of excitement or happiness and is frequently used to solicit play (see below).

Ferrets, like cats, can right themselves to land on their feet if they are dropped or fall from a height.

Ferret senses
Vision (see Chapters 3, 15)
Ferrets are highly efficient predators and are naturally nocturnal, thus have poor visual acuity and colour vision, and rely heavily on smell and auditory cues to detect prey. Studies have shown that their visual

system is very similar to the cat, with twelve cortical visual areas, and a cone-rich retina. They can detect red colour only, and are more sensitive to light *intensity* than colour. They are believed to be able to see best at dawn and dusk, and attention and predatory behaviour are triggered by rapid movement of objects – it has been demonstrated that they will preferentially follow objects moving at a speed similar to a running mouse (25–45 cm/s) (Apfelbach and Wester, 1972). Due to their poor eyesight they have poor perception of being at height and can fall from high shelves or balconies or through bannisters. They are also prone to bumping into objects or walls while running.

Hearing (see Chapters 3, 15)

Ferret hearing is also very similar to the cat, and is most sensitive in the range 4–15 kHz (Moore *et al.*, 1983). They lack the highly mobile pinna of the cat, but nevertheless can localise sound very accurately to detect and react to prey. The neuroanatomy of the ferret auditory system is thought to create a spatial 'map' in response to sound, enabling them to be highly efficient in locating prey in their environment. High-pitched squeaking sounds are useful for attracting a ferret's attention.

Smell and scent marking (see Chapter 3)

Smell is the most important of the senses to ferrets, not only for hunting, appetite and food preferences, but for social behaviour including breeding. Both jills and hobs define their territories by scent marking and behaviours associated with smell and scent marking are numerous and very noticeable. Ferrets can distinguish other individual ferrets and their sex and reproductive status by smell alone, mainly that produced by the anal sac secretions (Clapperton, 1988), but possibly also via the urine (Zhang *et al.*, 2005), and smell will undoubtedly be important in recognition of familiar and unfamiliar humans. The typical musty smell of ferrets is produced largely by the sebaceous glands of the skin, but the anal sacs, proctodeal glands in the rectum and preputial glands in the male are also important. Both sexes perform the 'anal drag', where the anus is lowered to the ground and the animal walks forward while wriggling its back end to spread the anal sac secretions, usually near the latrine site or litter tray (see Elimination behaviour).

Other scent-marking and wiping behaviours performed include the 'belly crawl', where the chest is lowered to the ground and the body pushed forward by the back legs, and the 'urogenital wipe', where the tail is raised and the urogenital area wiped over an object, with or without a leg raised and urination. This wiping behaviour is performed more by males and especially in spring when the breeding season begins (Clapperton, 1989). Ferrets will also rub and wipe their necks and flanks on the ground by rolling to spread scent, and this type of behaviour is often performed when two males meet. These scent-marking behaviours are typical of all mustelids, and are used to recognise individuals, whether they are potential mate or rival, and to announce territories and allow animals to avoid each other and conflict when moving around in the wild. Ferrets will also rub their chins backwards and forwards on objects at feeding sites. This may be related to food-stashing behaviour and serve as a cue to identify stored food sites, or warn other ferrets away from them (Clapperton, 1989).

Vocalisation

Ferrets use a wide variety of vocalisations. These include:

- 'Dooking' or 'the dook' – a chattering , chuckling or clucking sound made when excited or playing, or when new animals are introduced to each other.
- High-pitched chattering – an alarm call.
- Hissing – agitation, threatening/offensive behaviour, defensive behaviour, or play behaviour when dancing.
- Whimpering – made by females with young to encourage them to follow her.
- Muttering – low muttering or hooting under the breath, often performed when exploring.
- Screaming/squealing – indicative of pain or extreme fear, or defensive behaviour when fighting. Jills may also scream during mating. Deaf ferrets often squeal while playing, seemingly unaware they are vocalising.

Grooming

Ferrets have fastidious grooming habits and will groom themselves and other ferrets by licking (**Fig. 4.15**). Grooming by owners is not essential and

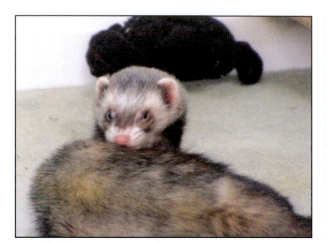

Fig. 4.15 Ferret grooming itself.

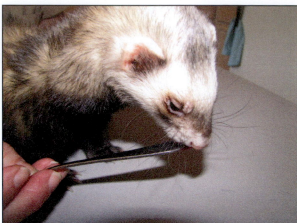

Fig. 4.16 Administration of a laxative gel.

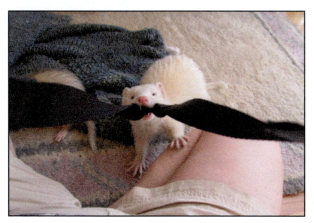

Fig. 4.17 Biting a strap and not letting go.

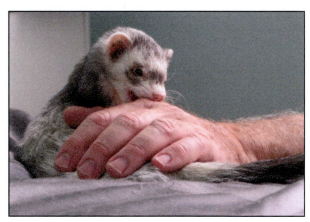

Fig. 4.18 Mouthing an owner's hand. This behaviour should be discouraged.

many healthy ferrets rarely stay still long enough to allow effective grooming anyway! However, ferrets can develop hair balls and grooming with a soft cat brush can be performed when the ferret is moulting (spring and autumn), and will enhance the pet–owner bond. If the ferret is ill or unable to groom itself for any reason, brushing by the owner may be required and appreciated. During the time of moulting it is a good idea to provide a laxative (a cat or ferret laxative gel) daily to prevent the formation of a trichobezoar (**Fig. 4.16**).

Investigative behaviour

Ferrets are by nature extremely inquisitive and investigate objects by mouthing or biting them (**Fig. 4.17**). This, combined with relatively poor eyesight, gives them a reputation for biting, but this is rarely true aggression (see behavioural problems below), although it can still be painful, and is a good reason to never place a ferret close to the face. Once bitten the instinctive attempt to immediately pull the ferret off frequently results in it gripping even harder, resulting in more serious wound. This behaviour and their tendency to chew also makes them at risk of ingestion of foreign bodies or injury from electric cables, etc., as well as being destructive to valued home items (**Fig. 4.18**).

Being naturally drawn to small openings reminiscent of rodent or rabbit burrows, any small gap is enthusiastically explored, which can be highly entertaining to watch but can get them into trouble or easily 'lost' in a home environment, disappearing into the smallest of spaces. Cupboards, drawers and the underside of sofas and beds are all highly desirable spaces, and there is no limit to a ferret's exploratory prowess (**Fig. 4.19**). Homes and veterinary consulting rooms should be thoroughly ferret-proofed before a ferret is let loose, to avoid embarrassing disappearances or access to harmful situations (see below). Ferrets also like to dig as part of their normal exploratory behaviour, and they can be destructive in a home environment as a result, damaging carpets, digging up plants in pots or the garden or digging under wire to escape.

Locating and recovering a lost ferret is best achieved by attracting their attention with a sound they associate with food and/or fun through previous positive reinforcement. Squeaking a familiar squeaky toy or rattling some food treats in a can or box usually works very well to lure them out of a hiding place and bring them running (**Fig. 4.20**).

Social, play and aggressive behaviour

Domestic ferrets are much more social than their solitary wild polecat ancestors, who will steer clear of each other to avoid conflict except during the breeding season. This is because domestication has resulted in retention of juvenile behaviours. As a result, pet ferrets should ideally be kept with other ferrets unless the owner can spend a lot of time playing and interacting with their pet, but they do have very individual temperaments, characters and preferences and some ferrets will be happier if kept alone. If kept together they will sleep together and perform some mutual grooming; however, it is important to be aware that ferrets do not exhibit complex cohesive social behaviours, such as seen in dogs, as this is not in their evolutionary profile (**Fig. 4.21**).

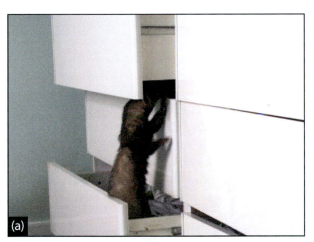
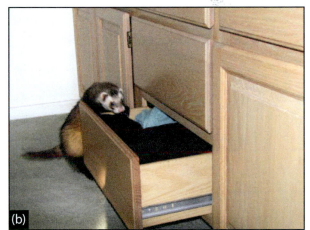

Fig. 4.19 (a, b) Exploring open drawers.

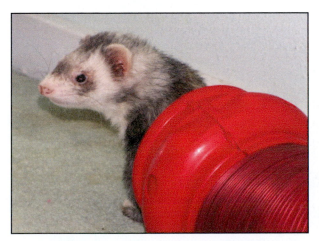

Fig. 4.20 Emerging from a tunnel when called.

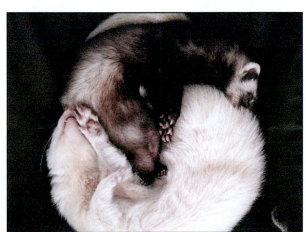

Fig. 4.21 Ferrets sleep together in a group.

As with all predatory mammals, it is believed that the aim of play is to learn and practice hunting and fighting skills that are needed by wild adults. Young ferrets play most, but play behaviour persists into adulthood and makes up an important part of social behaviour. Young ferrets begin to play from as early as 4 weeks, even when the eyes are still closed, but play is at its highest levels between 6 and 14 weeks. Ferrets will play on their own with a toy or object, particularly if it is novel (**Fig. 4.22**), but by far the best play stimulus for a ferret is another ferret. Toys such as balls will be 'dribbled' with the front feet or held in the front paws while the ferret scoots along or backwards with it.

Play in ferrets is very active and aggressive which can be alarming to inexperienced owners, but they very rarely harm each other. Play behaviour occurs when ferrets are relaxed and in a familiar environment without other distractions. Ferrets will play with food and water items and readily spill them and make a mess. Play behaviour includes:

- Locomotor play (see locomotion above):
  - Chasing and reciprocal chasing.
  - Ambushing.
  - Exaggerated approaching – 'back up then charge'.
  - Dancing.
  - Digging.
  - Stashing objects.
- Play fighting, or 'rough and tumble', involving:
  - Wrestling.
  - Mounting.

- Rolling.
- Mouthing, and an open-mouthed 'play face'– often used to initiate play.
- Inhibited biting, particularly neck biting.

During play, movements are loose and bouncy or jerky and galloping, and individuals may swap roles as aggressor or defender, with inhibited bites aimed at the neck and muzzle. Play between familiar ferrets can appear quite aggressive, but sustained neck biting, sideways attacking, defensive threats (arched back, raised head facing aggressor, bared teeth, hissing) and screaming usually indicate true aggression, which is uninhibited and has the purpose of establishing dominance and rank (Poole, 1966; Poole, 1973). Aggressive fighting can be prolonged and result in injury, especially between intact males in the breeding season. Surgical or chemical neutering of male ferrets has been shown to decrease aggressive behaviour, both when receptive females are present and when they are not (Vinke *et al.*, 2008).

Play will not occur or will stop if ferrets are placed in a novel environment (where exploratory behaviour will occur), if a prey item is detected (where chasing/hunting behaviour will occur) or if the ferret becomes fearful, where it will show escape behaviour or may become defensive. 'Brush tail' or 'bottlebrush tail', caused by piloerection of the tail hair, indicates a high state of arousal due to either anger, fear or excitement, and is usually seen in association with an arched back and hissing or screaming (**Fig. 4.23**). Sudden emptying of the anal sacs to release a large amount of foul-smelling secretions

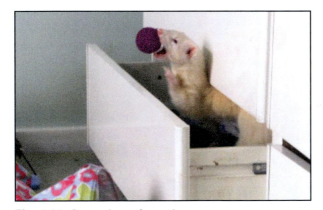

Fig. 4.22 **Capturing a favourite toy.**

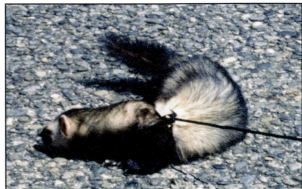

Fig. 4.23 **Bottlebrush tail occurring during excitement.**

can occur if the ferret is extremely alarmed, but this is unusual. Prophylactic removal of anal glands to prevent this event is illegal in the UK. Most ferrets in the USA are demusked at the time of neutering and the largest supplier to the pet trade does this at 5–6 weeks of age.

Sleeping

Ferrets will spend at least 12–18 hours a day sleeping, and prefer to sleep in a warm, dark, cosy, secluded area that mimics an underground nest burrow and makes them feel safe and secure (**Fig. 4.24**). Hammocks or fleece-lined enclosed cat beds are greatly enjoyed, but even a simple old towel or T-shirt that they can burrow under, placed in an old cardboard box, can work well (see Housing) (**Fig. 4.25**). Sleeping excessively or difficulty rousing are strong indicators that a ferret is unwell. As ferrets age they will sleep more, sometimes nearing 22 hours a day. Deaf ferrets may be difficult to rouse at any time and should not be startled from sleep, as the instinct may be to nip.

Feeding and stashing behaviour

Natural predatory behaviour involves stalking and then pouncing on prey such as rodents, small birds and rabbits, then biting and holding firm on the back of the neck to kill with the large sharp canine teeth. If food is provided *ad libitum* they have been shown to eat numerous small meals rather than fewer large ones – 9 or 10 per day in one study (Kaufman, 1980). Food preferences, based largely on olfaction, are established and imprinted at a young age, as is typical of other obligate carnivores. If not fed a variety of foods early on, introducing new diets to older ferrets can be challenging. Ferrets will tip over feed bowls so these need to be heavy to resist tipping or be secured to the side of the cage (see Husbandry) (**Fig. 4.26**).

Stashing, or caching, behaviour is normal, as wild polecats would bring a large prey item back to the den to store and eat frequent small meals from. Therefore owners must be aware to search for and remove decomposing food hidden in the cage or enclosure, or elsewhere in the home. As well as food, ferrets will also stash toys and other household objects, much to some owners' frustration when an essential item such as a mobile phone or pair of socks goes missing (**Fig. 4.27**)!

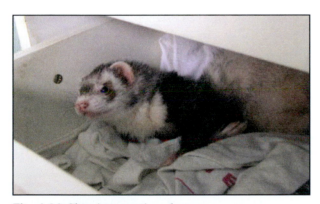

Fig. 4.24 **Sleeping spot in a drawer.**

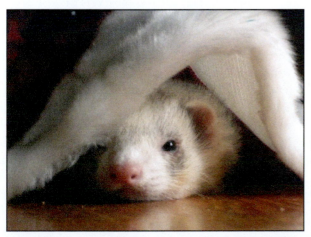

Fig. 4.25 **Ferret under fabric cover for a sleeping spot. (Courtesy of Vondelle McLaughlin.)**

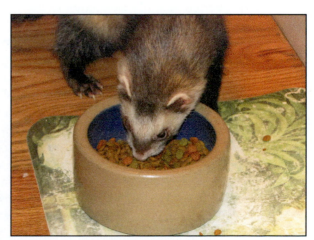

Fig. 4.26 **Heavy ceramic bowls for drinking and eating.**

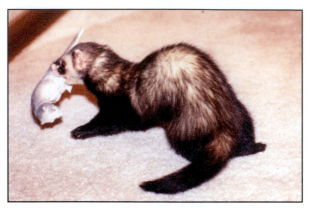

Fig. 4.27 Taking a toy to stash it in the cupboard.

Elimination behaviour and litter training (see also Husbandry)

Ferrets will naturally use specific latrine areas so it is easy to litter train them. They will usually urinate and defaecate at the beginning or end of periods of activity, or after eating. Latrines in the wild are multiple within the territory and usually near the den. Pet ferrets invariably select a corner of the cage, enclosure or room and will back up into this until their back end touches the walls, and lift their tail to defaecate by squirting their normally soft faeces upwards. It is best to let the ferret choose its preferred latrine area first and then place the litter tray there, rather than assume they will choose to use the area where a tray is placed. Ferrets do not bury faeces and will perform an anal drag after defaecating to scent mark. This often results in a little puddle of faeces a distance away from the full bowel movement.

Reproductive and maternal behaviour

Ferrets are naturally polygynous, so males will mate with many females. They reach sexual maturity at between 8 and 12 months (see Chapter 6). In males this is associated with increased sexual behaviours such as an interest in jills in oestrus, neck gripping and pelvic thrusting. In jills sexual maturity occurs with the onset of the first oestrus as days lengthen in early spring. Mating behaviour is a lengthy, noisy and aggressive affair where the hob grabs the jill by the back of the neck and drags her around. Receptive jills present their genital area repeatedly to the hob's head and will remain close and repeatedly crawl both over and under the hob. During copulation the female lies flat on the ground with the neck stretched forward and the male mounts, arches the back to bring the pelvis forward and performs multiple pelvic thrusts. Mating sessions can last from minutes to several hours but are usually about 1 hour in duration.

Pregnant jills should be separated from hobs, who play no role in rearing kits. After a 42-day gestation, parturition will occur in the nest area and should be complete within 2–3 hours, with an average of 8–9 (range 7–15) kits born. After birth the jill and litter should be left alone for a few days as disturbance may encourage cannibalism. She will eat the placentae and so tarry, black, loose faeces are a normal finding after parturition. The kits are altricial, born with eyes and ears closed, but can move using their front legs at birth and should start suckling almost immediately after birth. Initially they remain attached to the nipples for the majority of the time. Lactating jills have heightened orientation to the high-pitched frequency of kits' distress calls compared to non-lactating jills. Licking of the anogenital area by the jill is necessary to stimulate elimination. Eyes and ears open at about 4–5 weeks of age. Weaning starts from about 3 weeks of age when the jill will bring food to the nest for the kits, and from this time they will start to defaecate and urinate without licking stimulation from the mother. Weaning is completed by 5–6 weeks of age.

TRAINING AND DEALING WITH BEHAVIOURAL PROBLEMS

Ferrets are highly intelligent and are easily trained. Regular confident handling from a young age is vital in the socialisation process with humans, and for training. As with all animals, training by immediate positive reinforcement is essential, and training provides enrichment, mental stimulation and an enhanced ferret–owner bond and relationship (**Fig. 4.28**). Negative reinforcement or punishment of undesired behaviours by smacking, flicking, tapping on the nose or shouting does not work and only induces fear, which can lead to aggression such as biting. They can also be trained to accept a harness and lead for exercise, although parallels with dog training

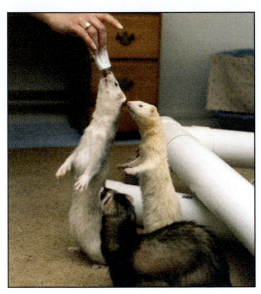

Fig. 4.28 **Training may require positive reinforcement with a treat.**

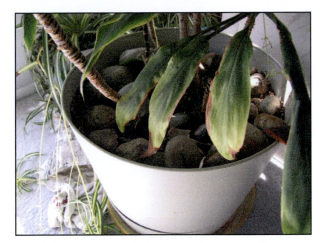

Fig. 4.29 **Ferret-proofed plant with large rocks to discourage digging.**

such as obeying 'sit, stay' commands are usually beyond the attention span, patience or interest of a typical ferret. Coming when called or when a toy is squeaked or rattled are usually easily trained using a food reward.

Biting/nipping is the commonest behavioural problem in ferrets (Bulloch and Tynes, 2010; Bradley Bays, 2012). Biting is part of normal play and exploratory behaviour, and young ferrets will often initiate attention or play by biting. Licking followed by a gentle nip can also be grooming behaviour, so licking of the owner should be discouraged to avoid progression to a bite. Similarly, owners should avoid provoking aggressive play with their hands or by instigating tug-of-war-type games. Behavioural modification should consist of passive correction of unwanted behaviour by distracting the ferret immediately with a favourite toy or treat, to redirect the unwanted overly aggressive behaviour. A firm 'stop/no' command and putting the ferret down or back in its cage for time out, to calm down if the distraction is ignored and the unwanted behaviour persists, can then be used. A hissing sound (to mimic the jill correcting unwanted behaviour of a juvenile) or high-pitched 'yip' combined with time out can also work. Consistency from all members of the family who interact with the ferret is essential, as well as positive reinforcement for non-biting desired behaviours. Unexpected onset or an increase in biting behaviour from a previously well-behaved ferret could indicate pain or illness and this should be investigated.

Destructive behaviour is normal and damage limitation can be achieved by ferret-proofing the environment, supervision at all times when loose in the house and provision of plenty of enrichment, toys and objects that the ferret is allowed to destroy in the areas it has access to. As ferrets like to dig, houseplants are often dug up. This can be prevented by placing plants where the ferret cannot get to them, placing large rocks on the top of the soil or by using screens over the soil (**Fig. 4.29**). It is advisable to have only non-toxic houseplants in case the ferret bites the plant during digging (Appendix 7).

INTRODUCING NEW FERRETS

It is always best to introduce ferrets when young and let them grow up together if owners want to have more than one. Introducing unfamiliar older ferrets to each other can be difficult and must be managed and supervised properly, otherwise serious aggression and fighting can occur. A neutral space is best with areas for escape and hiding. Sex and neutered status as well as age will affect success, and same-sex ferrets tend to fight more on introduction; two neutered males or a neutered male/female are least likely to be aggressive to each other. A younger ferret introduced to an older ferret that has previously lived alone or to a previously well-established group are situations that are likely to invoke fighting. On introduction there will be sniffing of the anal gland area, then some neck biting and a degree of fighting as the ferrets determine dominance. Contrary to expectations, caging two ferrets next to each other for a period before introducing them has been shown not to make any difference to the levels of aggression seen (Staton and Crowell-David, 2003). In rescue/shelter organisations, it has been found that introducing a new ferret first to the most friendly, sociable individual in a group and then slowly introducing the other group members can work well (Fisher, 2006). Distracting the ferrets by placing a tasty commercial paste-type or liquid treat (e.g. Ferretone™ [8 in 1, Islandia, NY] Nutri-Cal® [Vetoquinol US, Fort Worth, TX], Nutri-Plus® [Virbac US, Fort Worth, TX]) on the backs of their necks is also suggested as a way of decreasing aggression.

It is important to be aware that removing a ferret from a group or pair for as little as 2 days, for example for veterinary care or hospitalisation, can result in it being perceived as a stranger on reintroduction and lead to fighting. In a social group of ferrets, removing one may lead to stress and withdrawn behaviours in the remaining ferret(s). The owners need to be attentive to changes in appetite and stool associated with this stress.

SOCIAL INTERACTIONS WITH HUMANS AND OTHER SPECIES

Socialisation of ferrets with humans requires regular gentle handling from a young age. The critical time for socialisation is from 4 weeks when the eyes first open, until approximately 10 weeks of age.

Well-socialised ferrets will lick and groom their owner, run to greet them and exhibit great excitement, and will indulge enthusiastically in play behaviour with them, which is important in reinforcing the pet–owner bond (**Fig. 4.30**).

Ferrets can bond very closely with both cats and dogs in the same household (**Fig. 4.31**) and will play vigorously with them. These species should be introduced slowly, preferably when the ferret is still

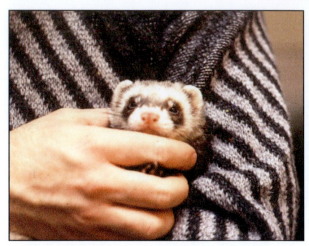

Fig. 4.30 **Ferrets bond closely with their owners and enjoy being held and cuddled.**

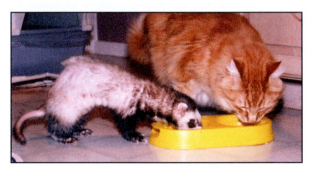

Fig. 4.31 **Ferret (adrenal disease present) eating from the same bowl as a cat.**

young, and always under supervision as the ferret's rapid activity may stimulate predatory behaviour in the other species. Even if well bonded, in general all interspecies interactions should be supervised, but this does depend largely on the temperament of the individuals involved and requires a common-sense approach.

It goes without saying that prey species such as rabbits or rodents should not be exposed to ferrets.

HOUSING AND HUSBANDRY

Ferrets can be housed indoors or outdoors depending on climate and intended use. The natural 'musky' body odour of ferrets, more prominent in non-neutered animals, is offensive to many and a key reason for being kept outdoors. Many pet ferrets have their housing outside but are regularly brought indoors to play and socialise; others are indoors permanently and are kept in apartments with no outdoor access.

Outdoor housing

Outdoor housing is traditional for working ferrets but is also used for pets. For outdoor ferrets the most important factor is to avoid overheating and heatstroke by not situating housing in direct sunlight. Traditionally for working ferrets a large, fully enclosed pit or 'court' is used with a weather-proof insulated house or nest box within it. Pets are more commonly kept in a wooden hutch-type housing unit, either with an exercise area integral to it or placed within a larger enclosure, or in a large, wire, aviary-type enclosure with an internal nest box (**Figs 4.32, 4.33**). Many options are possible but whatever is used must be secure and escape-proof, and the sleeping area dry and warm. Nesting areas should be raised off the ground to avoid damp. Hay or straw bedding are both suitable, as are towels

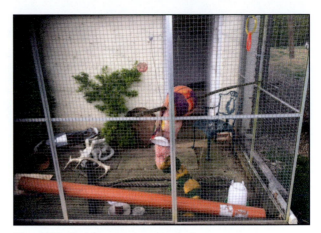

Fig. 4.33 Outdoor pen example 2.

or fleecy materials, without loose fibres that may be ingested. Chewing of wood or enclosure wire is not a major problem and wire mesh must be small enough so that the ferret's head cannot get trapped.

Outdoor latrines can be a soil or substrate area or a litter tray. They should be cleaned daily.

Indoor housing

Wire caging makes ideal ferret housing, and cages suitable for puppies/dogs are ideal as a safe enclosed area for when sleeping or when confinement is required (**Figs 4.34, 4.35**). Wooden housing can get easily soiled with urine and faeces. This should never be the sole accommodation and an opportunity to exercise and play for at least 2 hours a day is essential. Ideally a ferret-safe room or rooms should be provided for play and exercise without constant supervision. Owners need always to remember that anything chewable, e.g. training shoes and shoe inserts, clothing and books, is fair game for a ferret, so should be kept out of the way if valued (**Fig. 4.36**).

Ferret-proofing the home:

- Block off spaces under or behind cabinets, stoves, refrigerators and other appliances in kitchens and bathrooms – wire mesh or thin board can be used.
- Block off spaces under furniture in living and bedroom areas.
- Ensure any gaps in floorboards or skirting boards are closed off.

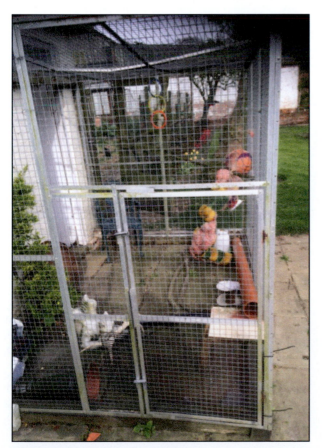

Fig. 4.32 Outdoor pen example 1.

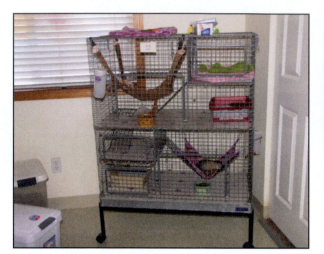

Fig. 4.34 Indoor housing example 1.

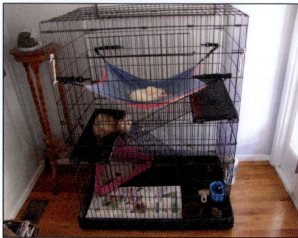

Fig. 4.35 Indoor housing example 2 showing corner-style litter tray and newspaper being used.

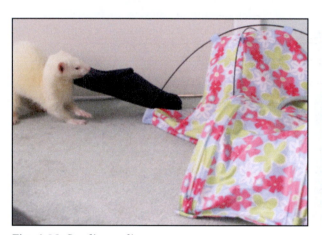

Fig. 4.36 Stealing a slipper.

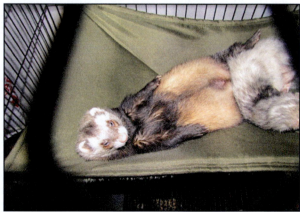

Fig. 4.37 Ferrets like to sleep in hammocks.

- Keep toilet lids down.
- Keep all cleaning supplies, chemicals, medications, etc., out of reach in firmly closed or locked cupboards.
- Keep all foam rubber or soft rubber items out of reach.
- Cover or encase electric wiring so it cannot be chewed.
- Keep house plants out of reach or cover the soil to prevent digging.
- Make sure the ferret is not inside a chair or couch/sofa before sitting down or using a reclining mechanism.
- Check washing machines and driers before closing the door and operating, particularly if clothing is already inside.

- Solid barriers, e.g. plexiglass or wood, can be used to block off rooms or areas that are out of bounds, or keep the doors firmly closed.

Nesting area

Ferrets like to sleep in dark enclosed areas. Hammocks (**Fig. 4.37**), slings or fleece-lined enclosed baskets, tents or tubes and other suitable nests or beds are widely available commercially. Alternatively, old towels or clothing in a box can be used. A selection of nest areas should be provided, and at least one for every ferret kept, although they will often all prefer to sleep together.

Litter tray

Although easily trained to recognise and use a litter tray, ferrets are not easy to truly housetrain. They have a short GI transit time and defaecate frequently, and so placement of multiple litter trays, at least one in each room that the ferret has access to, will help prevent accidents. Corner-shaped trays with low sides at the front and high sides at the back are best to protect walls, filled with a shallow depth of paper-based or pelleted litter, not the clumping or clay-based varieties. Thick layers of newspaper are also ideal and can be easily wrapped and removed daily (**Fig. 4.35**).

Toys and other enrichment

Environmental enrichment is important to stimulate natural behaviours and provide mental stimulation. Sufficient space to exercise vigorously, and other ferrets, humans or other pets to interact and play with are the priority. Tubing such as PVC drainpipes to mimic tunnels and burrows, ramps, platforms and boxes can all be used, and some owners go to great lengths to provide stimulating ferret play areas (**Fig. 4.38**). Changing the environment and introducing novel objects provides additional interest and stimulation. Water is also greatly enjoyed and shallow dishes or baths can be provided, as can digging boxes filled with clean soil or long-grain uncooked rice (**Fig. 4.39**). Ferret toys will always be chewed and so must be safe to avoid ingestion of foreign bodies that could cause GI obstruction. Hard rubber firm Kong®-type toys (The Kong Company, Golden CO), toys made of tightly braided rope or hard plastic or cloth cat or baby toys are suitable (**Fig. 4.40**). Soft latex rubber, foam rubber, Styrofoam, and furniture stuffing are all dangerous if chewed or ingested. *Box 4.2* lists items that can be used for play.

Food can be used as enrichment by hiding dry food items in playballs or in paper bags, etc., so the ferret has to work to find it. There are numerous commercial ferret treats that can be given directly or hidden somewhere in the ferret's play area. Olfactory enrichment in the form of food scents/favourings or safe essential oils (e.g. lavender, rosemary, clary sage, valerian) can add extra interest to objects.

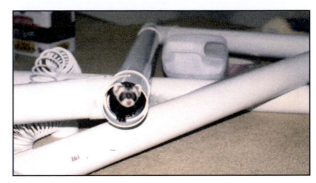

Fig. 4.38 **PVC pipes for tunnels.**

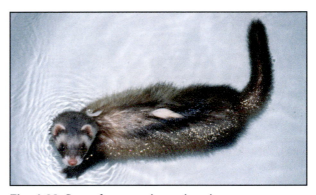

Fig. 4.39 **Some ferrets enjoy swimming.**

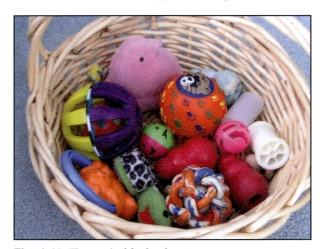

Fig. 4.40 **Toys suitable for ferrets.**

Bathing

Opinion is divided over the need to bathe ferrets. The main reason for bathing is to reduce the strong body odour that many find offensive, and that is perhaps the biggest negative aspect of ferret keeping. Neutering greatly helps to reduce this, and should be recommended for health

---

Box 4.2 Environmental enrichment for ferrets

- Wicker baskets (may also hide toys in the basket).
- Large plastic tub (like those used for feline litter trays) filled with uncooked rice (long-grain variety best). Let the ferret dig in it.
- Superchew Edible Toy. (Marshall Farms Pet Products: www.marshallpet.com/product-type/ferret/183/ superchew-edible-toy, available through online pet stores).
- Offer toys made for cats – fishing toys, bell toys, plush toys and plastic balls. Regularly wash and exchange the toys to maintain interest.
- Hide a toy in a different place each day for the ferret to find and take back to its favourite hiding place.
- Drill holes in flowerpots, and turn them upside down for exploration and to conceal treats for discovery and creative thinking.
- Use remote-control cars; some ferrets love to chase and 'kill' the car.
      Provide tubing and boxes in which the ferret can crawl or hide. Run tubing behind furniture and in various other places to keep the ferret stimulated. When multiple ferrets are out, tunnels make great play areas for mock 'battle' games.
- Fill a bathtub with 2–3 inches of water and add toys that float. Drape a wet towel over the side so the ferret can crawl in and out as it pleases.
      Place ping-pong balls inside a playpen-type enclosure for entertainment. Ping-pong balls can also be placed in a large plastic tub (like those used for feline litter trays) with other toys mixed in. The ferret then has to dig around to find the other toys.
- Offer whole mice (pre-killed or frozen/thawed) as a food item. These are excellent nutritionally, provide enrichment, and some ferret owners use them as part of the regular diet.
- Offer food in foraging toys. There are a number of excellent food-foraging toys made for dogs that are suitable for ferrets available on the market. (http://perfectpoochdogtraining.weebly.com/shop.html).

Adapted from Fisher P (2005) Environmental enrichment for ferrets. *Exotic DVM* **6(6)**:20.

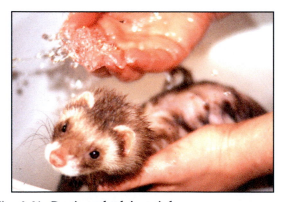

Fig. 4.41 Getting a bath in a sink.

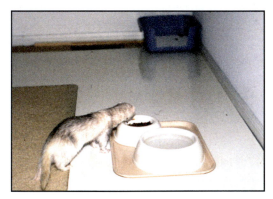

Fig. 4.42 Heavy dishes used for food and water. Note the corner litter tray in the background.

reasons unless breeding is desired (see Chapters 6, 9, 22, 25). Bathing is believed by some to strip the skin of oils and stimulate greater sebaceous oil production and hence odour, whereas others believe that bathing with a cat or ferret shampoo does keep odour under control. Most ferrets do seem to enjoy being in water and bathing, and a suggested interval is about every 4 weeks (**Fig. 4.41**).

Feeding (see Chapter 5)

Heavy bowls for food and water to prevent tipping should be used, and these can be fixed or clamped in place and removed for cleaning daily. Some ferrets will readily drink from a sipper bottle but some will not. Stashed or soiled food and water should be removed daily to prevent decomposition and pathogen build-up (**Fig. 4.42**). (All Figs except **4.32, 4.33** courtesy of Cathy Johnson-Delaney.)

CHAPTER 5

NUTRITION

Cathy A. Johnson-Delaney

INTRODUCTION

Ferrets are strict – or obligate –carnivores and they require high protein and fat levels. Their ancestor, the European polecat, feeds on birds and other small vertebrates. Their dentition and GI tract are adapted to this carnivorous diet (see Chapter 3). There are a number of commercial ferret diets that adequately meet the ferret's nutritional needs (**Fig. 5.1**).

Kibble is a popular food but the ferret's dentition is not really well suited to having to grind kibble. Kibble is crunchy and abrasive, a selling point to reduce dental calculus, but chewing kibble may cause structural changes to the tooth and underlying bony support (**Figs 5.2, 5.3**).

Nutritional diseases have been reported in ferrets, as seen in other species.

There are specific nutritional considerations for ferrets with insulinoma or who are geriatric.

WATER

Ferrets require approximately three times as much water as volume of dry matter food and should have fresh drinking water constantly available. They prefer to drink from a dish rather than a dropper bottle, and should be given this opportunity at least once daily, ensuring that their consumption of dry pellets is not limited by their water intake (**Fig. 5.4**). Heavy pots are the best water containers, as most ferrets rest their front feet on the edge of a dish as they drink, and may tip it over. Many pet ferrets also like to play in water. Fresh running water is also appreciated (**Figs 5.5–5.7**).

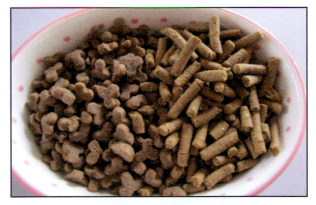

Fig. 5.1 **Two examples of commercial diets. Left, Totally Ferret® (Performance Foods); right, Premium Ferret Diet (Marshall).**

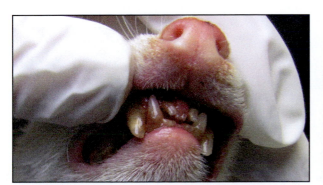

Fig. 5.2 **Dental wear from eating a kibble diet. Maxillary canine tooth is fractured and necrotic.**

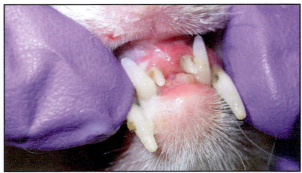

Fig. 5.3 **Dental wear and tooth loss from eating a kibble diet.**

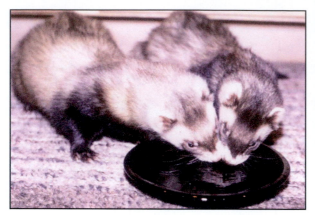

Fig. 5.4 **Drinking from a dish.**

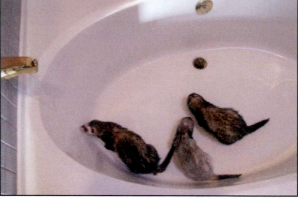

Fig. 5.5 **Drinking in a bathtub.**

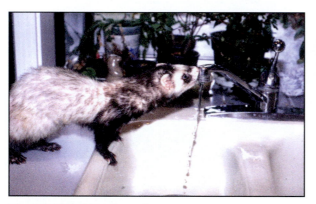

Fig. 5.6 **Drinking from the tap.**

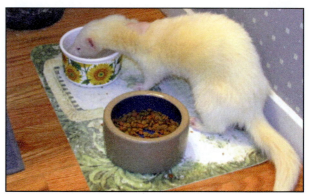

Fig. 5.7 **Drinking from a ceramic bowl.**

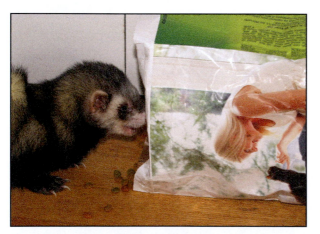

Fig. 5.8 **Eating cat kibble as a treat.**

COMMERCIAL DIETS

Years ago ranched ferrets were fed a mink diet, but pet ferrets usually do not like the fish flavour and instead prefer chicken flavour. Fish-source diets may cause vomiting in some ferrets. The stools also have a fishy odour, which is objectionable for a house pet. A whole-prey diet or a balanced fresh or freeze-dried carnivore diet may be most appropriate and such diets are currently fed in many areas of the world with great success. Clean sources of prey food such as chicks, mice and rats are now available in many areas thanks to the reptile market that uses these foods for carnivorous pets. If an owner does not want to feed a 100% whole prey, consider the occasional treat of a whole mouse or chick as valuable environmental enrichment. The stools of a ferret on a whole-prey diet are very firm and of low volume and odour.

Cat food kibbles are very palatable because of their coating of animal fat. Minimally stressed pet ferrets may get by on these foods for years, but nutritional deficiencies are quickly revealed in breeding animals or if the ferret becomes ill (**Fig. 5.8**).

The acid test of a complete diet is to feed it to a large group of young animals, then allow them to reproduce. Some premium dry cat foods and pelleted ferret diets have proved to meet all the ferret's nutritional requirements for growth and reproduction.

The most common type of diet fed to pet ferrets in the USA is in the form of dry kibble formulated for ferrets. A number of brands are available. *Table 5.1* lists analysis of several commercial diets that meet ferrets' needs for growth and reproduction.

Table 5.1 Analysis of commercial diets that support growth and reproduction

NUTRIENT	DIET A	DIET B	DIET C	DIET D
Crude protein %	36.5	38.0	39.8	39.0
Crude fat %	23.3	20.0	20.2	20.5
Crude fibre %	1.4	4.0	2.2	2.6
Moisture %	7.5	12.0	4.2	10.0
Ash %	6.5	7.5	7.4	6.5
Carbohydrate %	24.8	17.5	26.2	21.4
Metabolisable energy (ME) kcal/g	4.35	4.2	3.89	4.0
Fat				
Linoleic acid %	4.5	3.0	3.0	2.76
Amino acid profile				
Arginine %	2.4	2.5	2.52	2.05
Cystine %	0.44	0.56	0.45	0.59
Histidine %	0.95	0.75	0.91	0.61
Isoleucine %	1.30	1.40	1.67	1.44
Leucine %	2.55	2.60	3.09	3.20
Lysine %	2.40	2.20	2.74	2.02
Methionine %	1.05	0.80	1.18	0.85
Phenylalanine %	1.40	1.30	1.64	1.48
Tyrosine %	1.10	1.20	1.32	0.76
Threonine %	1.50	1.40	1.90	1.31
Tryptophan %	0.38	0.32	0.33	0.29
Valine %	1.72	1.70	1.99	1.77
Taurine %	0.24	0.52	0.25	0.24
Minerals				
Calcium %	1.28	1.4	1.2	1.4
Phosphorus %	0.88	1.30	1.05	1.25
Ca:P	1.45:1	1.08:1	1.14:1	1.12:1
Potassium %	0.68	0.70	0.75	0.56

(Continued)

Table 5.1 *(continued)* Analysis of commercial diets that support growth and reproduction

NUTRIENT	DIET A	DIET B	DIET C	DIET D
Minerals				
Magnesium %	0.09	0.10	0.10	0.12
Sodium %	0.42	0.40	0.55	0.40
Iron ppm (mg/kg)	240	305	360	320
Copper mg/kg	24	22	30	24
Manganese mg/kg	80	75	70	72
Zinc mg/kg	240	235	145	232
Iodine mg/kg	2.0	1.9	2.6	2.0
Selenium mg/kg	0.35	0.2	0.3	0.6
Vitamins				
A (IU/kg)	25,000	31,765	35,100	25,100
D3 (IU/kg)	1800	3560	2200	3700
E (IU/kg)	300	235	155	250
K (ppm, mg/kg)	2.0	3.0	1.2	3.2
Thiamin mg/kg	45	54	12.8	56
Riboflavin mg/kg	55	22	25	20
Niacin mg/kg	120	128	95	110
Pantothenic acid mg/kg	35	25	25	26.2
Folic acid mg/kg	3.0	4.4	1.5	4.3
Pyridoxine mg/kg	35	28	12.5	17.5
Biotin mg/kg	10.2	0.43	0.60	0.48

Ca: P, calcium to phosphorus (ratio)

Diet A: Totally Ferret® Active Show & Pet Formula (Performance Foods, Inc., Broomfield, CO).

Diet B: Mazuri® Ferret (PMI Nutrition International LLC, Brentwood, MO, www.mazuri.com/product_pdfs/5M08.pdf).

Diet C: Marshall Premium Ferret (Marshall Pet Products, North Rose, NY, www.marshallpet.com).

Diet D: Purina High Density Ferret Lab Diet 5L14 (Lab Diet, St Louis, MO, www.labdiet.com).

FOOD CONSIDERATIONS

To compensate for the inefficiency of its digestive tract, the ferret requires a concentrated diet that is high in protein and fat and low in fibre. The main source of calories should be fat. When fat is metabolised, it releases twice as much energy as either carbohydrates or protein. Diets with as much as 40% fat have been fed to ferrets without apparent injury, but 15–30% fat for pets is generally considered sufficient.

Most ferrets eat as much as they want without becoming pathologically obese. They normally increase their food intake by at least 30% in the winter, gaining a great deal of weight by depositing subcutaneous fat. Seasonal obesity is not harmful and should be considered normal (**Fig. 5.9**). As the hours of daylight increase in the spring, the ferret reduces its food intake, metabolises the extra fat and regains its long, slender shape. If the photoperiod does not vary seasonally, the natural physiological change may not occur. Some ferrets may remain either lean or plump all the time.

The rule of thumb is that an adult ferret will eat about 43 g/kg bodyweight of dry food per day. It will eat up to 10 meals a day if given feed *ad libitum*.

Ferrets require a higher protein level in the diet than most animals, probably owing more to the inefficiency of their digestive process, or to a need for certain amino acids in short supply, than to a greater protein requirement at the cellular level. The basic diet for adults should have a crude protein level between 30–35% and be composed primarily of high-quality meat sources, not grains.

Kits will not thrive on a diet containing less than 30% protein. Conception rate, litter size, and survivability of the kits improve when the protein concentration is increased to 35–40% of the breeding ferrets' diet (**Fig. 5.10**).

Protein quality is as important as concentration. The protein in the best-quality animal feeds is 85–90% digestible as compared with less than 75% in many supermarket cat foods. A food with 30% crude protein (CP) of 70% digestibility really only contains 21% available protein, and may be mainly cereals. The diet of an obligate carnivore like a cat or ferret must contain predominantly animal protein and fat. Infectious and metabolic diseases are prevalent in growing, gestating or lactating ferrets when grains are the major source of protein.

The only natural source of carbohydrates for mustelids is the gut content of their prey. Ferrets have a short intestinal tract, comparatively deficient in brush-border enzymes, and so are less able than cats and other species to make as much use of complex carbohydrates. The proportion of carbohydrate is higher in a grain-based diet than in a meat-based one. Grains are used to help the

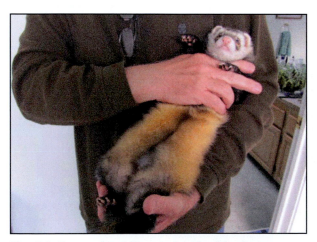

Fig. 5.9 Seasonal weight gain in a healthy ferret.

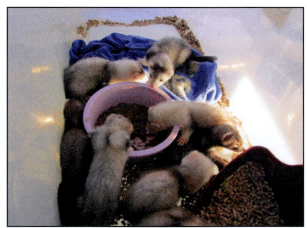

Fig. 5.10 Eight-week-old kits eating a soup made from kibble.

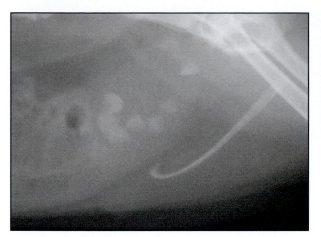

Fig. 5.11 **Urolithiasis possibly linked to inappropriate diet.**

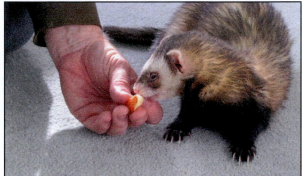

Fig. 5.12 **Offering a bit of apple.**

pellet hold its shape. Very high levels of plant proteins in the diet can lead to urolithiasis (see Chapter 22) (**Fig. 5.11**).

The nitrogen-free extract (NFE) in a chemical food analysis is made up of soluble, digestible carbohydrates (e.g. sugar or starch.) Insoluble carbohydrates are referred to as fibre. The digestibility of soluble complex carbohydrates is improved by cooking. However, fibre remains completely indigestible by simple-stomached animals. Fibre attracts fluid to the lumen of the gut, increasing stool volume and having a beneficial effect when natural laxative is required. Increasing dietary fibre causes the volume of stool to increase in ferrets as it does in dogs and cats, but it also induces a relative protein-calorie deficiency in the ferret. Ferrets cannot eat enough low-density food to meet their maintenance requirements. Simply, the ferret has little ability to digest fibre.

Pet ferrets sometimes develop a taste for high-carbohydrate or high-fibre foods such as fruits or vegetables, but they derive little nutritional benefit from them (**Figs 5.12, 5.13**). Treat foods consisting of cereals are likewise not digestible, but may be extremely palatable as they are sugary. A study looking at the sweet receptor gene (*Tas1r2*) and preference for sweet stimuli in species of carnivore has found that ferrets prefer fructose over other sugars. Ferrets do not respond to artificial sweeteners. They have an intact *Tas1r2* gene.

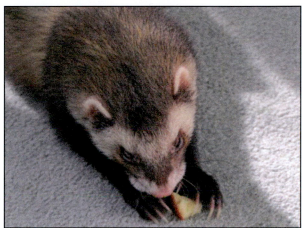

Fig. 5.13 **Relishing a small piece of apple demonstrating liking sweet foods. This particular ferret also likes sweetened ice tea!**

SPECIFIC NUTRITIONAL REQUIREMENTS

Although the exact nutritional requirements of ferrets have not been determined by feeding trials with defined diets as have been done for other animals, diets that have sustained reproduction and growth of generations of healthy kits must meet or exceed their minimum requirements.

Daily metabolisable energy (ME) intakes for ferrets have been estimated to range from 200–300 kcal/kg bodyweight. Energy intakes above maintenance are needed for growth, gestation and lactation. Examples of the nutritional content of several complete rations that support growth, gestation and lactation are shown in *Table 5.1*. These diets contain 3.9–4.58 kcal ME/g.

Table 5.2 Energy needs of ferrets (kcal ME/day) increase above maintenance for growth, reproduction, and lactation

MULTIPLES OF MAINTENANCE* (KCAL ME/DAY)

BODY WEIGHT (g)	1 (MAINTENANCE)	1.5 (MAINTENANCE, WINTER)	2.0 (GROWTH)	2.5 (REPRODUCTION)	3.0 (LACTATION)
600	150	225	300	375	450
700	175	262	350	438	525
800	200	300	400	500	600
900	225	338	450	562	675
1000	250	375	500	625	750
1200	300	450	600	750	900
1400	350	525	700	875	1050
1600	400	600	800	1000	1200
1800	450	675	900	1125	1350
2000	500	750	1000	1250	1500
2200	550	825	1100	1375	1650

* Maintenance is defined as the daily Metabolisable energy (ME) intake (kcal/day) of healthy adults in comfortable surroundings (250 [W]), in which W = body weight in kg.

Table 5.2 lists energy needs of ferrets in kcal ME/day with increases needed for differing calorie requirements. Ferret foods, or mink foods of similar analysis and quality of ingredients, may provide adequate nutrition for a breeding ferret and more than adequate nutrition for a pet. Palatability is a major concern when considering the benefits of any food for a ferret.

Table 5.3 lists nutrients provided by some of the ingredients found in ferret diets. *Table 5.4* lists examples of diets that failed to meet the nutritional requirements of breeding ferrets. These diets have a higher carbohydrate content and lower protein content than those in *Table 5.1*. Furthermore the protein is of lower quality, a fact that cannot be appreciated from either the analysis or the ingredients list, but which makes a significant difference to the animals. Low-quality meat or poultry meal contains too much indigestible protein (such as feathers or hooves), too much bone and too little muscle meat. The result is a diet deficient in essential amino acids.

The serious consequences of feeding poor-quality meat protein or too high a proportion of cereal protein to breeding ferrets include, but are not limited to, urinary tract, GI and respiratory infections, urolithiasis, reproductive failure and poor growth of kits.

Before the true requirements of ferrets can be known, purified diets must be tested on large groups of animals, so that a single nutrient may be varied and its effect analysed independent of other variables.

There are many gaps in what is known about ferrets' specific requirements. For example, arginine and methionine are limiting amino acids in the diets of other animals, and probably of ferrets, but their actual requirements in ferrets are unknown. An animal eats enough food to meet its requirements for the limiting amino acids, even if that means consuming two or three times more than the requirement amount of other amino acids. The excess is metabolised and used for energy, and the nitrogen is excreted by the kidneys. The high blood urea nitrogen of healthy ferrets suggests that they usually have an excess of protein, but their physical condition suffers when the diet contains less than 30% protein. Providing all of the limiting amino acids in the required concentrations in a lower-protein diet

Table 5.3 **Nutrients provided by some ingredients of ferret diets and supplements**

INGREDIENT OR SUPPLEMENT	CRUDE PROTEIN %	FAT %	FIBRE %	CARBOHYDRATE %	CALORIES/G	MOISTURE %	CALCIUM: PHOSPHORUS RATIO
Baby food chicken 10 mL	1.3 g	0.68 g	0	0	11	80%	Not listed
Ground beef	20.7	10.0	Not listed	3.5% calculated	1.8	68.3	1:19
Fresh liver (beef)	19.9	3.8	0.1	6.5	1.4	69.7	1:35
Liver meal	71.4	17.0	1.5	3.4	Not listed	8	1:2
Poultry by-product	58.7	13.1	2.3	3.6	2.8	7	1.9:1
Whole cooked egg (1egg, 50 g)	6.45	5.8	Not listed	Not listed	82	73.7	1:4
Whole milk (3.5% fat, 10 mL)	0.35	0.35	0	0.56	6.5	87.4	Not listed
Corn	10.9	4.3	2.9	80.4	NL	11	1:1
Soybean meal	42.9	4.8	5.9	30.4	Not listed	90	1:2.3
Rice	7.9	1.7	8.9	65.6	Not listed	89	1:4.7
Wheat	14.2	1.8	2.6	68.7	Not listed	89	1:10.5
Nutri-Cal® 1 tsp (6 g)	0.04 g	2.1 g	0.22 g	2.8 g	26.5	14	6:1
Ferrettone™ 1 mL	0	0.9	0	0	8.7	Not listed	Not listed
Raisins (6 small or 3 large yellow; 3 g)	0.1 g	0.02 g	0.2 g	2.4 g	9.5	Not listed	Not listed

Table 5.4 **Guaranteed analysis from the nutrition information on the packaging of two diets associated with poor reproductive performance in ferrets**

ANALYSIS (%)	DIET #1	DIET #2
Crude protein	30.0	31.0
Crude fat	8.0	16.0
Fibre	4.5	3.0
Ash	6.3	8.0
Moisture	12.0	11.0
Carbohydrate	39.2	31.0
First 8 listed ingredients	Whole kernel corn, soybean meal, corn gluten meal, poultry by-product meal, whole wheat, animal fat preserved with mixed tocopherols (source of vitamin E), brewer's rice, fish meal	Poultry by-product meal, ground wheat, ground yellow corn, soybean meal, wheat germ meal, animal fat preserved with BHA, meat and bone meal, salt

should make it possible to maintain the ferret in the same state of good health and productivity that presently necessitates that their diet contains at least 35% crude protein.

Taurine deficiency has been linked with dilated cardiomyopathy and retinal degeneration in cats. Although dilated cardiomyopathy and retinal degeneration are found in ferrets, there is no hard evidence that taurine deficiency causes either one. However, it is recommended that taurine be added to ferret diets at the same level as is present in premium cat foods. The author has used taurine supplementation in ferrets with dilated cardiomyopathy and has clinically seen improvement in the condition.

It is also assumed that arachidonic acid is an essential fatty acid for ferrets as it is for cats, because it is present only in animal tissues. Fish oil is a good source of arachidonic acid, hence the beautiful pelts grown by fitch ferrets that eat pelleted mink food. Meat-based diets usually are not deficient in either taurine or arachidonic acid.

MINERALS AND VITAMINS

Very little research has been done to evaluate ferret mineral requirements. Mink diets have been extensively researched, and their requirements appear to be similar to those of other animals, including cats. It is assumed that ferrets also have similar requirements.

The calcium–phosphorus ratio should be at least 1:1. Commercial formulations generally contain ratios 1.2:1 to 1.7:1. *Table 5.1* diets show the varying ratios and as all minerals have proved adequate for growing and lactating ferrets, the amount of each mineral in the food must be meeting or exceeding their requirements. Milk and meat meal that includes bone are well-balanced sources of calcium and phosphorus, but muscle meat or liver and grains are low in calcium.

A diet of meat alone induces a calcium deficiency and gross skeletal abnormalities. Signs of calcium deficiency include tooth loss, skeletal deformities in kits, and spontaneous fractures. Ferrets on ferret foods will not have mineral deficiencies unless they are persistently fed a supplement of a medication (e.g. tetracycline) that drastically unbalances the diet.

Commercial diets are considered adequate in iron, copper, sodium, chlorine, zinc, magnesium, iodine and potassium. Other microminerals are trace elements and include cobalt, chromium and molybdenum; these are usually combined with other nutrients and never added to the diet in pure form. Additionally, fluoride, nickel, vanadium, silicon and tin are necessary but in minute and organic form in the diet.

An interesting study looked at tobacco smoke induction of changes in the gastric mucosa of ferrets as a model for gastric cancer and found that lycopene effectively prevented the damage. In the author's opinion, this may have implications for its use in consideration of gastric health.

Vitamin A

Ferrets, unlike cats, are able to convert beta-carotene to vitamin A, and in the diet this conversion is stimulated by 1% taurocholate (cholic acid conjugated with taurine), 23% fat, 40% protein, and alpha-tocopherol (vitamin E) at physiological doses. However, ferrets convert beta-carotene to vitamin A inefficiently, and the diet should contain added vitamin A. Studies also have been done showing that ferrets had a higher bodyweight gain when supplemented with beta-carotene.

Oversupplementation of vitamin A in liver or concentrated nutritional products induces skeletal abnormalities in cats and has occurred in ferrets fed a diet of raw liver exclusively.

Vitamin D

Vitamin D requirements may depend on dietary concentrations of calcium and phosphorus or on the duration of exposure to ultraviolet (UVB) light. Other factors include dietary calcium to phosphorus ratio, physiological state of development and sex. Rachitic changes and abnormal bone development may occur when the diet is deficient in vitamin D, calcium or phosphorus, especially when exposure to UV light is minimised. Most pet ferrets receive little to no UVB light as they are kept indoors.

Commercial ferret diets generally have sufficient vitamin D, calcium and phosphorus in the appropriate ratios.

Vitamin E

Vitamin E is added to high-quality pet foods as an antioxidant. Ferrets fed extra fat (e.g. linoleic acid) might require more vitamin E, but deficiencies are unlikely to occur in pets fed pelleted diets. Vitamin E deficiency was a problem when ferrets were fed raw meat or fish that contained rancid fat. Steatitis has been seen in young ferrets fed diets containing an excessive amount of fish or horsemeat. The ferret foods listed in *Table 5.1* probably all contain an excess of vitamin E for normal animals. Other information on vitamin requirements of ferrets have been determined because of their use as laboratory research animals.

The natural source of vitamin E for a carnivorous animal is the liver of its prey. Studies have been done using the ferret as a model for lung cancer, and have found that the addition of beta-carotene, alpha-tocopherol (vitamin E) and ascorbic acid (vitamin C) have effectively blocked the formation of preneoplastic lung lesions and lung cancer tumour formation.

Vitamin K

Vitamin K metabolic need has not been established in the ferret, but it is likely that a dry diet concentration of 1.0 mg menadione/kg would sustain normal plasma prothrombin levels.

Vitamin K deficiency may result in hypoprothrombinaemia and haemorrhage.

Vitamin K toxicity has been linked with kernicterus and haemolytic anaemia in other species. This has not been documented in ferrets.

Thiamine

The thiamine concentration in commercially available ferret diets is generally considered adequate.

A diet of raw eggs may predispose ferrets to thiamine deficiency.

Thiamine deficiency disease has been reported on ferret farms in New Zealand that fed a diet of fish containing thiaminase. It was seen in weanling, growing and adult ferrets. It was characterised by anorexia, lethargy, marked dyspnoea, prostration and convulsions. Signs disappeared after parenteral injections of vitamin B complex (5 mg daily for 3 days).

Toxic doses of thiamine in excess of 200 mg/kg bodyweight may cause death caused by depression of the respiratory centre.

Riboflavin

Riboflavin needs are considered met with less than 3 mg/kg. Commercial ferret diets contain in excess of this amount.

Acute deficiency may result in decreased respiratory rate, hypothermia, weakness and coma. Chronic deficiency may result in anorexia, muscular weakness, dermatitis, microcytic-hypochromic anaemia, corneal vascularisation–opacification and reduced erythrocyte and urine riboflavin concentration.

B6 (pyridoxine)

A sufficient amount of pyridoxine is considered to be 1 mg of B6/kg dry matter. Commercial ferret diets contain eight times this level.

B6 deficiency in mink showed testicular atrophy, aspermia and degeneration. Absorption sterility occurs in females.

B12

B12 deficiency in other species has been linked with macrocytic hypochromic, macrocytic normochromic, normocytic hypochromic or normocytic normochromic anaemias. B12 deficiency has not been described in the ferret. Commercial diet amounts are considered adequate.

Folic acid

Folic acid synthesis by intestinal bacteria has not been studied in the ferret, but commercial diets are considered to have adequate amounts such that bacterial synthesis is not needed.

In mink, folic acid at 0.5 mg/kg of dry feed causes a remission of symptoms such as erratic appetite, poor weight gain, glossitis, leucopaenia and hypochromic anaemia.

Biotin

Biotin is provided in commercial diets upwards of 200 µg biotin/kg dry matter leading to 10 µg/kg bodyweight daily. This level is approximately twice the level required for optimal growth in dogs.

Deficiency of biotin may result in alopecia, hyperkeratosis, greying of fur, conjunctivitis and fatty liver.

Niacin

Niacin must be supplied although the metabolic conversion of tryptophan to niacin has not been systematically studied in the ferret. Mink cannot metabolise enough to meet requirements.

Commercial ferret diets provide several times the 20 mg/kg dry diet that is stated as a requirement for mink.

Deficiency in other species has been linked with anorexia, profuse salivation, diarrhoea, GI inflammation, haemorrhagic necrosis, dehydration and emaciation. High doses have been linked with vasodilation, pruritis and cutaneous desquamation in other species.

Pantothenic acid

Pantothenic acid requirements are probably about 500–750 µg/kg bodyweight based on the absence of deficiency signs in ferrets consuming a commercial ferret diet.

Deficiency in the ferret may result in poor appetite, slow growth, reduced blood cholesterol and total lipid levels, loss of conditioned reflexes, alopecia, vomiting, intermittent diarrhoea, GI disorders, convulsions and coma.

Choline

Choline requirements are linked with dietary concentration of methionine. Both choline and methionine may serve as methyl donors in metabolism, with the dietary supply of one tending to spare the need for the other. This interaction has not been systematically studied in ferrets.

Deficiency has led to elevated plasma phosphatase activity and blood prothrombin times. Toxicity may cause an increased alkalination of urine and decreased ammonia excretion.

SELECTING A COMPLETE DIET FOR A PET FERRET

Most pet ferrets are acquired either as kits or young juveniles from pet shops or from private breeders, or they are acquired as older juveniles or adults from shelters. A pet may come to its new owner with strongly established preferences for flavours and food textures. Once they have been accustomed to a diet, ferrets expect to find that food and no other in their dish every day. New owners must be educated on the basics of ferret nutrition and urged to continue with the balanced diet the ferret is already used to. However, if they are on a poor diet, conversion should be done on a gradual basis once the ferret has acclimatised to its new surroundings. The author recommends a 30-day period before diet change should be started (**Fig. 5.14**).

People buying a kit from a pet store may remain completely unaware of the animal's requirements, depending on what the pet shop staff tell them. A pet shop employee may suggest an expensive premium cat food rather than the ferret food currently being fed the kit. The owner may then decide that he can get by with a cheaper cat food, leading to malnourishment of the ferret. Most kits will readily accept cat food due to its high palatability, even though nutritionally it is not acceptable.

Even after selecting a good base diet, many ferret owners decide to give their ferret a taste of their own favourite foods. Ferrets end up snacking on bananas, raisins, apples, ice cream, crisps, peanut butter, carbonated drinks, beer, pizza, cereal, etc. Ferrets are utterly self-indulgent and will gorge themselves on anything they take a liking to. Left to themselves, they will eat only their favourite foods, eventually becoming grossly malnourished. Veterinarians who examine a pet shop ferret soon after purchase should advise the owner to select the ferret's diet carefully and limit snack foods that will unbalance it. Samples of different foods may be given out as a starter kit, along with instructions on how to make gradual food introductions.

Maintenance diets

A pet ferret's maintenance diet should be 30–35% crude protein and 15–30% fat. Meat or poultry, meat or poultry meals or their by-products should appear first in the list of ingredients and preferably several more times in the list as well. Other animal products such as liver and eggs are included in the highest-quality foods.

Although the most expensive commercial diet will not necessarily be the best for any individual ferret, the cheapest ones are certainly the worst.

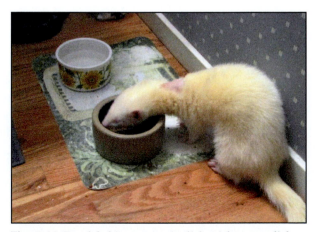

Fig. 5.14 **Food fed in a ceramic dish with water dish readily available. This ferret had a tumour removed from its neck hence the shaved area.**

Unsuitable diets leading to nutritional disease

Ferrets fed dog food eventually die, either directly of malnutrition or of GI or respiratory infections arising from poor immune function.

Serious health problems including alopecia, heart disease and overall muscle weakness have been directly or indirectly related to feeding a base diet of cheap cat food to ferrets. The list of ingredients for these foods usually starts with ground yellow corn. Metabolism of cereal proteins alkalinises the animal's urine, encouraging struvite urolith formation in ferrets and cats. (The normal pH of the urine should be less than 6.5.) When diets high in cereal proteins are fed to pregnant or lactating jills, 5–10% will have uroliths, and a significant number will require emergency surgery to remove large single or smaller multiple struvite uroliths.

Not only is the protein in cheap cat foods predominantly from cereals, there is too little of it for ferrets, and the proportion that comes from meat is usually of poor quality. Supplementing the ferret with the right balance of whole cooked egg, milk, and minced ground meat or liver will correct the amino acid deficiencies caused by a steady diet of generic cat food. However, fat must also be added, as generic cat foods contain only 8–10% fat, which is approximately half of what ferrets require; these foods also contain a high proportion of carbohydrate.

Young ferrets on protein-deficient diets grow poorly, and immune dysfunction makes them more susceptible to respiratory and GI infections. When poor nutrition is superimposed on stress and exposure to pathogens, ferrets develop respiratory infections, clinical coccidiosis, and heavy flea and ear mite infestations.

Juveniles raised on low-quality cat food are more likely to develop clinical *Helicobacter* gastritis and ulcers and proliferative colitis.

Nutritional steatitis has been described in ferrets fed a high level of dietary polyunsaturated fatty acids (PUFAs) and/or a diet deficient in vitamin E. A dietary supplement of 75–150 mg/ferret/day of vitamin E is advised when feeding ferrets a high-PUFA diet. The high level of selenium found in the liver of ferrets with steatitis did not reduce the toxicity of the high-PUFA content of the feed, although selenium does protect tissue against lipoperioxidases.

Recently grain-free diets have been made that utilise peas and sweet potatoes as their base rather than corn or wheat. Ferrets on these diets are prone to developing cysteine urolithiasis that requires cystotomy to remove the stones. It is recommended that radiographs be taken on any ferret presenting that is on one of these diets, as symptoms of urolithiasis may be difficult to observe unless the ferret experiences urinary tract blockage. Ferrets should also be switched over to another ferret diet. At this time it is theorised that the pea content is at the root of the problem (see Chapter 22).

Osteodystrophia fibrosa (nutritional hyperparathyroidism), mainly due to feeding an all-meat diet with no calcium supplementation, has been documented in ferrets.

True 'rickets' is defined as hypophosphorosis and/or hypovitaminosis D and has not been reported in ferrets. A bone disease similar to the clinical condition seen with rickets has been diagnosed predominantly in the young, although all ages are susceptible. Rapid growth predisposes ferrets to the disease if the diet is inadequate in calcium, phosphorus and vitamin D. Affected ferrets are reluctant to move, cannot support their own weight and the typical posture is abduction of the forelegs. The bones are soft, pliable and fractures may be present. This has been diagnosed predominantly in instances where a commercial ferret diet is not being fed. On necropsy, the bones are osteoporotic with typical lesions of osteodystrophia fibrosa. The parathyroid glands are hyperplastic.

Zinc toxicity has been reported in ferrets exposed to excessive levels of zinc leached from galvanised feeding pans and water dishes. All ages are susceptible. Affected animals have pale mucous membranes caused by anaemia. Posterior weakness and lethargy are seen. This problem was reported on two ferret farms in New Zealand.

Salt poisoning has been caused by feeding a diet of 100% salted fish. Clinical signs are typical of those seen in other species, particularly pigs, affected with the disease. Animals are significantly depressed and have periodic choriform spasms, seen 24–96 hours after ingestion of excessive salty diets. Death ensues shortly thereafter. Pathology is restricted to the brain, which is oedematous and shows coning of the cerebellum. A non-suppurative eosinophilic meningitis has also been found.

Switching to an optimal diet

A young ferret accustomed to a mixture of several premium cat or ferret foods will usually readily keep on eating just one brand of ferret food. Young ferrets imprint on food by smell at a very young age, and develop strong food preferences by the time they are a few months old. Therefore regardless of the diet strategy that is chosen, ferrets should be exposed to a variety of food tastes, textures and smells, and different protein sources as juveniles, so their diet will have more flexibility as an adult. This can be extremely helpful when ferrets experience medical conditions that may require altered diets. Older ferrets however, may be quite stubborn and difficult to switch from that lower-quality 'tasty' cat food.

Changing an adult ferret's eating habits can be frustrating and stressful for both the owner and the ferret. When a complete change is necessary, offer a smorgasbord of high-quality foods mixed with the diet that the ferret is used to. Some ferrets would rather fight than switch foods. They make a clear statement by digging all the new food out of the dish, or deliberately carrying it pellet by pellet into their litter tray. A sudden change is risky as some ferrets will fast to the point of starvation rather than eat the new food. Instead of giving up and allowing the pet to eat the generic kibble that it craves, feed it palatable, balanced supplements such as Nutri-Cal® (Vetoquinol USA, Inc., Fort Worth, TX) mixed into a soup of ground pellets (so that the new tastes are part of the powder), plus mix in some baby food chicken or turkey creating 'dook soup' (*Table 5.5*, Appendix 6) (**Figs 5.15, 5.16**). Gradually decrease the water content of the dook soup and increase the proportion of the correct diet in the ground powder until the ferret is converted.

Unfortunately using soup for conversion is also fraught with problems. Some ferrets decide that they would rather eat soup than kibble at all and will not switch back to kibble. Have kibble available always and make the soup more and more thick, and offer it only once or twice daily. Usually a healthy ferret will start back eating kibble, particularly if housed with more than one other ferret that has also been converted to a different kibble.

The ferret's weight should be checked at least every other day during conversion. If there is weight loss, instigate more frequent feedings of dook soup and increase the proportion of the good-quality food ground into the powder used as the basis for the soup.

Table 5.5 Commercial products used in dook soup

NUTRIENT	CARNIVORE CARE®	EMERAID® EXOTIC CARNIVORE	NUTRI-CAL®
Crude protein (min) %	45.00	37.80	0.68
Crude fat (min) %	32.00	34.00	28.14
Crude fibre (max) %	3.00	4.50	Not Listed
Moisture (max) %	10.00	9.00	14.21
Calories	6 kcal/g; 24 kcal/Tablespoon	Calculated, dry weight 5.14 kcal/g	60 kcal/Tablespoon
Calcium (min) %	1.40 (max 1.80)	1.00	0.0026
Phosphorus (min) %	1.20	0.67	0.0003
Omega 3 fatty acids (min) %	1.00	1.40	Not listed
Omega 6 fatty acids (min) %	7.60	11.00	Not listed

Analysis as listed on the package.
Emeraid® (Lafeber Company, Cornell, IL).
Carnivore Care® (Oxbow Animal Health, Murdock, NE).
Nutri-Cal® (Vetoquinol USA, Inc, Fort Worth, TX).

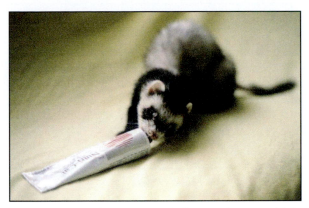

Fig. 5.15 **Ferret liking Nutri-Cal® supplement which is highly palatable.**

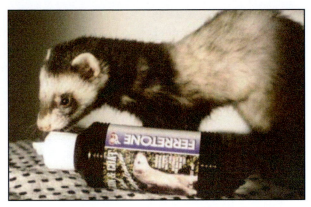

Fig. 5.17 **Ferret enjoying Ferretone™ supplement.**

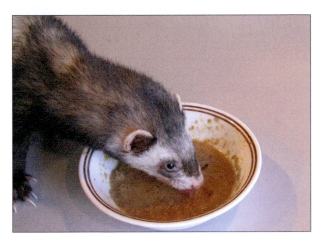

Fig. 5.16 **Ferret eating dook soup.**

High-fat supplements

A ferret on a good balanced diet, usually kibble, needs no supplementation.

Feeding coat conditioners that contain linoleic and other fatty acids adds 9 kcal/g of metabolised fat, causing the ferret to reduce its intake of the balanced diet. If only a few drops a day are fed as a treat, no harm will be done. The most common product used is Ferretone™ (8-in-1, Spectrum Brands, Inc., Islandia, NY, www.eightinonepet.com) (**Fig. 5.17**).

But, to give an example of the problems that can be caused: a 700 g jill requires approximately 200 kcal/day and will eat to her caloric requirement. If a teaspoon (5 mL) of Ferretone™ is given daily, she will reduce her intake by the approximately 40 kcal she acquires in the supplement, which is 20% of her caloric requirement per day. If she is on a good-quality ferret food, this added fat will probably only cause her to gain weight and have a thick coat. But what if she is on a marginal diet? A typical cat food contains 30% crude protein, 8% crude fat and 4.5% fibre and approximately 3.5 kcal ME/g. The jill was probably consuming approximately 60 g of that diet (18 g of protein). With the supplement she will reduce her intake of the dry diet by approximately 40 kcal or 11 g. And now she is eating approximately 50 g which is 15 g of protein. The jill's diet now contains approximately 27% protein, which is primarily from cereal grains and thus is less than 75% digestible. This ferret will have a poor coat, will be thin and abnormally susceptible to infectious diseases, and may even develop struvite urolithiasis.

High-carbohydrate supplements

High-carbohydrate supplements (treats) include carbonated drinks, biscuits, sweets and raisins. None of these help the ferret nutritionally and are not needed to augment a ferret's diet. Ferrets love raisins, which are very high in sugar and low in protein and fat. A few raisins a day for a normal ferret on an excellent diet will not cause a nutritional problem, and may pass largely through the GI tract with little digestion. But for a ferret on a generic cat food, a handful of raisins per day raises the carbohydrate intake enough to reduce the consumption of the dry food, inducing both protein and fat deficiencies. In some ferrets they may irritate the GI tract. As ferrets do not need sugars added to their diet, the author does not recommend feeding raisins.

Acceptable treats

Treats should be limited to no more than 10% of the daily caloric intake.

- 1 mL of Ferretone™ (9 kcal/mL) daily will not harm ferrets on good-quality ferret diets.
- Soft, moist meat or liver snacks manufactured for cats or ferrets make good treats: they contain 50–60% moisture and are balanced approximately like a good ferret diet. Check the label for the nutritional content and convert it to a dry matter basis.
- Other acceptable snacks are 1 inch (2.5 cm) of Nutri-Cal®, a teaspoonful of a high-protein, high-calorie human supplement; meat-based baby foods that contain no carbohydrates; egg yolk or whole cooked egg; or small amounts of raw meat or liver.
- Puréed raw liver or hamburger mixed with egg yolk and milk looks and smells disgusting to people, and to older ferrets raised on refined, pelleted kibble, but it is universally appealing to kits and contains amino and fatty acids that immediately correct the deficiencies of inadequate diets.
- Ferrets with sparse coats caused by nutritional deficiencies start growing hair within days. While some raw meat may contain bacteria or parasites harmful to humans, ferrets and other predators seem very resistant to such infections.
- Commercial ferret treats are marketed. These are usually soft, moist pellets, chunks or strips to encourage chewing behaviour (**Fig. 5.18**). Some are touted as dentifrices although the author has not seen evidence that those fed regularly have less build-up of plaque.

PHYSIOLOGICAL STATES THAT REQUIRE SPECIAL NUTRITION

Growth

Weaned kits require an excellent diet if they are to grow to their adult weight. Well-nourished male kits double their weight between 4 weeks (150 g) and 6 weeks of age (300 g) and double it again before they are 9 weeks old (700 g).

When fed generic cat foods exclusively, kits have poor hair coats, distended abdomens and a greater susceptibility to both respiratory and digestive diseases

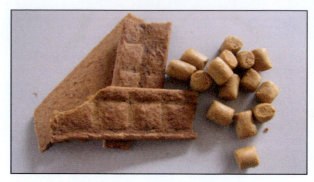

Fig. 5.18 **Commercial treats.**

than kits on high-quality ferret diets. This might not be noticeable to someone who has never seen well-nourished kits, but if weight and health records and photographs are compared, there are dramatic differences in litters on poor- and high-quality diets.

A meat-based dry diet with at least 35% protein and approximately 20% fat should be constantly available to growing kits. A palatable supplement to the dry diet for just-weaned kits is made by mixing the pellets with water and adding cooked eggs and animal fat (or fish oil) to give the resulting porridge the same concentration of protein and calories as the dry diet. Offer the soft food warm once or twice daily. The kits' intake of dry pellets will be limited by the availability of drinking water, which should be provided in a heavy bowl that will need to be cleaned and refilled at least 2–3 times a day. A water dropper bottle should also be available. Kits that are placed in pet stores are usually 6–8 weeks old, and are eating a kibble diet although most stores mix the kibble with water to keep it softened into a mash (**Fig. 5.19**).

Breeding and gestation

Jills intended for breeding do not need extra fat, but raising the protein to more than 35% improves conception rate. Jills on poor-quality protein have kits and litters that are smaller than average.

A pregnant jill increases her intake in the last trimester of gestation; because a large litter occupies most of the space in her abdomen, she has to eat frequently. Even a short fast a few days before her due date may induce life-threatening pregnancy toxaemia, which is essentially an energy deficit that causes fatty liver syndrome.

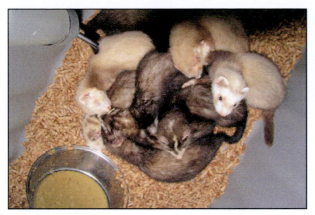

Fig. 5.19 **Soupy mash made from water added to the kibble fed to 8-week-old kits.**

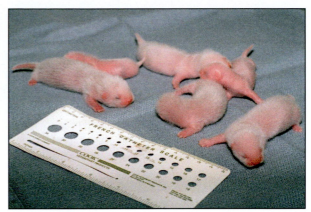

Fig. 5.20 **One-week-old kits.**

Extra dishes and water bottles should be provided so that unforeseen accidents will not restrict the jill's intake during the last week of gestation.

Lactating and weaning

Lactation is heavily dependent on nutrition.

A 700 g primiparous jill's litter of 10 kits weighs approximately 80 g at birth and 1000 g 3–4 weeks later (**Fig. 5.20**). After the third week of lactation, the jill daily produces an amount of milk that approaches 40% of her bodyweight, with a fat content of 10–20%. Her caloric requirement doubles if she provides the kits with enough milk to grow normally. A constant supply of high-quality food and unrestricted access to water will allow this tremendous expenditure of energy. The mash described above for weaned kits should be offered to the nursing jill 2–3 times daily, first a teaspoonful at a time then, after the litter is 3 weeks old, as much as she will eat. Jills seem to prefer the mash to their regular kibble: she will eat what the weaning kits are eating.

Jills nursing more than 8 kits lose weight no matter what they eat. Allowing the 3-week-old litter access to their mother's mash diet will have a sparing effect on her.

Three-week-old kits will drink a volume of milk replacer (20% fat) equivalent to 30% of their bodyweight daily, but they probably require less ferret milk, which is perfectly balanced to meet their requirements. Even before their eyes open at 30–35 days of age, kits are quite able to eat solid food, for their deciduous teeth come in at around 2 weeks of age. They may each consume 25 g food a day when they are only 3 weeks old. The more milk the jill has, the less solid food the kits will eat. After their eyes open, they will start eating the jill's pellets and any time after 5 weeks may be completely weaned.

Litters left with their mother until 6 weeks of age grow faster than early weaned kits.

Feeding ferret kits (*Box 5.1*)

If the jill rejects the kits or there are problems with her producing enough milk, supplementation or nursing will be required.

Illness

Any illness that causes anorexia requires nursing care. Anorexic ferrets may develop hepatic lipidosis and hypoglycaemia. Usually this means assist-feeding with foods high in protein and fat. Two commercial formulations are available that can be used alone or mixed into dook soup to get nutrition into the sick ferret. *Table 5.5* lists nutrients used in dook soup. A dook soup recipe is in Appendix 6 (**Fig. 5.21**).

- Emeraid® Exotic Carnivore ((Lafeber Company, Cornell, IL) is designed to be used by itself and can be delivered easily through a gastric tube if the ferret is refusing all oral administration (this includes syringing).
- Carnivore Care® (Oxbow Animal Health, Murdock, NE) can also be administered through a gastric tube or by syringing. It can be used solely for the ill ferret.

Box 5.1 **Feeding ferret kits**

- The formula to use is puppy or kitten milk replacer enriched with cream until the fat content is 20%.
- The formula that works well is three parts puppy milk replacer (Esbilac, Pet Ag, Hampshire, IL) to one part whipping cream.
- The kit will require teaching for the first few feedings.
- Wrap the kit in a towel, with its head protruding.
- Hold it at the angle it would naturally assume if suckling from the jill.
- With a drop of milk on it, coax the tip of a cannula (BD Interlink Cannula, Franklin Lakes, NJ) or small animal nipple very gently into the kit's mouth, slightly off centre. Be prepared to take plenty of time over the first feeding.
- If the bottle and nipple are not working, use a 1–3 mL syringe with a feeding tip or cannula.
- Dribble the liquid in very gradually and be extremely careful not to choke the infant.
- Kits will drink more if the milk is warm.
- Start by feeding about 0.5 mL per feed and increase to 1 mL per feed by the end of the first week. A rule of thumb, though, is to let the kit determine the amount.
- A puppy- or kitten-sized bottle and nipple can be used as the kit grows.
- Feed every 2–4 hours initially and gradually increase the time interval as the kit matures.
- At 3–4 weeks of age as the eyes open kits can be taught to drink from a low flat dish.
- In addition to the feeding, the kit will need to be stimulated to urinate and defaecate. This can be done by stroking the stomach and back legs. A cotton ball or moistened washcloth can be used to wipe its anogenital area very gently. Kits will start defaecating and urinating on their own at about 3 weeks of age.
- Mash can be introduced by 3–4 weeks of age. This is about the same time the kits move out of the nest box. The mash should be the ferret diet the jill is on, a commercial ferret food moistened with water.

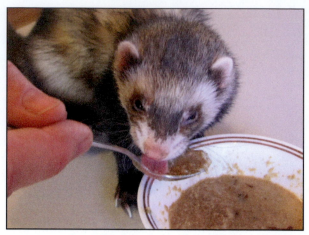

Fig. 5.21 Dook soup being fed to an ill ferret.

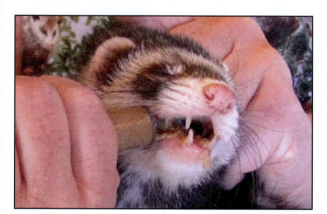

Fig. 5.22 Syringe feeding an ill ferret.

for the next 24–48 hours, then gradually mixing in the soaked ground regular diet that thickens up the gruel. It can all be puréed so that it can be administered through a syringe. Most ferrets will take syringing or hand feeding by dipping a finger in the mix and smearing it on their lips. Many ferrets will also take food off a spoon (**Fig. 5.22**).

Islet cell disease and dietary management

Insulin-secreting tumours may be benign (insulinomas or beta cell adenomas) or malignant (beta cell carcinomas). Whether histopathologically designated benign or malignant, these tumours secrete insulin and do not differ in their association with clinical signs and shortened life expectancy owing to repeated episodes of hypoglycaemia. Ferrets with

- Both powders can be used in combination with ground soaked kibble, baby foods, broth or water, and Nutri-Cal®.
- There are many formulations for dook soup, but all should maintain the ferret's weight or cause weight gain. The author's preference is to begin by using Emeraid® or Carnivore Care® alone for the first 24 hours, then to gradually introduce chicken baby food and Nutri-Cal®

islet cell disease present special problems because they are unable to regulate insulin production. Most affected ferrets have multiple pockets of neoplasia that secrete insulin persistently as well as in response to feeding (see Chapter 14).

Insulin both increases tissue uptake of glucose and decreases hepatic gluconeogenesis, effectively lowering blood glucose. The central nervous system depends on blood glucose for normal function.

Hypoglycaemia causes signs such as lethargy, nausea (shown by pawing at the mouth, hypersalivation, retching), confusion, weakness, convulsions and eventually coma. Repeated attacks of severe hypoglycaemia cause permanent brain damage.

The goal of treatment in ferrets with insulin-secreting tumours is to minimise the occurrence of clinical hypoglycaemia.

Absorption of glucose stimulates both normal and neoplastic beta cells to secrete more insulin, and blood glucose may then fall so low that the brain is unable to function normally, and the ferret is found unconscious or convulsing. Even when they appear to be completely unresponsive to other stimuli, hypoglycaemic ferrets will lick and swallow a glucose solution, 50% dextrose or Nutri-Cal® placed on their lips or gingiva or in the corner of their mouths, and rapidly recover consciousness. A glucose solution or 50% dextrose can also be given intrarectally (use about 0.5 mL of either).

Less severe levels of hypoglyaemia are associated with nausea or with weakness and unresponsive behaviour. Commonly the ferret seems confused soon after awakening or after a few minutes of active play. It either lies flat on its ventrum with eyes appearing glazed or it swims, dragging itself along with flipper-like leg movements. Ferrets showing any of these signs recover within a few minutes if given glucose or 50% dextrose, which immediately raises their blood sugar. However, administration of sugar also stimulates more secretion of insulin and a second episode of hypoglycaemia. Administering sugar alone as a treatment for hypoglycaemia or as a treat promotes peaks and valleys of blood glucose. Nutri-Cal® is a better treatment than a glucose source like corn syrup alone because in addition to sugar it contains fat, which is absorbed and metabolised slowly, maintaining blood glucose at a steady level. Emergency treatment with a sugar source or Nutri-Cal® should be followed by a snack of their regular food or dook soup. Most ferrets coming through an episode will be ravenous. Food should be placed in front of them!

Ferrets with islet cell disease should have constant access to food and should be encouraged to eat at least every 2–4 hours. It is advisable to get them to eat prior to a play period. The best medical care will not be successful in controlling hypoglycaemia unless it is combined with nutritional management. Owners should be advised not to give treats that are high in simple sugars including raisins, peanut butter, and any ferret supplements containing corn syrup or other sugar products. There has been discussion that the ferret should be on a diet high in protein and fats and very low in carbohydrates and fibre, but studies supporting the theory are currently lacking. Further scientific investigations are warranted before specific recommendations can be made. Most commercial ferret diets already fit this specification.

Geriatric ferrets

Ferrets become geriatric at 3–4 years of age (see Chapter 27). As they age, they establish their distinctive habits and food preferences, and changes imposed by humans become progressively more stressful. Thus it is essential to begin feeding a good diet when the ferret is young.

Lower-protein diets (under 35%) have been recommended for older ferrets to prevent chronic interstitial nephritis, although there has been no real evidence to suggest that a high-protein diet causes nephritis in ferrets or that feeding a lower-protein diet either alleviates the condition or stops its progress. Nephritis might actually be caused by unrecognised viral or bacterial infections or other dietary components present in all foods (see Chapter 22). However, the less active older ferret probably does not need more than 35% protein in his diet and may accept a lower-protein variety of his favorite food.

There are geriatric ferret diets on the market, but feeding trials looking at their effectiveness have not been done. And if switching foods is a struggle, the possible benefits of the change are outweighed by the stress of the conflict.

Some ferrets eat less and lose weight as they age, even when their teeth appear normal and no systemic disease is apparent. It may be that they are losing their sense of smell, because they will often eagerly devour their regular pellets mixed with warm water, either alone or with a favorite additive such as baby food or Nutri-Cal®.

Because more plaque will be deposited on their teeth as a result of the soft diet, geriatric ferrets' teeth need to be checked and cleaned twice a year. Daily tooth brushing is recommended.

Neoplasia

Ferrets with terminal cancer also need special attention to ensure that their nutritional needs are met. This may include extra meals and fortifying supplements.

The real secret of maintaining a good quality of life is the faithful care of an owner who is willing to hand-feed an old and/or ill ferret at any and all hours of the day or night.

CHAPTER 6

REPRODUCTION BIOLOGY

Cathy A. Johnson-Delaney

INTRODUCTION

Ferrets are easily bred and are produced in great numbers at commercial ferretries for the pet and laboratory animal trade. In the USA, most ferrets arrive in pet stores already demusked and neutered. Many practitioners will never see intact breeding ferrets. Elsewhere in the world ferrets are bred for hunting use, as well as for laboratory animals or pets. *Table 6.1* gives an overview of reproductive data for ferrets.

PHOTOPERIODS AND EFFECT ON REPRODUCTION

Many mustelids are seasonally monoestrus. In natural light conditions, ferrets breed from late March to August (northern hemisphere), with jills remaining in constant oestrus during this time unless bred (**Fig. 6.1**). This may result in a sometimes fatal anaemia (**Fig. 6.2**) (see Chapter 14).

In a short light cycle (less than 12 hours of daylight) the pineal gland secretes more melatonin. Both males and females grow thick winter coats with long guard hairs and pale fluffy undercoats. They can gain as much as 40% of bodyweight. Both sexes are sexually quiescent and it is possible to house hobs together and they will not fight (when in season, hobs fight and cannot be housed together). As the photoperiod increases, melatonin decreases and gonadotropins increase, inducing breeding behaviour. There is weight loss and coat change (loss of undercoat primarily).

In hobs, androgen levels begin increasing in midwinter during the short light cycle (December in the northern hemisphere), reaching peak in spring. Hormonally hobs are 1–2 months ahead of jills for the onset of the breeding season. Testicles increase in size, and there is an increase in oils in the skin

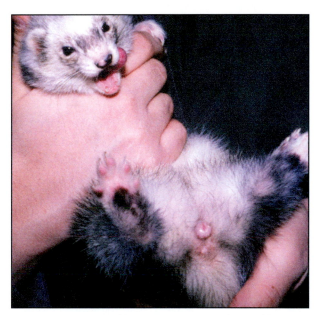

Fig. 6.1 An intact jill in oestrus. Note the swollen vulva.

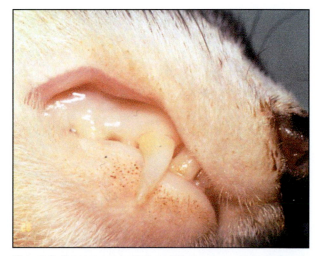

Fig. 6.2 Severe anaemia in a jill that was not bred and remained in oestrus.

Table 6.1 Reproductive data (adapted from Fox, Bell, Broome, 2014)

AGE AT PUBERTY

Jills (adult bodyweight 750–1500 g)	7–10 months (first spring)
Hobs (adult bodyweight 1000–2500 g)	8–12 months (first spring)
Oestrous cycle	Seasonally monoestrus (March–August northern hemisphere; September–February southern hemisphere)
Duration of oestrous cycle	Continuous until intromission
Mating time	10–14 days after onset of oestrus (signalled by vulvar swelling)
Type of ovulation	Induced by copulation
Ovulation time	30–40 hours after mating
Number of ova	12 (range 5–13)
Copulation time	Up to 3 hours
Sperm deposition site	Posterior os cervix
Ova capable of fertilisation	From 12 hours after ovulation, maximum 30–36 hours
Ovum transit time	5–6 days
Viability of sperm in female tract	36–48 hours
Cleavage to formation of blastocoele	Uniform rate
Implantation	12–13 days
Vulvar regression	3–4 days after mating, dries, regresses in size taking about 4 weeks
Gestation period	42 ± 1 day
Pregnancy validation	By palpation day 14 (fetus size of small walnut), ultrasonography day 12 (3–5 mm discrete non-echogenic spots). Jill may not show signs until day 30. Mammary development immediately before whelping
Hair loss	Loses coat approximately 10 days before whelping. Hair rings around teats
Implantation to parturition time	30 ± 1 day
Litter size	Average 8 (range 1–18)
Weight at birth	6–12 g
Weight at 10 days	30 g
Weight at 3 weeks	(Male) at least 100 g
Sexual dimorphism size	Apparent by week 7 and persists into adulthood
Return to oestrus	Next spring (dependent on light cycle season), occasionally postpartum oestrus
Pseudopregnancy	May occur if sterile mating. Vulva regresses. Duration approximately same as gestation period. 10–14 days following, vulva will enlarge, signalling oestrus
Weaning age	6–8 weeks
Weaning weight	Usually around 400 g
Solid food eaten	3 weeks, before eyes are open
Eyes open	34 days
Onset of hearing	32 days
Breeding life of jill	2–5 years
Breeding life of hob	5+ years
Breeding habits	One male to several females; in colony production

and in body odour with the increasing light cycle (**Figs 6.3, 6.4**). Hobs need to be cycled out in the autumn and receive a short light cycle of 8 hours or less for at least 6–8 weeks out of the year in order for them to cycle back to breeding status. With good nutrition and cycling, hobs may breed for most of their life.

In jills, oestradiol and progesterone levels start to rise in late winter (February in the northern hemisphere) (**Fig. 6.5**).

A rule of thumb for puberty is that jills reach reproductive status the following spring after birth. For example, a jill born in July will reach puberty the following March. A jill born in September will likewise reach puberty the following March. Hobs born the previous season will reach puberty the following December–January and be ready for breeding that spring.

BREEDING

- The mating process begins with genital and neck sniffing (**Fig. 6.6**).
- When the jill is receptive, she becomes flaccid and submissive, allowing the hob to grasp her nape with his teeth and grip her body by wrapping his forelegs around her ribcage.
- The hob repeatedly does pelvic thrusts lasting up to 3 minutes. Between thrusts there may be periods of rest in which he lies over the jill but still maintains the grip on her neck.

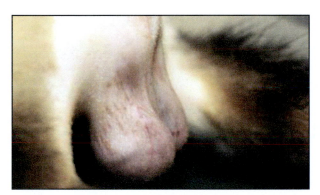

Fig. 6.3 **Testicles enlarged during season.**

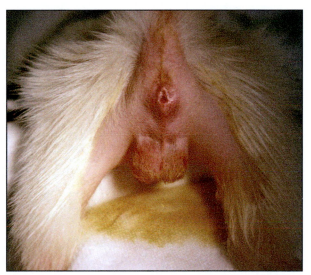

Fig. 6.4 **Testicles enlarged, in position for surgical castration.**

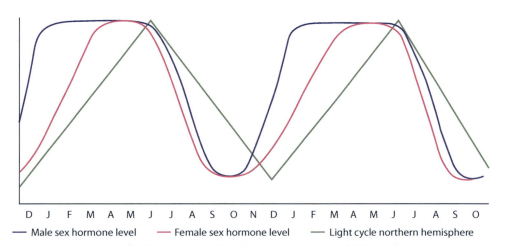

D J F M A M J J A S O N D J F M A M J J A S O

— Male sex hormone level   — Female sex hormone level   — Light cycle northern hemisphere

Fig. 6.5 **Representation of reproductive hormone levels in relation to the light cycle.**

- Total mating time is usually 1 hour, but can range from 15 minutes to 3 hours.
- There may be a lot of vocalisations.
- Ferrets are induced ovulators, with ovulation induced by pressure on the cervix.
- This leads to the endogenous release of luteinising hormone (LH). The LH surge causes the preovulatory follicles to begin maturation (average 12 oocytes, but can range from 5–13).
- Jills ovulate 30–40 hours after copulation.
- The ovary is encapsulated in a fatty bursa that prevents ovulated eggs from entering the abdomen. The gross structure of the ovaries and uterine horns resembles that of other carnivores (**Fig. 6.7**).

- Oocytes are capable of being fertilised up to 12 hours after ovulation, up to a maximum of 30–36 hours.
- Embryos enter the uterus over several days starting on day 5.
- Implantation is central.
- There is rapid invasion of the uterine epithelium by the trophoblast over a broad area that will become a zonary band of endotheliochorial placenta. The gravid uterus grossly resembles that of other carnivores (**Fig. 6.8**).
- The vulva starts drying and regressing in size 3–4 days after mating so that it is back to normal size within 4 weeks (**Fig. 6.9**).

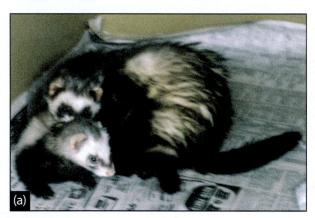
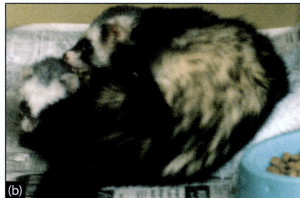

Fig. 6.6 (a) Mating begins with genital and neck sniffing; (b) the hob grasps the jill by the nape of the neck and grips her body.

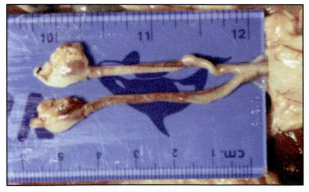
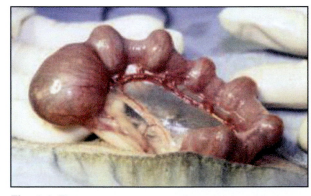

Fig. 6.7 Normal oestrus uterus and ovaries, necropsy picture.

Fig. 6.8 Pregnant uterus at surgery.

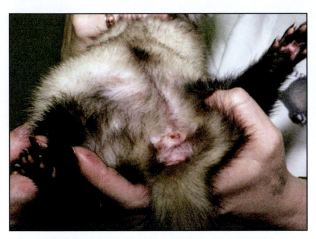

Fig. 6.9 Vulvar regression at 30 days postmating.

- Jills should be monitored closely for appetite or any changes in body condition, particularly late in gestation.
- Approximately 1.5 weeks before whelping, the jill loses her hair coat.
- Hairless rings develop around her teats.
- The jill should be fed a diet containing 36–40% animal-based protein and at least 20–30% fat. Food and fresh water should always be available. Many commercial diets are available that meet this need. The higher fat content is needed for weaning of the kits.

WHELPING

Place the pregnant jill's cage in a quiet area well before whelping. Jills should be housed separately for whelping and rearing of kits. The jill must be able to easily enter and exit the nest box without traumatising her mammary glands. The choices for whelping nest substrate include recycled paper bedding, small cloth towels or shredded hardwood shavings. Do not use large towels because kits can get lost in them.

Minimising stress is particularly important for the young, primiparous jill. This includes a decrease in handling of the jill. The risk of the jill being a poor mother increases with crowding or unusual noise and activity nearby. In addition the room should not be over 21°C. There should be a heat lamp over only part of the nesting box so that the jill and kits can select warmth as necessary.

Approximately 5 kits are born per hour, although it may take longer. Progress should be steady, with no outward signs of distress. The jill will not begin to nurse her litter until all are born. Once they are all born she will lie down in a semicircular position on her side.

If the jill becomes excited or stressed she may bury the kits in bedding or place them in a pile in a corner or in food or water containers. Some stressed jills will cannibalise the first few or all of their kits as they are born.

Later handling of kits does not appear to cause rejection.

Return to oestrus is 2 weeks after weaning if there is an appropriate long light photoperiod. If kits are removed at birth the jill will return to oestrus 8 weeks after mating. This is the same as pseudopregnant jills and those with resorbed fetuses. If a jill gives birth to a small number of kits (5 or fewer), she may return to oestrus during lactation (**Fig. 6.10**).

Diseases and problems with kits are covered in Chapter 26.

LACTATION

A properly lactating jill produces milk equivalent on bodyweight basis to a Holstein cow. Ferret milk has a higher fat content than cow milk. At parturition the milk is 8–10% fat, and at 3 weeks it is 15–20% fat. Lactating jills will become thin even when on a nutritionally fulfilling diet.

Milk production peaks when kits are approximately 3 weeks of age and are beginning to sample solid food. At this time it may be necessary to supplement the jill by blending the dry feed that contains less than 30% fat with water and a source of fat, e.g. linoleic acid, fish oil, or cooked chicken fat. This increases the fat content to roughly 30%. This mash is also offered to the kits. It is fed in increasing amounts twice daily as the kits grow and increase their intake. This supplementary feed reduces pressure on the jill to produce more milk. Kits will then start to eat dry pellets earlier, making weaning less stressful. If a commercial diet with at least 30% fat and 40% protein is fed, it may not be necessary to add in the supplementary fat.

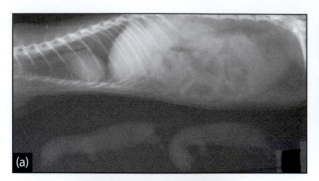

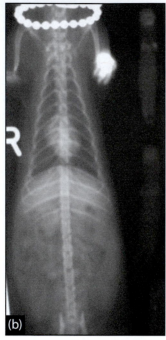

Fig. 6.10 (a) Lateral radiographs of a jill with large fetuses delivered via C-section; (b) ventrodorsal radiograph of jill and fetuses.

WEANING

Natural weaning is a gradual process beginning at about 3 weeks of age, although the eyes are still closed. Kits will begin exploring the nest at this age (**Fig. 6.11**).

Kits grow very quickly. They double their birth weight in 5 days, and triple it in 10 days.

- For the first week, kits gain 2.5–3.0 g daily.
- A 10-day-old average kit weighs 30 g.
- At week 2 they gain at least 4 g daily.
- At week 3 they gain at least 6 g daily.

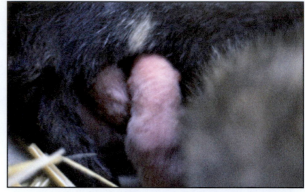

Fig. 6.11 Two-week-old kits with jill.

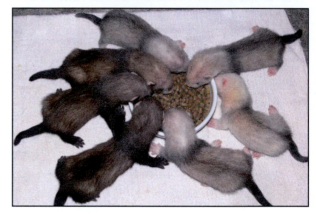

Fig. 6.12 Six-week-old kits. Kit at the 11 o'clock position is female; kit at the 2 o'clock position is male.

- Three-week-old kits have made a tenfold increase since birth weight. Males weigh at least 100 g.
- At 5–6 weeks, females should weigh 180–200 g, and males about 230–250 g.

Sexual dimorphism becomes obvious between 3–5 weeks of age. Male kits have broader heads and larger stature. Their weight is 8–16% greater than that of females (**Fig. 6.12**).

Kits weighing 200–250 g will eat about 30 g of a diet containing 30% fat, 40% protein and 66% moisture (about 13 g of dry matter) daily. Kits will drink 75–100 mL of water daily at that bodyweight.

Kits are best group-housed until mature, and social housing is recommended even then as ferrets are social animals. Room temperature can be 18.5–21.5°C as long as there is a snug nest for the kits to sleep in as a group. A single kit will need a supplemental heat source during and shortly after weaning.

CHAPTER 7

MEDICAL HISTORY

Cathy A. Johnson-Delaney

INTRODUCTION

A detailed medical history record should be created for every ferret in your practice (**Fig. 7.1**). The information should be included in the permanent computer record. **Fig. 7.2** is an example of a ferret history upon the first visit. At each visit, it is good to review the total health of the ferret. The owner can fill out a detailed list to update the pet's health information. This update helps both the owner and the vet to target the reasons for the day's visit. **Fig. 7.3** is an example of a form used for each visit.

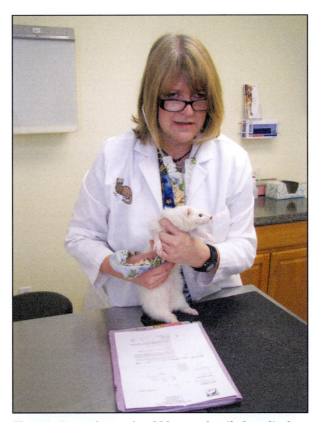

Fig. 7.1 **Every ferret should have a detailed medical record, updated at every consultation.**

Pet's name_____Weight_____

Variety (standard or angora)_____Microchip number_____

Sex: M__F__Neutered or spayed?_____Descented?_____Ear tattoo?_____

Deslorelin (Suprelorin) implant_____Date administered_____

Date of birth_____Coat colour_____Nose markings_____

Length of time in household_____

Acquired from_____Other ferrets in the household?_____

Other pets in household_____

Females only: How many litters?_____When was the last litter?_____

Lead/harness trained?_____

Housing

Does the ferret have access to the entire house?_____Garden?_____Exercise pen?_____

Time spent in cage_____h/day Time spent out of cage_____h/day Time unsupervised_____h

Type of caging/brand_____Multi-level?_____

Type of bedding/hammocks_____

Temperature in cage area: Day_____Night_____Air conditioning available?_____

Litter tray trained?_____Type of litter used_____How often is box cleaned?_____

Water source: Bottle_____Dish_____Other_____

Diet/Feeding

Pelleted diet_____% Canned food_____% Raw_____%

Brands used_____

Treats/supplements_____Amount and frequency given_____

Medical History

Please list briefly any previous health problems, including when they were noticed and when and how they were resolved.

_____

_____

_____

_____

_____

Adverse reactions to medications?_____Difficulty medicating?_____

Date of last distemper vaccine_____Date of last rabies vaccine_____

Has your ferret had a vaccine reaction?_____To which vaccination?_____

Date of last faecal check_____Date of last ear mite check_____

Date of last heartworm check_____Heartworm preventative used_____

Date of last heartworm medication given_____

Previous vet/veterinary clinic_____

Date of last veterinary visit_____Reason for visit_____

Fig. 7.2 **Example of a ferret registration form.**

Reason for today's visit_____

If your ferret is ill, how long ago did you notice symptoms?

A few hours or less_____1 day_____2–3 days_____1 week_____1 month_____Longer than 1 month_____

Has your ferret ingested:

Bones_____Toy or object_____Poison_____Chocolate/sweets_____Fertiliser_____Plants_____Rubbish_____Anti-freeze_____

Injuries: Fight wound_____Snake bite_____Insect bite_____

Head_____Eyes_____Front leg(s)_____Hind leg(s)_____Neck_____Back_____Rump_____Tail_____Abdomen_____

Please tick all that apply:

Vomiting_____Diarrhoea_____Constipation_____Seizures_____Muscle tremors_____Shaking_____

Salivating_____Paralysis_____Enlarged abdomen_____Difficulty giving birth_____Gagging/swallowing problem_____

Difficult or painful defaecation: Moderate_____Severe_____

Are your ferret's stools: Well formed_____Soft_____Liquid_____Bloody_____Other (explain)_____

Difficulty urinating: Yes_____No_____

Bloody urine: Yes_____No_____

Increased urination: Yes_____No_____

Increased drinking: Yes_____No_____

Changes in behaviour (please tick all that apply):

Circling_____Pacing_____Licking/eating non-food items_____Aggression_____Crying or whimpering_____

Decreased grooming or self-care_____Overgrooming_____Decreased play behaviour_____

Having problems with (please tick all that apply):

Breathing_____Hearing_____Seeing_____Rising and walking_____Increased stiffness_____

Weakness_____Uncoordinated movements_____Climbing_____

Coughing: Moderate_____Severe_____Frequency of coughing_____

Weakness during/after exercise: Moderate_____Severe_____

Decreased affection or interaction with owners: Yes_____No_____

Waking owners at night: Yes_____No_____   Vocalising during sleep: Yes_____No_____

Weight changes: Gain_____Loss_____Moderate_____Severe_____Seems to be seasonal_____

Appetite changes: Increase_____Decrease_____Moderate_____Severe_____

Decreased activity (sleeping more): Moderate_____Severe_____

Decreased awareness (gets confused or lost): Moderate_____Severe_____

Skin problems: Lumps/tumours_____Scratching_____Foul body odour_____Dandruff_____Scabs_____Hair loss_____

Dental problems (please tick all that apply):

Bad breath_____Difficulty chewing_____Inflamed/bleeding gingiva_____Broken tooth(teeth)_____

Discoloured tooth(teeth)_____Tartar buildup_____Loose tooth(teeth)_____

Ears: Excessive wax_____Odour_____Shaking head_____Sensitive to being touched_____

Eyes: Discharge from lids_____Redness_____Pupils gone white_____Squinting_____

Nose: Discharge_____Sneezing_____

Has your ferret been previously diagnosed with:

Heart disease_____Kidney disease_____Adrenal disease_____Insulinoma_____Lymphoma_____

Ulcer_____Ear mites_____Heartworms_____Other (explain)_____

Is your ferret currently on medication? Yes_____No_____

If yes, please list medications, dosage, frequency:_____

_____

_____

Fig. 7.3 Example of a ferret health information form.

CHAPTER 8

PHYSICAL EXAMINATION

John R. Chitty

INTRODUCTION

The fundamental part of any clinical investigation is the physical examination. Ferrets have an unjust reputation for being vicious and many vets may be nervous handling them. It is true that ferrets will often give a painful 'curiosity' nip. But this is principally due to their poor eyesight and can be overcome by careful handling. Certainly it is possible to perform a full physical examination on the majority of animals presented to the clinic without sedation.

One unusual aspect to ferrets is that they are particularly susceptible to influenza viruses (see Chapter 20). Therefore if vets or technicians/nurses are suffering from influenza (not common colds) then they should not handle ferrets. Facemasks and disposable gloves may help reduce risk to the ferret, but it is preferable not to risk passing on a potentially fatal (to the ferret) infection.

TRANSPORT

In terms of size, ferrets are easily transported and, fundamentally, any carrier suitable for a cat should be suitable for an adult ferret (**Fig. 8.1**). The two major problems are:

- Making a carrier escape proof.
- Making a carrier suitable such that it is easy to catch and restrain a ferret within.

Very calm trained ferrets may be transported on harness and lead. However, this is not ideal in a busy mixed-species veterinary clinic where ferrets may be frightened or even attacked by lead-restrained dogs. Even if not injured, it is not conducive to a calm physical examination to start with a scared ferret! Poorly fitting harnesses may also not prevent escape of a

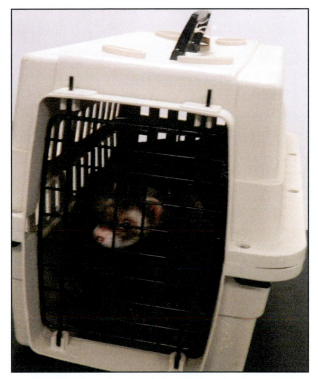

Fig. 8.1 **Ferret in standard cat carrier.**

startled ferret. Therefore, many vets will advise owners only to bring ferrets restrained in boxes. If ferrets are brought on leads, owners should be quickly ushered to a private waiting area away from other pets.

Working ferreters and some owners will often have special ferret travelling boxes. These are usually made of wood and have lift-up tops. Multi-ferret carriers with several compartments are available.

Otherwise, as stated above, cat carriers are suitable. These should have a small mesh size so the ferret cannot escape through or get stuck in the mesh (**Fig. 8.2**). Ideally top-opening boxes should be used rather than front-opening. Ferrets should be transported individually unless they are used to living together, in which case two or three may be brought

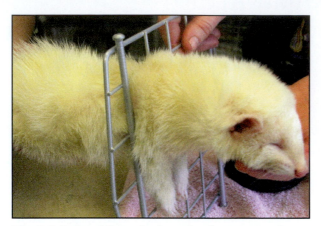

Fig. 8.2 Sedated ferret having wire door removed, after getting stuck. Ferrets will attempt to escape via the smallest gap in the wire door.

in the same carrier – however, this can cause difficulties when removing and replacing each animal in the carrier.

The transport box should be lined with paper, hay or straw. Paper is ideal as it is absorbent and does not litter the consulting room when the ferret is removed. Water bottles may be attached to the carrier for long journeys – these should not drip. Bowls are not appropriate.

It is rarely necessary to provide food for the journey, although owners are advised to carry a glucose supplement for longer journeys if the ferret is known or suspected to have an insulinoma. The carrier can be covered with a towel or blanket as darkened carriers may help calm the ferret. Overheating should be avoided, so ferrets should not be left in hot cars, and good ventilation is essential on hot days. Hypothermia is much less likely; however, on cold days the car should be 'prewarmed' before starting the journey.

Collapsed ferrets will become hypothermic very quickly due to their high surface area:volume ratio. They should therefore be wrapped in towels and placed on a hot water bottle (or hand warmer) during transportation.

HANDLING AND RESTRAINT

As stated earlier, the aim is to reduce stress on the ferret to minimise fearfulness and, hence, reduce risk of injury to ferret and handlers (and, of course, to increase the value of findings during the clinical examination). Ferrets should, therefore, not be kept waiting in noisy waiting areas with barking dogs. They should be seen as quickly as possible after arrival (especially emergency cases) and, in any case, wait in a quiet private waiting area.

Similarly, correct handling by the vet is vital to reduce patient stress. It also creates an excellent impression on the owner (who is often aware of ferrets' poor reputation!), especially one who may be visiting a practice for the first time. Certainly, heavy-duty handling gloves are rarely needed and certainly should not be immediately reached for unless the particular ferret is known to be difficult to handle, or the owner specifically advises it. In the UK, this is usually for certain working ferrets, especially wild polecat crosses. If gloves are used to capture the animal they should be discarded once the animal is restrained – bare hands are much more sensitive than gloves when handling.

Once secured, difficult animals can be tightly towel wrapped for injections or for certain more invasive examinations.

Most bites occur on removing the ferret from its box. This is mainly because the animal is fearful and because its poor eyesight may not distinguish a hand reaching in towards it.

As part of any examination, the ferret should always be observed prior to handling (see below). As well as giving clinical information, this also gives vital information about handling the animal. It should be noted if the ferret is blind or deaf so the approach to handling the ferret can be modified in order not to startle it. If it appears excited (very bright expression and may be moving in agitated fashion), is vocalising or has the classic 'bottlebrush' tail, then there is a greater chance that this animal may bite a handler. It is less likely to bite the owner than a stranger. However, it is not wise to ask an owner to reach into an agitated ferret as the vet will be liable for any injuries incurred in the examination room. Instead, the animal should be allowed to calm down before handling is attempted.

Handlers should never reach into the travelling box. Instead the door/lid should be opened and the ferret allowed to emerge from the box by itself so it can be grasped round the shoulders from above (**Fig. 8.3**). The ferret can then be held upright allowing the hind legs to dangle. Most ferrets appear relaxed in this position and

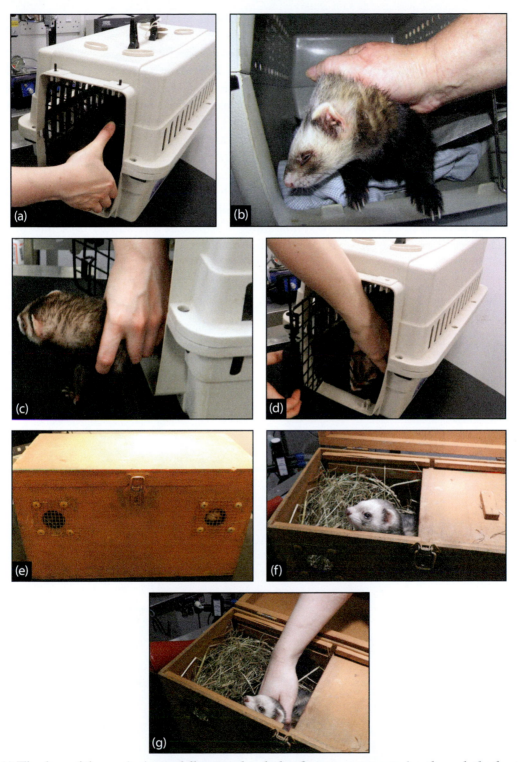

Fig. 8.3 (a) The door of the carrier is carefully opened such that fingers are not entering through the front (this can result in a bite); (b, c) the ferret sticks its head out and can then be grasped from above around the shoulders; (d) do not reach in and grab the ferret – unless the ferret is very calm this can result in a bite; (e) alternate type of ferret transfer box with opening on top; (f) ferret ready to be lifted; (g) ferret being extracted from the box.

will allow the majority of a clinical examination to be performed while 'suspended' (**Fig. 8.4**). More awkward animals may be scruffed (**Fig. 8.5**). Again, the hindlegs are allowed to dangle. An assistant (or the owner) may be asked to loosely hold the hind legs should the animal start to scrabble.

Another method of restraint uses a towel. Start by placing the towel at the ventrum neck and then wrap it around the ferret. It creates a kind of 'ferret burrito'. This may greatly facilitate an oral examination (**Fig. 8.6**).

Unlike cats and dogs, ferrets will become distressed if held horizontally against the examination table. Relaxed pet ferrets can be scooped up with a hand placed under the ventrum. However, even these animals often tolerate more procedures when held vertically.

More invasive examinations or sample taking or injections can be facilitated by an assistant giving a small quantity of a high-fat, high-protein nutritional gel, e.g. NutriPlus® (Virbac, Bury St Edmunds, UK), while the ferret is being held. The ferret is often so absorbed eating this (especially if smeared round the mouth, or slowly fed from the end of the tube or put on a tongue depressor or spoon) that it will tolerate a lot more (**Fig. 8.7**).

To release the animal back into its carrier, the box should be placed such that the opening is on

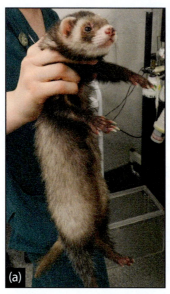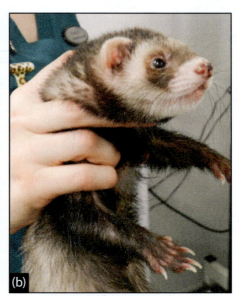

Fig. 8.4 (a, b) The ferret is held around the shoulders and allowed to 'dangle'.

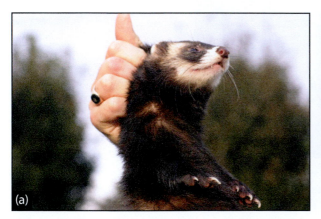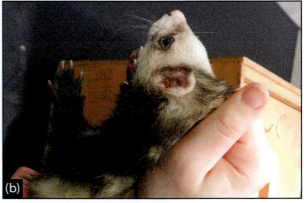

Fig. 8.5 (a, b) Scruffed ferret.

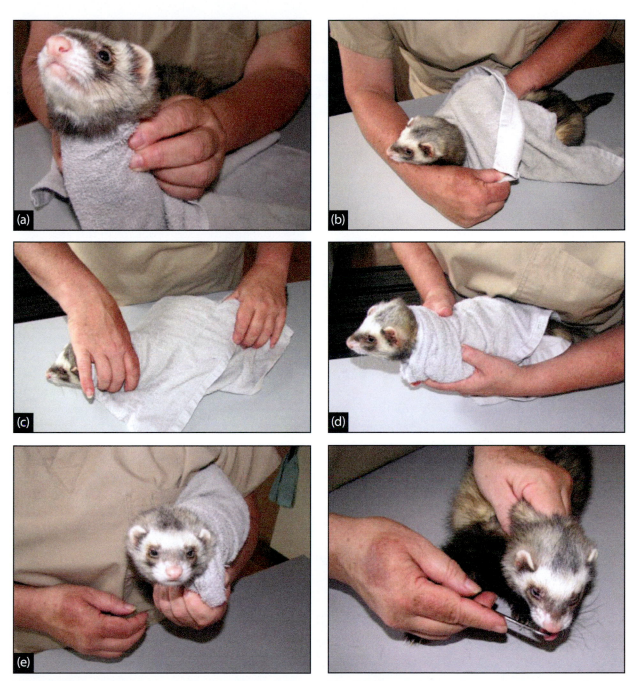

Fig. 8.6 Using a towel to wrap a ferret up for restraint. (a) The towel is positioned under the ferret and wrapped at the neck; (b–d) the sides of the towel are then wrapped snuggly around the body; (e) the ferret can now be held.

Fig. 8.7 Ferrets are much more cooperative and happy if they are fed some nutrient gel while being restrained. The gel may be placed on a tongue depressor or in a spoon for administration.

top (i.e. place front-opening carriers on their end – remove all loose food/drinkers/food carriers first) and lower the animal into the box. For nervous animals, or those that have just received an irritant injection, it greatly facilitates the rapid removal of the hand. For others, it enables the closing of the box lid before the animal escapes.

EXAMINATION

The principles of examination are similar for all species, so this section will simply emphasise those aspects particular to ferrets.

Prior to handling, the ferret's demeanour should be assessed (see above) in terms of whether it is bright and alert, collapsed, dyspnoeic, etc. This allows evaluation of handling risks, and the need for critical care (e.g. oxygen therapy) – i.e. how ill the animal actually is (**Fig. 8.8**). The second phase of initial assessment is to assess the ferret's response to being handled and whether or not the animal shows pain or distress.

The ferret's weight and body condition should be measured. It should be noted that ferrets' body-weight and condition will vary markedly through the year, the weight being much higher through winter and falling by up to a third by late spring. The situation may be a little different in intact hobs who will also lose body fat in late spring, but will

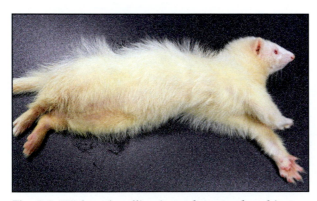

Fig. 8.8 Without handling it can be seen that this conscious ferret is alert; it is collapsed; the hind limbs are flaccid while the front legs are in rigid extension; and the hind feet are covered in urine. These findings indicate a likely severe spinal lesion in the thoracolumbar region (see Chapter 18).

gain muscle mass. These animals may not lose much *weight* but will lose *condition*; the hormonal signs of greasy coat and odour will indicate this is the likely situation. If in doubt, ask the owner what the normal body changes are for that ferret. Emaciation, though, is abnormal and it is important to check musculature over fore- and hindquarters as well as checking condition over the ribs and the lumbar spine.

Arthritis and joint problems are common and the finding of reasonable/good condition over the forequarters and lumbar area combined with muscle loss over the hips indicates problems in this area.

Lymph nodes should be checked – especially submandibular, axillary, inguinal and popliteal.

Skin should be picked up and 'dropped' to assess dehydration and protein status. Ferrets are like cats in that loss of skin elasticity may also show protein loss – the 'wetness' of mucous membranes should be assessed as well.

The normal body temperature of the ferret is 37.8–40°C. Body temperature may be measured with the careful use of rectal temperature probes or thermometers. However, it is this author's opinion that the risk of iatrogenic damage outweighs its usefulness in most ferrets and therefore should only be performed in collapsed ferrets as low temperatures may indicate a poor prognosis.

The coat should be checked for general character, i.e. colour, density, 'sheen', cleanliness, greasiness and odour. A dull coat, as in other species, is often a sign of general debility/illness. As with body condition, coat density will vary throughout the year, being thinnest in summer. Again, cyclical changes in coat should always be assessed in conjunction with what is normal for that ferret. Alopecia is common and may accompany coat changes. Areas of excoriation may indicate pruritus. Where hair appears broken off, a trichogram should be taken to see if the hair has been bitten off or has broken off. The hair should be parted looking for parasites and the skin surface examined looking for crusts, scabs and other lesions (e.g. papules, masses, discolouration) (**Fig. 8.9**).

The limbs and spine are readily palpated while the ferret is restrained. The spine is more mobile than in other species. Limbs are short and fractures unusual. Joints should be flexed and extended to assess range of movement. Recognition of areas of muscle loss should provoke further investigation of the joints in that region (**Fig. 8.10**).

The feet should be thoroughly checked as masses are common on the distal limbs, and claw loss or damage may be a cause of lameness.

Thorax

The initial examination of the chest should be to palpate it and to gently percuss it. The chest should feel 'springy' and not solid (may indicate presence of a mass). Percussing should produce a drum-like sound indicating presence of air, rather than a 'solid' sound. An enlarged heart may also be palpated. Grade 5 'thrill' murmurs are extremely rare.

Full examination should always be made with a stethoscope. Due to the small size of the ferret, an infant stethoscope is highly recommended. This should give audible soft air sounds.

Crackles and fluid sounds are abnormal and warrant further investigation. 'Dead' areas are similarly suspicious, especially if combined with a solid chest on palpation. Both sides should be auscultated and in various positions – these should correspond with the position of each lung lobe (**Fig. 8.11**).

The heart is positioned more caudally than in other species. Both sides of the heart should be auscultated as well as apex and base. Loud valvular murmurs are unusual. Instead, cardiomyopathy is common so soft murmurs may be significant. The heart may also be auscultated over a wider area or sound 'echoey'. Dysrhythmias may also be detected. Because pulses are not always obvious and the heart rate is rapid, simultaneous auscultation and pulse palpation is not helpful. If a dysrhythmia is suspected an ECG should be performed (see Chapter 12). If necessary an 8 mHz Doppler may be used to assess pulse separately (femoral or pedal – the latter may also be used in indirect blood pressure measurement). Audio Doppler is useful to pinpoint the valve or area of the heart where the murmur is being heard.

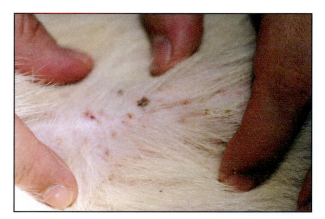

Fig. 8.9 **Close examination of coat and skin is always important.**

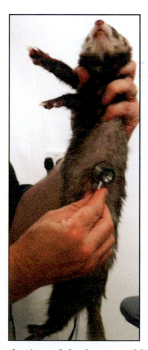

Fig. 8.11 **Auscultation of the heart and lungs. Note the use of an infant stethoscope. The heart is more caudal in ferrets than in dogs/cats, and when held in this manner may appear more caudal still.**

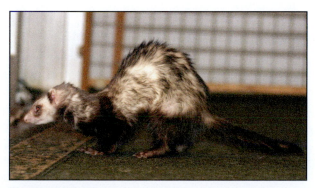

Fig. 8.10 **Muscle mass loss and hunched posture.**

Abdomen

Abdominal masses and organomegaly are common and the abdomen should always be thoroughly palpated. This should be done with care as the the visci may have fragile walls, for example the walls of a distended bladder. Percussion may reveal the presence of fluid, and this may be withdrawn for analysis (**Fig. 8.12**). It should be relatively easy to identify the kidneys, the spleen and the GI tract. It should be noted that splenomegaly may be normal in older ferrets (see Chapter 16).

- The kidneys may be palpated as irregular and/ or shrunken. In some cases of adrenal disease the enlarged gland(s) may be palpated slightly cranial to the kidneys.

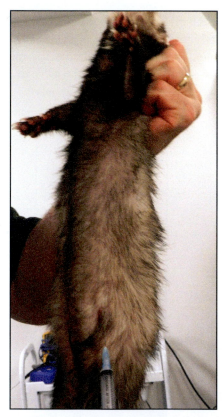

Fig. 8.12 Withdrawal of fluid from an ascetic ferret. The ferret is held dangling, the skin is cleaned with alcohol and the needle (1″ 23G) passed via the inguinal region (parallel to legs) into the abdomen. The hind legs may need to be held in some ferrets, or a small amount of local anaesthetic infiltrated at the injection site.

- The liver is rarely palpable unless markedly enlarged.
- The intestines may feel thickened in chronic diarrhoea cases and gas-filled loops may be found in the ileus or foreign body cases (see Chapter 13).
- Sublumbar and mesenteric lymph nodes should be assessed – they should not normally be palpable yet chains of masses may be found in lymphoproliferative disease (see Chapter 16).

Head

Some ferrets resent excessive handling around the head and many will bite if not handled carefully. For this reason, the head should be examined last as it may cause the most stress. Always perform a general look first, assessing discharges from eyes or nose and looking for evidence of hypersalivation. Then palpate for swellings or masses, including the submandibular lymph nodes. Swellings may be further investigated using fine needle aspirates (FNAs). It is usually necessary to sedate the ferret and use a local anaesthetic prior to doing FNAs as many ferrets will struggle and the procedure may be painful (see Chapter 24).

The ears should be examined with respect to their position, evidence of inflammation or swelling, and amount of cerumen emanating from the canal. Signs of hair loss or excoriation may indicate pruritus. The external ear should be checked for parasite. If possible, auriscopic examination should be performed and most pet ferrets will tolerate this while conscious (**Fig. 8.13**). However, it is often best performed using endoscopy while anaesthetised as this will also allow cleaning of the diseased canal. If there is evidence of disease and, in particular, ear mites (see Chapter 15), cerumen samples should be taken for cytology and culture.

The eyes should be assessed initially in terms of brightness, presence of discharges/fur staining, swelling (ocular and periocular) and colour (especially colour changes). It is hard to perform a full ophthalmological examination on such a small eye and use of a direct ophthalmoscope may increase the risk of being bitten (an indirect ophthalmoscope may help). A full examination under anaesthesia may be needed (**Fig. 8.14**).

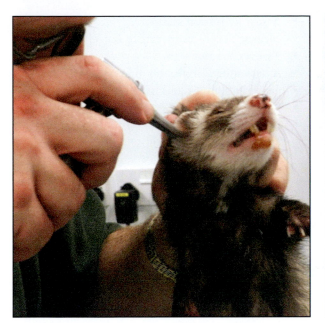

Fig. 8.13 **Auriscopic examination of the ferret.**

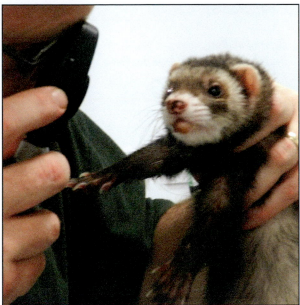

Fig. 8.14 **Direct ophthalmoscopy of a ferret. The need to get very close to the ferret may preclude this in some animals.**

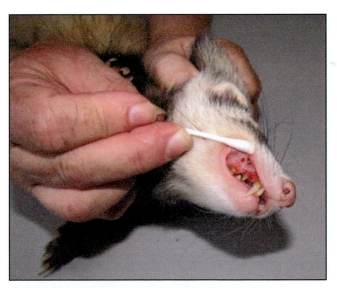

Fig. 8.15 **Oral examination facilitated by using a cotton bud.**

Examination of the mouth can be very difficult. The ferret should be well restrained, then carefully elevate the lips. This allows a basic examination of the teeth and gingiva as well as membrane colour (**Fig. 8.15**). It is not recommended to use a speculum to examine as these may cause damage. Instead, relaxed ferrets will often yawn, allowing some examination. The oral cavity should be checked for ulceration (see Chapter 19). Anaesthesia/sedation should be used if there is any oral pathology or if a thorough examination is not possible in the awake ferret.

CHECKLIST

Before handling:
- Is the ferret blind or deaf?
- Demeanour:
  - Alert? Aware?
  - Fearful?
  - Vocalising?
- Coat:
  - 'Bright' and shiny full, or dull?
  - Alopecia?
- Gait:
  - Standing/moving normally?
  - Walking normally?
  - Dragging hind limbs?
  - Swaying/wobbling on hindquarters?
  - All limbs at correct angle?
- Breathing – rate, effort, noise. Open-mouthed? Discharges from nose/eyes?
- Any obvious blood or blood loss?

On handling:
- Signs of pain? Vocalising; flinching; bite response? If so, where?
- Becomes distressed? Resents handling; open-mouthed breathing?
- Becomes dyspnoeic? Cyanotic? Open-mouth breathing?

Examination once restrained:
- Check bodyweight and body condition.
- Assess lymph nodes.
- Assess hydration status.
- Measure body temperature if deemed essential.
- Assess coat and skin.
- Assess spine, limbs and joints.
- Auscultate lungs and heart.
- Palpate abdomen.
- Head:
  - Discharges – eyes, nose.
  - Hypersalivation?
  - Swellings? e.g. malar abscess swellings under the eyes. Check submandibular lymph nodes.
  - Ears:
    - Position.
    - Excessive cerumen?
    - Signs of excoriation/hair loss around the ears.
    - Auriscopic examination.
  - Eyes:
    - Brightness and colour.
    - 'Colour' – note the difference between albino forms and non-albino forms.
    - Periocular/ocular swelling.
    - Ophthalmoscopic examination.
  - Mouth:
    - Teeth/gingiva.
    - Membrane colour.
    - 'Wetness' and amount of salivation.
    - Oral cavity looking for ulcers.

CHAPTER 9

FERRET PREVENTIVE CARE

John R. Chitty and
Cathy A. Johnson-Delaney

INTRODUCTION

The mantra of all medicine is that prevention is better than cure. This holds true for ferrets and in this chapter the authors will describe some of the medical regimes for preventive healthcare in ferrets. As may be expected, disease syndromes vary according to location, husbandry and life stage: there is no 'one size fits all' approach to preventive medicine. While contrasting the situations in the UK and the USA, these descriptions should not be taken as 'rules' for ferret preventive health plans that should be rigidly implemented. Instead they are more guidelines that can be recommended in part or entirety, depending on the needs of that ferret and its owner. The situation may vary in other countries and the reader is recommended to read Lewington (2007) where there is an excellent collation of experiences from ferret clinicians around the world.

It is also important that this chapter is not read in isolation. Preventive medicine is not simply about infectious disease control and neutering. To prevent disease, husbandry (see Chapter 4) and good diet (see Chapter 5) will arguably be far more important. As such, readers are recommended to read the relevant chapters in this volume in order to achieve a more balanced and holistic approach to disease prevention in pet ferrets.

REPRODUCTIVE CONTROL

The ferret's reproductive strategy is identical to its ancestor (*Mustela putorius*) and is well adapted to the life of a solitary hunter – both hobs and jills are seasonally monoestrous and ovulation is induced (see Chapter 6). In domesticated ferrets, there is still the release of pheromones and scent by both sexes when in season. Ferrets are usually purposely bred, unlike their wild ancestors who depend on chance meetings for inducing pregnancy. For the jill, this is one of the few situations in companion veterinary medicine where some form of reproductive control is essential for the pet's health. Throughout the season the jill will produce oestrogen from the ovaries – as season is controlled by light cycle, these oestrogen levels may start to rise in early spring and (if not mated) only fall in autumn (**Fig. 9.1**). The main consequence of this is an oestrogen-induced bone marrow suppression and, without intervention, fatal pancytopaenia, including anaemia and thrombocytopaenia (**Fig. 9.2**). In addition, ovarian tumours appear to be relatively common compared to other pet species in this author's experience (JRC).

There are various options available for reproductive control in the jill:

- Allow to breed each year.
- Use of a 'teaser' or vasectomised hob (V-hob). This strategy is useful for large groups of working animals, but less so for show or pet

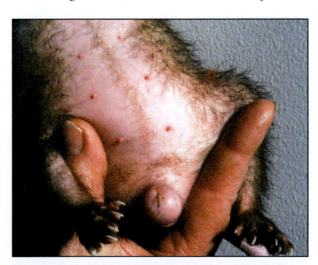

Fig. 9.1 **Female ferret in oestrus with swollen vulva.**

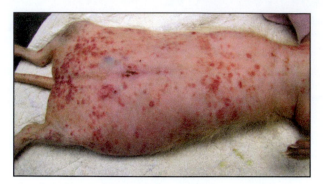

Fig. 9.2 Petechia seen with thrombocytopaenia.

animals as, by the end of the season, the jill has a thoroughly chewed neck from the repeated rough matings (being induced ovulators, mating is rough). It is also sensible that each owner has their own V-hob as loaning one between breeders increases potential disease transmission.

- Stimulation – some owners will stimulate the jill's vagina using a thermometer to mimic mating. Unless the owner is experienced, there is the potential for harm.
- Proligestone injections (also known as a 'jill jab') – 0.5mL Delvosteron (MSD, Hoddesdon, UK) can be given subcutaneously after onset of the season. This may last all season or need repeating at intervals depending on that year's light levels and weather cycles. This has always been one of the most economic options. However, changes in the product's UK licence mean that a bottle should be used with 24 hours of opening. Therefore, it is now only financially viable when injecting large numbers of ferrets – usually via a club or show. This drug is not effective if given before the onset of season. There is also a low risk of pyometra and skin changes (hair loss and pruritus at the injection site – even skin calcification after multiple doses) following injection. The injection is intensely irritant and many owners are put off by the jill screaming and biting when injected; owners should always be warned of this before giving this drug.
- Gonadotropin-releasing hormone (GnRH) agonist injections. Both buserelin (Receptal, MSD, Hoddesdon, UK) and leuprolide acetate have been used. In this author's (JRC)

experience buserelin has been effective for short-term use (a single dose of 0.001 mg buserelin is given intramuscularly) and postponement of breeding; it has not been effective for pet owners requiring season-long control. Leuprolide acetate 30-day formulation can take the jill out of oestrus and maintain her for at least 30 days, but this drug is not always easy to procure, and is expensive. However, it does have additional uses in the veterinary practice, so dividing the kit and freezing the drug may be cost effective. It is used in the treatment of adrenal disease (see Chapter 14). The introduction of deslorelin implants has greatly changed the approach to neutering of ferrets as they provide long-term control and appear to greatly reduce the risk of adrenal gland disease (AGD). See below.

- Surgical neutering. Traditionally this was the usual recommended route for long-term reproductive control in pet animals that would never be used for breeding. The technique is described in Chapter 25. Timing of neutering varies between countries. In the UK surgical neutering has been carried out either after the onset of their first season or, if prepubertal, in their first autumn when approximately 3–4 months old. However, the ferret's breeding cycle means that surgical neutering has emerged as the major cause of AGD (see Chapter 14). In the UK and many countries, surgical neutering is performed much less commonly and generally only for ferrets in rescue shelters or for owners who opt for this long-term control (without the need for regular hormone therapy) but are fully informed of the risks of AGD. Prepubertal neutering is almost never recommended in the UK as the timing of onset of AGD has been shown to be directly related to timing of neutering (Schoemacher *et al.*, 2000). Unfortunately in the USA, the vast majority of ferrets are neutered at 5–6 weeks of age, as well as demusked, to enter the pet trade at 7–8 weeks of age. There are a few private breeders remaining and with these the options above exist. It is usually recommended that all pet females be ovariohysterectomised, preferably following the timetable above.

For males, control is less about health and more about convenience: in-season hobs need to be kept individually and outside due to their sociability and smell. If an owner wants to keep multiple males, especially if they are to be housed indoors, then some form of neutering is essential.

There are fewer options than for the jill – essentially only surgical castration has been used (vasectomy will enable birth control, but no improvement in testosterone-linked traits) and this too carries the increased risk of AGD in hobs. Castration technique is discussed in Chapter 25.

Deslorelin implants

The high incidence rate of AGD in surgically neutered animals means that there is a need for an alternative to surgical neutering and the use of deslorelin implants (a GnRH agonist, refer to Chapter 14) has been of great assistance.

The 9.4 mg implants have been licensed in the UK for use in male ferrets within the last 3 years; however the 4.7 mg implants have been used successfully in UK ferrets for much longer. The 4.7 mg implant is licensed for use in ferrets in the USA (Suprelorin-F®, Virbac, Ft Worth, TX).

The following experiences relate, therefore, to the 4.7 mg implants, which these authors use rather than the 9.4 mg implants (**Fig. 9.3**).

- These appear to reduce hormone levels in both hobs and jills effectively, thus making them suitable for birth control. They reduce both the risk of oestrogen-induced pancytopaenia in jills, and undesirable testosterone-linked behaviours and scent in entire males.
- Initially they stimulate further sex hormone release, so any antisocial factors may increase. This lasts approximately 2 weeks (these authors have yet to see longer, though this has been described) after which hormonal signs vanish quickly. Out-of-season jills will come into season during this period, and implanted entire ferrets should not be mixed until all hormone-linked signs (vulval swelling, smell, sticky fur, testicular size) have reduced. For this reason, too, deslorelin cannot be recommended as part of the initial management of pancytopaenic jills.

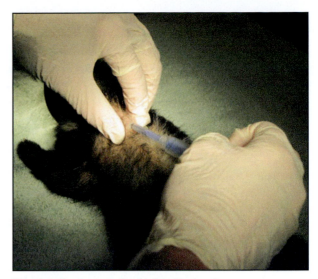

Fig. 9.3 **Insertion of a deslorelin implant.**

Instead, proligestone should be used to quickly reduce oestrogen levels.

- The implants appear to last 18–30 months. van Zeeland *et al.* (2014) recommend annual reimplantation as some animals in their studies returned to oestrus after less than a year (minimum 301 days). This has not been this author's (JRC) experience and in his clinic animals are implanted every 2 years. However, owners must be informed and told to watch for signs of oestrus before this period so the ferret can be returned earlier if necessary. The Suprelorin-F® (Virbac Animal Health, Inc. Fort Worth, TX) implant is licensed for annual reimplantation.
- The occasional implant is groomed out and lost (in spite of applying tissue glue or suture to the implant site). The implants are palpable in the scapular area and can be checked with palpation.
- Side-effects appear very few. While some do swell at the implant site, the only other adverse effect seen in this author's practice is a single jill that developed a pseudopregnancy (controlled with cabergoline (5 µg/kg q24h 5 days Galastop, Ceva, Amersham UK). Owners have reported good effects and response to implant reminders has been good.
- It is too early to definitively state that the deslorelin implants prevent AGD although studies

have shown this effect, and no cases have been seen by this author in implanted ferrets (see Chapter 14). Implanting already-neutered ferrets also appears of benefit, and owners who opt for surgical neutering, or who obtain surgically neutered animals from rescue shelters, can be offered this implant as AGD prevention.

- Normally ferrets are implanted while conscious – the implant and needle are large; however, the difference in ferrets' reactions when implanting deslorelin and injecting irritant proligestone is minimal (see above). The UK datasheet recommendation when using the 9.4 mg implant is to anaesthetise – although it is the same diameter as the 4.7 mm implant it is longer, so may be slightly trickier to place in the awake ferret. Certainly if the practitioner is unfamiliar at handling ferrets a short isoflurane anaesthetic should be considered. Anaesthesia is a good option if the practitioner prefers to close the injection site with a suture. Generally these implants are placed just distal to the scapular area subcutaneously (see **Fig. 14.17** in Chapter 14).

As stated, these experiences relate to the 4.7 mg implant. Under the prescribing cascade in the UK, the 9.4 mg implant should be the first consideration for *male* ferrets. However, clinical judgement does allow the clinician to use other choices if they deem them more efficacious in a particular case and this author continues to use 4.7 mg implants in both sexes as:

- Financially, the 9.4 mg implants are approximately twice the price of the 4.7 mg implants.
- While the 9.4 mg implants are licensed in the UK for a 16-month duration, it is likely that they will last much longer. This is a benefit in that longer duration means more owner convenience. However, it may mean increased likelihood of lack of owner vigilance at the end of implant life. One option is to automatically reimplant at a fixed period rather than wait for effects to wear off – there appears to be no indication that deslorelin overdosage is harmful, though whether this may apply to chronic overdosage is not yet

determined. Some degree of monitoring can be carried out in the clinic as ferrets should be presented annually for their distemper vaccination (see later in this chapter) – if this is timed for mid–late spring, reproductive status can also be checked.

VACCINATION

Vaccination needs should always be based on both susceptibility to disease and on risk of contracting that disease. These needs must then be balanced against any risks from vaccination itself.

The major infectious disease problem for which vaccination may be appropriate is canine distemper virus (CDV).

CDV

Ferrets are susceptible to this infection and it is invariably fatal to them (see Chapter 18). The source of virus is usually pet dogs in the same household (either direct transmission or a mechanical vector effect) but also, for ferrets who go outside, foxes form a continuing reservoir of virus.

Other ferrets may also act as a source of virus, especially in the short incubation period before signs develop. In both the UK and USA in recent years there have been outbreaks, especially in rescue shelters. Therefore all ferrets used for hunting, taken for walks in public places or taken to shows should be vaccinated.

Although in reality ferrets that do not get taken out generally would not require vaccination as long as any in-contact dogs are vaccinated and care is taken to prevent mechanical carriage of virus, that is problematic in areas where there are wild animal reservoirs and even pet dog immunity is unknown.

In the UK there is no licensed CDV vaccines specifically for ferrets, while there is one in the USA. As there have been reports of reversion to virulence from some live vaccines in other countries, this should always be discussed with owners. There are, however, good reports of use for most brands of CDV vaccine for dogs in the UK, although it is recommended to discuss this with your vaccine brand's manufacturer before use, especially as there are anecdotal unproven reports from the recent outbreaks that some vaccines may not have been protective.

The authors have used a half dose of Nobivac DHPPi (MSD, Hoddesdon, UK) or a full dose of Nobivac DP with solvent, rather than utilise the full dog vaccine with leptospirosis fraction (ferrets do not appear susceptible to leptospirosis), for many years with no obvious ill effects. The first dose is given after 12 weeks of age and repeated annually. A small-scale study has shown this dose does produce protective levels of antibody for a considerable period postvaccination (A. Raftery, personal communication). It should be noted that challenge studies have not been performed. However, anecdotal reports from the recent outbreaks have been that a full dose may be more protective – this is not yet proven, but may be requested by some ferret keepers (and certainly appears not to do any obvious harm). In the USA, it is recommended that a two-dose series of Nobivac DP be given starting after 12 weeks of age with the second injection 2–4 weeks later. Annual vaccination is recommended.

Rabies

Rabies vaccination is not required routinely in the UK but is mandatory for the Pet Passport scheme that also covers ferrets.

No vaccines for ferrets are licensed in the UK although all three UK-licensed rabies vaccines available have been used safely in ferrets. Nonetheless owners should be warned before use, and your vaccine manufacturer consulted before use. A full dog dose is given annually from 12 weeks of age. In the USA, the rabies vaccine is licensed for use in ferrets (IMRAB® 3, Merial, Duluth, GA, USA) and is recommended for the vaccination of healthy cats, dogs, sheep, cattle, horses and ferrets at 12 weeks of age and older for prevention of disease due to rabies virus. IMRAB® 3 contains the same virus strain that is used in the Pasteur Merieux Connaught human vaccine. Dogs, cats and sheep are protected for 3 years, following vaccination 1 year after their first vaccination. Ferrets, cattle and horses are protected for 1 year. There may be laws, regulations or recommendations for ferrets to be vaccinated against rabies. Ferret shelters may be required to provide vaccination for all ferrets leaving their facility.

ROLE OF HEALTH CHECKS AND ROUTINE TESTS

Another advantage of annual vaccination is that it allows an annual health check – physical examination is particularly important in picking up the early signs of heart, dental and adrenal disease. Particular attention can be paid to body condition as obesity is an increasing problem in pet animals. Inexperienced clinicians should always be aware that ferret weights fluctuate markedly (by up to 30%) between seasons. Therefore, significant weight loss in spring or significant weight gain in autumn is not necessarily pathological. Dental checks are also important as dental disease is seen increasingly regularly (see Chapter 19, **Fig. 9.4**).

For the majority of pet ferrets an annual health check may be sufficient. However, where the animal is suffering from chronic disease, e.g. cardiac disease or arthritis, more frequent checks may be necessary.

For animals with chronic disease and long-term medication it is clear that periodic haematology and serum biochemistry checks can be of great value. For more healthy animals the benefits of such tests may be more debatable, especially for animals that may be more difficult to handle or have very thick skin on the neck (common in the UK) that may require anaesthesia for venipuncture.

The value of regular infectious disease screening is also debatable. Some ferret clubs still insist

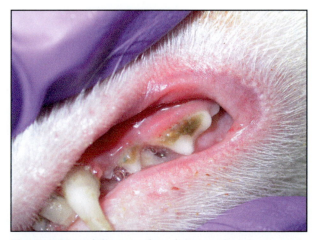

Fig. 9.4 Dental disease often diagnosed at the annual examination.

on annual blood or saliva testing of ferrets for Aleutian disease virus (ADV) antibodies (see Chapter 16).

Blood testing relies on the countercurrent electrophoresis test, which is quite insensitive and results in many false negatives so is not ideal as a screening test. The small volume of blood is traditionally taken by means of a toenail clip although this is deemed by the National Ferret Welfare Society to cause excessive pain. It is preferable to do a blood draw from the cephalic, cranial vena cava or jugular vein, but in some cases this may require sedation (see Chapter 10).

Saliva testing appears a more acceptable alternative but is very hard to perform without the ferret swallowing the swab. It does not seem to be much more sensitive than blood testing and has the similar disadvantage of being an antibody, rather than antigen, test.

It is clear in the UK that disease due to ADV is unusual in ferrets and the screening tests are not sensitive and may cause harm. Therefore many clubs are now abandoning their compulsory testing policies.

In the authors' experience this has not resulted in any increase in disease due to ADV and has had the added advantage that ferreters at shows have become more vigorous in their approach to biosecurity, thus reducing the chances of contracting more common diseases (e.g. coronavirus).

PET PASSPORTS (EUROPE)

Like cats and dogs, ferrets can be transported freely between European Union (EU) countries provided the owners have a Pet Passport for each animal.

The requirements for a ferret to travel under a Pet Passport are that:

- It is permanently identified by means of a microchip implanted subcutaneously between the shoulder blades.
- It is vaccinated against rabies.
- It cannot travel for 21 days from the date of first vaccination (or after a 'restarted' vaccine course if more than 1 year has passed between vaccinations).

- If entering the UK from an EU country, blood testing to check rabies antibody titres is not necessary. However, if entering from a non-EU country, an antibody titre must be established from a blood sample taken not less than 30 days postvaccination and submitted to an EU-approved laboratory.
- As from December 2014, antitapeworm treatment is not required for ferrets entering the UK.

Requirements do change from time to time so veterinarians licensed to issue or authorise Pet Passports are strongly advised to keep up to date with current requirements. In the UK, this can be checked on the Animal and Plant Health Agency website.

For other ferret exports or imports between countries not recognising the Pet Passport scheme, advice should be sought from the relevant animal health agency in each case prior to travel.

PARASITE CONTROL

Advice on parasite control is frequently sought, partly because some parasites (especially external parasites) are common in ferrets and partly because owners are particularly engaged with such prophylaxis, especially if they already own dogs or cats.

Internal

Endoparasitism is unusual in ferrets. The short small intestine with its extremely rapid transit time is not conducive to parasite colonisation. However, canine roundworm have been reported in ferrets, so where ferrets are kept in close proximity to dogs they should be included in roundworm control regimes. If ferrets are handled regularly there may be risks of larval disease from *Toxocara canis* infection, so regular deworming with fenbendazole, piperazine or imidacloprid-moxidectin (Advocate™, UK Bayer, Newbury UK; Advantage Multi™, BayerDVM; www.bayerdvm.com) is recommended. The latter is preferred as it is simple to use, licensed for ferrets in the UK and is also useful for flea control (see below). In the USA, products used in kittens such as selamectin (Revolution™, Florham Park, NJ, USA) have been used with good effect.

Otherwise, routine deworming is rarely needed and if concerned faecal checks should be performed rather than routine anthelmintic therapy.

Protozoal parasites may be of some significance with coccidia (**Fig. 9.5**) being a cause of enteritis in young animals and *Giardia* and cryptosporidiosis being reported occasionally in animals of any age. However, prophylactic therapy is not indicated unless:

- There is a disease outbreak and there is treatment of in-contacts.
- A breeder has a history of persistent problems in young ferrets.

Heartworm

Depending on location, ferrets may be exposed to heartworm. In endemic areas, ferrets can be tested using the canine test assays. Treatment is reviewed in Chapter 12. In the UK this may be of relevance for imported ferrets and it is advised that they are tested postimport if coming from endemic regions.

External

Ectoparasites are common in ferrets.

Flea infestation can be a major problem and the cat flea is commonly found on ferrets. All cats, dogs and ferrets in a household should be on a prophylactic programme. Advocate™ (imidacloprid & moxidectin, Bayer) is licensed in the UK for ferrets and can be applied monthly as a spot-on product. The same product is available in the USA as Advantage Multi™ for cats, and has been effective in ferrets using the kitten dosage. It is an extra-label usage however. This product is also efficacious in treating ear mites.

Generally outdoor ferrets rarely require prophylactic flea control, unless a flea infestation has become established in outdoor runs, hutches or courts and (as in dogs and cats) a combined on-ferret and environmental control is required. Where environmental control is required in outdoor ferret housing, Indorex™ (pyriproxifen-pyrimethamine, Virbac, Bury St Edmunds, UK) is effective outdoors following a full environmental cleaning with all bedding, flooring, substrate and furnishings removed and/or sprayed with an insecticide. The habitat should be thoroughly dry and aired prior to reintroduction of the ferret.

Ear mites (*Otodecteis cynotis*) (see Chapter 15) are frequently found in ferrets. These do not seem to cause pruritis, but do contribute to excessive wax build-up and in some cases otitis externa, media and/or interna. Screening can be by direct visual examination of the ear with an otoscope, or microscopically from a swab of the ear wax (**Fig. 9.6**).

Ticks are also a problem in ferrets in endemic locales. Adult ticks may be removed with hooks as in dogs and cats. Where these are a continuing problem

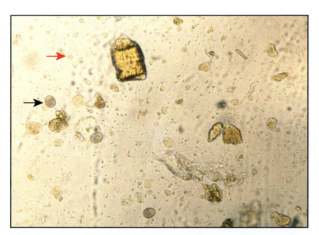

Fig. 9.5 Coccidia and cryptosporidia in a ferret with diarrhoea. Red arrow, cryptosporidia, black arrow, coccidian oocyte.

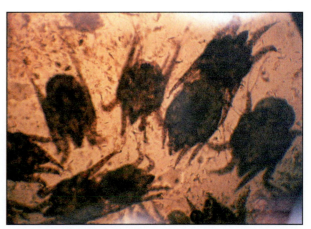

Fig. 9.6 Ear mites taken from an aural swab.

(especially with juvenile seed ticks) environmental control may also be required – again, pyriproxifen-pyrimethamine appears effective in the outdoor enclosure especially following a thorough environmental change.

Fipronil spray (Frontline™, Merial, Duluth, GA) may be used for on-ferret control of ticks – both as treatment and for limited prophylaxis (for prophylaxis, this should be applied weekly to affected areas, especially the ears and extremities). Cotton buds can be used to apply the spray to the ears and around the face.

Care must be taken when using the spray that the ferret is kept warm (but not near a naked flame) to avoid hypothermia from cooling effects of the alcohol-based spray, and that the ferret is not placed in an enclosed area until after the spray has dried in order to avoid intoxication from the alcohol vapour.

Sarcoptid mange (see Chapter 21) may also be found in ferrets but does not generally require prophylactic therapy.

BIOSECURITY

Another mainstay of disease prevention in any collection of animals is a biosecurity policy. This should apply to both new animals entering the group and to animals entering from shows. This should involve:

- Quarantine.
- Cleaning and disinfection.
- Where appropriate, disease screening, e.g. faecal screens for parasites or coronavirus.

The length of quarantine and the scale of precautions taken will depend upon:

- Age, number and type of ferret (e.g. pet, working, show).
- Likely disease risk.
- Type of disease risk.
- Source of animal.
- Health status of other ferrets.

In all cases it is important for keepers to request appropriate veterinary advice before importing or moving ferrets into their group. It is also important that ferret shows should also have a non-mixing policy and a biosecurity plan for likely infectious diseases. In the UK, the most important of these currently is coronavirus. The following is advice to those running a ferret show:

- Do not accept any ferret that is looking ill or has been ill (especially diarrhoea) in the week leading up to the show. It is worth asking owners to declare they have no ferrets with diarrhoea in the week prior to the show.
- All handlers should wash and use hand steriliser between ferrets. Tables must be washed down between each ferret and all faeces cleaned away as soon as possible.
- Ferrets from different owners should not be mixed and cages not put immediately next to each other. If in doubt it is worth requesting ferrets are kept in owners' vehicles when they are not being judged.
- Owners should be instructed not to handle each other's ferrets, and to wash/sterilise hands after handling theirs (see above – don't forget spread of virus via door handles and other fomites).
- Do not transfer bowls, equipment, etc. between owners.
- Owners should be instructed to keep ferrets coming to the show separate from their other ferrets for at least 7 days after returning. That way any problems should be limited to just those ferrets at the show. This is home quarantining and may be very difficult to do as it is usually not possible to separate out a room to have its own ventilation.

FERRET HOME HEALTH KIT

It is a good idea to have a home care kit assembled that is ferret specific. The items are listed in *Box 9.1*.

Box 9.1 **Ferret home health kit (Figs 9.7, 9.8)**

- Famotidine 10 mg tablets (generic, many brands).
- Pill cutter.
- Bismuth subsalycilate liquid (cherry flavour is favoured) (generic, many brands). (Tablets can also be used, but will need to be cut into eighths).
- Diphenhydramine oral solution (usually a children's strength, generic brands).
- Various sizes of syringes for oral administration of medications.
- Nail clippers.
- Cotton buds.
- Ear cleaner (see Box 15.1).
- Nutri-Cal® (Vetoquinol Care, Princeville, Quebec, Canada) or equivalent.
- Laxative (labelled for cats or for ferrets, several brands).
- Enzymatic toothpaste (such as C.E.T. Enzymatic Toothpaste, Virbac, Saint Lazare, Quebec, Canada) or equivalent.
- Haemostats or tweezers.
- Scissors.
- Brush (usually a cat brush).
- Ingredients for dook soup (Appendix 6) and a copy of the recipe.
- Carnivore Care (Oxbow Enterprises Inc., Murdock, NE) or equivalent.
- Chicken baby food.
- Veterinary clinic phone number and address.

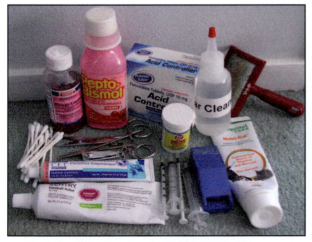

Fig. 9.7 Essentials of a home care kit.

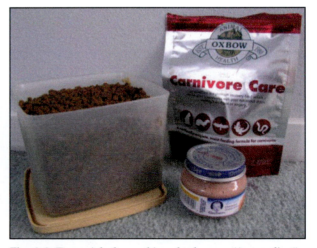

Fig. 9.8 Essentials for making dook soup (Appendix 6). This includes pulverised regular diet, baby food and a nutritional supplement designed for liquid feeding such as Carnivore Care® (Oxbow Animal Health, Murdock, NE).

CHAPTER 10

CLINICAL TECHNIQUES

John R. Chitty

INTRODUCTION

Without ignoring the importance of the clinical examination and history-taking (see Chapters 7, 8), it is fair to say that achieving diagnosis is unlikely without the performing of diagnostic tests. Similarly, proper dosing technique is required to medicate the ferret. This chapter will give a basic guide to diagnostic and therapeutic techniques in the ferret.

INJECTION TECHNIQUES

Subcutaneous

This route is suitable for most drugs and also fluid therapy (see Chapter 11). The usual site for subcutaneous injection of drugs is the scruff, between the shoulder blades. The ferret should be scruffed and the 'scruffing' hand used to tent up the skin – the needle is inserted caudal to this (**Fig. 10.1**).

The ferret may be more easily restrained if held up so it dangles (see Chapter 8). If an irritant injection is to be given, the ferret can be given some nutrient gel to distract it (**Fig. 10.2**).

Microchips should be inserted subcutaneously between the shoulder blades – a bleb of tissue glue or a single suture (in anaesthetised ferrets) may be used to close the insertion hole. One potential problem postmicrochipping is the grooming out of the microchip after implantation. Some clinicians like to manipulate the microchip away from the implantation site. However, care should be taken not to overmanipulate or there will be breakdown of the adhesions required to prevent microchip migration.

This is also the correct site and technique for hormone implant placement (**Fig. 10.3**).

Fluids may also be placed over the lateral abdomen. Although this is a more painful injection site,

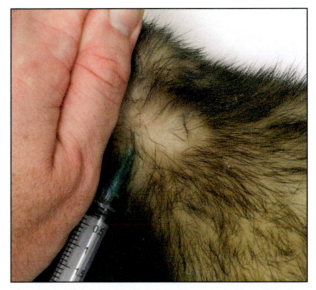

Fig. 10.1 The 'scruffed' ferret demonstrating the site for subcutaneous injections.

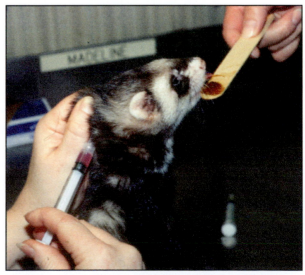

Fig. 10.2 The 'scruffed' ferret receiving a treat to distract it. This ferret is receiving a vaccination.

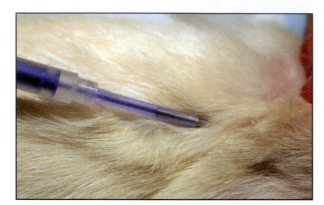

Fig. 10.3 Site and technique for hormone implant placement.

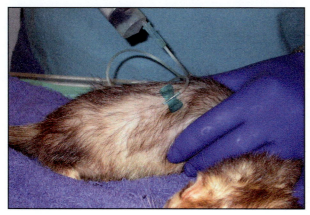

Fig. 10.4 Fluids can be given in the flank area as skin is loose and allows for large volumes.

there is more loose skin for larger volumes of fluid (**Fig. 10.4**).

Intramuscular

Few drugs (other than sedatives) need to be given intramuscularly, which is opportune as the muscle masses are relatively small in ferrets meaning that large volumes should not be given into them. Intramuscular injections frequently cause pain so the ferret should be well restrained with the hindlimbs held as well as the forequarters. Nutrient jelly should be given to distract the ferret.

Two muscle groups are suitable:

- Cranial thigh (avoid caudal thigh as there is a risk of irritant injections causing a neuropathy due to interaction with the sciatic nerve). However, muscle groups are very small and there

is a high risk of lameness following injection (**Fig. 10.5**).

- Epaxial muscles. Either the lumbar group (for very small volumes of 0.25 mL or less) or the cervical group in entire hobs that have larger muscle masses in this region. The lumbar spine may be grasped, the muscle mass palpated and the needle inserted such that it just enters the muscle mass (**Fig. 10.6**). In either site there is a risk of injection into fat deposits resulting in slow absorption. If injecting into the epaxial muscles, the ferret must be very well restrained. The intervertebral spaces are wide and there is a genuine risk of inadvertent injection into the spinal canal in a struggling ferret. Use of a short (5/8″) needle will reduce the chances of this occurring.

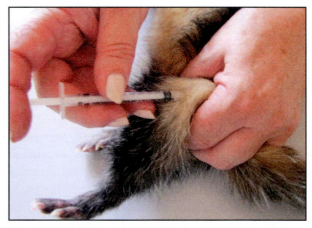

Fig. 10.5 Cranial thigh intramuscular injection site. Hold the femur, pressing the muscle onto the cranial surface of the thigh.

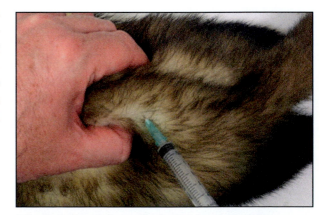

Fig. 10.6 Epaxial muscle site for intramuscular injection.

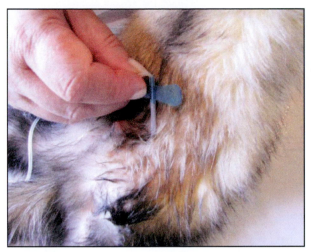

Fig. 10.7 **Intraperitoneal injection site. The skin is prepared with alcohol or surgical scrub. For abdominalcentesis, the fur should be clipped. The sheath on this needle was left on for demonstration purposes.**

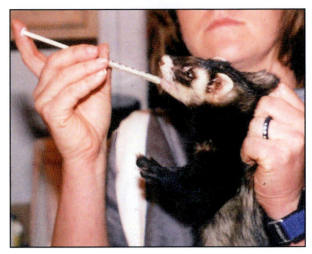

Fig. 10.8 **Liquid drugs given by syringe directly into the back of the mouth.**

Intraperitoneal

Suitable for fluids (emergency care, see Chapter 11) or for concentrated dextrose injections. The ferret is held vertically and the skin at the injection site prepared aseptically. The needle (typically 23G 1-1.5″) is inserted into the caudo-lateral abdomen at a 45° angle – the easiest route to follow is along the hindlimbs in the 'dangling' ferret; this allows entry via the inguinal canal.

After needle insertion negative pressure should be applied and any fluid noted. If fluid is aspirated, the needle should be withdrawn and the other side used instead (**Fig. 10.7**).

ORAL DOSING TECHNIQUES

For continued medication by the owner, the majority of drugs will need to be given orally. There are a number of techniques available.

Liquid drugs

These may be given by syringe directly into the back of the mouth (**Fig. 10.8**). Alternatively, the drug (if low volume) may be mixed with meat pastes or gels and taken freely or smeared around the mouth. Drugs should not be mixed with main feeds.

Tablets

These may be:

- Crushed in a small volume of water or pharmaceutical flavoured syrup such as Syrpalta™ (Humco, Texarcana, TX), syrups used to flavour coffee, or commercially available syrups (Flavorx™, Columbia, MD, USA) and given as above. This is considered veterinary compounding in the USA and comes under federal Food and Drug Administration regulation as listed in *Box 10.1*. Additionally powder can be mixed with a nutrient gel and given off a spoon. Be careful when doing this with sugar-coated tablets as it may affect absorption or cause hypersalivation if extremely bitter or irritating.
- Given directly (useful for sugar-coated medications) using a pill giver designed for cats.
- When feeding nutrient gel directly from the tube, the tablet may be placed on the nozzle of the tube and the ferret will often inadvertently take this.

Whichever method is used the ferret should always receive its favourite treat immediately afterwards – positive reinforcement is vital especially for long-term medication, or patient resistance and owner compliance will worsen.

VENIPUNCTURE

Blood sampling is an extremely useful tool in ferret medicine. However, they can be very hard to bleed even though they have a number of accessible veins. The main problems are restraint and skin thickness. Ferrets, especially intact males and working ferrets, have very thick skin around the neck and shoulder area and this can make jugular and cranial vena cava (CVC) venipuncture difficult, even when the ferret is anaesthetised. The thick skin causes the needle to 'blunt' as it passes the skin, making entry to the vein more difficult.

To reduce this problem narrow gauge needles should be used. The author will generally use 23G or 25G needles (if difficulties are encountered, always change to a narrower gauge needle). In extreme cases, jugular cutdown techniques may be utilised. In the USA, CVC is routinely used as being safe and easy. Neutered ferrets do not have as thick a skin and even when bulked up in winter, rarely is it a problem. A 22 gauge ¾ inch needle is adequate for most ferrets.

Restraint

The ferret can be restrained by the scruff and if held vertically may often relax (see Chapter 8). Distracting the ferret with treats may assist. However, in most cases, unless extremely debilitated, some anaesthesia or sedation is required when taking blood samples. As radiographs are often needed when investigating a sick ferret (see below), it is often appropriate to do all testing together. If using gaseous anaesthesia, hypotension can be an issue in making venipuncture more difficult – this can be partly reduced by taking the samples as early as possible after induction or by using midazolam and/or buprenorphine as a premedicant to reduce the isoflurane dosage.

Samples

As with most species, it is possible to collect up to 2% bodyweight as sample – i.e. for a healthy 1 kg ferret, up to 20 mL blood may be withdrawn (obviously, unhealthy animals can only tolerate smaller volumes of blood being taken). Most commercial laboratories can perform a comprehensive profile on 1–2 mL blood. However, larger volumes may be required for more specialised tests (e.g. hormone panels or serology) or for transfusion.

Blood should be taken into:

- Ethylenediamine tetraacetic acid (EDTA) – haematology.
- Heparin – biochemistry (note, if electrolytes are not being measured patient-side, heparin gel tubes should be used and the tubes spun as soon as possible).
- Serum – biochemistry, serology, hormone panels.
- Fluoride-oxalate – glucose.

- Air-dried smears – two smears should always be made from blood that has not been in contact with anticoagulant. This means that cytology can be evaluated without any potential cytological changes due to EDTA or heparin.

If in doubt it is worth asking your lab before sampling; anticoagulants can have effects on various parameters (a good example of this is insulin) and different laboratories may utilise different analysers and/or methodologies. Better results will be obtained if using the method of their choice.

Sites

Previously, claw trims have been used for collecting small volumes of blood, e.g. for Aleutian disease (AD) serology. However, this does cause pain and serial sampling of a claw will induce claw dystrophy. It is therefore no longer recommended.

For serial glucose sampling, skin pricks can be used. However, the author has found the pinnae to be poor for this (unlike cats and dogs) and prefers to use a foot pad.

For larger diagnostic samples, the following sites may be used:

Jugular vein

Ferrets have a well-developed jugular vein on both sides of the neck. While this is an excellent vein for sampling, problems with neck skin thickness and restraint mean that this vein can be quite difficult to enter even when the animal is anaesthetised. However, it is still first choice vein for sampling.

- The ferret is restrained or sedated/anaesthetised.
- The side of the neck over the vein is clipped and prepared aseptically (usually the right side, but either jugular can be used).
- The head is extended and flexed slightly away from the phlebotomist (**Fig. 10.9**).
- A 5/8″ 23G or 25G needle is used with a 2–5 mL syringe.
- The vein is then entered in similar manner to jugular venipuncture in a dog or cat (**Fig. 10.10**). After withdrawing the needle, digital pressure is applied to the site for a minute or two.

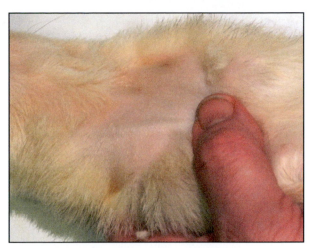

Fig. 10.9 **For jugular blood draw, the head is extended and flexed slightly away from the phlebotomist.**

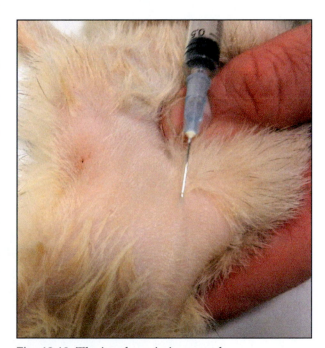

Fig. 10.10 **The jugular vein is entered.**

Cranial vena cava (CVC)

This is the author's preferred vein in the anaesthetised/sedated animal as skin thickness appears less of a problem when using the CVC. However, this vein should only be used in the anaesthetised/sedated or debilitated patient as the positioning may be distressing and struggling may cause laceration of the vein. It is also difficult to apply pressure on the venipuncture site after sampling, which can be a problem for animals with a coagulopathy. The anatomy of the site is presented in **Figs 10.11** and **10.12**.

- The ferret is laid in dorsal recumbency with the head hanging over the edge of the table allowing access to the thoracic inlet (**Fig. 10.13**).
- Either side of the thoracic inlet is clipped and prepared aseptically.

- A 2–5 mL syringe with a 23 gauge 1″ needle is used.
- The needle is inserted either side of the thoracic inlet and the 'notch' between 1st rib and manubrium. This is inserted at a 45° angle aimed towards the opposite (right) hindleg (**Fig. 10.14**).

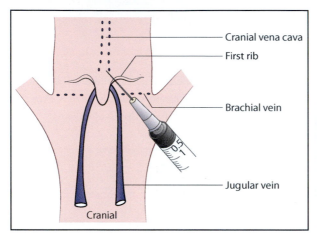

Fig. 10.11 CVC site diagram.

Cranial vena cava
First rib
Brachial vein
Jugular vein
Cranial

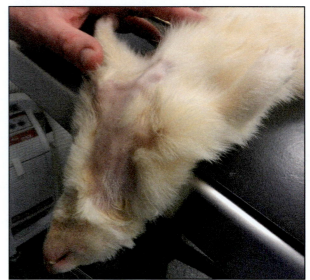

Fig. 10.13 The ferret is laid in dorsal recumbency with the head lowered over the edge of the table allowing access to the thoracic inlet.

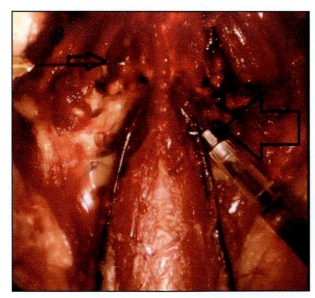

Fig. 10.12 The dissected anatomy for the CVC site. Small arrow is the first rib, large arrow is the site of entry.

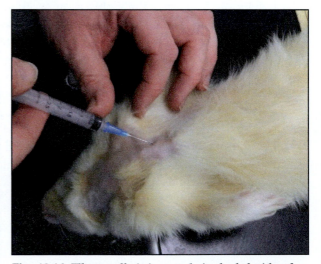

Fig. 10.14 The needle is inserted via the left side of the thoracic inlet at the notch between the first rib and manubrium at a 45° angle aimed towards the opposite hindleg.

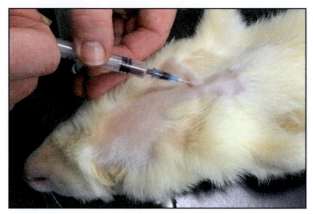

Fig. 10.15 **As soon as the skin is penetrated, negative pressure is applied to the syringe and the needle is slowly advanced until blood is withdrawn.**

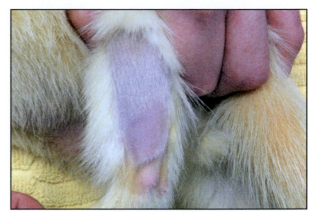

Fig. 10.16 **The lateral saphenous vein raised for venipuncture.**

- As soon as the skin is penetrated, negative pressure is applied to the syringe and the needle is slowly advanced until blood is withdrawn (**Fig. 10.15**).
- As soon as the needle is withdrawn, pressure is applied to the venipuncture site for 1–2 minutes.

Lateral saphenous vein

This is a smaller vein that can be used for collection of smaller blood volumes. It is easier to access in the conscious ferret than the other veins.

- The lateral hind limb is clipped between stifle and hock.
- It is prepared aseptically.
- The vein is raised by an assistant gripping around the stifle (**Fig. 10.16**).
- A 1 mL syringe and 25G 5/8″ needle are used.
- After withdrawal of the needle, pressure needs to be applied to the site for several minutes as large haematomas may form.

Cephalic vein

This may be accessed in the conscious ferret but is probably easier in the sedated animal. It is only suitable for withdrawal of small volumes of blood, but is useful for catheter insertion (see later).

- The vein is clipped and prepared aseptically.
- The vein is raised by an assistant gripping (or application of a tourniquet) around the elbow (**Fig. 10.17**).

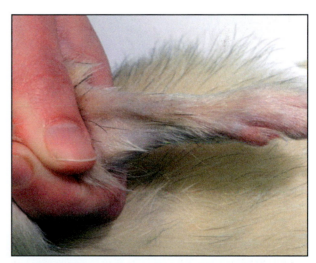

Fig. 10.17 **The cephalic vein raised for venipuncture.**

- A 1 mL syringe and 25G 5/8″ needle are used.
- After withdrawal of the needle, pressure needs to be applied to the site for several minutes.

Tail vein

The ventral tail vein may be used for small volumes. It can be accessed in the conscious ferret, usually being provided a treat during the procedure.

- The ventral surface of the tail is clipped 3–6 cm from the anus and prepared aseptically.
- The vein is raised by digital pressure just caudal of the anus.

- A 1 mL syringe and 25G 5/8″ needle are used.
- The needle is inserted approximately 3 cm and on the midline, and at an approximately 30–45° angle. The needle may prick the bone, then withdraw slightly to get blood flow (**Fig. 10.18**).

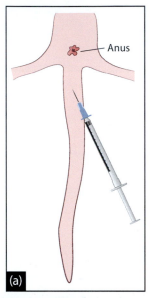

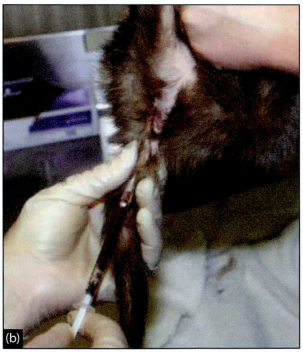

Fig. 10.18 (a) Diagram of tail vein venipuncture; (b) demonstration of blood collection from the tail vein.

INTRAVENOUS CATHETERISATION

Intravenous catheters may be placed in the cephalic veins (or the lateral saphenous, though it is harder to maintain catheter patency in this vein). Catheterisation is useful for both fluid therapy and intravenous drug therapy, especially chemotherapy.

Sedation greatly facilitates placement, although debilitated or very tractable animals may be catheterised conscious.

The technique is essentially that used in cats (and as described for venipuncture, above). A 24G catheter is normally used – over-the-needle catheters being easiest to place. In very dehydrated and/or thick-skinned animals, a cutdown technique may be used using a hypodermic needle or No15 scalpel blade to make a small incision in the skin.

Once placed, the catheter should be plugged and taped in place (**Fig. 10.19**). Use of a T-connector greatly facilitates needle-free repeat dosing via the catheter.

Intravenous catheters should be well protected as ferrets are very good at removing them.

INTRAOSSEOUS CATHETERISATION

Intraosseous catheters (typically 1–1.5″ 21–18G hypodermic needles or spinal needles, depending on size of ferret) can be inserted into the proximal femur.

The ferret is anaesthetised or sedated. Alternatively, in debilitated animals, a bleb of local

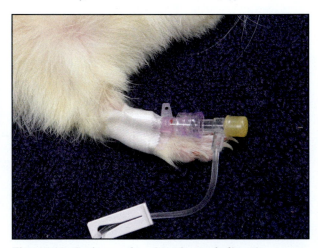

Fig. 10.19 Catheter placed in the cephalic vein.

anaesthetic may be injected at the insertion site. The skin is clipped and prepared aseptically. The femur is grasped and the space between the joint and the greater trochanter is located.

The needle is inserted through the skin and the bone penetrated at this site (**Fig. 10.20**). A drilling action may be required to assist piercing of the bone cortex. The needle can usually be 'felt' within the bone medulla. However, a small amount of saline may be injected and the leg checked for swelling. If the needle has blocked on entry, it should be removed and replaced with another of the same size.

If in doubt, placement can be checked using radiography.

A syringe pump or Springfusor™ spring-loaded syringe infuser (Admedus, Malaga, Western Australia) is essential whether using this route for fluids or for chemotherapy.

The advantages of this route over the intravenous route is that the needles are faster to place and easier to maintain. The needle is normally welltolerated (especially if local anaesthesia has been used).

BLOOD TRANSFUSION

A donor ferret is needed along with a standard blood transfusion set that has a filter in it. The recipient ferret should be catheterised as described above. Depending on the size of recipient, the decision to use 20–40 mL volume should be decided. The recipient ferret may be sedated or anaesthetised depending on physical condition. If a cephalic or intraosseous catheter is already in place, sedation is not necessary. The donor ferret should be anaesthetised and have either the jugular or the CVC site aseptically prepared. The blood is withdrawn into the blood transfusion collection syringe (that contains an anticoagulant). Once the blood is in the transfusion kit, it is administered slowly, either manually or using a syringe pump, into the recipient via a catheter. In emergencies, it can be transfused directly into an anaesthetised recipient via the jugular or CVC (**Fig. 10.21**).

SALIVA COLLECTION

This is used in ADV testing where ELISA antibody testing for saliva has been developed. It appears to

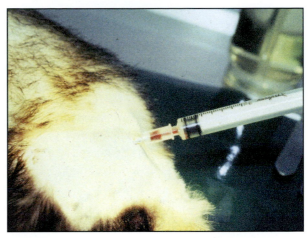

Fig. 10.20 Site for intraosseous catheterisation of the femur. The needle is directed into the space between the joint and the greater trochanter. The needle penetrates the bone at this site into the femur medulla. This is identical to the location used for bone marrow aspiration.

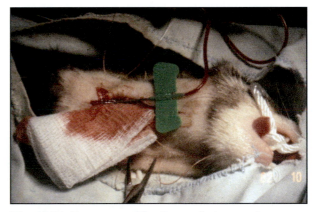

Fig. 10.21 Emergency blood transfusion can be done injecting the blood into the jugular vein using a butterfly catheter.

be less invasive than blood testing. However, the test available in the UK recommends insertion of a swab into the mouth for 60 seconds. This means there is a high risk of foreign body ingestion – the ferrets normally resent the process and restraint is not easy. In a small study by this author, saliva testing appeared less sensitive than serology, presumably due to difficulties in sampling.

Anaesthesia or sedation may be utilised, but will usually result in reduced saliva production.

IMAGING

For many investigations, imaging is essential. In practice radiography and ultrasonography are routinely used although advanced imaging techniques such as computed tomography (CT) or magnetic resonance imaging (MRI) are increasingly indicated. Normal anatomy must be known and understood before imaging, and various texts are recommended to assist with this (see Further Reading).

Ultrasound

Ultrasonography is indicated for imaging of soft tissues where there is no air present. It is particularly useful in the presence of ascites and when investigating abdominal organomegalies, and is essential in cardiac investigations (**Fig. 10.22**).

The following equipment requirements are needed for ferret ultrasonography:

- Small footplate.
- 7.5–12.5 MHz.
- Rapid image turnover.

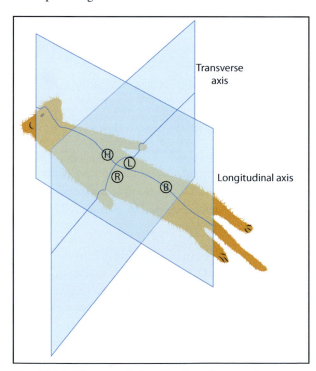

Fig. 10.22 Planes and visualisation diagram for ultrasonography. Key: H, heart; R, right kidney; L, left kidney; B, bladder.

- Colour Doppler and M-mode needed for cardiology investigations (colour Doppler is also useful when imaging adrenals as the vena cava may be located and the adrenal glands found near or on this).

Positioning is as dictated by the views required.

While sedation makes the process much easier, it is possible to scan conscious ferrets especially if they are tractable (**Fig. 10.23**). However, if guided biopsy is required then sedation will be needed.

For abdominal ultrasound, the author will generally restrain ferrets in the vertical position, clipping the ventral abdomen before application of spirit and ultrasound gel.

For cardiac ultrasound, imaging may be performed in dorsal recumbency, with direct placement of the probe over the heart from either the ventral or lateral positioning. Typically the left side is prepared and the ferret placed in left lateral recumbency such that the probe may be placed from the ventral approach. Cutaway ultrasound tables used for small animal ultrasound are very useful. Both long and short axis views should be obtained.

Radiography

Radiography is a key diagnostic tool in almost all disease investigations. The advent of digital radiography has made imaging much simpler in that the basic 'ferretogram' can be utilised for assessment of all regions rather than needing different settings for thorax,

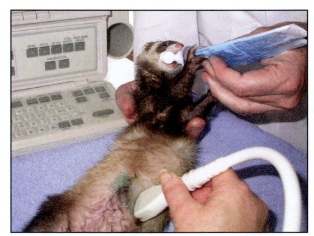

Fig. 10.23 Ultrasonography can usually be done in the conscious ferret while providing a treat.

abdomen, etc. Settings should always be guided by those recommended firstly for that machine and secondly by clinical experience within that clinic.

The two basic body views are:

- Dorsoventral. The ferret is placed in ventral recumbency and the guideline aligned with the spine. The legs are positioned symmetrically on either side (**Fig. 10.24**). Alternatively, ventrodorsal can be utilised.
- Lateral. The forelimbs are extended cranially, and the hind limbs extended caudally. Foam should be placed under the ventral thorax and between the limbs (left and right) to reduce rotation (**Fig. 10.25**).

Specific views will be required for orthopaedic issues with the limbs and in neurological investigations of the spine.

Contrast techniques may also be used in ferrets:

- Barium – gastro-intestinal disease. Generally given by stomach tube at 2–5 mL/kg, but may also be given as a swallow when investigating oesophageal disease.

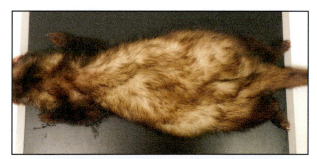

Fig. 10.24 Dorsoventral positioning on an X-ray plate.

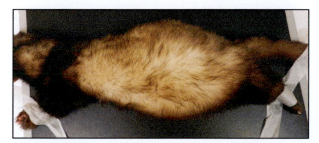

Fig. 10.25 Lateral positioning on an X-ray plate.

- Angiography – imaging of heart, blood vessels and kidneys.
- Contrast cystography – positive, negative and double techniques may be used in investigating bladder disease.
- Positive contrast canalography in investigation of aural disease
- Water-soluble iodine may be injected into sinus tracts to ascertain their path prior to surgery.
- Contrast myelography using an iodine based agent introduced usually in the ventral subarachnoid space at the most caudal lumbar vertebra. The ferret should be fully anaesthetised and intubated, and methylprednisolone sodium succinate at 30 mg/kg by slow IV infusion may be administered prior to the injection of the contrast agent to prevent an anaphylactic reaction. As with other species, it may be advised to have anticonvulsive drugs on hand to use if indicated.

Routes, techniques and dose rates are as used in feline radiography.

Dental radiography units do have uses in ferret radiography in investigation of dental disease and also in imaging the extremities. Advances in digital technology mean these images are much better quality and more diagnostic than previously obtained.

Endoscopy
Endoscopy is probably under-utilised in ferret medicine, but does have a range of uses.

Rigid endoscopy
- Ears (see below) – 4 mm otoendoscope or 2.7 mm endoscope.
- Nose – investigation of nasal discharge; 1.2 mm needlescope.
- Pharynx and larynx – investigation of swellings, cough and swallowing disorders; 2.7–4 mm endoscope.
- Trachea – investigation of cough; 2.7 mm endoscope.
- Oesophagus – investigation of regurgitation; 4 mm endoscope.

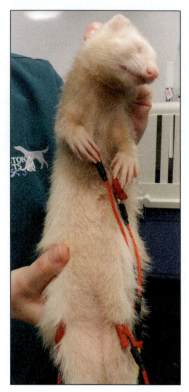

Fig. 10.26 Positioning of leads for ECG.

Flexible endoscopy

- Bronchoscopy – investigation of cough, possible foreign body, obtaining lung samples; 2 mm endoscope.
- Gastroscopy – investigation of vomition, foreign body retrieval, biopsy; 4 mm endoscope.

In general, endoscopy will require anaesthesia. Video-endoscopy is of great help as it provides better image quality and magnification.

Use of appropriate biopsy grabs enables samples to be obtained and foreign bodies to be grasped and removed.

Electrocardiography (ECG) (see Chapter 12)

With cardiac disease being relatively common, ECG is a useful technique as it is non-invasive, does not require sedation (this is contraindicated), and provides the following information:

- Heart rate.
- Heart rhythm.

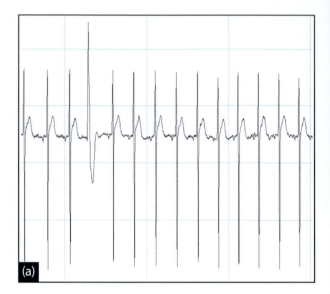

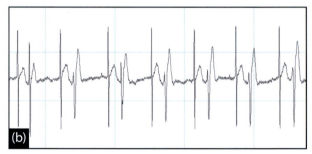

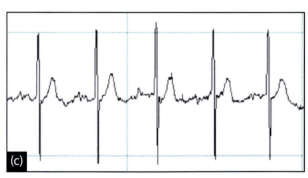

Fig. 10.27 Examples of ferret ECGs (vertical line = 1 mV; horizontal line = 1 s). (a) Single ventricular premature complex. Large complexes with deep S waves and S-T slurring indicative of cardiomegaly (lead II); (b) ventricular bigeminy in a case of cardiomyopathy (lead II); (c) normal lead II ECG in a manually restrained ferret. (Normal values may be found in Malakoff *et al.* [2012] and Bublot *et al.* [2006]).

- Heart size – though it should be noted that this is by inference and is not as accurate as radiography or ultrasonography. However, if the ferret is ECGed in the same position each time it does give a good measure of *changes* in heart shape.

The author will usually perform an ECG with the ferret held in the typical vertical dangling position (**Fig. 10.26**). The ferret may be fed nutrient gel during the procedure. The procedure is facilitated by use of:

- Atraumatic clips or pads (though the author has found the latter to give very poor connection in ferrets).
- Application of alcohol via swab rather than spray or bottle. This should be applied prior to applying clips as they usually resent the cold alcohol and will struggle, displacing the clips.
- Digital ECG. This allows more sensitive assessment and manipulation of ECG traces, which is vital in small animals with small complexes and rapid heart rates. It also enables measurement of the ECG in one 'run' over 20–30 seconds rather than a paper trace, which will require measurement of each lead in turn as well as a longer lead II rhythm strip.

Some examples of ferret ECGs are shown in **Fig. 10.27**.

BONE MARROW BIOPSY

Bone marrow biopsy is infrequently indicated other than where there is:

- Suspected bone marrow tumour, e.g. production of aberrant white cells in blood samples.
- Persistent non-regenerative anaemia.
- Splenomegaly to assess bone marrow haematopoiesis.

Bone marrow may be harvested via the proximal femur using the same approach as for intraosseous catheter placement (see above). It may also be harvested from the wing of the ilium and the head of the humerus. In older ferrets it is recommended to try more than one site as the femur marrow is often replaced by fat as the ferret ages.

Collection of bone marrow is painful and should always be done under anaesthesia.

- Essentially, the needle is placed in the femur.
- A 20 mL syringe is attached and negative pressure applied forcefully until a small amount of bloody fluid appears in the syringe. Air-dried smears (thick) should be made from this and the remainder placed in an EDTA blood tube and submitted for cytology.
- The needle is withdrawn and the skin closed with tissue glue. Analgesia should be given.

ABDOMINOCENTESIS

Indications
Abdominocentesis is indicated in cases where there is abdominal fluid (**Fig. 10.28**). This may be to take small volumes for analysis (some should be collected in EDTA; some in a standard clotted blood tube; and air-dried smears made) or to provide therapeutic drainage of fluid.

Procedure
- Fluid may be drawn using the site and technique as described above for intraperitoneal injection. This is usually performed in the conscious ferret and is normally well tolerated. Where providing therapeutic drainage, a larger (21G) needle should be used.

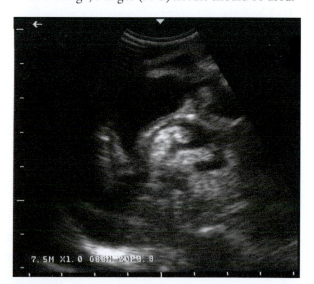

Fig. 10.28 **Ultrasonogram showing fluid within the abdomen.**

- In all cases the skin is prepared aseptically prior to insertion of a needle.
- Most dependent part of the abdomen. In some cases where large masses are present the fluid may be compartmentalised.
- If unsure of what may be within the abdomen and unwilling to risk blind injection/aspiration, the ferret may be sedated (to reduce chances of accidental injury through struggling) and ultrasound used to guide.

Catheters should not be used (especially over-the-stylet) as there is a risk of part of the catheter being severed and remaining within the abdomen should the animal struggle.

URINE COLLECTION

Urinary disease is common and urinalysis is an under-used tool in ferret medicine. While free catch may be suitable for some tests (for litter-trained ferrets, the kits available for urine collection from cats are appropriate), cystocentesis is often needed.

It should be remembered that the bladder may be fragile if overdistended. Nonetheless, very tractable or debilitated individuals may allow samples to be taken while conscious. Others should be anaesthetised or sedated.

- The ferret is restrained by scruff and hindlegs (extended caudally) on its side. The bladder is palpated and fixed in position.
- The ventral midline area over the bladder is aseptically prepared.
- A 23G 1.25″ needle is then inserted into the ventral midline and directed caudally into the bladder.
- Alternatively, ultrasound may be used so the process may be carried out under direct visualisation.

Urethral catheterisation

This is rarely used to collect urine, but is commonly required to relieve urethral obstruction (see Chapter 11).

In jills, endoscopic guidance is of great help in urethral guidance; however, this is rarely required.

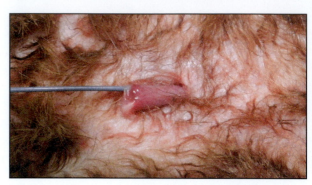

Fig. 10.29 **J-shaped os penis with urinary catheter placement. (Previously published in BSAVA Manual of Rodents and Ferrets.)**

In hobs the procedure is greatly hindered by the J-shaped end of the penis (**Fig. 10.29**).

Anaesthesia is essential to enable the penis to be exteriorised allowing access to the urethral opening. End-opening silicone catheters (e.g. Slippery Sam, Global Veterinary Products, Seaforth QLD, Australia) are ideal – the gauge should be dictated by the size of urethra with the widest gauge possible being used.

Expression of urine

This should not be attempted as a general means of obtaining a urine sample as there is a high chance of iatrogenic damage, especially in animals with a functioning bladder sphincter. However, for ferrets with spinal damage urine expression is often an essential part of their nursing when they cannot void urine voluntarily.

This is carried out in the same way as for cats, with the bladder located in the caudal abdomen and gently squeezed cranial to caudal. If the bladder is overdistended and urine is not readily voided, a small amount (5–10 mL) should be removed by cystocentesis prior to expression.

CEREBROSPINAL FLUID (CSF) COLLECTION

CSF collection is indicated in many neurological diseases. Where it is to be combined with myelography, the site for CSF collection/injection of contrast medium should be selected on the basis of the major area required for radiography (this is decided on the basis of presenting signs and a full neurological examination). Where CSF collection is the major interest, cisterna puncture allows easier collection of larger volumes of fluid.

Cisterna magna

The ferret is anaesthetised, placed in lateral recumbency and the head flexed at 90° to the neck (excessive flexion may increase intracranial pressure thus increasing the potential for cerebellar herniation). The fur is clipped on the dorsal head/neck and the site surgically prepared. With the head flexed, the needle (23G 1.25″) is inserted in the dorsal midline approximately midway between the external occipital protuberance and the craniodorsal tip of the dorsal spine of the C2 (axis) vertebra, just cranial to the cranial wings of the C1 (atlas) vertebra. Although a spinal needle may be used and reduces chances of extradural leakage, placement involves use of a stylet and repeated stabilisation and checking for CSF during placement. This author prefers use of a hypodermic needle due to the lack of space in a small species.

The needle is slowly introduced until the subarachnoid space is entered. This may be felt as a sudden loss of resistance or when CSF is seen within the hub of the needle. CSF may then be passively collected into tubes (plain and EDTA) and dropped onto a clean glass slide. Alternatively gentle aspiration using a 1 mL syringe may be used to collect a larger sample, but great care must be taken not to place excessive pressure and induce cerebellar herniation. No more than 0.25 mL CSF should be collected from an average-sized ferret and this should be collected over no less than 10 seconds.

Lumbar puncture

The ferret is anaesthetised and placed in ventral recumbency. The fur is clipped over an area cranial to the pelvis, which is prepared surgically. A 23G 1.25″ hypodermic needle is introduced almost perpendicular to the spine just cranial to the 6th lumbar vertebra (aiming for the L5–6 space). The needle is inserted slowly until CSF is seen in the hub – it will probably only be possible to collect a drop or two of fluid for cytology from this site. Negative pressure should not be used to aspirate CSF from this site.

BRONCHOALVEOLAR LAVAGE (BAL) (SEE CHAPTER 20)

This is another under-utilised tool, but is of immense value when investigating lower airway disease, especially where the changes are diffuse (focal lesions should be investigated and sampled using endoscopy; see above).

The ferret should be anaesthetised and intubated. It is placed in ventral recumbency (or where lesions are unilateral, placed in lateral recumbency with the affected side lowermost). A sterile 6 French gauge urinary catheter is premeasured and fed into the endotracheal tube (after removal of the anaesthetic circuit) to the level (approximately) of the division of the trachea.

Warmed sterile saline (5 mL/kg) is gently washed via the catheter several times. A very small cloudy sample should be obtained.

This should be submitted for cytology and culture.

EAR CLEANING

Ear cleaning is often required as aural disease is common in ferrets. Cleaning is useful for two reasons:

- As part of therapy – allowing better penetration of both topical and systemic therapies, and to provide symptomatic relief.
- To facilitate examination, especially where there is excess cerumen production and it is required to check for the presence of tumours and to assess the integrity of the tympanic membrane. Cerumen should also be checked for the presence of ear mites.

Cleaning is generally carried out under general anaesthesia (sedation is rarely adequate) and utilising either an auriscope with the smallest size examination cone, or endoscopy. The latter gives much better image quality and, when utilised with video capability, better magnification. In larger animals a 4 mm otoendoscope is ideal as these also have a channel for instruments. Otherwise, a standard 2.7 mm rigid endoscope may be used.

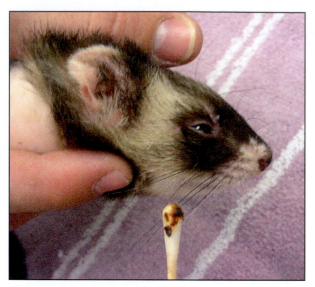

Fig. 10.30 **Excess cerumen can be removed from the external meatus for cytology.**

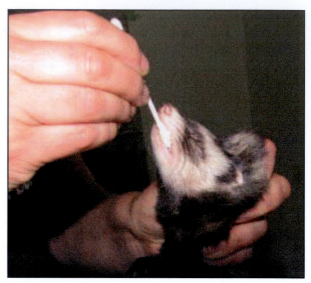

Fig. 10.31 **Using an enzymatic pet toothpaste on a cotton bud for brushing teeth.**

To clean, a Spreull needle (or small avian crop tube) is used. Saline is washed into the ear canals and then aspirated. Larger lumps of cerumen may be removed using endoscopic grabs. As the integrity of the tympanum is usually not known at this stage, agents that may be ototoxic should never be used.

Samples of cerumen should always be retained for cytology and bacteriology.

Once cleaned, the canal should be thoroughly checked endoscopically and any suspicious masses may be biopsied by means of fine-needle aspirate or pinch biopsy.

For longer-term therapy, owners may clean the ears on a regular basis. Squalene-based cleaners are generally well tolerated and less likely to cause ototoxicity. The cleaner is placed in the ear canal as per other species. The canal may then be gently massaged. The external auditory meatus and pinna are then cleaned using a cotton bud to remove excess cerumen (**Fig. 10.30**). The cotton bud should not be pushed into the ear canal as this will result in impaction of cerumen in the proximal part of the canal.

TEETH CLEANING (SEE CHAPTER 19)

Dental disease is common. Where this is diagnosed and treatment required, the ferret should be anaesthetised and intubated.

- The teeth and gingivae are thoroughly examined including the periodontal regions.
- Dental tartar may be removed using standard small animal ultrasonic scalers. After descaling, teeth should be polished using mechanical polishers with a prophy cup and paste.
- Dental disease can be prevented to some extent by regular toothbrushing/cleaning by the owner. Toothbrushes and toothpaste marketed for cats are suitable and the technique of brushing is similar. An enzymatic toothbrush on a cotton bud works well (**Fig. 10.31**). As with medicating (see above), positive reinforcement is essential in maintaining compliance in the long term.

This author has also used dental diets marketed for cats (e.g. Hill's Feline t/d) to successfully reduce recurrence of dental disease in ferrets, although nutritional adequacy over time on these diets is unknown.

NAIL TRIM

Nail trimming is a common request from pet owners. The ferret's feet are long as are the claws, which can affect handling, or can mean claws, getting caught in carpets/ furnishings (**Fig. 10.32**).

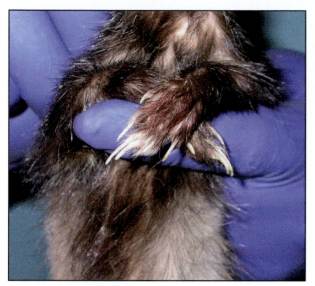

Fig. 10.32 **Overgrown toenails that can catch in fabric, carpet.**

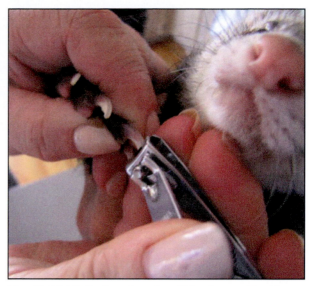

Fig. 10.33 **Nail trimming should be done with side-to-side clipping.**

Declawing is not an ethical procedure in the UK or the USA.

- Claws are simple to cut and any clippers suitable for cats may be utilised (**Fig. 10.33**).
- The claws are normally white so the quick is normally visible. The clippers should be applied 1–2 mm below the end of the visible quick and the nail squeezed side to side to minimise bleeding should the quick accidentally be cut.
- If cut, the quick may be cauterised using potassium permanganate, silver nitrate or a haemostatic powder.

(**Figs 10.2, 10.4, 10.5, 10.7, 10.8, 10.12, 10.18b, 10.20, 10.23, 10.27, 10.31–10.33** courtesy of Cathy Johnson-Delaney.)

CHAPTER 11

EMERGENCY CARE

*John R. Chitty and
Cathy A. Johnson-Delaney*

INTRODUCTION

Ferrets are frequently presented in a critical state. It is important in these cases to be as prepared as possible before the animal's arrival and to have sufficient facilities to accept the case. For non-specialised practices, an understanding is needed of how to stabilise a critical ferret and then where to refer to for further investigation, treatment and hospitalisation (**Fig. 11.1**).

TRIAGE

As ever, a key to successful emergency care is the initial triage. The word triage derives from the French 'trier' (to sort) and is the process whereby cases are prioritised according to their urgency – in other words, recognising an emergency is an emergency! Triage can be categorised into different phases:

1. The owner – recognising that their ferret is ill as early as possible. Ideally many emergencies can be prevented from reaching that stage simply by picking up early signs of disease. Good education of owners in recognising signs of illness as well as good ownership in terms of knowing their own pet are needed to achieve this. However, accidents, injuries and acute disease do occur and so emergencies will happen – again, good education is essential in teaching owners to recognise when they really need to call the vet.
2. Receptionists – this is the first point of contact for any owner. Failure to recognise an emergency case will result in a delay in that patient being seen and, at best, damage to the practice's credentials. At worst it may result in patient death while waiting for an appointment.

Reception training is essential so they can prioritise the urgency with which a patient is seen; for non-specialised practices assess whether the case should come to that clinic, or to a specialised or emergency care clinic; and to know to alert clinical staff as to the imminent arrival of a critical case. Where cases arrive unannounced reception must understand how to assess the immediate needs of the animal and owner, and how to contact relevant staff in the practice.

3. Clinical staff – not all emergencies are pre-announced and so clinical staff also need to recognise an emergency case; this is especially important for veterinarians less experienced with ferrets. It is also important when an emergency case is imminent that clinical staff are aware of clinic protocols and that equipment and critical care needs are prepared and ready for use as the animal arrives.

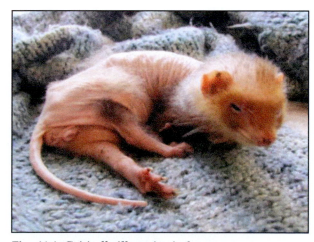

Fig. 11.1 **Critically ill, geriatric ferret.**

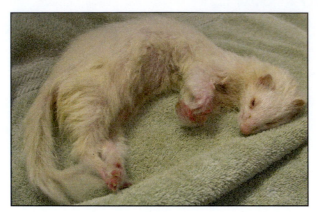

Fig. 11.2 **Ferret having a seizure, pawing at the mouth.**

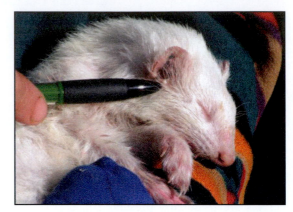

Fig. 11.3 **Non-responsive ferret nearing death.**

The following is a list (though not exhaustive) of clinical signs that warrant an emergency or very urgent appointment depending on severity:

- Continuous haemorrhage:
  - From wound, especially if arterial bleed.
  - Present in urine/faeces.
  - From eyes/nose/ears.
- Collapse.
- Loss of consciousness.
- Overt pain signs/distress – disorientation, vocalising, falling.
- Seizures.
- Persistently pawing at the mouth (**Fig. 11.2**).
- Tachypnoea/dyspnoea/open-mouth breathing.
- Persistent vomition.
- Unproductive straining to pass urine/faeces.
- Known trauma.

EUTHANASIA

It is always important to appreciate the needs of both owner and ferret. For some working ferrets, there may be little in the way of owner–animal bond (though this should never be assumed), while with others there may be a close owner–pet bond and the euthanasia must be managed accordingly. In all cases, the animal should not be allowed to suffer during the procedure and owner needs should be provided for in a sympathetic manner (**Fig. 11.3**).

Pentobarbital via intravenous (IV) or intracardiac routes is the recommended choice for euthanasia although it may be technically difficult. The latter route should never be utilised in the conscious animal as it is considered painful.

Choice of route will depend on the owner's desire to be present or not and the degree of urgency for the animal. If the owner does want to stay with their pet, it is recommended to sedate the animal and then give pentobarbital IV. This maybe done via catheter or needle. Ideally the ferret should not be removed from the owner prior to euthanasia (e.g. to place a catheter) as this may interfere with the bond between pet and owner at an important time. It is therefore essential that euthanasia consultations are appropriately scheduled giving sufficient time and, ideally, in a space away from the usual consulting room which may be too stark and clinical for many.

Where owners do not wish to remain with their ferret, the animal may be anaesthetised or sedated and pentobarbital given IV or intracardiac.

BASIC NEEDS (*BOX 11.1*)

Fundamentally, emergencies in ferrets can be stabilised using the same first principles as in other species, and if in doubt, treat as you would for cats!

When preparing to receive an emergency case (especially if the type of emergency is unknown or reported signs are non-specific) the following should be prepared:

- Heat pads/mats/lamps or even just hot water bottles.
- Oxygen and mask/chamber.

- Sedation/anaesthetic – including endotracheal tubes, laryngoscope, endoscope.
- Fluid therapy – including fluids, catheters, infusion pumps/syringe drivers.
- Critical care unit – warmed and humidified.
- Crash drugs – respiratory/cardiac stimulants
- Anticonvulsives.
- Prepare radiography and ultrasonography facilities.

- Venipuncture equipment and laboratory facilities to measure glucose, electrolytes, acid–base, ionised calcium.
- Blood pressure measurement equipment.
- Operating facilities.

SEDATION

Some cases will require sedation in order to stabilise or to facilitate examination. Inhalant anaesthetic such as isoflurane via face mask is simple and effective but may induce excessive hypotension in some cases. If used, blood pressure should always be monitored. It is important to remember that isoflurane is not analgesic. In the emergency situation this author prefers not to use alpha-2 agents or ketamine. Instead, if not using gaseous anaesthesia, midazolam at 0.25 mg/kg IM with 0.3 mg/kg butorphanol IM can be used if necessary. Oxygen should always be provided via facemask to all sedated ferrets.

FLUID THERAPY

Fluid therapy is often the mainstay of critical care. Various routes may be used and the pros and cons are summarised in *Table 11.1*.

TREATMENT OF SHOCK

Fluids indicated should be based on need, and a patient-side electrolyte monitor is invaluable as is the ability to monitor haematocrit/packed cell volume (PCV) and plasma proteins.

In general, any of the routine isotonic fluids used for dogs and cats may also be used via any of the routes outlined above.

Hypertonic dextrose solutions may also be required in cases of hypoglycaemia – these may be given IV, intraosseously (IO), or intraperitoneally (IP) (**Fig. 11.5**). Diagnosis of hypoglycaemia should be confirmed prior to administration, and dosage and flow rate closely monitored to prevent overdosing.

Colloids should be used in cases where there is blood or plasma loss and there is hypotensive shock. They should be given by the IO or IV routes and must be carefully monitored. Regular/continuous assessment of blood pressure is essential in determining

Table 11.1 **Fluid therapy routes**

ROUTE	SITE	SUGGESTED VOLUMES AND FLUID TYPE	PROS	CONS
Oral	Water should always be offered. Use bowl/drinker depending on what that animal is used to. Can also be given via pharyngostomy or nasogastric tube, or syringed carefully into the mouth/throat	Hypotonic (i.e. plain water) or isotonic rehydration formulae	Should always be given or offered. Can be done at home by an informed owner	For semi-collapsed animals, bowls should be used with care as may collapse in the bowl resulting in drowning. For severely ill animals, oral fluids unlikely to be sufficient
Subcutaneous	Between shoulder blades, or over lateral abdomen	Up to 30 mL/kg. Isotonic solutions only	Easy and fairly atraumatic. Useful for perioperative fluids in routine surgeries	Relatively slow absorption means this route is not suitable for the collapsed animal. Repeated doses may be resented
Intraperitoneal	Intra-abdominal – usually via the inguinal region	Up to 30 mL/kg. Generally isotonic solutions though hypertonic solutions (especially glucose) may be given on non-dehydrated animals. Crucial that these be of appropriate temperature	Easy and a wider range of fluid solutions may be used. Also suitable for peri-/postoperative use. More rapid absorption than subcutaneous	Repeated boluses may cause resentment. Struggling may increase risks of iatrogenic damage. Not to be used where there is abdominal fluid or likely abdominal pathology
Intravenous	Cephalic vein/ lateral saphenous	All solution types (provided sterile) suitable depending on needs. Rates calculated on needs – fluid infusors or syringe drivers are invaluable. Fluid warmers should be used in hypothermic, shocked or postsurgical cases (**Fig. 11.4**)	Method of choice for intensive cases	May be difficulties in placing and maintaining catheters. Sedation or anaesthesia usually required for catheter placement
Intraosseous (**Fig. 11.5**)	Proximal femur	As intravenous. Syringe driver essential	Easier to place and maintain than intravenous. Uptake same as intravenous	Risk of iatrogenic fracture

when to stop colloid use. Indirect blood pressure may be 10–30 mmHg difference from direct, but it monitors trends in the blood pressure. A blood pressure cuff and Doppler can be done on the tail, or in larger ferrets from the forelimb, medial surface. Remember that only 25% of crystalloids administered remain in the intravenous circulation (IVC) after 30 minutes.

In ferrets, shock is considered decompensatory. Blood pressure will measure less than 90 mmHg, and many times will be less than 40 mmHg. Crystalloids should be first given at 10–15 mL/kg along with a colloid such as hetastarch (Novation LLC, Lake Forest, IL) at 5 mL/kg. Bolus as many times as needed until blood pressure equals 40 mmHg. Aggressive warming is needed at this stage if body temperature is below 36.6°C. The plan is to get the ferret to 36.6°C within 1 hour. Use of warming systems such as the Bair Hugger® forced warm-air heating blanket is one of the best ways for overall warming. Fluids also need to be administered warm (**Fig. 11.6**).

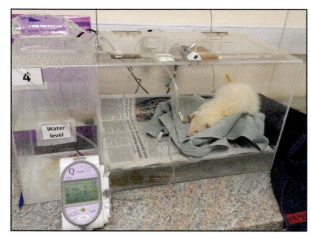

Fig. 11.4 Critical case in warmed, humidified unit. Fluid is given via an IV catheter using an infusion pump.

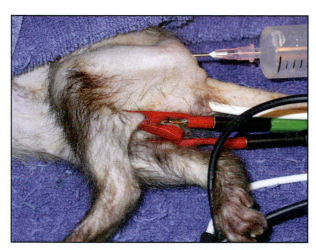

Fig. 11.5 Intraosseous administration of fluids.

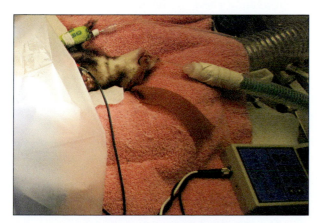

Fig. 11.6 Use of a forced-air warming blanket, with ferret provided oxygen and ECG monitoring.

When the blood pressure reaches 40 mmHg switch to crystalloids at 3–4 mL/kg/hour. Continue warming slowly and check the body temperature at least every 15 minutes. When the body temperature is 36.6–37.2°C, but blood pressure is still less than 90 mmHg, increase the crystalloids to 10–15 mL/kg and hetastarch at 5 mL/kg. Bolus until blood pressure is greater than 90 mmHg systolic.

In cases of anaemia or blood loss where the PCV has fallen below 10%, blood transfusion or Oxyglobin (Biopure, Cambridge, MA) may be considered. Oxyglobin has oxygen-carrying capacity. If there has been no response to hetastarch at a total dose of 20 mL/kg and crystalloids at 40–50 mL/kg, Oxyglobin may boost the blood pressure. Bolus it at 2–3 mL/kg along with hetastarch at 5 mL/kg. Blood transfusions can be utilised if a suitable donor is available and also can help stabilise the blood pressure. As ferrets are all one blood type, multiple transfusions can be done safely, and there is no need to cross-match.

Blood can be collected from a donor at a rate of approximately 3–4% bodyweight and is collected in a heparinised or citrated syringe before being transfused slowly into the recipient (see Chapter 10).

In view of possible disease risks and the need to anaesthetise the donor, this author prefers the use of Oxyglobin in spite of the additional expense. It is important to remember that diagnostic blood samples should be taken before giving Oxyglobin and that this compound will affect the ability to monitor electrolytes and PCV.

Whether blood or Oxyglobin are used by IV or IO routes, a syringe driver should always be utilised in order to control flow more accurately. Total volume has to be based on blood pressure measurement with cessation of colloid when systolic pressure has returned to over 90 mmHg.

EMERGENCY DRUG DOSES

The following is not an exhaustive list, but does provide a guide to what may need to be available in a crash or emergency kit (*Table 11.2*).

Table 11.2 Emergency drugs

DRUG	DOSE RATE	INDICATION
Aminophylline	4 mg/kg IV	Bronchodilation; respiratory stimulant
Atropine	0.02–0.04 mg/kg IM (higher dose for organophosphate toxicity; see below)	Bradycardia
Butorphanol (2 mg/mL)	0.2 mg/kg SC	Analgesic, sedative
Dexamethasone sodium phosphate	1–2 mg/kg IV 4–8 mg/kg IV shock	Anti-inflammatory
Dextrose 50%	0.25–2 ml/kg IV bolus 1.25–5% IV infusion	For hypoglycaemia
Diphenhydramine HCL injectable	1.0–2.0 mg/kg IM, IV	Antihistamine
Dobutamine	0.01 mL/ferret IV	Cardiac stimulant
Doxapram	1–11 mg/kg IM, IV	Respiratory stimulant
Epinephrine (adrenaline)	0.02 mg/kg IV or intratracheal	Cardiac arrest; vaccine anaphylaxis
Famotidine injection (10 mg/mL)	2.5 mg/ferret	For acute gastric distress to reduce acid reflux, ulceration
Furosemide	1–4 mg/kg IM, IV	Diuretic; cardiac failure
Lidocaine 2% (20 mg/mL)	1 drop topically to inhibit laryngospasm for intubation; for arrhythmia, 2 mg/kg slow IV infusion. May dilute this	IV: anti-arrhythmic, titrate to effect
Mannitol	0.5–1 mg/kg IV given over 20 min	Cerebral oedema
Metoclopramide	0.2–1 mg/kg IM, SC	Antiemetic
Nitroglycerine ointment 2%	1–6 mm per animal applied to skin (shaved inner thigh)	Vasodilation
Prednisolone sodium succinate	22 mg/kg IV	Anti-inflammatory

Key: IM, intramuscular; IV, intravenous; SC, subcutaneous.

SPECIFIC SYNDROMES

Certain presentations are seen more regularly, and although the usual clinical adage of 'Treat a ferret as you would a cat' holds fairly true in the emergency situation too, it is useful to have some emergency protocols for these common situations. The following are some of those used in the author's clinic. It is always valid to remember that these provide a framework to guide the clinician. In all cases, protocols should be amended with respect to the individual circumstance, both in terms of the animal's immediate welfare needs and the owner's resources (financial and otherwise). Where suffering cannot be controlled then euthanasia is indicated (see earlier).

Collapse (Fig. 11.7)

Immediately check if the ferret is having a cardiac event, such as third-degree block, erratic beats, bradycardia or arrest. Get the heart stabilised with indicated drugs such as dobutamine or atropine, and commence ECG monitoring (**Fig. 11.8**). Cardiac massage for arrest is indicated (**Fig. 11.9**). If the ferret has a normal heartbeat on auscultation, proceed to general care.

- Provide oxygen – intubate, ventilate and give sedation or minimal concentration isoflurane as necessary.
- Check rectal temperature.
- Provide heat – via heat pad or overhead lamp. Monitor body temperature throughout – hyperthermia should be avoided.

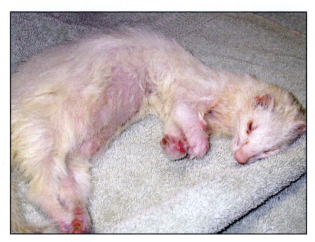

Fig. 11.7 **Collapsed ferret.**

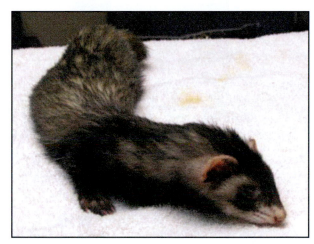

Fig. 11.8 **Ferret presented with bradycardia and marked arrhythmia, suspected of having a cardiac event. Patient was stabilised with oxygen and dobutamine and atropine IV.**

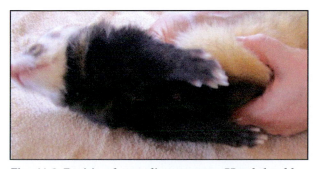

Fig. 11.9 **Position for cardiac massage. Hand should be holding the heart and compressing the chest laterally.**

- Perform physical examination.
- Perform (see Chapter 10):
  - Radiography – whole body; 2 positions.
  - Bloods – immediate: blood glucose. Then electrolytes, PCV, blood smear for differential count and cell morphology, ionised calcium, acid–base.
  - ECG and cardiac ultrasound if cardiac silhouette enlarged.
  - Blood pressure measurement.
- Fluids – ideally by IV/IO routes. Choice and volume dictated by blood and blood pressure results.
- If hypoglycaemic consider IV glucose and/or glucagon drip.
- Further therapy given as indicated.

Dyspnoea

- Provide oxygen:
  - If collapsed – place head in face mask. If distressed add isoflurane in minimal concentration until the animal is immobilised. Alternatively midazolam may be given. If less distressed, an oxygen chamber may be used.
  - CHECK AIRWAYS.
- Check improvement in membrane colour.
- Check breathing pattern – has it improved?
- Once improved, perform physical examination. If breathing worsens place back in oxygen, stabilise and reperform examination under anaesthesia or sedation. Chest radiography should be performed as soon as possible (see below).
- If stable, then provide antibiosis, anti-inflammatories and monitor. Look to perform further diagnostics after a few hours.
- As soon as practicable:
  - Perform chest radiography.
  - Drain any pleural effusion (**Fig. 11.10**).

Dysuria

- Examine and gently palpate abdomen to assess bladder size.
- If empty, consider possibility of cystitis – give antibiotic and anti-inflammatory, then monitor. Try to obtain urine sample by free catch (if let down on the floor, may urinate in a corner. Can have plastic sheet in corners to catch).

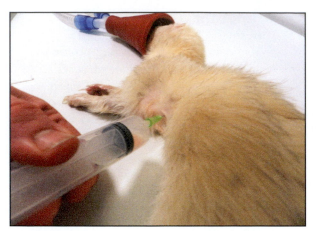

Fig. 11.10 Emergency chest drain. The ferret is placed in right lateral or ventral recumbency. The skin is clipped, prepared aseptically, and a 21G 1″ needle on a syringe is passed into the ventral thorax via rib space 3–4 on the left side. Fluid is aspirated – when no more can be aspirated, the needle is withdrawn while still applying negative pressure on the syringe.

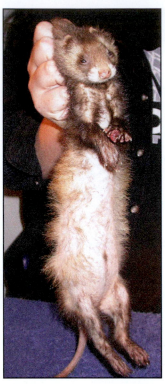

Fig. 11.11 Weak ferret with poor body condition. Depressed mentation.

- If full, anaesthetise.
- Reduce pressure by withdrawing proportion of urine (not all) by cystocentesis.
- Perform urinalysis.
- Perform radiography and ultrasonography – always assess prostate size and morphology in neutered males. If uroliths are present, cystotomy is probably indicated unless the only stones present are in the urethra and can be managed by catheterisation and flushing.
- Catheterise bladder and flush.
- Assess blood electrolytes and renal parameters – provide fluids as indicated.
- Further surgical/medical intervention as required (see Chapter 22).

Hindlimb weakness and spinal damage
- Assess spinal, proprioceptive and hindlimb reflexes (see Chapter 18).
- Assess consciousness and awareness of pain in hindlimbs – be prepared to assess deep pain response.

- Assess body condition – weakness may appear similar to paresis (**Fig. 11.11**).
- Assess bladder size and tone of rectal/bladder sphincters.
- If reflexes diminished/lost perform spinal radiography (plain films) as soon as possible in order to establish prognosis. Anaesthesia or sedation are indicated to ensure appropriate positioning.
- If history of acute injury, then ultra-short-acting corticosteroids may be of some use, though their use is always controversial. May be best avoided with non-steroidal anti-inflammatory drugs (NSAIDs). Covering antibiosis and benzodiazepine may be better options than using corticosteroids. Analgesics are probably indicated.

Hypersalivation and pawing at the mouth
This suggests nausea and the primary differential is insulinoma and hypoglycaemia (**Fig. 11.2**).

- Assess blood glucose using a haematocytometer.
- Check mouth for foreign body/ulceration/dental disease/irritation.
- Measure serum insulin levels if necessary, although this test may not be practical in acute cases.
- If hypoglycaemic consider IV glucose and/or glucagon drip.
- If insulinoma ruled out then investigate as per acute vomition (see below).

Hyperthermia

The ferret will usually feel hot and weather conditions/history will probably confirm suspicions. Continued elevated body temperature following the below treatments would suggest pyrexia of systemic diseases such as disseminated idiopathic myositis (see Chapter 17) or ferret systemic coronavirus (see Chapter 16).

- Stabilise in an oxygen chamber (the added advantage is that oxygen flow is usually cold). Midazolam may be given if distressed.
- Measure rectal temperature – digital units are best as the probe can be inserted rectally allowing continuous monitoring.
- Cover in wet cloths – do not use cold water or ice packs to avoid induction of shock.
- Give broad-spectrum antibiotic and NSAID.
- Monitor lung and cardiac function.
- When rectal temperature normal – place in cool hospitalisation unit (**Fig. 11.12**).

Seizure/syncope

If not currently having a seizure then treat as 'routine'. If having a seizure:

- Stabilise seizure – benzodiazepine may be given – e.g. diazepam per rectum; midazolam IV or IM. Isoflurane and oxygen may stabilise long enough to allow placement of an IV catheter.
- Take blood – glucose, ionised calcium, PCV, electrolytes, acid–base.
  - Also, urea, creatinine and liver parameters if possible.
- Provide glucose or calcium if indicated.

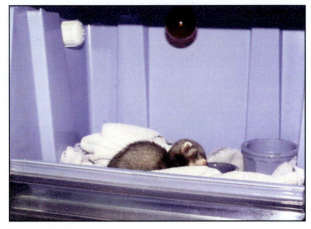

Fig. 11.12 Intensive care unit constructed from a storage container with a clear front panel. Unit has an oxygen port in the front section (not pictured).

- If hypoglycaemic consider IV glucose and/or glucagon drip.
- Fluids – based on blood results. Give by IV, IO or IP routes depending on perceived need and whether or not fluid to be given continuously or as bolus.
- Observe as recovers from anaesthesia or sedation – if seizures reoccur consider use of longer-acting drugs, e.g. phenobarbital.
- Further diagnostics should be performed as soon as practicable and as indicated by primary tests.

Vomition (acute, haemorrhagic)

- Collapsed?
- Assess hydration status.
- If so, place IV catheter – assess electrolytes, acid–base, glucose.
- Start IV fluids. Then continue as below.
- If not collapsed – palpate abdomen: masses, foreign body?
- Abdominal radiography – foreign body?
- If suspected, then perform exploratory surgery or gastric endoscopy under anaesthesia once the patient is stable.
- If no evidence of foreign body – assess bloods for renal/liver function.
- Perform abdominal ultrasonography (**Fig. 11.13**).
- Perform gut barium study if still suspicous and/or vomition continues.

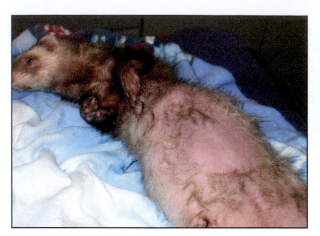

Fig. 11.13 **Prepped for abdominal ultrasound.**

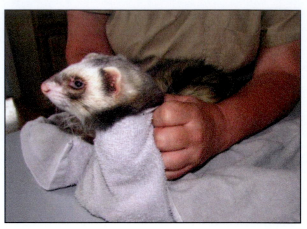

Fig. 11.14 **Ferret wrapped in a towel to prevent ingestion of a topical toxin, prior to bathing to remove the toxin.**

- Consider gastric biopsy/wash.
- If sure no foreign body then may use antiemetic drugs e.g. metoclopramide (0.2–1 mg/kg IM, SC).
- If no response and test results inconclusive consider exploratory laparatomy.

Toxicities

Toxicoses appear unusual in ferrets (see Chapter 18, Chapter 23). Some may present after known ingestion of a toxin and this may occur before clinical signs occur. It is recommended to be a member of the Veterinary Poisons Information Service (http://vpisglobal.com) as they hold a large database relating to poisons across a wide range of species and this database is continuously updated.

If it is suspected that a ferret has ingested a toxin, it is vital to know what it may have had access to and how much has been ingested. If owners are not sure then request that they bring the animal along with the packet (or product name) of what it has or may have ingested.

If the toxin has been ingested recently, then basic decontamination may be considered:

- Dermal decontamination – the initial response to a toxin on the skin should be prevention of ingestion of the toxin. Wrapping the ferret in a towel may be appropriate (**Fig. 11.14**). Care should be taken that the toxin is not rubbed onto other animals or people. As soon as possible the toxin should be washed off. Warm water, mild detergents or degreasing

detergents may be appropriate. Care should be taken not to induce hypothermia. Organic solvents should never be used.

- Ocular decontamination – the affected eye should be washed with copious amounts of warm water or 0.9% saline. This may be done at home, but should still be examined subsequently, as the degree of corneal damage must be assessed.
- Gastric decontamination:
  - Gastric evacuation – contraindicated if the ingested substance is caustic, corrosive, petroleum-based or volatile, or if it was ingested more than 2–3 hours previously. This can be performed in 2 ways:
    - Induction of emesis. In addition to the above contraindications this should not be done if the patient has severe CNS depression; respiratory distress; or if it has ingested a substance likely to cause seizures. Induction of emesis can be performed using apomorphine (0.7 mg/kg SC) or sodium carbonate (washing soda crystals) given orally. A small crystal should be sufficient.
    - Gastric lavage – if it is not safe to induce emesis. The patient should be anaesthetised and intubated. A large-bore stomach/feeding tube is placed carefully via the mouth into the stomach and warmed saline (10 mL/kg) instilled. The stomach is gently massaged and the fluid drained

via the tube with the patient's head lowered. This should be repeated until the fluid returns clear.

- Administration of adsorbents – should be used where gastric evacuation is unsafe or after gastric evacuation. Typically activated charcoal is given at 1–4 g/kg PO q 4–6 hours. However, these agents should not be given in the presence of orally dosed antidotes.

Where clinical signs are occurring, or ingestion was not recent, the following basic stabilisation may be considered:

- Specific antidotes:
  - Coumarols – Vitamin K1: initially give 2.5 mg/kg SC. The follow-up treatment and dosing regime depends on the specific coumarol ingested and specialist advice should always be taken.
  - Organophosphates – 5–10 mg/kg atropine IM, SC.
  - Heavy metal toxicosis – calcium EDTA 20–30 mg/kg SC q12h.
  - Copper toxicity – penicillamine 10 mg/kg PO q24h.
- Supportive care:
  - If no signs:
    - Administration of specific antidote if needed.
    - Fluid therapy as indicated according to severity of signs/need for renal support.
    - Gastric protectants such as famotidine for agents likely to cause gastrointestinal ulceration.
    - Observation.

- If signs:
  - Fluid therapy.
  - Gastric protectants for agents likely to cause gastrointestinal ulceration.
  - Antiemetics if vomiting.
  - Adsorbents if likely further toxin will be absorbed in the gut.
  - Benzodiazepines/anticonvulsants if neurological signs.

Vaccine reaction

It is recommended that ferrets receive 0.5–1 mL of a children's diphenhydramine syrup (12.5 mg/5 mL) 15–30 minutes prior to vaccination. It is advisable not to give distemper and rabies at the same time, because if a reaction occurs it is impossible to tell which vaccine triggered it for future vaccination status.

A vaccine reaction may occur anytime but usually starts up to 30 minutes after vaccination. It is recommended that the ferret stays under observation for 20–30 minutes postvaccination. Discuss this with the owner – in fact it should be told to the owner when the appointment is made. A vaccination appointment may be for an hour: first 30 minutes waiting after diphenhydramine, then 30 minutes postvaccination observation.

Signs of a reaction are listed in *Table 11.3* and may include any or all of the following, in varying degrees of severity.

It is a good idea to have a vaccine reaction kit along with the protocol at the ready. This kit should contain small vials of drugs listed below as well as syringes so that one does not have to try to gather the medications at the time (*Box 11.2*) (**Figs 11.15–11.17**).

Table 11.3 **Signs of a vaccine reaction (Fig. 11.2)**			
Hypersalivation	Vomiting, may be haemorrhagic	Retching	Pawing at mouth
Bottlebrush tail	Piloerection	Rash and flushing	Erythema of nose, skin, feet
Explosive diarrhoea, may be haemorrhagic	Frantic behaviour	Coughing, sneezing	Dyspnoea

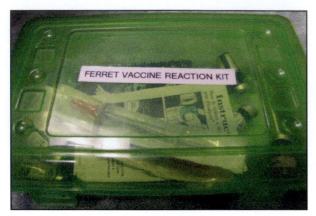

Fig. 11.15 **Vaccine reaction kit made from a pencil box.**

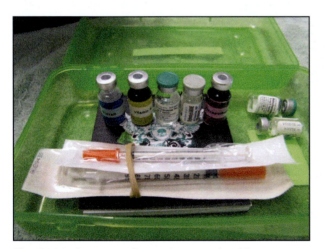

Fig. 11.16 **Contents of a vaccine reaction kit.**

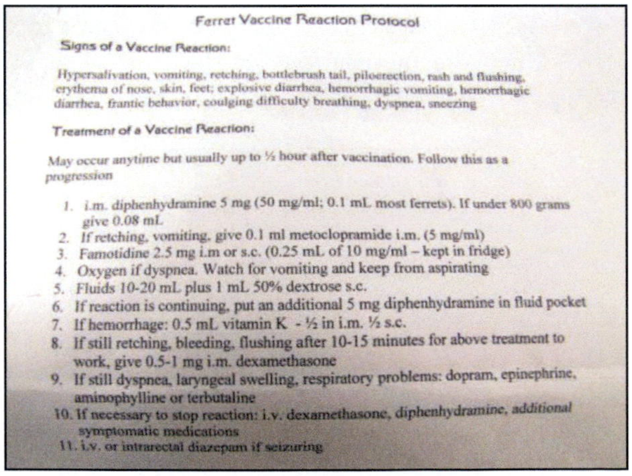

Box 11.2 **Treatment of a vaccine reaction: This is a progression**

1. Diphenhydramine IM 5 mg (50 mg/mL; 0.1 mL most ferrets). If under 800 g, give 0.08 mL.
2. If retching, vomiting, give 0.1 mL metoclopramide IM (5 mg/mL).
3. Famotidine 2.5 mg IM or SC (0.25 mL of a 10 mg/mL commercial solution).
4. Oxygen if dyspnoea. Watch for vomiting and keep from aspirating.
5. Crystalloid fluids 10–20 mL plus 1 mL 50% dextrose SC.
6. If reaction is continuing, put an additional 5 mg diphenhydramine in fluid pocket.
7. If haemorrhage give 0.5 mL vitamin K (half in IM, half in SC).
8. If still retching, bleeding, flushing after 10–15 minutes for above treatment to work, give 0.5–1 mg dexamethasone IM.
9. If still dyspnoeic, laryngeal swelling, respiratory problems: give dopram (1–5 mg/mL IM), epinephrine (0.02 mg/kg IM, IT, IV, SC), aminophylline (5 mg/kg IM, IV) or terbutaline (2.5–5 mg/kg PO).
10. If necessary to stop reaction: IV dexamethasone, diphenhydramine, additional symptomatic medications.
11. IV or intrarectal diazepam if seizuring (1–2 mg/kg).

CRITICAL NUTRITION

Hospitalised ferrets should be provided with their usual food bowls and/or water bowls or bottles – otherwise the clinic's own should be used but they should be of the same design as used by the owner. Bowls should be heavy duty to avoid tipping.

As a matter of course ferrets should be offered their usual food (type and brand). Even where dietary deficiency is suspected as a part of the disease, the priority is to encourage the ferret to eat before converting to a more desirable ration (**Fig. 11.18**).

Critical nutrition may also be required in severely ill animals. The following are used by this author.

- Nutrient gels – these may be given directly to the sick ferret or may be smeared on (or mixed with) other foods to encourage eating.

Fig. 11.17 **Protocol is taped to the lid.**

- Critical care diets suitable for cats are usually suitable for ferrets as they should be high in protein and fat and low in carbohydrate/fibre. These can be given by syringe into the mouth or via nasogastric/pharyngostomy tube. Quantities to be given can be calculated in the same way as for cats.
- More specialised critical care diets are now available – e.g. Emeraid Carnivore Diet (Lafeber, Cornell, IL) or Oxbow Carnivore Care Diet (Oxbow Animal Health, Murdock, NE). Manufacturers' instructions should be followed in terms of mixing and feeding quantities.
- For short periods more general critical care mixtures may be used, e.g. Critical Care Formula (Vetark, Winchester, UK). However, this should only be short term as many of these are more carbohydrate-based than protein-/fat-based.
- Homemade diet dook soup can be made (Appendix 6) and has successfully been used in nursing care.

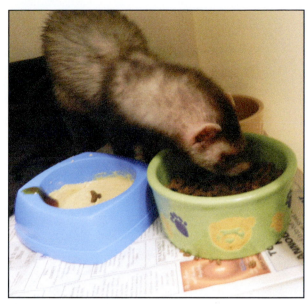

Fig. 11.18 **Hospitalised ferret offered choice of own food, critical care diet and water. All in heavy ceramic bowls. (Brown material in the blue bowl is nutrient gel.)**

DISORDERS OF THE CARDIOVASCULAR SYSTEM

Yvonne R.A. van Zeeland and Nico J. Schoemaker

INTRODUCTION

Cardiac disease is relatively common in pet ferrets, particularly in middle-aged to older ferrets, and may comprise problems with conduction, contractility and/or outflow. Cardiac disease encompasses a wide range of anatomical and physiological disorders of varying causes, which may be classified by various characteristics, including: presence at birth or not (i.e. congenital versus acquired heart disease); cause (e.g. infectious, degenerative, genetic, neoplastic); duration (i.e. chronic or acute); clinical status (e.g. left, right or bilateral heart failure); tissue type that is involved (i.e. endocardium, myocardium or pericardium); type of anatomical malformation (e.g. ventricular septal defect); or type of electrical disturbance that is present (i.e. arrhythmias and conduction disturbances resulting in tachycardia or bradycardia or arrhythmias, e.g. atrial fibrillation, second-degree AV-block, or sinus arrhythmia).

Heart failure is often the end result of severe (systolic and/or diastolic) cardiac dysfunction and may give rise to a variety of clinical signs that are either the result of increased venous pressure and congestion (i.e. *backward failure*), or result from low cardiac output and poor tissue perfusion (i.e. *forward failure*). Heart failure may only occur if severe cardiac disease is present. In contrast, cardiac disease can be present without the ferret ever developing heart failure.

CLINICAL PRESENTATION

Clinical presentation of cardiac disease in the ferret greatly depends on the severity and type of cardiac disease. Ferrets may be presented as completely asymptomatic (when cardiac disease is an incidental finding) to showing signs of fulminant heart failure.

Many of the clinical signs that may be observed are non-specific and may include lethargy, exercise intolerance, weight loss and anorexia. Weakness in the hindlimbs and syncopes (the latter specifically in bradyarrhythmic animals) may be noted as well (**Fig. 12.1**). In ferrets with left- and/or right-sided heart failure, pleural effusions, hepato- and/or splenomegaly, ascites, coughing and dyspnoea may be seen. Many ferrets with cardiac disease will present with an increased respiratory rate, especially if thoracic effusions or lung oedema are present. Some ferrets will also cough. Pale or cyanotic mucous membranes with a prolonged capillary refill time (CRT) may also be noted as a result of reduced cardiac output (**Fig. 12.2**), as well as a weak or irregular pulse (**Fig. 12.3**). Heart murmurs (common in dilated cardiomyopathy, congenital heart disease and valve insufficiency), bradycardia, tachycardia, arrhythmias and/or muffled heart sounds (e.g. in case of pericardial or pleural effusion) may be heard upon auscultation of the heart (**Fig. 12.4**). Auscultation of the lungs may reveal moist rales or crackles, muffled lung sounds or increased bronchovesicular sounds.

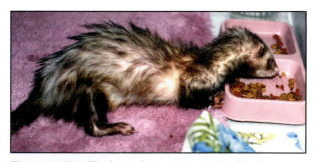

Fig. 12.1 **Hindlimb weakness, as seen in this ferret with dilative cardiomyopathy, is one of the signs of cardiac disease. (Courtesy of Cathy Johnson-Delaney.)**

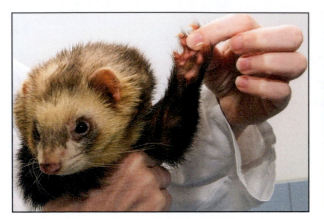

Fig. 12.2 The capillary refill time (CRT) can best be determined in ferrets by pressing on the unpigmented foot pads.

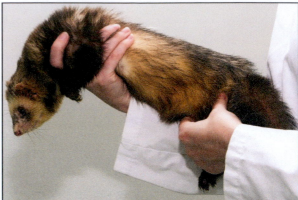

Fig. 12.3 By placing the ferret along the lower arm it will usually remain calm enough to determine the frequency and quality of the pulse. Just as in other companion animals, the femoral artery is the preferred location.

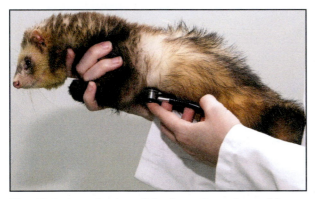

Fig. 12.4 Auscultation of the heart is performed in a similar fashion as in other companion animals. Due to the small size of the heart in ferrets, it is difficult to determine the origin of a murmur, when present. Note that the thorax of ferrets is very elongated and that the heart is located more distal (ribs 6–8) than one may expect.

DIAGNOSTIC TESTING FOR DISEASE

Based on the history and physical examination, cardiac disease may be suspected. To confirm the diagnosis a diagnostic work-up, which may include an echocardiogram, thoracic radiographs, ECG, blood pressure measurement, blood work (CBC + biochemical profile) and/or urinalysis, may be required. Testing for heartworm (*Dirofilaria immitis*) may be indicated in those cases in which clinical signs are suggestive of infection, especially in areas where

heartworm is endemic. If pleural effusion or ascites is present, thoraco- or abdominocentesis may be performed to alleviate the associated dyspnoea and discomfort (**Figs 12.5, 12.6**). Cytological, biochemical or bacteriological examination of this fluid may provide further insight into the cause of the effusion (**Fig. 12.7**).

The initial choice of diagnostic modality is based on the findings during the physical examination. When abnormal sounds are auscultated an echocardiogram is the first-choice diagnostic technique. In case of coughing, tachypnoea and/or dyspnoea a radiograph is the first choice. An echocardiogram may be required if pleural effusion or an enlarged heart is seen on the radiograph. An ECG is considered useful when an abnormal rhythm or pulse frequency is detected.

Echocardiography

Echocardiography is the preferred diagnostic tool when attempting to identify structural and/or functional abnormalities of the heart. Echocardiography may be performed both in awake and sedated ferrets (**Fig. 12.8**). For accurate M-mode registrations and for colour flow Doppler examinations, however, anaesthesia is required for which the use of short-acting injectables (e.g. midazolam) and/or inhalant anaesthetics (e.g. isoflurane or sevoflurane) is recommended. Another advantage of performing

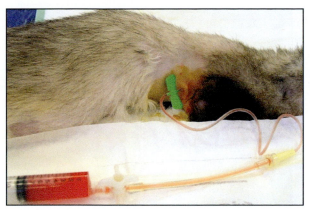

Fig. 12.5 Thoracocentesis is frequently performed under ultrasound guidance. It can also be performed 'blind' whereby it is important to insert the needle in the lower third of the thorax in an area where no lung sounds are auscultated. To avoid puncturing the heart it is best to insert the needle caudal to the heart, which is located between the 6th and 8th rib. Insertion of the needle should be as parallel to the ribs as possible, with the opening of the needle pointing medially.

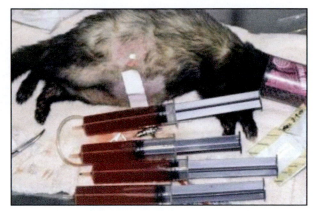

Fig. 12.6 Abdominocentesis in a ferret with severe ascites. Using a butterfly needle makes draining of the fluid a lot easier as syringes can easily be switched without having to remove the needle during aspiration of the fluid. (Courtesy of Cathy Johnson-Delaney.)

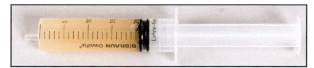

Fig. 12.7 Abdominal effusion obtained from a ferret with cardiac disease. In case of cardiac disease, the produced transudate usually has a clear appearance with low protein content.

echocardiography in sedated ferrets is that measurement is easier, as the animals do not move.

The echocardiogram is performed with the ferret in both right and left lateral recumbency using imaging planes similar to those obtained in other species. Reference ranges for common cardiac measurements are summarised in *Table 12.1*. Aside from two-dimensional echocardiograms (B-mode), which are used to assess cardiac size, check valves and function (**Fig. 12.9**), M-mode measurements and Doppler echocardiography may be performed. With the M-mode measurements the chamber dimensions, wall thickness and systolic function are determined (**Fig. 12.10**). Doppler ultrasonography may be useful to assess the velocity of the blood flow and check whether turbulence (indicative of e.g. valvular regurgitation) is present (**Fig. 12.11**). Ultrasonography may furthermore reveal presence of effusion in the pericardium, thorax or abdomen, as well as hepatomegaly or splenomegaly due to congestion (**Fig. 12.12**). Liver congestion is often associated with dilation of the major vessels throughout the liver (**Fig. 12.13**).

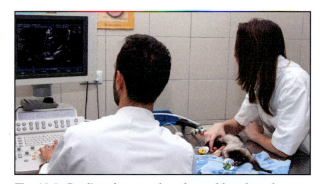

Fig. 12.8 Cardiac ultrasound performed by a board-certified cardiologist. Although anaesthetics may influence the cardiac measurements, ferrets are frequently so mobile that performing a proper echocardiography is not possible without sedation. For this purpose the use of short-acting injectables (e.g. midazolam) and/or inhalant anaesthetics (e.g. isoflurane or sevoflurane) is recommended. Just as in other companion animals, ultrasound should best be performed on both sides of the thorax. However, in case of severe dyspnoea, it may be best to place the ferret in sternal recumbency.

Table 12.1 Echocardiographic reference values obtained in 29 ferrets anaesthetised with isoflurane (derived from Vastenburg et al., 2004)

PARAMETER	MEAN ± SD	RANGE	MEDIAN
IVSd (mm)	3.4 ± 0.4	2.5–4.4	3.4
IVSs (mm)	4.4 ± 0.6	3.3–5.4	4.4
LVIDd (mm)	9.8 ± 1.4	6.8–12.7	9.6
LVIDs (mm)	6.9 ±1.3	4.5–9.7	6.9
LVWd (mm)	2.7 ± 0.5	1.8–3.7	2.7
LVWs (mm)	3.8 ± 0.8	2.4–5.9	3.8
FS (%)	29.5 ± 7.9	13.9–48.7	28.0
Ao (mm)	4.4 ± 0.6	3.3–6.0	4.2
LAAD (mm)	5.8 ± 0.9	3.2–7.3	5.7
LAAD/Ao	1.3 ± 0.2	1.0–1.8	1.3
EPSS (mm)	1.2 ± 0.6	0–2.2	1.2

Key: Ao: aorta diameter; EPSS: E-point to septal separation diameter; FS: fractional shortening; IVSd and IVSs: interventricular septum thickness in diastole and systole; LAAD: left atrium appendage diameter; LVIDd and LVIDs: left ventricular internal diameter in diastole and systole; LVWd and LVWs: left ventricular wall thickness in diastole and systole; SD: standard deviation.

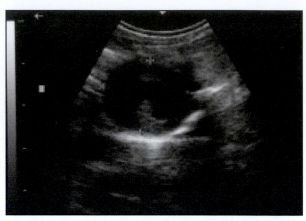

Fig. 12.9 B-mode ultrasound of a ferret in which no cardiac abnormalities were found. The B-mode produces a 2D image of a cross-sectional view of the heart. The most commonly used scanning directions of the heart are the right and left parasternal long axis 4-chamber view. (Courtesy of Cathy Johnson-Delaney.)

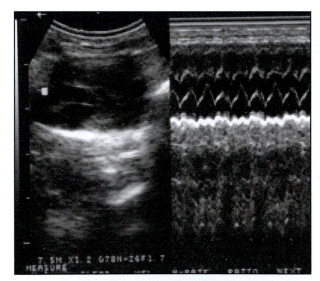

Fig. 12.10 M-mode ultrasound (right) of a ferret with minor signs of cardiomyopathy. The M-mode, or motion mode, is a 1D analysis of the heart in motion. In this mode the valve motion, chamber sizes, aortic root size, wall thickness and ventricular function can be assessed. (Courtesy of Cathy Johnson-Delaney.)

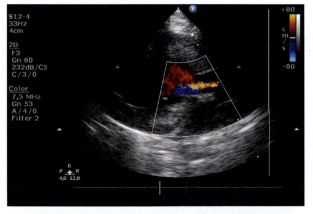

Fig. 12.11 Colour-flow Doppler can be used to assess the velocity of the blood flow and potential presence of turbulence, indicative of e.g. valvular regurgitation. Flow towards the transducer is depicted in red while flow away from the transducer is shown in blue. In case of turbulent flow both colours are mixed, as can be seen in this ferret with an aorta valve insufficiency.

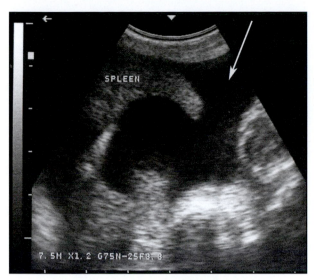

Fig. 12.12 **Effusion, indicated by the hypoechogenic area (arrow), can easily be identified with ultrasound. As the ultrasound shows homogenous fluid, it most probably is transudate. (Courtesy of Cathy Johnson-Delaney.)**

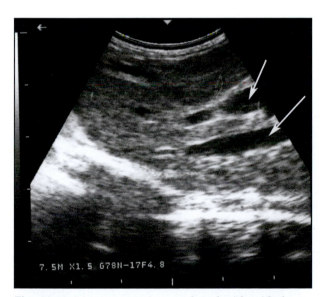

Fig. 12.13 **Liver congestion can best be identified during an ultrasound examination by presence of clearly dilated hepatic veins (arrows). (Courtesy of Cathy Johnson-Delaney.)**

Radiography

Radiographs are considered useful for determining presence of signs of congestive heart failure (especially lung oedema or pleural effusion) (**Fig. 12.14**). Standard two-view thoracic radiographs may be obtained by physically restraining the ferret or sedating/anaesthetising it with short-acting sedatives or inhalant anaesthetics. It should be realised that with sedation the inspiratory volume is decreased,

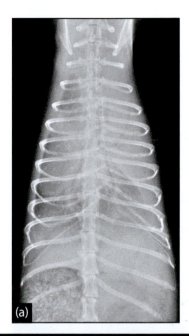

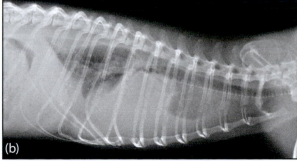

Fig. 12.14 **Dorsoventral (a) and lateral (b) radiographs of a ferret with severe pleural effusion. Fluid accumulation obscures the heart shadow and compresses the lungs, which – similar to the trachea – show up as radiolucent structures dorsal in the thorax, due to the presence of air.**

thereby hindering accurate evaluation of the lungs. As the ferret's thorax is long and flat, care should be taken to include the entire thorax in the radiographs. When the abdomen is included, hepato- and/or splenomegaly or signs of ascites may also be noted (**Fig. 12.15**).

Radiographs may furthermore be used to determine cardiac size (**Fig. 12.16**). For this purpose, a modified vertebral heart score may be calculated. Different methods have been described to relate cardiac dimensions to those of thoracic vertebrae. Although these methods correct for differences in size between ferrets, no distinction can be made between cardiomegaly and pericardial effusion, nor does radiography distinguish between dilated and hypertrophic cardiomyopathy. The authors

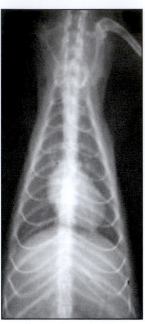

Fig. 12.16 **Ventrodorsal radiograph of a ferret with a cardiomegaly. The apex of the heart is broadened and displaced towards the left, indicating a dilation of the left ventricle. (Courtesy of Cathy Johnson-Delaney.)**

therefore see no added value in using these, often complicated, methods of measuring cardiac dimensions over the use of echocardiography.

Electrocardiography

With ECG electrical activity of the heart is recorded. Electrical activity, however, only indicates where potential abnormalities within the heart may be found, and does *not* provide any information on cardiac contractility. The ECG is primarily used to identify arrhythmias or conduction disturbances and should be obtained in any ferret suspected of an abnormal heart rate or rhythm. An ECG may furthermore assist in the diagnosis of cardiac chamber enlargement, pericardial and/or pleural effusion, and monitoring the progression of cardiac disease and effects of cardioactive drugs as well as cardiac function during anaesthesia or surgery.

Ideally, the ECG is performed in an awake animal placed in right lateral recumbency (**Fig. 12.17**). Since this is seldom possible, a good alternative is to keep the animal in an upright (dorsoventral) position. The reference values described in *Table 12.2* have been obtained in this position. A variety of

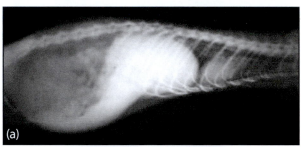

(a)

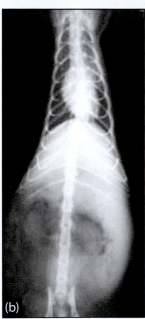

(b)

Fig. 12.15 **Lateral (a) and ventrodorsal (b) radiographs of a ferret with obvious hepatosplenomegaly. (Courtesy of Cathy Johnson-Delaney.)**

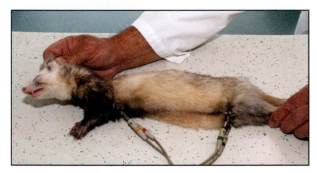

Fig. 12.17 **While scruffing a ferret an ECG may be made in right lateral recumbency.**

Table 12.2 **ECG reference values obtained in 20 awake ferrets placed in dorsoventral position (derived from Zandvliet, 2004)**

PARAMETER		MEAN ± SD	RANGE
Heart frequency		220	175–265
Heart axis		88.5° ± 5.5°	85°–102°
Measurements in lead II	P duration (s)	0.019 ± 0.003	0.01–0.02
	P amplitude (mV)	0.11 ± 0.04	0.09–0.2
	PR interval (s)	0.049 ± 0.009	0.04–0.07
	QRS duration (s)	0.026 ± 0.006	0.02–0.04
	QRS amplitude (mV)	2.9 ± 1.2	1.4–4.4
	QT interval (s)	0.14 ± 0.02	0.11–0.16
	ST segment (mV)	0.03 ± 0.01	0.02–0.05
	T duration (s)	0.084 ± 0.018	0.06–0.11
	T amplitude (mV)	0.26 ± 0.08	0.15–0.4

Key: SD, standard deviation.

different (physiological and pathological) arrhythmias have been identified in ferrets, including sinus brady- and tachycardia, atrial and ventricular premature contractions, atrial fibrillation, first-, second- and third-degree atrioventricular (AV) blocks.

In cases of a bradycardia or bradyarrhythmia it may be important to exclude underlying metabolic causes (e.g. hypo- or hyperkalaemia, hypoglycaemia) as well as a vagally-mediated decrease in heart rate. In this latter instance, a so-called atropine response test can be performed, during which atropine is administered IV, IM or SC at 0.02–0.05 mg/kg.

In case of a vagally-mediated bradycardia, increases in heart rate and/or improved SA and AV node conduction may be noted within 15–30 minutes following administration (**Fig. 12.18**). In case an incomplete response is observed, the above mentioned steps may be repeated.

Relationship between ECG deflection and electric activity of the heart

To understand each deflection of the ECG (**Fig. 12.19**), an understanding of the normal pattern of electric activity in the heart is necessary. Electric activity starts in the sinoatrial (SA) node, which is located close to the entrance of the cranial vena cava. The cells of the SA node have the highest rate of discharge and therefore set the pace of the cardiac contractions. Depolarisation of the SA node initiates atrial depolarisation, which is reflected in the ECG as the P-wave. The initial part of the P-wave represents the right atrial depolarisation, whereas the last part represents the depolarisation of the left atrium. Atrial repolarisation is not identified in the ECG as this coincides with ventricular depolarisation.

The electrical impulse in the atrium is conducted to the AV node, which is located close to the right AV valve. The transmission of the impulse is delayed in the AV node, which is recorded as an isoelectric period called the PR-segment. The combined P-wave and the PR-segment are referred to as the PR-interval. The electrical impulse then continues from the AV node via the His bundle to the cardiac apex and both ventricles. Both ventricles contract simultaneously, which can be seen in the ECG as three distinct phases referred to as the QRS-complex. The first negative deflection following the P-wave is by definition the Q-wave, followed by a positive R-wave and finally the S-wave which also has a negative deflection. The Q-wave corresponds to contraction of the middle and apical portions of the ventricular septum; the R-wave to depolarisation of the ventricular free wall and the S-wave to depolarisation of the basal part of the septum and ventricles. Following the QRS-complex, a short period of electrical inactivity may be noted, referred to as the ST-segment. Finally, a (positive) T-wave may be noted, which represents ventricular repolarisation.

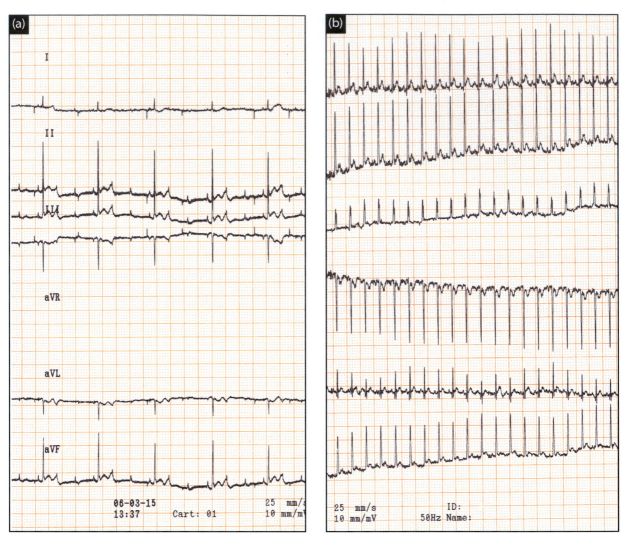

Fig. 12.18 (a) An electrocardiogram of a ferret with a second-degree type II AV block. In type II blocks the PR interval is constant and there is a fixed relationship between the atrial and ventricular rate of, e.g. 2:1, meaning two P-waves to every QRS complex; (b) 20 minutes after administration of atropine (0.05 mg/kg IM), the block disappeared and a fully normal ECG was seen.

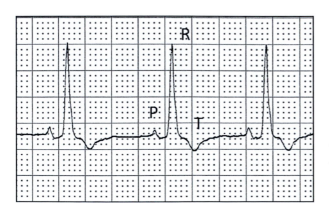

Fig. 12.19 Ferret lead II ECG showing the P-wave, QRS-complex and T-wave (50 mm/s, 10 mm/mV). The P-wave represents the depolarisation of the atria; whereas the QRS-complex and T-wave represent the ventricular depolarisation and ventricular repolarisation, respectively.

ECG interpretation

For the interpretation of the ECG, a standardised protocol may be followed, whereby most measurements are collected using lead II.

First, the heart rate is calculated. If a paper speed of 25 mm/s is selected, the heart rate can be calculated by counting the number of QRS-complexes over a length of 7.5 cm (equalling 3 seconds) and multiplying the number of complexes by 20 to determine the heart rate in beats per minute (bpm).

Next, the heart rhythm is assessed. For this purpose, the ECG should be evaluated for (1) regularity of the rhythm; (2) presence of P-waves; (3) presence of QRS-complexes; and (4) presence of a relationship between the P-waves and following QRS-complexes. Regularity of the rhythm may be checked by using a piece of paper to mark four R-waves. The paper may subsequently be moved alongside the ECG, whereby the marks should continue to correspond to any of the R-waves that are present. A variation of 10% is considered acceptable. Next, the presence of P-waves and QRS-complexes may be assessed. To accurately assess the configuration, uniformity and regularity of the complexes, it may be necessary to increase the sensitivity of the ECG. Finally, it needs to be determined: a) whether each P-wave is followed by a QRS-complex; and b) whether each QRS-complex is preceded by a P-wave.

After the rhythm has been established, the duration and amplitude of each of the complexes and intervals are determined. For this purpose, lead II is used. Reference ranges for the different measurements can be found in *Table 12.2*.

Last, the mean electrical axis (MEA) is determined. This can be done most accurately by measuring net deflections in two leads (most often leads I and III) and marking these off from the zero point in the triaxial system. Next, perpendicular lines are drawn originating from the end points of the deflections until they intersect. A connecting arrow is then drawn between the origin and the point of intersection (**Fig. 12.20**). The MEA is subsequently determined as the angle between the lead I axis (horizontal plane) and the connecting arrow.

Once all aforementioned measurements are completed, the results will subsequently need to be evaluated before conclusions may be drawn.

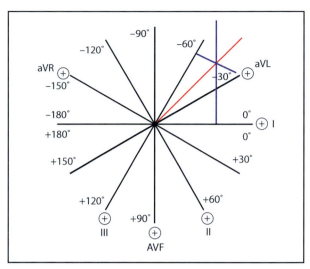

Fig. 12.20 The mean electrical axis can be determined by drawing perpendicular lines (blue) to, for instance, the lines representing lead I and III. The distance along these lines to the centre of the axis is similar to the height of the R-wave in the two leads. At the junction of these perpendicular lines another line (red) may be drawn from the centre of the axis. The angle between this line and lead I is the mean electrical axis (reference 85° to 102° for ferrets).

GENERAL MANAGEMENT OF CARDIAC DISEASE

In general, therapeutic intervention for cardiac disease in ferrets follows the same guidelines as those applied in dogs and cats. For many of the drugs used, no specific pharmacokinetic or pharmacodynamic data are available on ferrets. Feline doses are therefore often used as a starting point for therapy. An overview of the different drugs that may be used in ferrets with cardiovascular disease, including the recommended dosing regimen, can be found in *Table 12.3*.

Therapy for acute congestive heart failure often focuses on three aspects: 1) improving oxygenation by placing the animal in an incubator with supplemental oxygen; 2) reduction of the preload by giving diuretics (e.g. furosemide, thiazide, spironolactone) or nitroglycerin (a venous dilator); and 3) reducing the afterload by giving angiotensin-converting enzyme (ACE) inhibitors that induce vasodilatation

Table 12.3 **Drugs to be used in the treatment of cardiovascular disease in ferrets**

DRUG	ACTION	DOSAGE
Amlodipine	Calcium antagonist; afterload reduction	0.2–04 mg/kg PO q12h
Atenolol	Beta-blocker for treatment of HCM	3.125–6.25 mg/kg PO q24h
Atropine	Parasympathicolytic drug for treatment of bradycardia	0.02–0.05 mg/kg SC/IM
Benazepril	ACE inhibitor; vasodilator	0.25–0.5 mg/kg PO q24h
Captopril	ACE inhibitor; vasodilator	$^1/_8$ of 12.5 mg tablet/animal PO q48h
Digoxin	Positive inotropic drug for treatment of DCM	0.005–0.01 mg/kg PO q12–24 h
Diltiazem	Calcium channel blocker for treatment of HCM, AF or SVT	1.5–7.5 mg/kg PO q12h
Dobutamine	Sympathicomimetic drug used in treatment of heart failure and cardiogenic shock	5–10 µg/kg/min IV (canine dose)
Enalapril	ACE inhibitor; vasodilator	0.25–0.5 mg/kg PO q24–48h
Furosemide	Loop diuretic for treatment of congestion	1–4 mg/kg PO/SC/IM/IV q8–12h
Hydroclorothiazide	Diuretic for treatment of congestion; may be combined with spironolactone	1 mg/kg PO q12–24h (cat dose)
Isoproterenol	Sympathicomimetic drug for treatment of 3rd-degree AV block	40–50 µg/kg PO/SC/IM q12h
Ivermectin	Broad-spectrum antiparasitic avermectin for treatment of heartworm	0.02 mg/kg PO/SC (preventive) or 50 µg/kg SC q30d (treatment)
Melarsomine	Arsenical; adulticide used to treat heartworm disease	2.5 mg/kg IM at day 1, 30, 31
Metaproterenol	Sympathicomimetic drug for treatment of 3rd-degree AV block	0.25–1 mg/kg PO q12h
Milbemycin oxime	Broad-spectrum antiparasitic milbemycin; prevention of heartworm disease	1.15–2.33 mg/kg PO q30d
Moxidectin	Broad-spectrum antiparasitic avermectin; used to treat heartworm (adulticide)	0.1 mL SC (single dose); use every 6 months as preventive treatment
Nitroglycerin	Vasodilator	$^1/_{16}$ – $^1/_8$ inch/animal of a 2% ointment q12–24h, applied to shaved inner thigh or pinna
Pimobendan	Phosphodiesterase inhibitor; increase cardiac contractility in patients with DCM	0.5–1.25 mg/kg PO q12h
Propanolol	Beta-blocker for treatment of HCM	0.2–1 mg/kg PO/SC q8–12h
Propanthelin	Long-acting parasympathicolytic for treatment of sinus bradyarrhythmia	0.25–0.5 mg/kg PO 8–12h (canine dose)
Selamectin	Broad-spectrum antiparasitic avermectin; used as preventive treatment for heartworm	18 mg/kg topically
Spironolactone	Diuretic for treatment of congestion	1–2 mg/kg PO q12h
Theophylline	Methylxanthine drug, which serves as a bronchodilator (relaxation of bronchial smooth muscles) and also has positive inotropic and chronotropic effects	4.25 mg/kg PO q8–12h

Key: ACE, angiotensin-converting enzyme; AF, atrial fibrillation; AV, atrioventricular; DCM, dilated cardiomyopathy; HCM, hypertrophic cardiomyopathy; IM, intramuscular; IV, intravenous; PO, per os; SC, subcutaneous; SVT, supraventricular tachycardia.

and decrease water and salt retention (thereby also reducing the preload). In case of significant pleural effusion, thoracocentesis may be performed to alleviate dyspnoea (**Fig. 12.5**). Once the animal has been stabilised, digoxin and/or pimobendan may be added to the treatment regimen to enhance inotropy.

Beta-blockers (e.g. atenolol) or calcium channel blockers (e.g. diltiazem) may be used to reduce the heart rate and treat supraventricular and ventricular arrhythmias. In case of ventricular tachycardias, intravenous lidocaine may also be titrated to effect, whereas atropine may be indicated if bradycardia or bradyarrhythmia is present. As this drug only results in a short-term effect, long-acting parasympatholytic drugs (e.g. propanthelin) may be used to increase the heart rate. Sympathicomimetic drugs such as metaproterenol or isoproterenol have also been used in the medicinal therapy of third-degree heart block. As these drugs do not always result in a clinical effect, pacemaker implantation may be considered as an alternative.

CONGENITAL HEART DISEASE

Definition/overview
Congenital heart disease comprises abnormalities in cardiovascular structures that occur before birth. Defects may involve: 1) the heart valves, i.e. stenosis or insufficiency, which respectively impede forward blood flow, or result in leakage; 2) the septum between the atria or ventricles, i.e. atrial or ventricular septal defects, which result in abnormal mixing of oxygenated and unoxygenated blood between the right and left sides of the heart; 3) heart muscle abnormalities that may result in heart failure. In ferrets, congenital heart defects have only been described since the last decade. Thus far, case reports have been published on atrial and ventricular septal defects (n = 1 for both), and tetralogy of Fallot (n = 2). Tetralogy of Fallot comprises a congenital heart defect that is classically understood to involve four anatomical abnormalities of the heart, i.e. 1) a ventricular septal defect; 2) an overriding aorta; and 3) pulmonic stenosis associated with 4) right ventricular hypertrophy.

In addition, the occurrence of patent ductus arteriosus in ferrets has been mentioned in literature.

Although no other congenital defects have been reported thus far, it is expected that these do occur in ferrets, similar to other animals. In general, however, congenital heart disease should be considered rare.

Aetiology/pathophysiology
Congenital heart disease should be considered a birth defect, resulting from an abnormal development of the heart during the embryonic phase. Although the exact aetiology is currently unknown, it is likely that causative factors are similar to those described in man and other animals (e.g. single or multi-genetic defects and/or exposure to infections or environmental toxins).

Clinical presentation
Congenital heart disease has been diagnosed in both young and adult animals up to 6 years of age. Dependent on the size and type of defect, animals may either show no symptoms at all (thereby leaving the disease undetected until it is found by coincidence), or die before or shortly after being born. If symptoms are present these may include growth retardation, exercise intolerance, cyanosis, dyspnoea and (sporadic) cough. Animals may also develop signs of congestive heart failure, resulting in pulmonary oedema, pleural effusion, hepatomegaly and/or ascites, which may result in the animals presenting with a dyspnoea, tachypnoea, cough, muscle wasting and/or distended abdomen (**Fig. 12.21**). On physical examination a (holodiastolic, holosystolic or continuous) cardiac murmur will often be audible. In addition, a tachycardia, faint pulse, cyanotic or pale mucous membranes and/or prolonged CRT may be detected.

Differential diagnosis
The differential diagnosis of congenital heart disease includes other congenital abnormalities as well as other types of cardiac disease (e.g. cardiomyopathy, myositis), diseases that may be associated with exercise intolerance, dyspnoea and/or cough (e.g. primary pulmonary disease), pleural effusion or congestion (e.g. hypoalbuminaemia due to protein-losing nephropathy or enteropathy, liver cirrhosis, trauma).

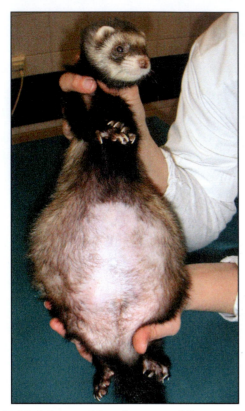

Fig. 12.21 A 2-year-old, male castrated ferret presented with a severely distended abdomen due to ascites resulting from an atrial septal defect.

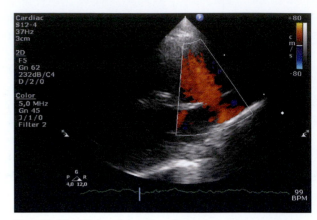

Fig. 12.22 With colour-flow Doppler, a direct blood flow between both atria could be seen in this ferret with an atrial septal defect. (Previously printed in *Journal of Exotic Pet Medicine* 2013;22 (1):70–77.)

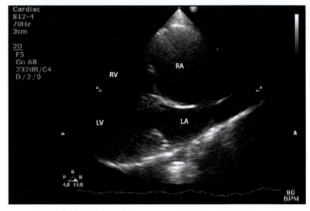

Fig. 12.23 Right parasternal long axis view of the heart of a ferret with an atrial septal defect. Severe eccentric hypertrophy of the right atrium and ventricle can be seen. LA, left atrium; LV, left ventricle; RA, right atrium; RV, right ventricle. (Previously printed in *Journal of Exotic Pet Medicine* 2013;22 (1):70–75.)

Diagnosis

Prior to the introduction of ultrasound, non-selective angiocardiography was needed to exclude or confirm congenital cardiovascular lesions. Nowadays, echocardiography is the preferred technique to be used for diagnosing congenital heart abnormalities. Colour Doppler ultrasonography may be useful to detect abnormalities in blood flow (e.g. left-to-right or right-to-left shunting, turbulent blood flow due to stenosis, valvular insufficiencies) (**Fig. 12.22**). Dependent on the type of defect that is present, secondary cardiac changes (e.g. atrial dilatation, concentric or eccentric ventricular hypertrophy) may also be noted (**Fig. 12.23**).

Radiographs may be performed in case congestive heart failure is suspected. These may reveal an enlarged cardiac silhouette and signs of congestive heart failure (e.g. pulmonary oedema, pleural effusion ascites).

Management/treatment

Treatment is dependent on the severity of the congenital heart disease. Mild congenital heart defects in asymptomatic ferrets may not require any treatment at all. Others may require treatment, which may include the use of drugs to treat congestive heart failure (e.g. furosemide, enalapril, pimobendan, digoxin, atenolol) or surgical intervention (e.g. preoperative donated autologous blood [PDAB]). Thus far, surgical intervention for congenital heart disease has not been described in ferrets.

Regardless of the type and severity of congenital heart disease, regular monitoring of the patients is recommended so that developing congestive heart failure can be caught early and treated promptly. Prognosis depends on the severity and type of congenital defect that is present. Small defects may often go undetected and not result in clinical disease, whereas larger defects may quickly result in death following birth. If congestive heart failure is present, prognosis is usually guarded, although treatment may help to alleviate clinical signs for up to several months or years.

ACQUIRED HEART DISEASE

Among the acquired heart diseases, dilated cardiomyopathy and acquired valvular disease (endocardiosis or myxomatous valvular degeneration) are the most common diseases to be encountered in ferrets. Other, less frequently reported, cardiac conditions include infectious diseases (such as fungal or bacterial myo-, endo- or pericarditis, toxoplasmosis (see Chapter 18), heartworm disease or dirofilariasis, and Aleutian disease (see Chapter 16), neoplasia (e.g. lymphoma, lymphosarcoma, see Chapter 16), hypertrophic cardiomyopathy and pericardial effusion.

DILATED CARDIOMYOPATHY

Definition/overview

The most common acquired cardiac disorder to be encountered in ferrets is dilated cardiomyopathy (DCM), which is characterised by an increased diastolic dimension and systolic dysfunction of the left and/or right ventricles (**Fig. 12.24**). As a result of the decreased contractility and diminished cardiac output the renin–angiotensin–aldosterone system (RAAS) is activated, which subsequently will lead to sodium retention, fluid accumulation and volume overload. This will result in an eccentric hypertrophy (dilatation) of the ventricle, valvular insufficiency and – once the disease progresses – signs of congestive heart failure (e.g. pulmonary oedema, pleural effusion, ascites). Histologically, DCM is characterised by multifocal myocyte degeneration and necrosis, myofibre loss and replacement fibrosis. Occasionally, inflammatory infiltrates may be present.

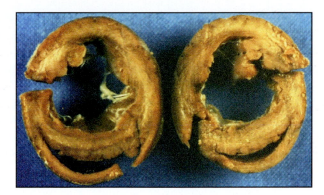

Fig. 12.24 **Transsections of the left and right ventricle of a ferret heart with dilated cardiomyopathy. Note the wide lumen of the left ventricle. (Courtesy of Michael Garner, Northwest ZooPath.)**

Aetiology/pathophysiology

DCM is most common in middle-aged to older ferrets, with no sex predilection reported. The exact aetiology is not known (i.e. idiopathic). Associations with taurine or carnitine deficiencies, as seen in cats and dogs, have been made, but cannot thus far be confirmed in ferrets. Other causes might include pre-existing endocrine disease, intoxications or infectious disease (e.g. viruses). In one ferret, DCM was reported in association with a cryptococcal infection. Similar to humans, cats and dogs, a genetic origin may also be present.

Clinical signs

Clinical signs are similar to those observed in dogs and cats. Ferrets may initially appear asymptomatic but once the disease progresses, clinical signs such as lethargy, weakness, anorexia, weight loss, exercise intolerance and respiratory distress (tachypnoea, dyspnoea, cough) may be seen. Further physical examination may reveal a weak pulse, pulse deficit, hypothermia, pallor, cyanosis, prolonged CRT, posterior paresis, hepato-/splenomegaly and/or ascites. Upon heart auscultation, a tachycardia (>250 bpm), (systolic) heart murmur, gallop rhythm or arrhythmia may be identified. In case of pleural effusion, the ferret may show increased respiratory effort with muffled heart and lung sounds heard on auscultation. Although the size of the ferret may be a limiting factor, thoracic percussion may be useful to detect and delineate pleural effusion by presence of respectively resonant and dull sounds, dorsal and ventral to the horizontal line of effusion. Pulmonary oedema may also be present and will result in moist rales, crackles and increased respiratory sounds to be heard during auscultation.

Differential diagnosis

Differential diagnoses for posterior paresis may include metabolic disease (in particular hypoglycaemia due to insulinoma), anaemia (e.g. due to hyperoestrogenism-related pancytopaenia, chronic renal failure, leukaemia, blood loss in the GI tract), neurological or neuromuscular disease (e.g. spinal cord trauma, herniated disc) or generalised weakness.

Differential diagnoses for tachy-/dyspnoea include primary lung disease (e.g. influenza, canine distemper virus, bronchitis, pneumonia, pulmonary haemorrhage, neoplasia), pleural effusion (e.g. due to chylo-, haemo- or pyothorax, mediastinal lymphoma or other type of neoplasia), pneumothorax, diaphragmatic herniation (e.g. due to trauma), upper airway disease (e.g. obstruction due to foreign body), hyperthermia, stress and/or pain. Differential diagnoses for ascites may include hypoproteinaemia (e.g. due to protein-losing enteropathy or nephropathy), liver cirrhosis, renal disease, ruptured bladder (uroabdomen), haemoabdomen (e.g. due to trauma), (septic) peritonitis, abdominal neoplasia (e.g. mesothelioma, lymphoma) and congestive heart failure due to other cardiac disease.

Diagnosis

A definite diagnosis is usually made using echocardiography. Characteristic findings are similar to those observed in other species and include thin ventricular walls, dilated left ventricle with increased end-systolic and end-diastolic dimensions, enlarged left atrium and reduced fractional shortening (**Fig. 12.25**). Outflow tract velocities of the left ventricle may be normal or reduced, as can be seen with pulsed-wave or continuous-wave Doppler. In case of involvement of the right side of the heart, the right ventricle and atrium may also be dilated. In advanced stages of the disease, mitral valve and tricuspid insufficiency and regurgitation may be seen upon the use of Doppler ultrasound. During the ultrasound, signs of congestion

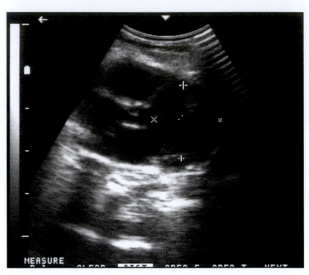

Fig. 12.25 Cardiac ultrasound of a 6-year-old ferret with dilated cardiomyopathy. The inner diameter of the left ventricle was 1.7 × 1.6 cm (reference <1.3 cm in ferrets). In addition to a dilated ventricle, a decreased wall thickness and decreased FS may also be observed. (Courtesy of Cathy Johnson-Delaney.)

(e.g. pleural effusion, liver congestion, ascites) may also be observed.

Radiographs may reveal an enlarged, globoid cardiac silhouette (**Fig. 12.26**). Moreover, radiographs can be useful to identify presence of signs of congestive heart failure such as pleural effusion or pulmonary oedema (**Fig. 12.14**), or to rule out mediastinal lymphoma (in dyspnoeic ferrets). If the abdomen is included in the radiograph, hepato- and/or splenomegaly, or ascites may also be detected (**Fig. 12.15**).

ECG may identify a variety of abnormalities, including atrial and ventricular premature contractions, atrial or ventricular tachycardia, atrial fibrillation and first- or second-degree heart block. Similarly, ECG may reveal signs of left atrial or ventricular enlargement (e.g. broadened P-wave, reduced voltage and/or widened QRS-complexes; **Fig. 12.27**). Often, however, the ECG will appear normal, thereby not aiding in the diagnosis.

In humans, dogs and cats, b-type natriuretic peptide (BNP) and N-terminal pro-b-type natriuretic peptide (NT pro-BNP) levels were found to be increased in individuals with cardiomyopathy. Renal insufficiency may, however, also result in increased levels. Although similar findings may

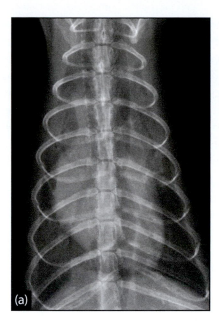

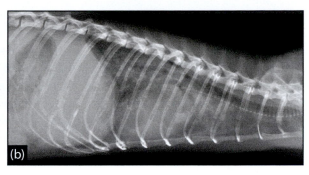

Fig. 12.26 Radiographs of a 6-year-old male castrated ferret with dilated cardiomyopathy. The dilated heart will result in an enlarged cardiac silhouette, as can be seen in both the dorsoventral and lateral views. Moreover, the trachea is displaced dorsally, as can be seen on the lateral view. Based on radiographs, a pericardial effusion cannot be ruled out.

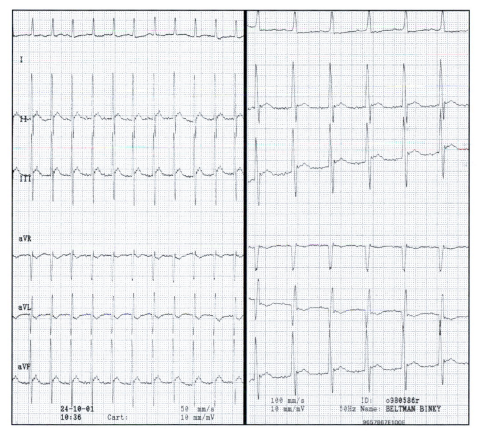

Fig. 12.27 ECG of a ferret with dilated cardiomyopathy showing an increased heart rate (350/min; reference 175–265/min), and a left rotation of the heart (MEA 60°; reference 85° to 102° for ferrets), indicative of an enlargement of the left ventricle. The other cardiac measurements were within normal limits. (Previously printed in *Seminars in Avian and Exotic Pet Medicine* 2005;14(1):34–51.)

apply to ferrets with cardiomyopathy, the aforementioned blood tests currently appear to be of limited clinical use to the practitioner. Routine blood tests and urinalysis will generally not reveal abnormalities unless there is presence of severe heart failure resulting in prerenal azotaemia, hyponatraemia and increased alanine aminotransferase (ALT) concentrations, or concurrent disease. Similarly, therapy may induce biochemical changes (e.g. hypokalaemia, hypochloraemia induced by diuresis).

If pleural effusion or ascites is present, thoraco- or abdominocentesis may be performed. Cytology, culture or chemical analysis may be performed on the collected fluid to identify its origin (i.e. transudate, exudate, chylus, etc.).

Management/treatment

Therapy for acute clinical congestive heart failure includes oxygen therapy, administration of diuretics (e.g. furosemide, 1–4 mg/kg q8–12h IV or IM), nitroglycerin (2% ointment, $^1/_{16}$–$^1/_8$ inch topically on the hairless skin q12–24h), and thoracocentesis (if pleural effusion is present). External heat (e.g. incubator or heating pad) may be provided if the animal is hypothermic. The response to this initial treatment always needs to be monitored closely. This can best be done by regularly evaluating the respiratory rate and effort and auscultating lung sounds. Handling of critically dyspnoeic ferrets should, however, be minimised as too much stress may result in death of the animal.

After the ferret's condition has stabilised, therapy may be initiated with diuretics (e.g. furosemide, 1–2 mg/kg q8–12h PO), ACE inhibitors, and pimobendan and/or digoxin. The dose of diuretics should be reduced to the lowest dose that prevents reaccumulation of pleural effusion and pulmonary oedema, as overzealous administration of diuretics may result in dehydration and hypokalaemia. ACE inhibitors (e.g. enalapril, 0.25–0.5 mg/kg q24–48h PO) are recommended for long-term therapy as these may be useful to reduce pre- and afterload, which helps to improve cardiac output and reduce congestion, respectively. Care should, however, be taken to prevent overdosing with ACE inhibitors as ferrets are suggested to be sensitive to their hypotensive effects, thereby quickly becoming weak

and lethargic. Pimobendan (0.5 mg/kg q12h PO) and digoxin (5–10 µg/kg q12–24h PO) may be used to increase ventricular contractility. For severe systolic dysfunction, a combination of both drugs may be beneficial. Aside from acting as a positive inotrope, pimobendan acts as a vasodilator, thereby helping to reduce pre- and afterload. Digoxin, on the other hand, may be useful in ferrets with atrial fibrillation, as it slows down the heart rate. It may be given for this indication with or without propranolol (0.2–1.0 mg/kg q8–12h PO) with the intended goal to slow down heart rate to 180–250 bpm in resting state. Since digoxin has a narrow therapeutic window, careful monitoring of serum concentrations (therapeutic range: 1–2 ng/mL 6–12h following oral administration) and clinical signs of toxicity (e.g. tremor, nausea, emesis, diarrhoea, collapse, arrhythmia, dyspnoea) is recommended, especially in patients with renal insufficiency. Long-term management may furthermore include periodic monitoring of the patient (including a physical examination, thoracic radiographs, echocardiography, ECG, blood pressure measurement and plasma biochemistry, including urea or BUN and electrolytes), feeding the ferret a low-salt diet and restricting exercise, as these have been suggested to be beneficial in the management of heart failure. The latter two measures may, however, be difficult to institute in practice. Although in dogs and cats, carnitine or taurine supplementation were found capable of reversing the disease, in ferrets thus far no clinical improvement has been reported following taurine supplementation. Currently, the amount of available data is too limited to provide an accurate estimation of the prognosis of ferrets with DCM. If the disease is diagnosed in an early stage, prognosis generally appears fair, with ferrets often responding well to therapy and living a good quality of life for several months up to 2 years. In more advanced stages of the disease, the prognosis should be considered more guardedly. Sudden death may occur due to life-threatening arrhythmias.

DIROFILARIASIS (HEARTWORM DISEASE)

Definition/overview

Dirofilariasis or heartworm disease is an uncommon disease in ferrets, caused by an infection with

Dirofilaria immitis. The susceptibility and life cycle of *D. immitis* have been studied extensively in ferrets and were found to be similar to those in dogs. However, because of the ferret's small size, the clinical presentation more closely resembles that of infected cats. Worms may reside in the right ventricle, cranial vena cava, or main pulmonary artery and cause villous endarteritis. Although natural infections with worm burdens of up to 21 worms have been reported, ferrets may already develop severe heart disease by the presence of a single worm, due to the small size of the ferret's heart (**Fig. 12.28**). As few as two adult heartworms may result in fatal

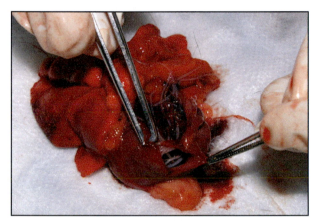

Fig. 12.28 **Postmortem image of a heart of a ferret infected with heartworm. Note the large amount of worms present in this heart, as even one or two worms may be fatal in ferrets. (Courtesy of Natalie Antinoff.)**

right-sided heart failure, especially if the worm's presence causes a mechanical obstruction of the blood flow (e.g. due to the presence of worms in the right ventricle or pulmonary artery).

Aetiology/pathophysiology

D. immitis is a filarial parasite that is transmitted by mosquitoes, which serve as a vector and intermediate host for the parasite. Microfilaria are ingested by mosquitoes and become infective in the third stage, at which they migrate subcutaneously to the thorax and vascular system following their deposition onto the skin when the mosquito feeds. Microfilaria can be found within the small pulmonary arteries of as many as 50–60% of infected animals. Dogs are considered the primary reservoir, but heartworms may also infect other animals such as ferrets, which are considered aberrant hosts. Ferrets that live in or originate from heartworm-endemic areas (i.e. along the Atlantic and Gulf coast, in tropical and semi-tropical areas; **Fig. 12.29**), especially those that are kept outdoors, are considered most at risk to develop disease.

Clinical presentation

Clinical signs of heartworm disease in ferrets are similar to those observed in the dog, and may range from asymptomatic individuals to sudden death, most probably resulting from pulmonary artery obstruction. Other clinical signs that have been

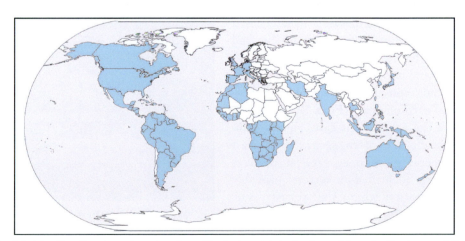

Fig. 12.29 **Worldwide distribution of canine *Dirofilaria immitis* infections (blue shading) as published on http://creatureclinic.com (with permission). Ferrets that live in these areas are at an increased risk of becoming infected and should therefore regularly receive preventive medication.**

reported include anorexia, lethargy, weakness, depression, dyspnoea, tachypnoea, cyanosis, coughing, pale mucous membranes, abdominal distension, and (rarely) melena. Further physical examination may reveal laboured breathing, crackles and moist rales in case of pulmonary oedema, or shallow breathing, decreased chest compliance and muffled heart and lung sounds in case of pleural effusion. Ascites, hepato- and splenomegaly may also be present in case of right-sided heart failure. Upon heart auscultation, a tachycardia and/or heart murmur may sometimes be heard. Occasionally, arrhythmias (most commonly atrial fibrillation) may also be present. Caval syndrome, frequently leading to haemoglobinaemia, haemoglobinuria, and haemolytic anaemia, as well as renal and hepatic dysfunction, has been reported in ferrets and may be life threatening. Aberrant larval migration, with associated CNS signs, has also been documented in one ferret with a *D. immitis* infection.

Differential diagnosis

Differential diagnoses include other causes of heart failure (e.g. dilated cardiomyopathy), mediastinal lymphoma, and other systemic or pulmonary diseases resulting in dyspnoea, tachypnoea and/or cough.

Diagnosis

Due to the rapid progression of the disease, it is important to diagnose heartworm as early as possible. Diagnosis of heartworm disease is usually based on clinical signs, combined with radiographic and echocardiographic findings, and testing for circulating microfilariae and heartworm antigen.

Thoracic radiographs may reveal pleural effusion, ascites and cardiomegaly (**Figs 12.14–12.16**). Enlargement of the caudal vena cava, right atrium and right ventricle are often seen. In contrast to dogs, peripheral pulmonary arterial changes are not commonly identified in ferrets, probably because of the location where the worms reside (i.e. in the right side of the heart and pulmonary arteries versus the lung arterioles and lung parenchyma). Angiography may reveal right-sided heart enlargement and filling defects in the right side of the heart, pulmonary artery and vena cava.

Its clinical usefulness is, however, limited due to the need for specialised equipment and experience with the technique. Echocardiography may be extremely useful in the diagnosis as the adult worms may be visualised in the pulmonary artery, right ventricle and/or right atrium as parallel, linear echodensities (**Fig. 12.30**). Right atrial and ventricular dilation may also be noted. Doppler echocardiography may be useful to confirm the presence of pulmonary hypertension.

A modified Knott's test may be performed to detect circulating microfilaria. However, peripheral microfilaraemia may only be observed in approximately 50% of affected animals, thereby limiting the usefulness of this test. Low worm burdens (<5 worms) and single-sex infections will commonly result in false-negative results. Serological tests that identify adult *D. immitis* antigen (**Fig. 12.31**) appear to have higher diagnostic usefulness, although little is known regarding its sensitivity and specificity. Since the test (an enzyme-linked immunosorbent assay, ELISA) will only detect antigen that is shed by the adult female heartworms, false-negative results may occur in ferrets with low worm burdens. Tests that detect circulating antibodies to immature and adult heartworm antigen may be of use but, similarly as for antigen tests, further studies are needed to evaluate the sensitivity and specificity of these tests in ferrets. A complete blood count and biochemistry

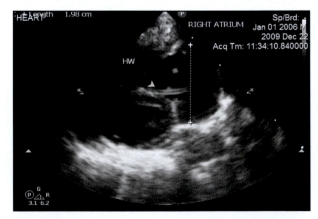

Fig. 12.30 Cardiac ultrasound image of a male ferret infected with *D. immitis*. The small arrowhead points towards the heartworm which can be recognised as two hyperechoic parallel lines. (Courtesy of Natalie Antinoff.)

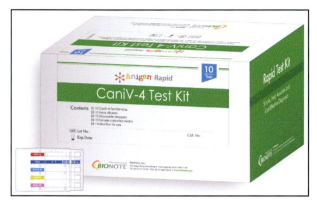

Fig. 12.31 A serological test to detect *D. immitis* antigens is commercially available. However, the sensitivity and specificity of this test in ferrets is currently not known.

profile will often be normal although mild to moderate anaemia may occasionally be noted. Eosinophilia and basophilia, which are often associated with parasitic burdens, are generally not seen in ferrets with heartworm disease.

Management/treatment

Treatment options for ferrets with heartworm disease include adulticide therapy combined with symptomatic treatment to alleviate the clinical signs that result from the right-sided heart failure. The currently recommended treatment protocol for ferrets with heartworm disease includes ivermectin (0.05–0.1 mg/kg q30d SC), which needs to be administered until clinical signs resolve and microfilaraemia is no longer present. Other treatment protocols include the use of adulticides such as melarsomine (Immiticide, Rhone Merieux; 2.5 mg/kg IM followed by two injections 24 h apart 1 month later) and thiacetarsamide (0.22 mL/kg q12h IV for 2 days). If the ferret is microfilaria positive, a microfilaricide therapy may be initiated 4–6 weeks following adulticide therapy. Microfilaricides that have been used include dithiazanine iodide (6–20 mg/kg PO), ivermectin (0.05–0.1 mg/kg q30d PO) or milbemycin oxime (1.15–2.33 mg/kg q30d PO) although therapeutic efficacy of the latter two has not been clearly documented. Transvenous heartworm extraction is nowadays also considered a viable option, especially since adulticide therapy has fallen out of favour because

of adverse reactions that were observed, which anecdotally have included sudden death and myositis at the injection site. Moxidectin (0.1 mL SC) has anecdotally also been suggested as an effective and safe adulticide.

Treatment for heartworm disease carries a risk of complications from worm emboli. As a result, prednisone (0.5–1 mg/kg q12–24h PO) is often initiated concurrently with the adulticide treatment and continued for at least 4 months. Strict cage rest and restriction of exercise is also advised for at least 4–6 weeks following adulticide therapy.

Symptomatic ferrets may require stabilisation and treatment for heart failure (including oxygen, furosemide, enalapril and theophylline) prior to initiating adulticide treatment. Thoracocentesis may be indicated in ferrets with pleural effusion. Whether pre-treatment with doxycycline for *Wolbachia* (a bacteria that lives in symbiosis with *D. immitis* and contributes to renal and pulmonary pathology) will enhance the efficacy of heartworm therapy in ferrets, similar to dogs, is currently not known.

A follow-up ELISA for heartworm antigen may be performed approximately 3 months after initiating therapy, following which testing may be repeated on a monthly basis until results are negative (usually 4 months following successful adulticide therapy). Further diagnostic tests (e.g. radiographs, echocardiography) may be warranted in case test results remain positive. To prevent reinfection, appropriate prophylaxis is needed. Control is best achieved through monthly administration of a heartworm preventive to ferrets in heartworm-endemic areas. This may include the administration of ivermectin (0.05 mg/kg q30d PO or SC), milbemycin oxime (1.15–2.33 mg/kg q30d PO), selamectin (18 mg/kg topically) or moxidectin (0.1 mL [single dose] SC, repeat every 6 months). Therapy should start 1 month before and continuing until 1 month after the heartworm season. Housing ferrets indoors, particularly during the mosquito season, may also help to minimise exposure.

Prognosis is considered fair to guarded for ferrets with asymptomatic infections. For ferrets with moderate-to-severe infections, postadulticide pulmonary complications (e.g. pulmonary thromboembolism) are likely.

ENDOCARDITIS

Overview/definition

An endocarditis is characterised by an inflammation of the endocardial tissues. This may include the valves (endocarditis valvularis), but the wall (endocarditis parietalis) and chordae tendineae (endocarditis chordalis) may also be affected.

Aetiology/pathophysiology

To date, one case report described the presence of non-bacterial endocarditis of the aortic valvular leaflets in a 4-year-old male ferret. Aside from non-bacterial endocarditis, bacterial endocarditis (due to haematogenic spread of bacteria resulting from bacteraemia or infections elsewhere in the body) may potentially also be found in ferrets, similar to other animals. Thus far, however, no reports have been found to confirm the presence of this disease in ferrets.

Clinical presentation

Clinical signs that may be observed are similar to those described in dogs and cats and may include lethargy, anorexia, weight loss, lameness and pyrexia. Haemorrhage may also occur if the animal develops disseminated intravascular coagulation (DIC). Moreover, a cardiac murmur may be heard upon auscultation. In the ferret with non-bacterial endocardiosis clinical signs included hindlimb ataxia and weakness, which both developed shortly after diagnosis of a bite wound-associated cellulitis. A high-intensity cardiac murmur was not heard at that time, but was noticed during a recheck 2 weeks after the ferret's initial presentation.

Differential diagnosis

Differential diagnoses for endocarditis include endocardiosis and other types of heart disease such as DCM.

Diagnosis

Establishing a final diagnosis can be difficult. In dogs, a presumptive diagnosis is usually made on the finding of two or more positive blood cultures in addition to echocardiographic evidence of vegetations or valve destruction, or the documented recent onset of a (regurgitant) cardiac murmur. However, negative cultures do not rule out the possibility of bacterial endocarditis, and structural abnormalities and vegetations visualised during echocardiography will be difficult to differentiate from endocardiosis. A haematologic profile may sometimes reveal neutrophila and monocytosis as well as thrombocytopaenia or prolonged clotting times (if the animal has developed DIC). Hypoalbuminaemia, hypoglycaemia, proteinuria and pyuria may also be found. Radiographs and ECG are often unremarkable, although occasionally signs of congestive heart failure (e.g. pleural effusion) or ventricular arrhythmias may be noticed.

In the ferret with non-bacterial endocarditis, echocardiography revealed an irregular thickening of the valve leaflets, with normal chamber dimensions and normal systolic function. As the ferret's condition rapidly deteriorated, the ferret was euthanased. Postmortem examination revealed myxomatous degeneration of the aortic valves, with ulceration and vegetative lesions. As no bacterial aetiological agent could be identified upon culture and histopathology, a final diagnosis of non-bacterial thrombotic endocarditis was made.

Treatment and prognosis

Thus far, no treatment has been described in ferrets. In the case of bacterial endocarditis, prolonged antibiotic treatment (over the course of at least 4 weeks) will often be required. For this purpose, either a broad-spectrum antibiotic or an appropriate antibiotic based on culture and sensitivity results can be used. Further treatment will generally be symptomatic and aimed at alleviating the clinical signs.

In other animals, long-term prognosis is considered guarded to poor, with animals often succumbing to complications associated with endocarditis (e.g. septic shock, DIC, congestive heart failure and embolisation of other organs).

HYPERTROPHIC CARDIOMYOPATHY

Definition/overview

Hypertrophic cardiomyopathy (HCM) is a rare condition in ferrets. HCM is characterised by concentric hypertrophy (i.e. increased wall thickness)

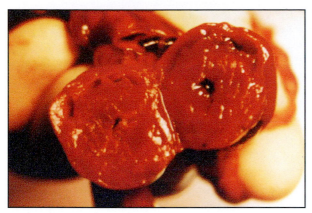

Fig. 12.32 Severe concentric hypertrophy (i.e. increased wall thickness) of the left ventricular wall and interventricular septum in the heart of a ferret with hypertrophic cardiomyopathy. (Courtesy of Michael Garner, Northwest ZooPath.)

of the left ventricular wall and interventricular septum (**Fig. 12.32**). The increased wall thickness results in lack of compliance and impaired filling of the ventricle (diastolic dysfunction), with subsequent increases in ventricular filling pressure and enlargement of the left atrium. Secondary to these changes, pulmonary venous hypertension and pulmonary oedema may develop. In addition, mitral valve insufficiency and/or biventricular failure may occasionally be seen. Histologically, HCM is characterised by hyperplasia of the individual myofibres, primarily of the left ventricle.

Aetiology/pathophysiology

HCM is suggested to occur more commonly in younger ferrets, although it is difficult to provide accurate accounts of any predisposing factors due to the low incidence of the disease. The aetiology is currently unknown. Genetic abnormalities have been reported in humans and cats, but have thus far not been studied in ferrets. Similarly, no association has been found with hyperthyroidism or hypertension (as has been diagnosed in cats).

Clinical presentation

Due to the low incidence of HCM in ferrets, little is known about the classical clinical presentation of the disease. It is, however, likely that the clinical course follows a similar pattern to that in cats, remaining silent until the onset of heart failure, thromboembolism or sudden death. Clinical presentation may thus range from an asymptomatic ferret to sudden death (especially during anaesthesia) without pre-emptive signs. If clinical signs are seen, these may be linked either to the reduced cardiac output resulting from the impaired ventricular filling (e.g. weakness manifesting by paresis posterior, ataxia) or to the increased filling pressure in the left ventricle that results in pulmonary congestion (left-sided heart failure) and clinical signs of tachypnoea and dyspnoea. A further physical examination may reveal a weak or irregular pulse, tachycardia, (S3 or S4) gallop rhythm, arrhythmias and/or systolic heart murmur. In case of pulmonary congestion, increased respiratory sounds, moist rales and/or crackles may be heard.

Differential diagnosis

Differential diagnoses are similar to those reported for DCM. In addition, hypovolaemia may cause the heart wall to appear thickened, thereby mimicking HCM.

Diagnosis

Similar to DCM, echocardiography is the most commonly used technique to diagnose HCM in ferrets. Ultrasound may reveal (generalised or local) gross thickening of the interventricular septum and/or left ventricular free wall, and decreased left ventricular dimensions (**Fig. 12.33**). Fractional shortening may be normal or increased. In addition, left atrial enlargement or systolic anterior mitral valve motion (associated with interventricular septum hypertrophy) may be seen. Doppler echocardiographic evaluation may furthermore reveal turbulence in the left ventricular outflow tract secondary to dynamic obstruction and mitral regurgitation (**Fig. 12.34**).

Similar to DCM, radiographs may reveal a normal to increased cardiac silhouette or – in case of (left-sided) heart failure – signs of pulmonary oedema or pleural effusion. Electrocardiography may reveal sinus tachycardia (>280 bpm) and – occasionally – atrial or ventricular premature contractions. In addition, widened QRS-complexes of increased amplitude, as well as signs of atrial enlargement (i.e. broadened P-wave) may be noted.

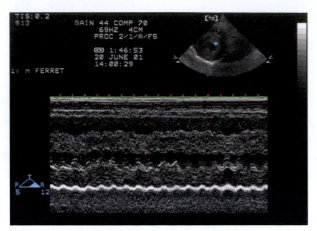

Fig. 12.33 M-mode ultrasound of a 1-year-old ferret with hypertrophic cardiomyopathy. The left ventricular wall diameter during diastole (LVWd) was 20 mm (reference 1.8–3.7 mm) and the LVWd during systole was 22 mm (reference 2.4 –5.9 mm). (Courtesy of Robert A. Wagner and Donald Brown.)

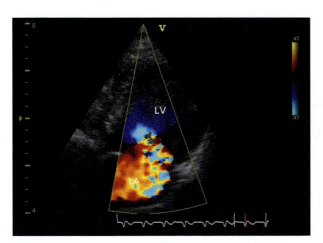

Fig. 12.34 Doppler echocardiogram revealing turbulence around the mitral valves, which may be secondary to a dynamic obstruction. (Courtesy of Robert A. Wagner.)

Haematology and biochemistry will generally be normal, although signs of prerenal azotemia (i.e. increased urea) may be noted.

Management/treatment

Treatment for ferrets with HCM is aimed at eliminating heart failure (if present) and – following stabilisation – improving the diastolic filling of the ventricles. Beta-blockers, e.g. propranolol (0.2–1.0 mg/kg q8–12h PO) or atenolol (3.125–6.25 mg q24h PO) are commonly recommended to reduce heart rate and correct atrial and ventricular arrhythmias. In addition, calcium channel blockers (e.g. diltiazem, 3.75–7.5 mg q12h PO) may be administered to reduce heart rate, improve diastolic relaxation and ventricular filling and induce vasodilatation, which may help to reduce pre- and afterload and increase myocardial perfusion (through vasodilatation of the coronary arteries). Combined, the two drugs help to reduce myocardial oxygen consumption and increase cardiac output, but care should be taken to prevent overdosing as this may result in significant bradycardia, hypotension, lethargy and/or inappetence. Drugs are titrated to effect, i.e. until an effective reduction in heart rate and clinical improvement is seen.

If clinical signs of heart failure are present, treatment with diuretics and ACE inhibitors may be considered. Positive inotropic drugs should be avoided. Aspirin or heparin therapy is not considered necessary due to the rare incidence of arterial thromboembolism in ferrets.

Therapeutic monitoring follows similar guidelines as those for ferrets with DCM.

Due to the low incidence of the disease, reliable information regarding prognosis is lacking. Ferrets with HCM are generally considered to have a guarded to poor prognosis, with survival times estimated to be only a few months following the time of diagnosis, and sudden death occurring in various patients.

MYOCARDITIS

Definition/overview

Myocarditis is a focal or diffuse inflammation of the myocardium with myocyte degeneration and/or necrosis, which results in reduced myocardial function, arrhythmias, and – in the end stages – replacement fibrosis (**Fig. 12.35**). The condition is rarely diagnosed in ferrets.

Aetiology/pathophysiology

Myocarditis can have various causes, and may occur as part of a systemic vasculitis, autoimmune disease,

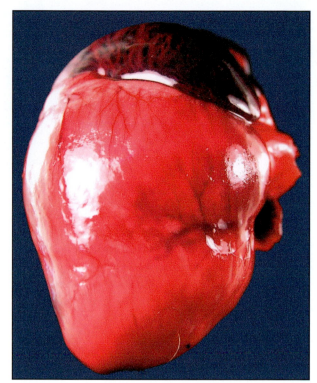

Fig. 12.35 **Heart of a ferret with disseminated idiopathic myofasciitis (DIM). The white streaks of the myocardium are signs of myocarditis. (Courtesy of Michael Garner, Northwest ZooPath.)**

intoxication (e.g. doxorubicin cardiotoxicosis), traumatic injury (e.g. cardiac puncture or ischaemic events) or parasitic, bacterial, fungal or viral infection. In addition, myocarditis may occur secondary to an endocarditis or inflammatory process elsewhere in the body.

A *Toxoplasma*-like organism has been described as causing multifocal myocardial necrosis in ferrets. Similarly, Aleutian disease (a parvoviral infection, see Chapter 16) may cause fibrinoid necrosis and mononuclear cell infiltration in interstitium of the subepicardium, subendocardium and myocardium. Inflammatory lesions in the myocardium have furthermore been observed in hearts of ferrets with bacterial or fungal sepsis.

Clinical presentation

The clinical signs to be observed in ferrets with myocarditis are generally the result of the systolic dysfunction or pathological arrhythmias that occur.

These may result in classic signs of congestive left or right heart failure (e.g. dyspnoea, tachypnoea, ascites) or sudden death due to onset of ventricular tachycardia or ventricular fibrillation. Other signs that may be noted include lethargy, anorexia and fever. A heart murmur, resulting from mitral or tricuspid valve regurgitation, may be audible upon auscultation, as well as an irregular heart rhythm.

Differential diagnosis

Differential diagnosis includes other causes of congestive heart failure and arrhythmias, as described elsewhere.

Diagnosis

The gold standard for the diagnosis of myocarditis is histological evaluation of the myocardium. Because of the difficulty in obtaining cardiac biopsies, antemortem diagnosis is difficult. Thus, the clinical diagnosis of acute myocarditis is usually presumptive and based on exclusion of other causes of cardiac disease. Atrial fibrillation is commonly seen during ECG, but ventricular or atrial premature complexes may also be seen. Echocardiography may reveal chamber dilation and poor contractility of the ventricles with essentially normal valves. A haematological and biochemical profile may reveal leucocytosis, neutrophilia and hyperfibrinogenaemia. Cardiac isoenzymes (creatinine kinase, lactate dehydrogenase and troponin) are often increased. Particularly serum cardiac troponin T (cTnT) and I (cTnI) are considered to be sensitive and specific indicators of myocardial damage (e.g. due to ischaemia or inflammation) in humans and other animals, and may therefore also be of use in the ferret. Reference ranges for normal ferrets (i.e. 0.05–0.10 ng/mL) are, however, found to be below the detection limit of a commercially available assay. Combined with a lack of clinical trials or controlled studies this currently limits the clinical use of cTnT and cTnI in ferrets.

Management/treatment

Treatment of myocarditis should be aimed at eliminating the primary cause and symptomatic treatment of congestive heart failure and arrhythmias. Pimobendan or digoxin may be used to improve contractility, whereas furosemide may be indicated to control signs of pulmonary oedema, pleural effusion or ascites. In case an infectious agent is deemed unlikely, the use of corticosteroids may be considered.

Prognosis is dependent on the cause and may be favourable in patients that can be treated in an early stage of the disease. Most often, however, diagnosis will only be made *post mortem.*

NEOPLASIA

Definition/overview
Neoplasia involving the myocardium or pericardium has thus far not been reported in ferrets. The authors have, however, diagnosed a ventricular sarcoma in a 5-year-old male ferret that was presented with a sudden onset of dyspnoea. A gallop rhythm was heard on auscultation. In addition, a pleural effusion was found. The ferret died shortly after presentation in the clinic, thereby enabling the diagnosis only to be made at postmortem examination.

Neoplasia within the cranial mediastinum has, however, been reported in ferrets more often, and will be described below.

Aetiology/pathophysiology
Cranial mediastinal or thoracic masses frequently involve lymphomas or lymphosarcomas, one of the most commonly reported neoplastic diseases in ferrets (**Fig. 12.36**). The disease is often seen in younger ferrets ranging from 10 months to 2 years. Although these tumours do not directly involve the cardiovascular system, they may result in clinical signs resembling cardiac disease as the result of compression of the cardiovascular structures within the thoracic cavity.

Clinical presentation
Ferrets with cranial mediastinal or thoracic masses may clinically present with mild to marked dyspnoea associated with the presence of pleural effusion or the mass-associated effect of the tumour. In addition, anorexia, lethargy, weight loss, generalised lymphadenopathy and/or hepatosplenomegaly may be present. Clinical signs will furthermore vary depending on the organ involvement (e.g. liver, spleen, kidney, intestines) in the disease process.

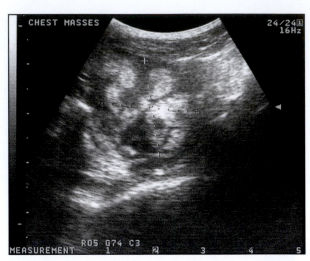

Fig. 12.36 Cranial mediastinal or thoracic masses frequently involve lymphomas or lymphosarcomas, one of the most commonly reported neoplastic diseases in ferrets. (Courtesy of Cathy Johnson-Delaney.)

Differential diagnosis
Important differential diagnoses for mediastinal lymphoma include thymoma, pleuritis/pleuropneumonia, abscesses or granulomas and cardiovascular disease.

Diagnosis
Radiography will often reveal a pleural effusion accompanied by the presence of a radio-opaque mass in the mediastinal area. Ultrasonography may also be useful to rule out the presence of cardiac disease and to visualise the mass (if obscured by the pleural effusion). Fine-needle aspirates of the mass, or cytological examination of the pleural effusion, can be used to establish a definite diagnosis.

Management/treatment
Although chemotherapy protocols for lymphoma have been published, prognosis is generally considered poor, especially since lymphoma will commonly involve other organs (e.g. liver, spleen). Aside from chemotherapy, palliative treatment using prednisolone may be considered, as well as symptomatic treatment to alleviate the clinical signs.

RESTRICTIVE CARDIOMYOPATHY

Definition/overview

Restrictive cardiomyopathy, which is defined as a clinically normal-appearing left ventricle combined with left atrial enlargement, is rare in ferrets, with only two cases reported in literature. Restrictive cardiomyopathy is a disease in which the heart muscle is stiffened and does not expand, preventing normal filling of the ventricles (i.e. diastolic dysfunction).

Aetiology/pathophysiology

As with cats, the cause of restrictive cardiomyopathy is unknown, although scar formation following inflammation and/or ischaemic events may play a role.

Clinical presentation

Clinical signs, diagnosis and treatment follow that of HCM.

Differential diagnosis

Differential diagnoses are similar to those for HCM and DCM.

Diagnosis

Definite diagnosis requires documentation of diastolic dysfunction during ultrasound (e.g. using tissue Doppler imaging) or histological evaluation of cardiac tissue.

Management/treatment

Treatment follows similar guidelines to those described for HCM. In cats, prognosis of restrictive cardiomyopathy appears guarded to poor, with animals rarely surviving for long periods of time following the diagnosis and responding poorly to therapy. Prognosis in ferrets is likely to be similar.

VALVULAR DISEASE (ACQUIRED) OR ENDOCARDIOSIS

Definition/overview

Acquired valvular disease (AVD) or endocardiosis is recognised with increasing frequency in ferrets. Valvular endocardiosis is characterised by degenerative changes and depositions of proteoglycans and glycosaminoglycans in the subendocardial valve leaflets and chordae tendineae. These changes subsequently lead to progressive valvular dysfunction, regurgitation of blood across the closed valve, and – in the final stages – congestive heart failure. The aortic and mitral valves appear most commonly affected, whereas changes to the tricuspid and pulmonic valves are observed less frequently. Gross lesions include opaque nodular thickening and shortening at the free edge and base of the valve leaflets. Mitral and aortic valve regurgitation may lead to secondary dilatation of the left atrium and ventricle. Isolated aortic valve regurgitation is often an incidental finding and rarely gives rise to congestive heart failure as a result of volume overload. In case of concurrent mitral valve regurgitation and/or other abnormalities (e.g. third-degree heart block), left-sided heart failure (e.g. pulmonary oedema, pleural effusion) may develop. In case of tricuspid valve regurgitation, right atrial and ventricular dilatation and subsequent right-sided heart failure (e.g. hepatosplenomegaly, ascites) may be seen.

Aetiology/pathophysiology

Endocardiosis is most commonly observed in middle-aged to older ferrets. Its cause is currently unknown.

Clinical presentation

Clinical signs are highly variable and depend on the severity of the underlying disease. Mitral valve regurgitation may result in a systolic murmur to be heard over the left apical region, whereas tricuspid valve regurgitation may be best auscultated in the right parasternal location. Aortic insufficiency, which may present as a diastolic murmur, is rarely heard upon auscultation. With significant aortic regurgitation, femoral pulses may be hyperdynamic, but often the pulse remains normal. If congestive heart failure is present, a weak pulse may be palpated. In addition, these ferrets may show dyspnoea, tachypnoea, increased respiratory sounds and moist rales or crackles during lung auscultation as a result of pulmonary oedema. Heart and lung sounds may also be muffled if pleural effusion is present. Coughing may be present due to presence of lung oedema and/or atrial enlargement. Ferrets with right-sided heart failure may furthermore display abdominal distension resulting from hepatosplenomegaly and/ or ascites.

Differential diagnosis

The primary differential diagnosis of chronic valvular heart disease in ferrets is DCM. Ultrasonography is essential to distinguish the two diseases.

Diagnosis

Echocardiography is considered the most valuable technique to diagnose valvular disease. Echocardiographic findings consistent with valvular disease include cardiomegaly, atrial and/or (mild) ventricular dilatation, thickening of the valves and a normal to increased fractional shortening with normal ventricular contractility and wall thickness (**Fig. 12.37**). Valvular regurgitation may be identified and quantified using colour flow and/or pulse wave Doppler (**Fig. 12.34**). Small regurgitant jets of blood may, however, also occur in clinically healthy ferrets and should not be mistaken as cardiac pathology during echocardiography. In most of these ferrets, no cardiac murmurs are heard.

Apart from echocardiography, thoracic radiographs may also be useful, as these may help to evaluate cardiac size and establish whether signs of congestive heart failure (pulmonary oedema, pleural effusion, ascites) are present. ECG is often unremarkable but may include signs of atrial enlargement (i.e. broadened P-wave) or atrial arrhythmias.

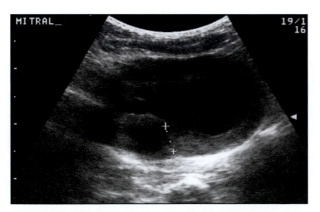

Fig. 12.37 Ultrasound valvular disease. Markers denote the mitral valve that appears thickened and irregular. (Courtesy of Cathy Johnson-Delaney.)

Management/treatment

Therapy is not recommended as long as ferrets are asymptomatic. If signs of congestive heart failure are present, treatment may be initiated with furosemide and ACE inhibitors such as enalapril. This will alleviate the neurohormonal activation of RAAS that occurs with advanced cardiac disease and congestive heart failure. In case of impaired systolic function and/or supraventricular arrhythmias, positive inotropic drugs, such as pimobendan and digoxin, may be given as soon as the ferret has been stabilised.

Currently, no scientific data are available to predict the prognosis in ferrets with congestive heart failure due to degenerative valvular disease. In dogs, 75% of patients are considered to have died within a year following diagnosis. Several factors may, however, influence the prognosis of ferrets with endocardiosis, including heart rate and rhythm, renal function and presence of concurrent disease.

PERICARDIAL EFFUSION AND PERICARDITIS

Definition/overview

A pericardial effusion is characterised by the presence of an abnormal amount of fluid between the heart and the pericardium. Dependent on the amount of fluid present in the pericardial sac, clinical signs may be totally absent or indicative of significant disease, resulting from impaired filling of the ventricles after effusion-associated compression of the ventricle (i.e. cardiac or pericardial tamponade). Pericardial effusions may occur as a primary condition or secondary to other medical conditions (e.g. cardiomyopathy or right-sided heart failure). Primary pericardial effusion without concurrent disease has thus far not been reported in ferrets.

Aetiology/pathophysiology

Pericardial effusions may be caused by inflammation of the pericardium (i.e. pericarditis). As the pericardium becomes inflamed, extra fluid is produced, leading to a pericardial effusion. In humans and other animals, viral or bacterial infections, neoplasia, uraemia, autoimmune disease, trauma, coagulopathies, hypoalbuminaemia and congestion (i.e. right-sided heart failure) may all result in pericardial effusion and/or pericarditis. If no cause can be identified, the pericardial effusion is referred to as being idiopathic.

Clinical signs

Clinical signs often result from an impaired cardiac output caused by compression of the pericardial effusion. If the pericardial effusion builds up slowly, the left ventricular function often remains intact and only signs associated with right-sided heart failure (i.e. hepatomegaly, ascites, pleural effusion with concurrent dyspnoea, tachypnoea and cough and exercise intolerance) will develop. A rapidly developing pericardial effusion may compromise both left and right ventricular outflow, thereby resulting in severe shock, syncopes and potentially death. In case of minor to moderate pericardial effusion, animals can remain asymptomatic, with the pericardial effusion only noted as a coincidental finding during echocardiography. Upon physical examination, a weak pulse and so-called pulsus paradoxus (a drop in arterial blood pressure concurrent with inspiration) may be detected. In addition, muffled cardiac sounds and tachycardia may be heard upon auscultation.

Diagnosis

Pericardial effusion is often diagnosed using echocardiography, which reveals the presence of excess fluid surrounding the heart. ECG may also be helpful, and reveal low-voltage QRS-complexes and pulsus alternans (i.e. changing amplitude of the QRS-complexes). Radiographs may reveal an enlarged cardiac silhouette, suggesting that a pericardial effusion may be present (**Fig. 12.38**). Definite diagnosis cannot, however, be made using radiography alone.

To identify the cause of the pericardial effusion, pericardiocentesis may be performed, following which the fluid may be submitted for cytological or biochemical analysis, or (bacterial) culture.

Treatment/management and prognosis

Treatment and prognosis depend on the severity and cause of the pericardial effusion. Small pericardial effusions in asymptomatic animals often require no special treatment. For pericardial effusion due to pericarditis or secondary to other diseases, treatment should be aimed at the initiating cause. If severe

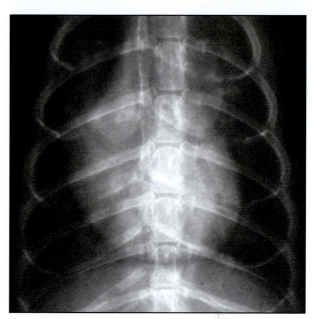

Fig. 12.38 **Radiograph of a ferret with an enlarged cardiac silhouette, suggestive of a pericardial effusion. (Courtesy of Cathy Johnson-Delaney.)**

pericardial effusion and cardiac impairment are present, the pericardial effusion should be drained using pericardiocentesis. In case of recurrence and/or idiopathic pericardial effusion, pericardiectomy may also be considered (although this has not yet been described in ferrets).

CARDIAC ARRHYTHMIAS AND CONDUCTION DISTURBANCES

Definition/overview

Cardiac arrhythmias and conduction abnormalities occur due to problems with the electrical conduction system of the heart. These may subsequently result in abnormalities in the heart rate (brady- or tachycardia), rhythm (arrhythmias, originating from the sinus, atria or ventricles) or impulse conduction (e.g. first-, second- or third-degree AV blocks). A (respiratory) sinus arrhythmia, sinus tachycardia and second-degree AV block have been reported to occur physiologically in healthy ferrets.

Aetiology/pathophysiology

Cardiac arrhythmias and conduction abnormalities may be physiological or pathological in origin.

Sinus arrhythmia is the most common abnormality to be noted, and may be caused by an increased vagal tone. Following exercise or administration of a parasympatholytic drug (e.g. atropine, glycopyrrolate), the sinus arrhythmia will often resolve. Similar to other animals, pathological arrhythmias may result following a variety of different causes including stress, pain, hyperthermia, hypoxia, shock, electrolyte or metabolic disturbances (e.g. hypercalcaemia, hypo- or hyperkalaemia), infections (e.g. sepsis), intoxications (e.g. digoxin), anaesthesia, endocrine disease (e.g. hyperthyroidism), anaemia and cardiac abnormalities (e.g. dilated cardiomyopathy, myocarditis).

Clinical presentation

Many cardiac arrhythmias and conduction abnormalities may go undetected and can be found as coincidental findings during routine auscultation or ECG. Second- and third-degree AV blocks are the most common conduction disturbances and may cause (life-threatening) bradycardia (<120 bpm) (**Fig. 12.18a; Figs 12.39–12.44**). As a result, clinical signs such as lethargy, weakness, exercise intolerance and syncope may be noted. Congestive heart failure and hypoperfusion may develop once the heart rate consistently drops below 80 bpm. In animals with severe tachycardia (>300 bpm), similar clinical signs may be noted. Due to impaired cardiac filling and output, the pulse will often be weak. Severe tachycardia, especially when ventricular in origin, may be life threatening and can quickly result in death if not treated promptly. Dependent on the type of arrhythmia or conduction disturbance that is present, irregular pulse waves or pulse deficits may also be palpated.

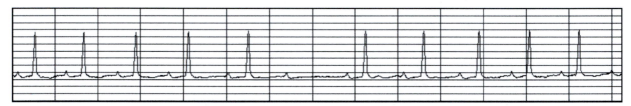

Fig. 12.39 Normal sinus rhythm. A single second-degree, Mobitz type II AV-block (absence of a QRS-complex following a P-wave), which is frequently seen in ferrets without further health implications, may also be seen in the middle of the ECG.

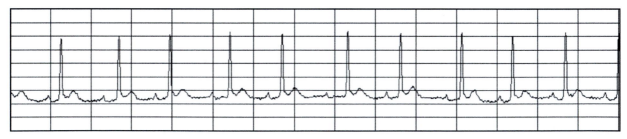

Fig. 12.40 Respiratory sinus arrhythmia, which is a physiologic phenomenon characterized by a mild alteration in the heart rate (i.e. acceleration and slowing) concurrent with the respiration.

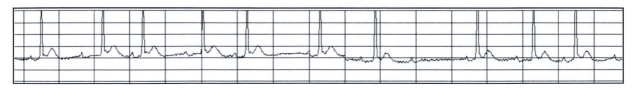

Fig. 12.41 Second-degree AV-block, Mobitz Type 1 or Wenkebach block, which is characterized by a progressive prolongation of the PR interval on consecutive beats until conduction of the P-wave finally fails (i.e. a 'dropped' QRS complex). After the dropped QRS complex, the PR interval resets and the cycle repeats.

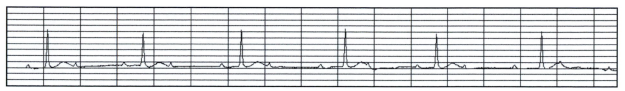

Fig. 12.42 Second-degree AV-block, Mobitz Type II or Hay block, which is characterized by a constant PR interval and intermittent non-conducted P-waves. Usually, there is a fixed number of non-conducted P-waves for every successfully conducted QRS complex, and this ratio is often specified in describing Mobitz II blocks. For example, in this ECG for every one QRS complex there are two P-waves, thereby referring to this AV-block as a '2:1 Mobitz II block'.

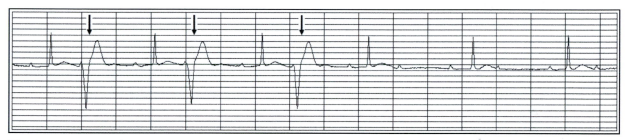

Fig. 12.43 ECG of the same ferret as in (**12.42**). In between the normal QRS complexes, ventricular premature complexes (VPCs; arrows) are present, which can be identified as wide QRS complexes of an abnormal configuration that is not preceded by a P-wave followed by a T-wave with an amplitude in the opposite direction compared to that of the QRS complex. In contrast to ventricular escape beats, which have a similar configuration and may be seen following a long pause, VPCs usually appear soon after a normal QRS complex. Potential underlying causes include, for example, hypoxia and underlying heart disease, such as dilated cardiomyopathy.

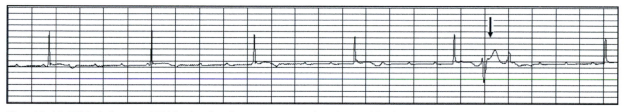

Fig. 12.44 Third-degree AV block, also known as complete heart block. Characteristic for this block is the absolute absence of conduction of the atrial impulses to the ventricles. Because the impulse is blocked, an accessory pacemaker in the lower chambers will typically activate the ventricles (i.e. an escape rhythm). Since this accessory pacemaker also activates independently of the impulse generated at the SA node, two independent rhythms can be noted on the ECG, i.e. (1) the atrial rhythm, as represented by the regular P-P intervals; (2) the escape rhythm, as represented by the regular R-R intervals, which may either be junctional (resulting in normal complexes as seen here) or ventricular (resulting in QRS complexes of abnormal configuration). A hallmark of complete heart block is the complete dissociation between the P-waves and QRS complexes. Typically, patients with a third-degree heart block experience bradycardia, as can also be seen in this ferret, demonstrating a heart frequency of 73 bpm. For junctional escape rhythms the frequency is often higher compared to the ventricular escape rhythm. At the end of the ECG, a ventricular premature complex (arrow) can be identified.

Differential diagnosis

Differential diagnoses include other causes of weakness and exercise intolerance, including metabolic disturbances (particularly hypoglycaemia due to insulinoma), neuromuscular disease (e.g. myasthenia gravis), anaemia (e.g. due to blood loss in the GI tract, impaired erythropoiesis in case of renal failure, lymphoma or hyperoestrogenism-related pancytopaenia), hypoxia resulting from primary pulmonary disease (e.g. influenza) or other types of cardiac disease (e.g. cardiomyopathy, myocarditis), hypovolaemia/shock or generalised weakness (e.g. due to sepsis, generalised infection).

Diagnosis

ECG is required to establish a definite diagnosis and identify the type of arrhythmia or conduction disturbance that is present. In case a bradycardia is detected, an atropine response test may be performed to determine whether parasympathicolytic drugs can be used in the treatment. Other diagnostic tests (e.g. echocardiography, radiography, haematology and biochemistry) may be performed to rule out underlying disease.

Management/treatment

Management of cardiac arrhythmias and conduction abnormalities is dependent on the severity and the cause, and follows similar guidelines to those established in dogs and cats. In case of tachycardia or tachyarrhythmia, antiarrhythmic drugs such as lidocaine, digoxin or beta-blockers (e.g. propranolol, atenolol) may be administered to lower the heart rate. In case of ferrets with clinical signs resulting from high-grade second-degree and third-degree AV block, anticholinergics (e.g. propantheline), beta-adrenergics (e.g. terbutaline, isoproterenol) and phosphodiesterase inhibitors (e.g. aminophylline, theophylline) may be beneficial (particularly if the ferret showed an increased heart rate in response to atropine administration). In animals that show little response to the aforementioned medications, pacemakers may be implanted to effectively treat a clinical bradycardia. Treatment may furthermore be aimed at treating the clinical signs resulting from the cardiac arrhythmia, as well as eliminating the underlying cause, if possible. The prognosis is dependent on the type of cardiac arrhythmia or conduction abnormality that is present, as well as the underlying disease that may be present. Most ECG abnormalities that have been identified in ferrets are discovered by coincidence and will not affect the animal in any way. Profound bradycardia (<80 bpm), as can be seen with high-level second- or third-degree AV block, carries a poor prognosis, with ferrets often dying within a few months due to congestive heart failure. To prevent this, ferrets with severe bradycardia must therefore be treated promptly.

HYPERTENSION

Hypertension is defined as a chronic increase in systolic arterial blood pressure (i.e. systemic arterial hypertension). Systemic arterial hypertension often develops secondary to an underlying disease, such as renal failure, cardiac disease or endocrine neoplasia (i.e. aldosterone producing adrenal tumours or norepinephrine-secreting phaeochromocytomas). Although these conditions are commonly seen in ferrets, clinical reports documenting hypertension in ferrets are thus far lacking. Clinical signs that may be observed in ferrets are suspected to be similar to those reported in cats with hypertension, and may include ocular changes (e.g. retinal ablation, hyphema), neurological signs, renal failure and cardiac changes (i.e. concentric hypertrophy). To confirm the diagnosis, blood pressure measurements may be needed. Although considered the gold

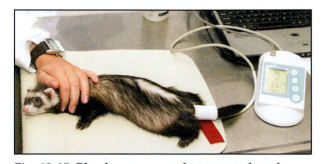

Fig. 12.45 Blood pressure can be measured on the forelimb, hindlimb and tail. The forelimb and tail are the preferred locations. This ferret was lightly sedated with midazolam and butorphanol allowing for an accurate blood pressure measurement by means of high definition oscillometry.

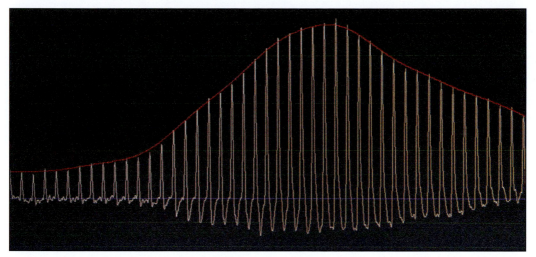

Fig. 12.46 Successful measurement of blood pressure using high-definition oscillometry, showing optimal representation of arterial opening behaviour during blood pressure measurement as indicated by an initial slight, followed by a more dominant increase in height:relaxation of the arterial wall ratio (SAP) up to a maximum (close to MAP) due to turbulence caused by an increase in blood flow, a subsequent decrease in amplitude size due to a change from turbulent to laminar blood flow (DAP) and finally a complete opening of the artery.

standard, direct arterial blood pressure measurement is only feasible in ferrets in an experimental setting (i.e. using the carotid artery) due to the relative inaccessibility of peripheral arteries. Studies have shown normal systolic and diastolic blood pressure ranges from 140–164 mmHg and 110–125 mmHg respectively. Indirect systolic blood pressure measurements may be obtained using a Doppler and pressure cuff placed around the forelimb, hindlimb, or tail (**Fig. 12.45**). Proper cuff size, i.e. approximately 40% of the circumference of the extremity, is important, as too large cuff sizes may result in underestimation of actual blood pressure. Recently, a study was performed to establish the accuracy and precision of indirect arterial blood pressure measurement using high-definition oscillometry (**Fig. 12.46**), which showed the method to be feasible and reproducible in ferrets. Bias was found to be the lowest

when the cuff was placed around the tail or forelimb. Blood pressure measurement was, however, found to be complicated due to the animal's liveliness and lack of compliance. Two follow-up studies were therefore performed to establish a minimal sedative dose needed to be able to perform the blood pressure measurements. Using the established dose (i.e. butorphanol and midazolam, 0.2 mg/kg each), reference ranges were subsequently established at 95–155, 69–109 and 51–87 mmHg for systolic, mean and diastolic arterial pressure in healthy, minimally sedated ferrets (n = 63).

In case of confirmed hypertension, treatment may be initiated using arterial vasodilators (e.g. amlodipine; 0.2–0.4 mg/kg q12h PO), which help to reduce arterial blood pressure. Treatment should furthermore be aimed at eliminating the underlying cause, which also affects the animal's prognosis.

CHAPTER 13

DISORDERS OF THE DIGESTIVE SYSTEM AND LIVER

David Perpiñán and
Cathy A. Johnson-Delaney

INTRODUCTION

Disorders of the gastrointestinal (GI) system are frequently observed in ferrets, particularly foreign bodies and chronic gastroenteritis. The intestine of the ferret is a particularly reactive organ, and tends to develop a significant inflammatory response in front of a variety of causes. Veterinarians should be aware of the GI diseases affecting ferrets and should know how to work-up two of the main symptoms observed: vomiting and diarrhoea.

ANATOMY OF THE DIGESTIVE SYSTEM (SEE CHAPTER 3)

Adult ferrets have 34 teeth, being the dental formula 2(I3/3, C1/1 P3/3 M1/2). For young ferrets, the formula of deciduous or baby teeth is 2(I3-4/3, C1/1, P0/0, M3/3), for a total of 28–30 teeth. Ferrets are born with most deciduous incisors, but those do not generally erupt and are rarely noted; they undergo intragingival resorption before the adult incisors erupt. The rest of the baby teeth erupt between 20 and 30 days (3–4 weeks), and the definitive teeth start replacing milk teeth at about 6–7 weeks. This process occurs earlier in females than in males. Deciduous and definitive canines can be seen in position at the same time, but this is not a pathological condition in ferrets. Premolars have two roots, except for the upper third premolar that has three, as have all molars.

The remainder of the digestive anatomy is similar to other small carnivores such as the dog or the cat. The stomach is quite distendible and has a capacity of about 100 mL. The small intestine measures about 2 m, while the large intestine measures about 10 cm. The caecum is absent in ferrets, and the ileocolic junction can only be detected on histology.

The pancreas is divided into right and left lobes, united by a body that lies close to the pylorus. The liver is relatively large and has six lobes and a gallbladder. Finally, there are two anal sacs with ducts emptying in the external sphincter; with the animal in dorsal recumbency, the openings of the anal sacs are at about 4 and 8 o'clock position.

PHYSIOLOGY OF THE DIGESTIVE SYSTEM

Digestive physiology in ferrets is similar to that of cats (and even to that of dogs), and only a few differences or interesting facts for the veterinarian will be mentioned. Fasting gastric pH is 1.5–3.5. GI transit time is 2.5–4 hours in adults on a meat-based diet, but it is just about 1 hour in milking kits. Intestinal flora are simple and are not commonly affected by the use of antibiotics.

VOMITING AND DIARRHOEA

Vomiting and diarrhoea are two clinical signs that occur frequently in ferrets with GI diseases, and therefore they will be covered in more depth.

Vomiting

The mechanism of vomiting is similar to that found in dogs and cats. Before vomiting, ferrets can show a behaviour characteristic of nausea, which includes salivation, sticking the tongue out, teeth grinding, scratching or touching the chin and mouth with the forelimbs, walking backwards and closing the eyes (**Fig. 13.1**). Signs of tearing at the mouth can also occur if a piece of food is wedged against the roof of the mouth, and in cases of hypoglycaemia. Ferrets are relatively resistant to the emetic effects of different drugs, but vomiting can be induced consistently with the use of high doses of

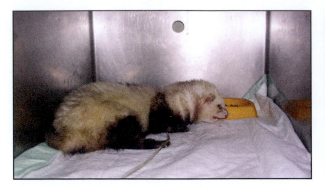

Fig. 13.1 Ferret showing nausea. (Courtesy of Ferran Bargalló.)

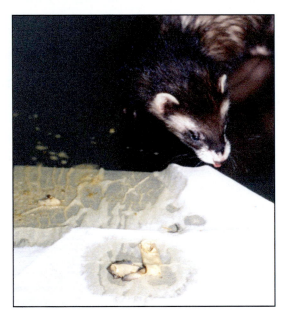

Fig. 13.2 Projectile vomiting.

apomorphine (0.1 mg/kg SC). Conditions that can produce nausea/vomiting include gastritis and gastroenteritis (*Helicobacter* gastritis, bacterial enteritis, eosinophilic gastroenteritis, epizootic catarrhal enteritis (ECE), inflammatory bowel disease, etc.), gastric hair balls, gastrointestinal foreign bodies, gastrointestinal lymphoma, chemotherapy and radiotherapy (**Fig. 13.2**). It is important to separate regurgitation from vomiting. Regurgitation (the ejection of food after only a few minutes of ingestion) is typical of megaoesophagus; in these cases, the ferret does not show nausea and can continue eating immediately after regurgitation. Radiography is one of the most important diagnostic tests in the investigation of vomiting.

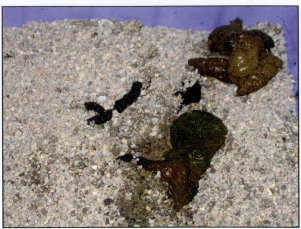

Fig. 13.3 Diarrhoea.

Diarrhoea

The morphological characteristics of diarrhoea in ferrets can progress depending on the degree of involvement of the gastric or intestinal mucosa, and can be brown-yellowish, green, dark, etc. No type of diarrhoea is specific or pathognomonic of a particular disease (**Fig. 13.3**). Lethargy and dehydration are commonly associated with diarrhoea. Anorexic ferrets can produce dark, green faeces (bile) that can look like melena. Unlike other animals, in ferrets it is difficult to tell if the diarrhoea originates in the small or large intestine. Other than haematology, biochemistry and radiology, obtaining intestinal biopsies is very useful in the investigation of diarrhoea in ferrets, particularly the chronic cases. Most common conditions that can produce diarrhoea in ferrets include coronavirus enteritis, inflammatory bowel disease, intestinal lymphoma, coccidiosis, giardiasis, Aleutian disease and eosinophilic gastroenteritis. Grey diarrhoea with some undigested food is typical of bacterial overgrowth, but the possibility of an exocrine pancreatic insufficiency should also be considered.

OTHER CLINICAL SIGNS

Other clinical signs that can be seen with GI diseases include weight loss, fever (acute bacterial enteritis or hepatitis, coronaviral enteritis, septicaemia, perforating gastrointestinal ulcer with peritonitis), melena (Aleutian disease, bacterial enteritis, gastric or duodenal ulcers, inflammatory bowel disease,

Helicobacter gastritis, gastrointestinal lymphoma), proctitis (chronic diarrhoea), thickened intestinal loops on palpation (lymphoma [relatively common], eosinophilic gastroenteritis [uncommon], proliferative bowel disease [extremely rare]) and rectal prolapse (uncommon with chronic enteritis, more common as a complication after removing anal glands at a very early age). Mesenteric lymph nodes in ferrets are very reactive and become enlarged with many GI conditions (lymphoma, eosinophilic gastroenteritis, Aleutian disease, systemic coronaviral disease, and peritonitis [due to pancreatitis or perforating GI ulcers]).

BACTERIAL GASTROENTERITIS

Definition/overview
Gastroenteritis (most commonly enteritis) is caused by gram-negative bacteria, mainly *Campylobacter*, *Escherichia coli* and *Salmonella*. Recently there was a report of kits with mucoid diarrhoea due to *Staphylococcus delphini*.

Aetiology
Campylobacter spp., *Escherichia* spp., *Salmonella* spp., *Staphylococcus delphini*.

Pathophysiology
Stress, overpopulation and lack of hygiene can predispose to infection and disease. Uncooked meat, particularly if intestines are included, can also be a source of infection. There are ferrets that are asymptomatic carriers of any of these bacteria, so they can also be a source of infection. Up to 80% of ferrets in some populations can be carriers of *Campylobacter jejuni*. *Staphyloccus delphini* induced a hypersecretory diarrhoea with colonisation of the small intestine. The culture *in vitro* showed the potential of producing enterotoxin E.

Clinical presentation
Common clinical signs include diarrhoea (mucoid, watery, bile-streaked, bloody), lack of appetite, lethargy and dehydration (**Figs 13.4, 13.5**). A dirty perineum can be observed on physical examination. If the condition progresses, fever, muscular trembling, haemorrhagic diarrhoea, anorexia,

abortion and abdominal pain can be seen. Diarrhoea caused by *Campylobacter* is generally self-limiting in youngsters with appropriate maternal antibodies; appropriate immunity does not prevent infection but does prevent development of clinical disease. Campylobacteriosis is seen in ferrets younger than 6 months and it is rare in adult animals. Colibacilosis has also been described as being more common in young ferrets. In cases of *E. coli* or *Salmonella*, duration, severity, consistency and presence/degree of haematochezia in the diarrhoea is strain-dependent, and septicaemia with systemic signs is more common than in cases of campylobacteriosis.

The incubation period is less than 24 hours with *Campylobacter* and a few days with the other bacteria.

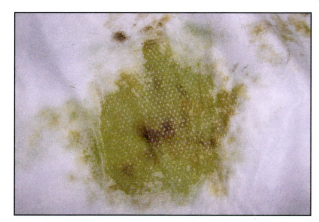

Fig. 13.4 **Diarrhoea associated with *E. coli* gastroenteritis.**

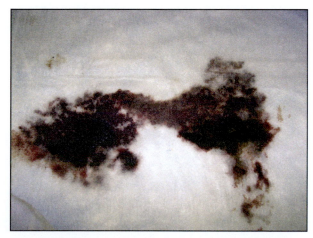

Fig. 13.5 **Haemorrhagic diarrhoea associated with *E. coli* gastroenteritis.**

In cases of campylobacteriosis, diarrhoea can persist for more than 4 weeks and can be intermittent. Diarrhoea caused by *Salmonella* or *E. coli* can progress quickly to severe dehydration, haemorrhagic gastroenteritis and septicaemia/toxaemia, and animals may die within just 24 hours of the start of clinical signs. Disseminated intravascular coagulation can be seen in some cases (**Fig. 13.6**).

Differential diagnosis

Any other cause of diarrhoea, such as proliferative bowel disease, eosinophilic gastroenteritis, rotavirus, coronavirus, inflammatory bowel disease, etc.

Diagnostic testing

Campylobacter has particular characteristics on culture (slow growth, microaerobic conditions), *E. coli* grows in aerobic culture and *Salmonella* grows readily in enrichment media, such as selenite broth and others, before being transferred to a routine culture media. PCR is increasingly being used for diagnosis of these infections, as it avoids the special culture needed for *Campylobacter*, can determine the presence of virulent factors in *E. coli* and can determine the species of *Salmonella*. Growth from organs such as liver, blood or urine is more diagnostic that growth from intestinal contents, as it should be remembered that ferrets can act as asymptomatic carriers, and the mere culture of these bacteria from intestine does not equal disease.

Haematological and biochemical abnormalities are usually present only in animals with severe clinical illness, and include non-regenerative anaemia, thrombocytopaenia, toxic leucocytes (in cases of systemic disease and endotoxaemia), hypoproteinaemia and electrolyte abnormalities. Necropsy can show redness of the GI tract, with bloody, mucoid or watery intestinal contents.

Diagnosis

Identification of bacteria in organs that should be sterile (liver, spleen, kidney, etc.) is diagnostic. Isolation from intestine is indicative, but other pathogens need to be ruled out. The use of PCR to determine virulent factors is also useful for a definitive diagnosis.

Management/treatment

Although *Campylobacter* is a self-limiting disease, antibiotics shorten the course of the disease and can prevent mortality in outbreaks involving a large number of ferrets. Cases of salmonellosis or colibacillosis should be aggressively treated to avoid the rapid progression of the disease. Erythromycin is the antibiotic of choice in campylobacteriosis, although other antibiotics are also generally effective such as aminoglycosides, tetracyclines, chloramphenicol, furazolidone and clindamycin. Resistance to *E. coli* is common, but isolates are commonly susceptible to amikacin, gentamicin, ciprofloxacin, florfenicol, chloramphenicol, enrofloxacin, ceftiofur, ceftriaxone, amoxicillin with clavulanic acid and imipenem. Routine antibiotics reported to be effective against *Salmonella* include chloramphenicol, trimethoprim-sulphonamide and amoxicillin.

When a bacterial enteritis is suspected, samples for culture and sensitivity should be obtained. In the meantime, antibiotic treatment should be started before the results become available: chloramphenicol seems the most appropriate choice as it is effective against all three species of bacterium. As oral chloramphenicol is not readily available in some countries, the combination of amoxicillin/clavulanic acid + aminoglycoside or quinolone should be considered as a first-line treatment. The use of amoxicillin without clavulanic acid is generally not recommended due to the frequency of resistance. Supportive treatment (particularly with fluids and easily digestible food) is always indicated.

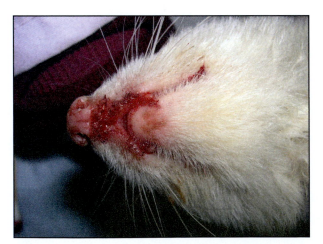

Fig. 13.6 Disseminated intravascular coagulation seen in this case of *E. coli* enteritis.

During treatment, the possibility of reinfection should be avoided through frequent bedding changes. Cultures after treatment will confirm the elimination of the bacteria. Ferrets infected with either of these bacteria pose a zoonotic risk, particularly to children and immunosuppressed people.

COCCIDIOSIS

Definition/overview
Diarrhoeal disease caused by a variety of species of *Isospora* and *Eimeria*. The condition is generally asymptomatic, but outbreaks producing severe enteric disease and even death have been described in high-density populations.

Aetiology
Eimeria furonis has been linked to more severe disease. Other species of *Isospora* and *Eimeria* have also been reported in ferrets (**Fig. 13.7**).

Pathophysiology
Coccidia has a host-specific, direct life cycle. Oocysts shed in the faeces undergo sporulation (2–5 days at 24°C in *E. furonis*) to become infectious. Infection occurs by ingestion of sporulated oocysts.

Clinical presentation
Ferrets of any age group can be affected, although in private practice it is more commonly seen in recently purchased young ferrets. Coccidiosis is generally considered a subclinical disease with low numbers of parasites present in faeces. However, outbreaks have been described in shelters and breeding facilities, with high numbers of parasites affecting the intestinal mucosa. Foul-smelling diarrhoea, ranging from pasty/gelatinous to melena and frank blood, has been observed in clinical cases (**Fig. 13.8**). Lethargy, rectal prolapse, perineal staining, tenesmus, weight loss, dehydration, anorexia and weakness can also occur. Dehydration can be evidenced by sunken eyes, tenting of the skin, dry mucous membranes and capillary refill times higher than 2 seconds. The course of the disease is 5–10 days, after which the animal recovers or the condition progresses to death. Coccidiosis can be observed together with other enteric diseases and can therefore be responsible for part of the clinical signs. Hepatic (biliary) coccidiosis, affecting mainly the biliary system and producing blood changes compatible with liver disease (elevated liver enzymes, hypoalbuminaemia, hyperbilirubinaemia), has rarely been observed in ferrets, although it has been seen in a case of chemotherapeutic immunosuppression.

Differential diagnosis
Infectious causes of diarrhoea are more common in recently purchased young ferrets and in ferrets from shelters or breeding facilities. This may include rotavirus, enteric coronavirus, bacterial gastroenteritis or proliferative bowel disease.

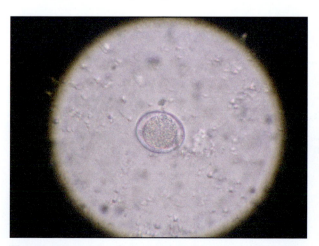

Fig. 13.7 Coccidia from a ferret. (Courtesy of Ferran Bargalló.)

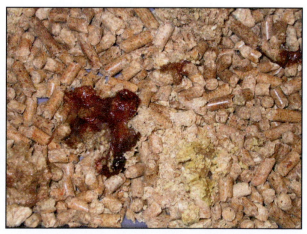

Fig. 13.8 Frank blood in a stool with Coccidia.

Diagnostic testing

Bloodwork can indicate dehydration and regenerative anaemia. Routine faecal tests (fresh smear and flotation) yield inconsistent results in ferrets with coccidiosis; therefore, the results of faecal tests may not reveal the true extent of the disease, and false negatives are common with these tests. Sporulated oocysts of *E. furonis* are spherical, measure approximately 13 μm in diameter, and contain four sporocysts with two sporozoites in each sporocyst. Other species have different sizes and morphology. Unsporulated oocysts can also be seen on faecal tests. Necropsy may show dilated and thin-walled intestines. Splenomegaly and hepatic lipidosis, both indicative of unspecific disease, may also be observed on gross postmortems (any condition leading to anorexia can rapidly progress to hepatic lipidosis in ferrets). Histopathology can reveal oocysts and intestinal lesions.

Diagnosis

Finding large numbers of coccidia in the presence of clinical signs is indicative of the disease, particularly if no other cause is found for the diarrhoea. Histopathology is commonly necessary for a definitive diagnosis.

Management/treatment

Treatment can be challenging in the face of an outbreak. Sulphadimethoxine (usually combined with trimethoprim and given at 30 mg/kg PO SID for 2–3 weeks) has been reported to be only partially effective in the face of an outbreak. Amprolium can also be given at 20 mg/kg PO SID, but efficacy is unknown. Newer antiparasitic drugs, such as ponazuril, have been suggested at doses of 30 mg/kg PO SID.

The disease can spread rapidly through contact with faeces or fomites. Environmental cleaning should be done using bleach, quaternary ammonium compounds or heat.

CRYPTOSPORIDIOSIS

Definition/overview

Cryptosporidium is an apicomplexan protozoan. *Cryptosporidium* oocysts are 4–6 μm in diameter and exhibit partial acid-fast staining that may or may not be species specific and therefore regarded as zoonotic.

Aetiology/pathophysiology

Cryptosporidia causing diarrhoea is often expressed due to stress and immunosuppression. It is transmitted via faecal–oral route and appears to be highly contagious in stressed animals. It causes damage to the small intestinal mucosa resulting in diarrhoea. It is shed in the faeces (**Fig. 13.9**). It is usually self-limiting in 2–3 weeks.

Clinical presentation

Diarrhoea. Anorexia, weight and condition loss also seen.

Differential diagnosis

Coccidiosis, giardiasis, bacterial gastroenteritis including *Helicobacter mustelae* infection, inflammatory bowel disease, neoplasia, viral gastroenteritis (ECE, rotavirus), dietary indiscretion – i.e. any cause of diarrhoea.

Diagnostic testing

Wet mount direct smear, faecal flotation, ELISA, PCR.

Diagnosis

Positive identification of the organism in the faeces.

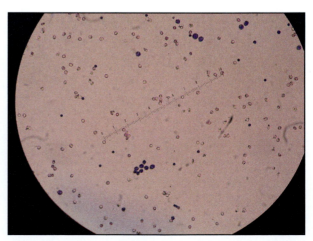

Fig. 13.9 **Cryptosporidia (unstained) in faeces during an outbreak at a shelter.**

Management/treatment

There is no treatment although paromomycin has been tried. It is usually self-limiting in 2–4 weeks so supportive care (fluids, dook soup, B-complex vitamins) may help. It is potentially zoonotic so gloves and mask should be worn while cleaning the cages and handling the ferrets. Frequent cleaning of litter trays may prevent additional transmission. Bleach is effective for environmental cleaning. As immunosuppression plays a role, determining the stressors and eliminating them may help speed up self-limiting time.

EPIZOOTIC CATARRHAL ENTERITIS (ECE, FRECV)

Definition/overview

Highly contagious diarrhoeal disease of ferrets. Reduction in severity of disease has been observed over the last years.

Aetiology

It is caused by the ferret enteric coronavirus (FRECV), a group I coronavirus closely related to the ferret systemic coronavirus (FRSCV).

Pathophysiology

Original descriptions from the 1990s reported ECE as a highly contagious diarrhoeal disease affecting sometimes 100% of ferrets, particularly in situations of high density and close contact between animals (shelter, breeding facility, household). Despite this high morbidity, mortality was low, with less than 5% of affected ferrets dying. Currently, prevalence of infection continues to be high in some ferret populations around the world, but the disease has become enzootic and rarely results in clinical signs.

The virus is shed in faeces and saliva, and is transmitted through the faecal–oral route. Shedding can be intermittent and reinfection may play a significant role in maintaining infection in large ferret populations. Ferrets can reactivate excretion of the virus after a stressful situation.

Clinical presentation

Initial outbreaks affect mainly adult animals (with severe clinical signs and higher mortality rates), while young ferrets develop mild subclinical disease.

Clinical signs consist of lethargy, hyporexia or anorexia and vomiting, followed by (in the early stages) a profuse, foul-smelling, bright green watery diarrhoea with high mucus content, leading also to dehydration (**Fig. 13.10**). Later on in the course of the disease, the destruction of the enteric villi produce maldigestion/malabsorption and faeces contains undigested material with a grainy consistency resembling bird seeds (**Fig. 13.11**).

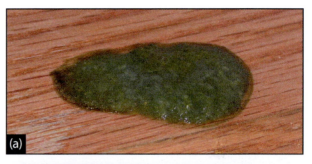

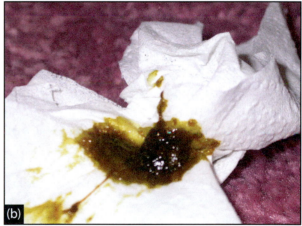

Fig. 13.10 (a) Green faeces associated with ECE; (b) mucoid diarrhoea associated with ECE.

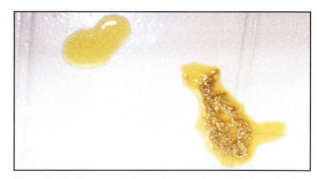

Fig. 13.11 Faeces with undigested material typical of ECE.

Physical examination reveals lethargy, mesenteric lymphadenopathy, dehydration and diarrhoea. Although green diarrhoea is mentioned as a characteristic of this disease, many other GI diseases of ferrets can produce green diarrhoea. Melena can be observed in some cases that develop gastric ulcers.

During the original outbreaks, the clinical history often reveals that the disease occurred in adult animals after the introduction of a new, young ferret (asymptomatic carrier) in the population. Following initial infection, the disease spreads easily in adult ferrets. Currently, the enzootic condition of the disease produces less severe and often intermittent disease in severely stressed young ferrets.

Differential diagnosis

Any enteritis/gastroenteritis, particularly the initial stage of FRSCV disease, bacterial enteritis, intestinal coccidiosis, etc.

Diagnostic testing

Bloodwork is usually unspecific and may reveal changes compatible with dehydration, such as increased PCV and proteins. Intestinal biopsies may show grossly hyperaemic intestinal loops and histological changes consisting of diffuse lymphocytic enteritis with villus atrophy. The virus can be detected on faeces and saliva using RT-PCR, which can differentiate FRECV from FRSCV. Currently available RT-PCR to detect feline coronavirus (FCoV) will not detect ferret coronaviruses. Other ways to detect infection consist of using electron microscopy of faeces to visualise coronaviral particles, immunohistochemistry in tissues, *in situ* hybridisation and serology, but these tests will generally not differentiate between FRECV and FRSCV, although it is advisable to contact the laboratory for further information. The interpretation of serological results is complicated.

Diagnosis

A combination of history, clinical signs and diagnostic tests can be used in the diagnostic approach of ECE. Additionally, histology is needed to confirm the diagnosis, as the demonstration of virus in faeces/intestine only supports a diagnosis of infection, but not of disease. The best area for an intestinal biopsy is jejunum and ileum.

Management/treatment

Treatment should include broad-spectrum antibiotics, aggressive fluid therapy and supportive care. Additional treatment with a short course of steroids (prednisone 1 mg/kg PO q12h × 14 d) and changing the diet to an easily digestible/absorbable food may speed recovery and reduce future problems of malabsorption due to villi destruction. Metronidazole has anti-inflammatory and antibiotic effects and can improve stool consistency (20 mg/kg PO q12h), but palatability for ferrets is usually poor except for metronidazole benzoate, which is recommended as it has virtually no flavour and can be purchased as a powder. An alternative antibiotic combination is enrofloxacin (5 mg/kg PO q12h) and amoxicillin/clavulanic acid (10–20 mg/kg PO q12h).

Coronaviruses are RNA viruses that do not persist for a long time in the environment. Therefore, close contact among animals or their faeces is necessary to spread the infection, which can become highly contagious and easily transmissible in situations of overcrowding and poor hygienic conditions. The affected animals are commonly isolated, although this may not be that important in an enzootic situation. Coronaviruses are easily inactivated with many commonly used disinfectants.

EOSINOPHILIC GASTROENTERITIS

Definition/overview

Gastroenteritis produced by the accumulation of eosinophils in the GI mucosa. The condition is also named eosinophilic granulomatous disease as it may affect other organs, including mesenteric lymph nodes and, less frequently, liver and lungs.

Aetiology/pathophysiology

Aetiology is unknown. Parasites or food allergy have not been found to be related.

Clinical presentation

There is no age or sex predilection. Clinical signs include chronic diarrhoea and weight loss. Anorexia, lethargy and dehydration are less common. Vomiting is inconsistent and may be more common with gastric involvement. Eosinophilic granulomatous disease can sometimes develop in mesenteric lymph nodes, producing mesenteric lymphadenopathy.

The occurrence of the disease is rare, and it should be suspected when peripheral eosinophilia or thickened intestinal loops/mesenteric lymphadenopathy is detected.

Differential diagnosis

Any gastroenteritis, including inflammatory bowel disease (IBD), Aleutian disease, proliferative bowel disease, or *Helicobacter* gastroenteritis. Gastrointestinal foreign bodies can also produce similar clinical signs. Mesenteric lymphadenopathy can also be found in lymphoma, Aleutian disease and systemic coronaviral disease. Lymphoma and proliferative bowel disease can produce thickened intestinal loops.

Diagnostic testing

Bloodwork commonly shows eosinophilia, with eosinophils being 10–35% of total leucocytes. Cases without eosinophilia have also been described. Hypoalbuminaemia can also be observed. Abdominal palpation may reveal thickened intestinal loops and, sometimes, enlarged mesenteric lymph nodes. As the condition can produce malabsorption, dehydration and electrolyte imbalances can be found. On laparotomy (or necropsy), affected intestinal loops may be bright red and thickened, and occasionally cystic structures (lymphangiectasia) can be observed in the serosa. Intestinal (or mesenteric) biopsy is necessary to diagnose the disease. When in doubt, other tests should be done in order to rule out other diseases: faecal tests to rule out parasites; serology and antigen detection for Aleutian disease (in combination with biopsy); rectal cultures for bacterial gastroenteritis.

Diagnosis

Definitive diagnosis is made by GI biopsy. Sometimes, biopsy of enlarged mesenteric lymph nodes can also yield a diagnosis.

Management/treatment/prognosis

Treatment is similar to IBD and consists of long-term use of corticosteroids (prednisone 1.25–2.5 mg/kg PO q24h) or azathioprine (0.9 mg/kg PO q24h), lowering and adjusting the dose based on response to treatment. A protocol of 1.5 mg/kg of prednisolone PO q24h for 1 week and then 0.8 mg/kg PO q24h or less long term has been reported. Supportive care with a soft, easily digestible, high-calorie diet may be needed. Severely affected lymph nodes and parts of the intestine may be removed in order to control (or even solve) the disease. Treatment with ivermectin has been reported useful in one case (0.4 mg/kg SC and repeated in 14 days). Allergen-restricted diets have not been successful in treating this condition, although that does not rule out completely the possibility of food allergies. Assessment of peripheral eosinophils may be an adequate method to monitor progression or remission of the disease.

GASTRIC DILATATION VOLVULUS (GDV)

Definition/overview

Rotation on the axis of the stomach. It is also called stomach torsion.

Aetiology/pathophysiology

GDV involves rotation on the mesenteric axis (longitudinal). It becomes severely distended with gas or fluid. Usually the stomach rotates clockwise between 90° and 360°. It causes obstruction. Predisposing factors include family history, stress, increased thoracic depth, exercise, diet and concurrent disease. Torsion may also occur with the spleen and result in congestion.

Clinical presentation

Acute onset vomiting mucus. Respiratory distress. Lethargy, dehydration. The ferret may be hypothermic. There is pain on palpation. Abnormal serum chemistry include hyperglycaemia, hyponatraemia and hypokalaemia. There may be peritoneal effusion. The spleen may be enlarged.

Differential diagnosis

Peritoneal effusion may come from peritonitis, haemorrhage, lymphatic obstruction, hypoalbuminaemia and neoplasia. Splenomegaly may be due to extramedullary haematopoiesis, neoplasia (i.e. lymphoma) and inflammation. Gastric pain and shock condition can also be associated with foreign body ingestion and obstruction in the GI tract.

Diagnostic testing
Radiographs, CBC, serum chemistry.

Diagnosis
Radiographic findings of the torsion. Exploratory laparotomy will be definitive.

Management/treatment
An analgesic is warranted as this is a painful problem. Fluid therapy should start as well as warming the ferret. Blood pressure should be closely monitored and fluids adjusted accordingly to keep the blood pressure stable and greater than 90 mmHg (see Chapter 10, Chapter 12). Surgery is indicated as soon as possible as the torsion may have led to necrosis of the stomach. Splenectomy may also be indicated. Prognosis is guarded to poor but depends on how long the stomach had been under torsion.

GASTRIC HAIR BALLS/TRICHOBEZOARS

Definition/overview
A trichobezoar is a mass found in the GI system formed from the ingestion of hair. Ferrets are prone to developing gastric trichobezoars.

Aetiology/pathophysiology
The ingestion of hair is necessary for the formation of trichobezoars. Predisposing factors for the formation of trichobezoars include previous GI surgery, GI hypomotility, gastroenteritis, pruritic skin conditions, flea infestation and excessive moulting.

Clinical presentation
Trichobezoars are more common in older ferrets (while GI foreign bodies are more common in young ferrets). Ferrets older than 4 years are considered at higher risk, as well as ferrets with predisposing conditions. As the formation of a trichobezoar is a progressive condition, clinical signs can vary from none (incidental finding on palpation or radiographs) to nausea, lethargy, loss of appetite and progressive weight loss. Vomiting is not very frequent, and diarrhoea and melena could be uncommonly observed due to irritation of the stomach.

Differential diagnosis
GI foreign body, oesophageal foreign body, gastritis and gastric neoplasia. When the trichobezoar has been able to pass the stomach and block the intestine, then other differential diagnoses that should be included are enteritis, intestinal foreign body and intestinal intussusception.

Diagnostic testing
Diagnosis can be done at palpation, but the location of the stomach (very cranially and between the ribs) makes the identification of trichobezoars difficult; however, the stomach of most ferrets can be fully palpated with patience (**Fig. 13.12**) The trichobezoar may also pass into the intestine causing a blockage (**Fig. 13.13**). Localised pain or discomfort can be elicited on palpation.

Radiographs should include abdomen, thorax and, if possible, oesophagus. The trichobezoars can sometimes be clearly visualised on radiographs, and other findings will appear when there is obstruction (gaseous distension of stomach or intestines) (**Fig. 13.14**). Contrast studies (with barium, iodine

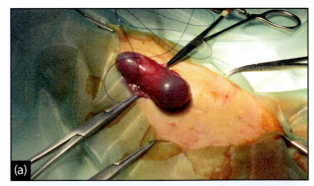

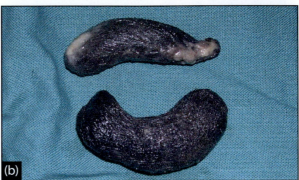

Fig. 13.12 (a) Two gastric trichobezoars; (b) removed gastric trichobezoars.

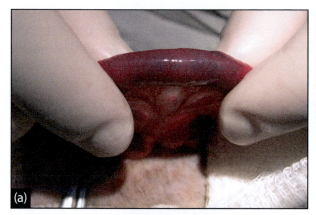

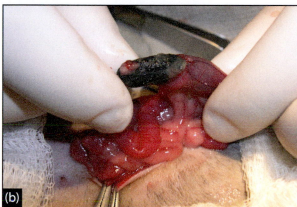

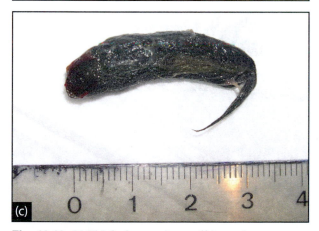

Fig. 13.13 (a) Trichobezoar in small intestine; (b) removal of trichobezoar; (c) removed trichobezoar.

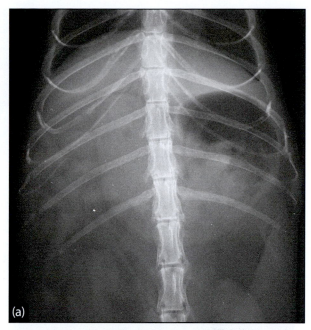

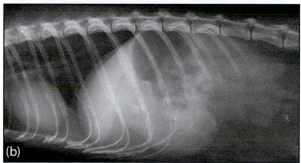

Fig. 13.14 (a) Dorsoventral (DV) radiograph showing gastric trichobezoar; (b) lateral radiograph showing distention of the stomach with the trichobezoar.

of trichobezoars, particularly those located in the intestine.

Exploratory laparotomy is also a possibility for the diagnosis and treatment of trichobezoars. Bloodwork is generally unspecific for the diagnosis of this condition.

Diagnosis
A final diagnosis is made by direct or indirect visualisation of the trichobezoar.

Management/treatment/prognosis
Ferrets do not generally vomit trichobezoars (something that cats can do) and therefore surgery

compounds or air) can be performed for better visualisation, although they are seldom needed. Ultrasound is helpful in detecting both gastric or intestinal trichobezoars, and it can also assess GI motility. Endoscopy can also be used for the diagnosis of gastric and small intestinal trichobezoars. Finally, CT scan is also useful for the diagnosis

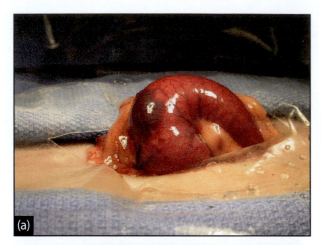

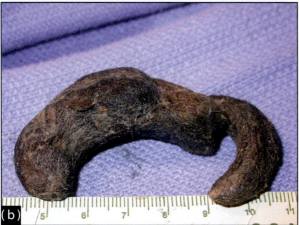

Fig. 13.15 (a) Gastric trichobezoar at surgery; (b) Trichobezoar may have a portion that extends into the pylorus.

within the stomach; these ferrets usually represent in a few weeks or months with worsened symptomatology, which is usually resolved by surgery. When medical treatment is attempted, the ferret should be closely monitored to assess efficacy of therapy and the possibility of intestinal blockage. Only small trichobezoars should be treated medically. Endoscopic fragmentation and the use of Coca-Cola® has been effective in the treatment of other types of bezoars in people, but they are not effective with trichobezoars.

Cat hairball laxatives can be given to prevent the condition in any ferret, but particularly those that have already developed trichobezoars. Prevention is more important in ferrets with predisposing factors to develop trichobezoars. Laxatives can be given at feline doses, although a dose of 1–2 mL every 2–3 days has been suggested. If the trichobezoar is caused by poor gastric motility, prokinetic drugs may be used for prevention. Predisposing conditions such as skin disease should be treated or controlled. Gastric ulceration is common with trichobezoars, so affected animals should be treated with antacids (ranitidine, famotidine, omeprazole) and gastric protectants (sucralfate). Brushing moulting ferrets also prevents the development of trichobezoars, particularly at the seasonal coat change.

GASTROENTERITIS BY *HELICOBACTER MUSTELAE*

Definition/overview
Chronic gastritis (sometimes with duodenitis) and ulcers caused by the spiral bacteria *Helicobacter mustelae*. The disease has many similarities with gastritis in humans caused by *Helicobacter pylori*. The ferret has been use as an animal model for *Helicobacter*-associated illness.

Aetiology
H. mustelae is a gram-negative and curved bacteria, better visualised using silver stains such as the Warthin-Starry stain. Prevalence of infection is variable, and some research facilities in the USA have reported a prevalence of 100% in adult animals, while only a few ferrets younger than 6 weeks were infected; this is indicative of infection after weaning

(gastrotomy) is usually necessary and is the treatment of choice. Careful examination of the full GI tract is necessary during surgery, as it is not unusual to find more than one trichobezoar (**Fig. 13.15**). When surgery reveals there was not a trichobezoar or foreign body, gastric and intestinal biopsies should be collected to investigate the origin of the clinical signs.

Treatment with cat laxatives is rarely completely effective when the condition is fully developed, as it can facilitate the passage of the trichobezoar into the intestine and cause intestinal obstruction; in this situation, the condition should be treated as an obstructive foreign body, requiring immediate surgery. Medical treatment can produce temporal improvements due to relocation of the trichobezoar through the mother, that persists for the life of the ferret. Other authors have reported much lower prevalences in other countries.

Pathophysiology

Koch's postulates have been fulfilled, and the oral administration of *H. mustelae* to ferrets free of this bacterium produces colonisation, chronic gastritis and a raise in anti-*H. mustelae* antibiotic titre. Histological changes consist of superficial mononuclear gastritis in the body of the stomach and diffuse mononuclear gastritis in the pyloric antrum. The highest number of bacteria is usually found in the pyloric antrum. Ferrets free of *H. mustelae* do not have these lesions. Severity of gastritis is correlated with the number of organisms (**Fig. 13.16**). In addition, some authors state that disease is more frequently seen in older animals, while other authors believe stressed young (3–5 months old) animals are more susceptible to the disease.

Infection by *H. mustelae* produces auto-antibodies, which can contribute to the development of gastritis. It is possible that these auto-antibodies could also be implicated in the reactivity of spleen and mesenteric lymph nodes, although lymphoid tissue (particularly mesenteric) reacts significantly in ferrets with any inflammation. The infection is also associated with hypochlorhydria and hypergastrinaemia, and it has been observed that the hypochlorhydria caused by the administration of omeprazole increases faecal excretion of the bacteria. Hypergastrinaemia is linked to the development of gastric ulcers. Due to

the faecal excretion, the faecal–oral route seems the most important route of transmission.

However, it should be noted that the results of experimental infections do not necessarily correlate with clinical results of ferrets infected spontaneously. While experimental infections have demonstrated Koch's postulates, have detected 100% infection in some populations and have directly linked the bacteria with the development of chronic gastritis, clinical experience indicates that the disease is not that prevalent in pet ferrets and many infections are asymptomatic. Differences in experimetal vs. spontaneous infections can be caused by some characteristics of infection, such as use of pathogen-free animals for research studies, and infecting animals with high doses of bacteria, with more pathogenic strains or through unusual routes, etc. An Australian author indicated that, based on gastric biopsies and histopathology, less than 50% of ferrets with gastritis had *Helicobacter*, and that only 2% of cases of gastritis (without generalised enteritis) may be caused by *Helicobacter*. This author also indicated that many cases of gastritis also have generalised enteritis, and those cases cannot be linked to *Helicobacter* infection, as it has only been demonstrated that the bacteria affects stomach and duodenum.

Clinical presentation

Most infected animals are asymptomatic. Clinical cases may have gastritis, duodenitis and gastric and duodenal ulcers, which can produce clinical signs such as melena, nausea, vomiting, anorexia (total or partial), chronic weight loss, bruxism and lethargy (**Figs 13.17, 13.18**). The disease is generally chronic. Some owners may misinterpret signs of nausea for respiratory symptoms. Physical examination may show pale mucous membranes, weight loss and dehydration. Splenomegaly and mesenteric lymphadenopathy may occur, but these findings are unspecific in ferrets and may occur in many other GI diseases. Other species of *Helicobacter* have been associated with hepatobiliar disease in ferrets and have produced clinical signs such as weight loss, anorexia, lethargy and diarrhoea.

Chronic gastritis can lead to preneoplastic changes, and infection with *H. mustelae* has been associated with gastric adenocarcinoma and lymphoma.

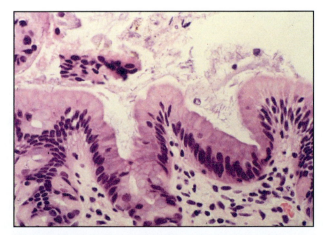

Fig. 13.16 *Helicobacter* organisms present in ulcer.

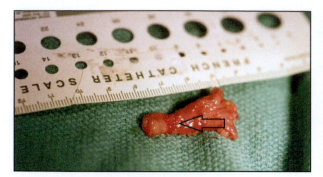

Fig. 13.17 *Helicobacter* pyloric ulcer (arrow).

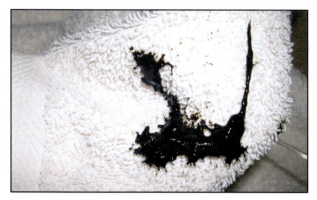

Fig. 13.18 **Melena associated with GI ulceration.**

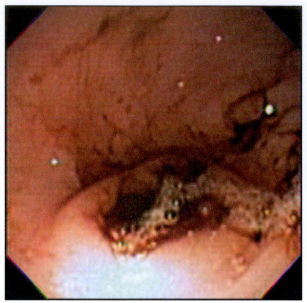

Fig. 13.19 **Gastric ulcer found on endoscopy.**
(Courtesy of University of Georgia.)

In people, it has been speculated that gastric lymphomas appear after decades of antigenic stimulation by chronic infections by *H. pylori*. These gastric lymphomas can disappear with treatment for *H. pylori*; a similar situation could happen with ferrets infected by *H. mustelae*. Clinical signs of gastric neoplasia are similar to those observed in GI foreign bodies: vomiting, anorexia and weight loss.

Differential diagnosis
Gastritis (eosinophilic gastritis, any other gastroenteritis), gastric foreign body, trichobezoar.

Diagnostic testing
Anaemia is the only haematological or biochemical change that can be seen in cases with GI ulceration. Serologically, immunoglobulins against *H. mustelae* can be used to assess the degree of infection over time and they correlate well with the results of other diagnostic tests. High levels of antibodies do not protect from the disease. Antibodies increase with age and with chronicity of infection. Antibody

levels start to decrease 4 months after elimination of *H. mustelae* with treatment.

Endoscopy with gastric biopsy is another good method of diagnosing the problem. *Helicobacter* is most commonly found in the pyloric antrum, but lesions in other parts of the stomach and in the duodenum can also be found (**Fig. 13.19**). Histological analysis of those biopsies should include silver stains (Warthin-Starry) to improve the visualisation of *Helicobacter*. The degree of proliferation of the bacteria can be seen on histology. Biopsies can also be collected through laparotomy, but the endoscopic approach is preferred.

Samples for bacterial culture can be collected from faeces, gastric biopsies or gastric swabs or washes. A stomach tube with a culture swab can be passed into the anaesthetised ferret and the stomach manually swabbed (**Fig. 13.20**). *Helicobacter* has special requirements for growth. PCR can also be performed from those samples. As infection is widespread but clinical disease only occurs in some cases, the use of these techniques is not an effective way to assess problems related to *Helicobacter* in ferrets, although these antigen-detection techniques can be used to assess bacterial elimination after treatment.

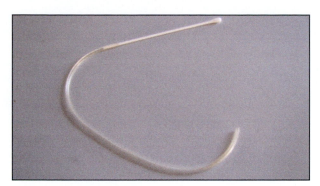

Fig. 13.20 Stomach tube with culture swab attached for gastric sampling.

> **Box 13.1 Treatment regimen for *Helicobacter mustelae* clinical infection**
>
> **Treatment of Choice (For 3–4 Weeks)**
> - Clarithromycin (12.5 mg/kg PO q 8–12 h)
> - Metronidazole (20 mg/kg PO q 8–12 h)
> - Note: use metronidazole benzoate as it is palatable
> - Bismuth subsalycilate (17.5 mg/kg or 0.5 ml) (Pepto Bismol, Proctor & Gamble, Cincinnati OH) PO q 8–12 h. Note: Cherry flavoured seems to be preferred

Diagnosis

Similar to other diseases with high infection rates and low clinical disease prevalence (e.g. Aleutian disease), the mere demonstration of bacteria in faeces or samples from the stomach is not enough for a diagnosis, as it will only confirm infection and not disease. Therefore, a definitive diagnosis is usually done by endoscopy, biopsy and histology.

Response to treatment is not a good way to diagnose the problem, as many other GI disorders may improve with antibiotic treatment (due to the control of intestinal bacterial overgrowth). In addition, there may be other GI problems associated with infection by *Helicobacter*, and therefore biopsy plus histopathology is extremely useful in these cases to assess whether *Helicobacter* is a primary agent or just an incidental finding.

Management/treatment/prognosis

Treatment (*Box 13.1*) consists of a combination of different drugs to prevent the development of resistance.

This treatment eliminates the bacteria in 70–100% of infected animals. Other effective treatments are modifications of this one, such as changing clarithromycin for amoxicillin or amoxicillin/clavulanic acid (30 mg/kg PO q12h) or change (or add) bismuth subsalycilate (not available in some countries) with omeprazole (0.7–4 mg/kg PO q24h), sucralfate (25–100 mg/kg PO q8h), ranitidine (2.5–3.5 mg/kg PO q8h), famotidine (0.25–0.5 mg/kg PO q24h) or cimetidine (10 mg/kg PO q8h). The combination of enrofloxacin (5 mg/kg PO q12h) plus bismuth subsalicylate (6 mg/kg PO q12h) has also been effective. Sucralfate should be administered on an empty stomach to avoid interference with the absorption of other drugs. It is important to select palatable drugs in other to have the compliance of the owner; therefore, metronidazole (use metronidazole benzoate as the usual form is extremely bitter) can be changed for amoxicillin or amoxicillin/clavulanic acid. Bleeding ulcers can be treated endoscopically by cauterisation of topical application of epinephrine.

The infection can be eliminated with an appropriate treatment, but reinfection can occur at any time, as previous infection does not protect against future infections. If treatment does not work, *Helicobacter* may not be the main problem and there may be other aetiologic agents, *H. mustelae* being just an incidental finding.

Drugs increasing gastric pH have been commonly used in the treatment of *Helicobacter* gastritis; however, faecal excretion of the bacteria increases with omeprazole. In addition, the use of antacids or other drugs that inhibit gastric acids causes elevation in the production of gastrin, already elevated due to infection by *H. mustelae*. Gastrin elevation can produce gastric ulcers. However, these data do not seem to correspond with what is seen in clinical cases, where antacids have been mentioned to be effective to help eliminate the bacteria and reduce gastritis.

Prognosis is generally good, although it can be guarded in those cases with ulcers and significant anaemia.

GASTROINTESTINAL FOREIGN BODIES

Definition/overview

The presence of an ingested object that irritates or obstructs (partially or completely) the GI tract.

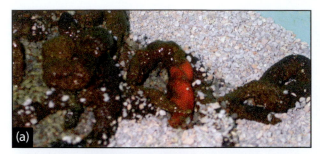

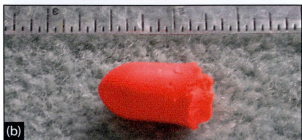

Fig. 13.21 (a) Foreign material seen in stool. In this case the foreign material passed; (b) corresponding foam ear plug identified as the material.

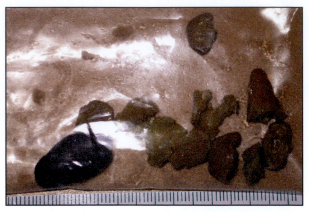

Fig. 13.22 Material removed at enterotomy proved to be pieces of a rubber toy.

Aetiology/pathophysiology

Ferrets are inquisitive and like to chew on different objects, particularly those made of rubber, sponge or foam; these materials are easily ingested but poorly digested (**Fig. 13.21**). Foreign bodies are commonly ingested by ferrets, and those ferrets that roam free in the house and have unsupervised access to toys or other objects are predisposed to it (**Fig. 13.22**). Bone may act as a foreign body in those animals feeding on diets containing bones or whole animals. Linear foreign bodies are uncommon in ferrets (**Fig. 13.23**). Most foreign bodies are identified in the stomach and jejunum, followed by the duodenum and oesophagus.

Clinical presentation

No age or sex predisposition has been detected, although some authors believe foreign bodies are more common in young ferrets. Clinical signs include anorexia, lethargy, diarrhoea, melena, absence of faecal production, weight loss, weakness and signs of nausea such as bruxism, ptyalism and face rubbing. Vomiting is uncommon. When a GI foreign body is suspected, the presence of lethargy, inappetance and absence of defaecation indicates an emergency laparoscopy.

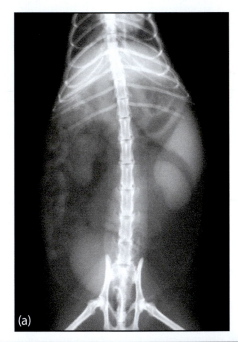

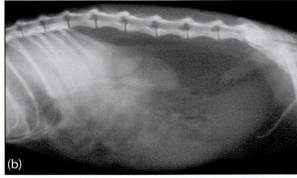

Fig. 13.23 (a) DV radiograph showing linear foreign material in intestine; (b) lateral radiograph depicting linear foreign material.

Differential diagnosis

Similar to trichobezoars, including GI tumours, inflammation or intussusception.

Diagnostic testing

Similar to trichobezoars, but symptomatology may be more severe and acute in cases of foreign bodies, and therefore physical examination is more likely to show dehydration, pale mucous membranes and weight loss. Also similarly to trichobezoars, foreign bodies in the intestine are generally palpable, as the ferret abdomen is very easy to palpate. However, inability to palpate a foreign body (particularly if it is located in the stomach) does not rule out its presence. Palpation can also detect gas and fluid-filled intestinal loops or bloated stomach.

Diagnostic imaging techniques (radiography, ultrasound, endoscopy, CT scan) are explained as in trichobezoars. In obstructing foreign bodies, gas will be visualised in the GI lumen anterior to the obstruction. Contrast radiography is useful in some cases (**Fig. 13.24**). In some cases the foreign body will be radio-opaque. Bloodwork is unspecific but may provide information on prognosis; however, increased lipase and globulins may indicate enteritis.

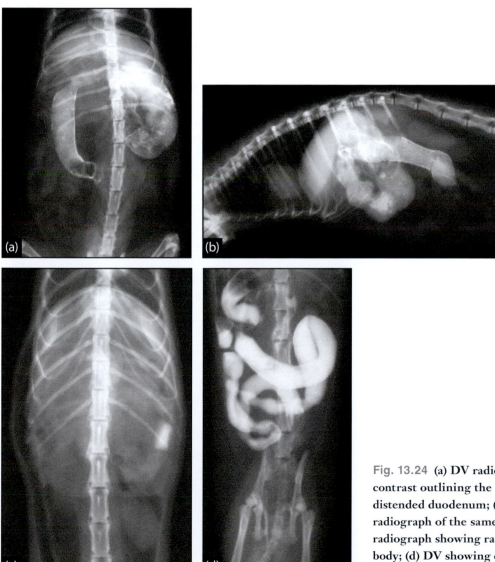

Fig. 13.24 (a) DV radiograph with contrast outlining the stomach and distended duodenum; (b) lateral radiograph of the same case; (c) DV radiograph showing radiodense foreign body; (d) DV showing distended bowel loops indicative of obstruction.

Diagnosis
See trichobezoars.

Management/treatment/prognosis
Medical treatment (with cat laxatives and fluid therapy) should only be attempted with small and non-obstructive foreign bodies. For other foreign objects surgery is generally indicated, and an emergency exploratory laparotomy is often required (**Fig. 13.25**). Multiple foreign bodies may require more than one enterotomy. Surgical prognosis is very good. Some foreign bodies may be removed with endoscopy. Subclinical cases (non-obstructive foreign bodies) may develop gastritis. Hepatic lipidosis may be seen when the ferret has been without eating for a few days. Prevention includes supervision of the ferret when outside its pen/cage. Ferret-proofed toys should be used.

GIARDIASIS

Definition/overview
Giardia sp. protozoa that belongs to the phylum Sarcomastigophora. *Giardia intestinalis* (syn. *Giardia duodenalis*) has been isolated. Clinical cases have not been reported although cysts and trophozoites are occasionally found on routine faecal examination. Giardia is considered zoonotic.

Aetiology/pathophysiology
The organism can disrupt intestinal mucosa causing diarrhoea. It is shed in the faeces. Transmission is faecal–oral.

Clinical presentation
Diarrhoea, sometimes bloody, but in many it is asymptomatic.

Differential diagnosis
Any cause of diarrhoea.

Diagnostic testing
Wet mount direct microscopy, ELISA on faeces (**Fig. 13.26**).

Management/treatment
Clinical management is similar to that used in dogs and cats. Metronidazole at 25 mg/kg PO q24h for at least 5 days has been used. Sanitation of the premises should be done; bleach is effective as a disinfectant. As this may be zoonotic, gloves and masks should be worn during cleaning and handling of affected animals.

INFLAMMATORY BOWEL DISEASE (IBD)

Definition/overview
A relatively common cause of gastroenteritis. It is inflammation of the intestinal tract.

Aetiology/pathophysiology
Cause is unknown although it has been thought to be related to dietary intolerance, hypersensitivity reaction or another aberrant immune response. On histopathology the inflammation is usually lymphoplasmacytic. It tends to occur in young or middle-aged adults and surprisingly in multi-ferret households although only one animal may be affected.

Clinical presentation
Diarrhoea that looks grainy. There may be substantial melena or haemorrhage (**Fig. 13.27**). The ferret may have bouts of nausea and vomiting intermittently, weight loss, and weakness as it progresses. Signs may be subtle and chronic and include generalised lethargy.

Differential diagnosis
Coronavirus diarrhoea (ECE), dietary indiscretion and helicobacterial-associated gastroenteritis, intestinal lymphoma.

Diagnostic testing
On palpation the intestines may feel thickened. Radiographs, ultrasonography to look at thickness of intestinal walls. CBC and serum chemistry. Full-thickness biopsies of the intestines and stomach are the definitive test.

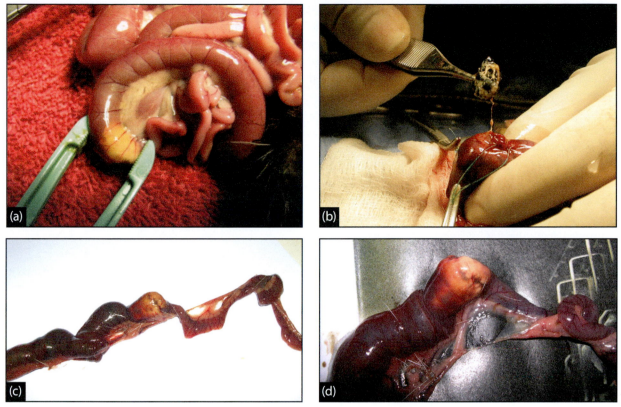

Fig. 13.25 (a) Surgical removal of foreign material; (b) obstructing foreign body; (c) necropsy image showing foreign body in intestine; (d) necropsy image showing obstructing foreign material.

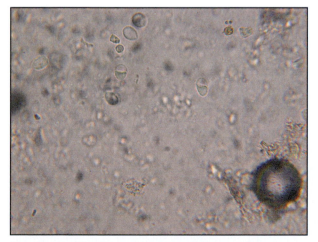

Fig. 13.26 Giardia on a wet mount from a dog.

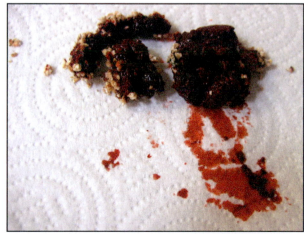

Fig. 13.27 Haemorrhagic stool seen in a case of inflammatory bowel disease confirmed on biopsy.

Diagnosis

Thickened intestinal walls confirmed with biopsy and results of lymphoplasmacytic inflammation. Liver enzymes and plasma globulins may be elevated. There may be lymphocytosis. Anaemia may be present if there have been gastrointestinal haemorrhages.

Management/treatment

Treatment is aimed at suppressing the immune response in the gut. Dietary management has been proposed by switching to a novel protein diet such as one containing turkey, venison and lamb; this is a commercially available ferret food (Performance Foods, Broomfield, Colorado, US). Switching diets in ferrets may be met with resistance and may take time. Prednisone at 1 mg/kg orally q12–24h has been tried, but many do not respond. Azathioprine at 0.9–1 mg/kg orally q24–72h seems to aid in limiting the disease. The author concurrently treats with famotidine if vomiting is present, and other supportive care such as encouraging extra meals with dook soup to combat the weight loss. Many ferrets go on to develop intestinal lymphoma found at necropsy.

MEGAOESOPHAGUS

Definition/overview

Megaoesophagus is a term to describe the dilatation of the oesophagus, which is believed to be a consequence of oesophageal hypomotility.

Aetiology

Unknown. It is believed that megaoesophagus in ferrets is not a congenital disease, as it is seen in adult animals.

Pathophysiology

Unknown. Loss of oesophageal motility could be caused by conditions affecting oesophageal nerves or muscles. Some cases are believed to be related to gastritis and gastric reflux; however, it is not clear if gastric reflux is a cause or a consequence of megaoesophagus. A case of mild megaoesophagus associated with myasthenia gravis has been described.

Clinical presentation

Clinical signs include regurgitation (after a few minutes of ingesting the meal), difficulty in swallowing (dysphagia), stretching the neck just after eating, ptialism, bruxism, reduced appetite and lethargy. The physical examination may reveal loss of body condition, weakness, dehydration and respiratory noises. Cough and respiratory problems can be a sign of aspiration pneumonia.

Differential diagnosis

When vomiting and regurgitation cannot be clearly told apart, then all causes of vomiting listed previously should be considered, particularly gastric foreign body and gastritis. Oesophageal foreign bodies are rare but should be included in the differential diagnosis. Dysphagia can also occur in cases of oral ulcers. Bruxism may be associated with gastric pain. Ptialism may be seen in dental disease, but also with oral growths or even with oral pain. Reduced appetite and lethargy (as well as loss of body condition, weakness and dehydration) are unspecific clinical signs common to many other diseases. When respiratory problems occur, conditions such as influenza or distemper should be taken into account.

Diagnostic testing

Imaging studies are necessary to investigate this condition (**Fig. 13.28**). Plain radiographs (lateral and ventrodorsal views) should include neck, thorax and abdomen, and may show dilated oesophagus with intraluminal food or gas, ventral displacement of the thoracic trachea, gastric gas or pneumonia. Contrast radiographs are better at outlining the lumen of the oesophagus, and contrast should be administered at 5–10 mL/kg; both barium or iodine-based contrast media can be administered, but barium should be avoided if the ferret is likely to have regurgitation and aspiration. To avoid this complication, radiographs can be taken holding the ferret vertically. Contrast radiographs should be taken immediately after administering the contrast media. Anaesthesia is better avoided for radiology studies, as it can induce a temporal oesophageal dilatation; if anaesthesia is to be used, the patient should be properly intubated to avoid aspiration pneumonia. Abdominal radiographs are taken to rule out other conditions.

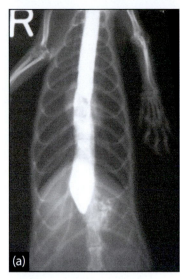
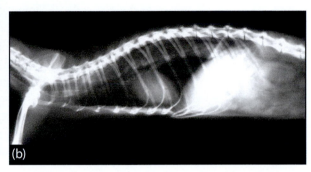

Fig. 13.28 (a) DV view with contrast of megaoesophagus; (b) lateral view of megaoesophagus.

Fluoroscopy (with or without contrast) is very useful to assess oesophageal diameter and motility. Endoscopy may reveal congestive, eroded or ulcerated oesophageal and gastric mucosa; endoscopic biopsies are recommended in cases of gastric involvement. Palpation of the left cervical area can provide additional information.

Diagnosis
A definitive diagnosis is obtained based on clinical signs and the radiological observation of oesophageal dilatation. Generally, the oesophageal diameter in affected cases is 1 cm cranially to the heart and 1.5–2 cm around the diaphragm.

Management/treatment
Prognosis is poor and most affected ferrets die or are euthanased soon after diagnosis due to weakness, hepatic lipidosis or aspiration pneumonia, although necropsy may also show gastritis and oesophagitis. However, some ferrets may live for months or years after the diagnosis. Treatment is therefore palliative and may include prokinetics such as metoclopramide (0.2–1 mg/kg PO or SC, q8h), which stimulates oesophageal motility and also helps to prevent vomiting. Mucosal protectants (100–125 mg of a solution of sucralfate PO q8–12h) and antacids such as ranitidine (doses of 1–2 mg/kg PO q8h and 3.5 mg/kg PO q12h have been reported) should be administered

if oesophagitis is suspected; famotidine or cimetidine could also be used. Antibiotics should be administered if aspiration pneumonia is suspected. When myasthenia gravis is the cause of the megaoesophagus, treatment with pyridostigmine bromide (1 mg/kg PO q8h) is indicated. The affected ferret should be placed on a soft/liquid, energetic diet administered in small amounts 4–6 times a day; the ferret should be maintained in a vertical position for 10–15 minutes after feeding. In severe cases, the placement of an oesophagostomy tube is indicated.

PROLIFERATIVE BOWEL DISEASE

Definition/overview
Bacterial disease producing diarrhoea and thickened intestinal loops (proliferative enteropathy), particularly those of the colon. The disease was described in 1983 in a research facility, but it has been poorly reported after that, and it is actually a very rare disease in clinical practice.

Aetiology
It is caused by the intracellular bacterium *Lawsonia intracellularis*.

Pathophysiology
The infection produces epithelial hyperplasia and inflammation of the colonic mucosa. Faecal–oral

transmission is suspected. Exposure to other animal species (or their faeces) may be a potential source of infection, but this has not been proved.

Clinical presentation

Young animals from 4–6 months old are most commonly affected. Chronic and intermittent diarrhoea and weight loss is observed. Faeces are mucous and contain red (blood) or green (bile) discolouration. Partial rectal prolapse, thickened intestinal loops and weight loss can be found during physical examination. Enlarged and palpable mesenteric lymph nodes can also be found due to general inflammation or extension of the proliferative epithelium into regional lymph nodes. Duration of illness can range from 3–18 weeks.

Differential diagnosis

Lymphoma, systemic coronavirus infection and eosinophilic gastroenteritis can produce thickened intestinal loops and enlarged mesenteric lymph nodes. Clinical signs of chronic diarrhoea and weight loss can be seen after suffering ECE (due to malabsorption), with IBD, *Campylobacter*-associated diarrhoea or with foreign bodies producing partial obstruction.

Diagnostic testing

Palpation may reveal thickened bowel loops, particularly colon. PCR from faeces can detect *L. intracellularis*. Colonic biopsy can be performed, followed by histology, PCR, silver stains or fluorescent antibody tests specific for *L. intracellularis*.

Diagnosis

Histology of terminal colon showing hyperplastic mucosa with intracytoplasmic organisms (demonstrated with silver stains) is diagnostic. The use of fluorescent antibody techniques and immunoperoxidase monolayer assay can also be used in tissues from biopsies or necropsies to provide a diagnosis. Faecal PCR can detect the organism, but it is not clear if all infected ferrets develop the disease.

Management/treatment

Treatments with chloramphenicol (20–50 mg/kg PO BID for 10–14 days) or metronidazole (20 mg/kg PO BID for 10–14 days) have been effective, although some animals may die. Supportive treatment with fluids and easily digestible food is recommended.

RECTAL PROLAPSE

Definition/overview

Rectal tissue is prolapsed out of the anus. This is most commonly seen in kits although it can be seen in older ferrets that develop tenesmus or severe haemorrhoids (**Fig. 13.29**).

Aetiology/pathophysiology

Most commonly there is disruption to the anal sphincter due to the demusking procedure (see Chapter 25). Too much tissue is taken from the anus and sometimes from the rectal muscle itself. There can be local nerve disruption. Severe intestinal infection with coccidia, cryptosporidia, giardia, gastroenteritis or bacteria dysbiosis and diarrhoea may contribute to tenesmus and irritation to the rectum/anus resulting in a prolapse. Rectal prolapses are most often seen in young ferrets.

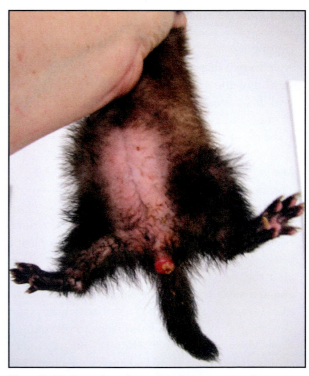

Fig. 13.29 Rectal prolapse in a kit as a sequelae to anal sacculectomy.

Clinical presentation

There is protrusion of rectal tissue. It may be desiccated, scabbed, erythematous or congested, with faeces adherent. It is painful upon touching the tissue. There may be faecal staining of the perineum and fur of the ventral tail (**Fig. 13.30**). There may be some haemorrhage from the tissue.

Differential diagnosis

Straightforward anatomical presentation. Underlying cause must be found. Rule out results of anal sacculectomy, parasitic, bacterial, inflammatory bowel disease, neoplasia.

Diagnostic testing

For ruling out causes (faecal flotation, cytology, PCR for ECE, radiographs).

Diagnosis

Visual presentation.

Management/treatment

Surgical correction of the prolapse is necessary (see Chapter 25). The author has found that purse-string sutures are not as effective as doing a wedge removal to decrease the anal orifice (**Fig. 13.31**). To help shrink the tissues prior to surgery, topical application of lidocaine (diluted 2% into 2 mL physiological saline) or ophthalmic proparicaine; 50% dextrose, 0.1 mL injectable dexamethasone 2 mg/mL, then saline should be irrigated over the prolapsed tissue. Antibiotic therapy is usually initiated, as is an analgesic. Any underlying disease needs to be addressed. Prognosis is good with surgery, provided the underlying cause is resolved.

ROTAVIRUS

Definition/overview

The ferret rotavirus is categorised as ferret rota C-MSU. Rotaviruses are 55–70 nm non-enveloped, double-stranded RNA viruses in the family Reoviridae. Rotaviruses are divided into seven major serogroups designated A to G based on antigenic properties and RNA migration patterns in polyacrylamide gels. All groups are serologically unrelated containing their own distinct antigen. Group A are called 'typical rotaviruses' and share a common antigen within the inner virion capsid layer. There are anecdotal reports of a Group A causing diarrhoea in ferrets. Group C are in the group designated as 'atypical' that do not contain the common antigen present in group A viruses. The ferret rotavirus is a Group C, species-specific rotavirus. It primarily causes disease in young ferrets although older ferrets may experience a mild form. Outbreaks can occur throughout the year in breeding facilities although it is more common in colder months.

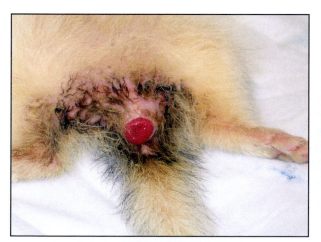

Fig. 13.30 Rectal prolapse with accompanying diarrhoea and soiling of the perineum.

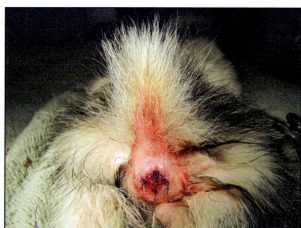

Fig. 13.31 Wedge resection to decrease the anal orifice.

Aetiology/pathophysiology

Ferret rota C-MSU is transmitted by faecal–oral route, via contact with contaminated fur or skin, objects and surfaces. It has also been suggested that it may be transmitted by the respiratory route. Large numbers of infectious viral particles are shed in faeces, although it takes fewer than 100 of these particles to transmit disease. Transmission to the kit is usually from the jill or the environment. Infected jills may harbour the virus for long periods in their fur. Reinfection is a common occurrence in breeding facilities. Once the virus is ingested it is resistant to gastric pH and digestive enzymes. It adheres to epithelial cells along the tips of the intestinal villi. It enters cells by receptor-mediated endocytosis. Once in the cell it replicates in the cytoplasm. Infected cells of the epithelium undergo structural and functional changes, resulting in the clinical signs of diarrhoea.

Clinical signs also include enlarged abdomen and dehydration. Gross lesions are thin-walled small intestines, often distended with gas and fluids. Microscopically the small intestine has superficial atrophic enteritis. Villous tips are degenerating and necrotic, which results in loss or sloughing of the affected epithelial cells into the intestinal lumen. In more chronic cases there may be mild blunting and fusion, as well as bridging of affected villi with moderate to severe lymphoplasmacytic infiltrate in the lamina propria. There may also be calcified casts within renal tubules secondary to severe dehydration.

Clinical presentation

Rotaviral disease primarily occurs in kits younger than 8 weeks of age and most commonly at 1–3 weeks of age. Diarrhoea is yellowish, soft and watery. The kit may quickly dehydrate and die. The perianal region as well as the fur on much of the body can be matted or stained by faeces. There may be erythema of the anus and perineum. Morbidity is highest in litters of primiparous jills. It can reach 90% of the infected kits in the first litter but tends to decrease to 10–20% with each subsequent litter. The abdomen is commonly distended by gas and fluid-filled intestines. Older infected ferrets may only exhibit mild, transient diarrhoea.

Differential diagnosis

Epizootic catarrhal enteritis (intestinal coronavirus), coccidiosis, cryptosporidiosis, giardiasis, systemic illness of the jill and/or mastitis that is passing bacteria to the kit through nursing, weaning with diet change. Bacterial diarrhoea.

Diagnostic testing

Faecal parasitic examination to rule out coccidian. ELISA testing for giardia, cryptosporidia (athough these may be picked up with microscopic faecal examination). PCR for cryptosporidia is available commercially. Full examination of the jill. PCR of faeces to rule out coronavirus. Culture of the faeces to rule out bacterial diarrhoea, dysbiosis. RT-PCR on faecal samples or sections of small intestine at necropsy.

Diagnosis

Positive identification on RT-PCR. Transmission electron microscopy is used in some laboratories to detect the characteristic viral particles in faeces. The commercially available ELISA test for group A rotaviruses will not detect ferret rota C-MSU.

Management/treatment

There is no treatment other than trying supportive care for the individual. Once established in a breeding colony it is difficult to eradicate as it is resistant to common disinfectants. Viral particles are stable in faeces. Emphasis should be on prevention. Household bleach or sodium hydroxide are the most effective means of disinfection. There is currently no commercial vaccine available. There are anecdotal reports that describe controlling the diarrhoea by force feeding stool from affected juveniles to pregnant jills. Then colostral antibodies may protect the next litter from the diarrhoea but not the infection itself. Ferret kits receive all their IgA from the milk, which appears to be important to protect them from disease.

SYSTEMIC DISEASES PRODUCING GASTROINTESTINAL SIGNS

A number of systemic diseases may affect the GI tract (including the liver) and produce GI clinical signs.

Many of these diseases will be covered more extensively in other chapters of this book, and only a short review of their gastrointestinal implication will be mentioned here.

Disseminated idiopathic myofasciitis (DIM) (see Chapter 17)

The disease consists of a pyogranulomatous inflammation affecting muscle and fascia, characterised clinically by fever, neutrophilic leucocitosis, muscle weakness, pain, lack of response to treatment and eventually death. When the disease affects the oesophagus, dysphagia can be observed, with the ferret having difficulty swallowing or drinking.

Lymphoma (see Chapter 16)

In certain ferret populations, lymphoma is the third most common neoplasia after adrenal tumours and insulinoma. Lymphoma can occur in adult and young animals. Neoplastic infiltrates usually affect spleen, liver and mesenteric lymph nodes. The intestinal wall can also become affected and produce maldigestion, malabsorption and partial or total obstruction. The stools may be abnormal with melena or haemorrhage (**Fig. 13.32**). Hypoalbuminaemia is common in these cases, and the intestinal wall can be felt thickened on abdominal palpation. Gastrointestinal signs, such as diarrhoea and vomiting, are usually seen together with other systemic signs. Liver disease can be expected when significant neoplastic infiltrates affect the hepatic parenchyma.

Other neoplastic conditions

Some neoplastic conditions (squamous cell carcinoma, osteoma) can grow on the head and interfere with mastication. Chronic infections with *Helicobacter mustelae* have been associated with the development of gastric adenocarcinoma. Invasion of the intestine from islet cell carcinomas has been observed (**Fig. 13.33**).

Aleutian disease (see Chapter 16)

Infection with ADV may produce deposition of immune complexes in the stomach and intestine, leading to clinical signs such as chronic weight loss and melena due to haemorrhagic enteritis (**Fig. 13.34**). These clinical signs are usually associated with other systemic signs (neurological signs, renal failure, etc.). ADV has also caused hepatitis characterised by bile duct hyperplasia and periportal fibrosis.

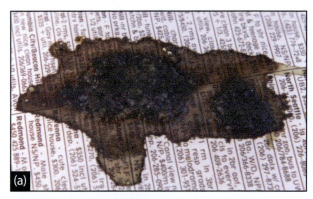

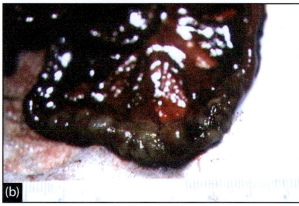

Fig. 13.32 **(a) Melena in stool with intestinal lymphoma; (b) necropsy section of intestine with lymphoma.**

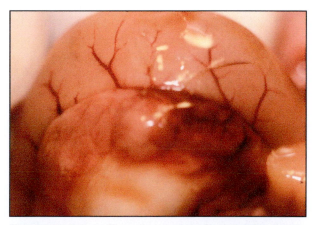

Fig. 13.33 **Islet cell carcinoma invading the duodenal wall.**

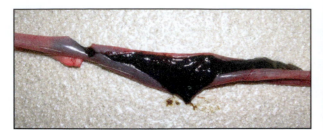

Fig. 13.34 Haemorrhagic enteritis with Aleutian disease.

Ferret systemic coronaviral disease (FRSCV, see Chapter 16)

This is a systemic disease with histopathological changes very similar to those observed in feline infectious peritonitis in cats. One of the early clinical signs is diarrhoea. Later in the course of the disease, granulomas develop in different organs, particularly in mesenteric lymph nodes, kidney, spleen and liver, but also in intestine. Hepatic and GI clinical signs can be seen.

Pancreatitis

Although uncommon, serious pancreatitis can occur after pancreatic surgery to remove insulinomas. When severe pain or lethargy is observed after insulinoma surgery, pancreatitis should be suspected. In some cases of pancreatitis, the adjacent intestine will be necrotic.

Gastric and intestinal ulceration

Gastric ulcers have been reported in this chapter associated with gastritis, *Helicobacter mustelae* infection or gastric foreign bodies. Gastric ulceration can also be observed with renal failure due to azotaemia. Ulcers may also appear in the intestine (**Fig. 13.35**). Ulcerogenic drugs (such as ibuprofen) can produce gastric ulceration in ferrets, although this toxicity will also produce other serious clinical signs such as neurological signs, depression, weakness and recumbency.

LIVER AND GALLBLADDER

The liver may be affected by conditions of the GI tract. This includes non-specific hepatitis, hepatic lipidosis (seen any time there has been prolonged

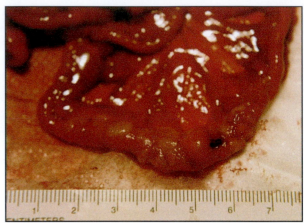

Fig. 13.35 Ulceration in the wall of the small intestine.

anorexia), metastatic neoplasia (lymphoma, islet cell carcinoma), hepatomegaly (particularly with right heart disease), even trichobezoars or foreign bodies that may obstruct bile ducts as they enter the small intestine. ADV causes hepatitis characterised by bile duct hyperplasia and periportal fibrosis.

Gallbladder disease

Definition/overview

Cholangitis, cholelithiasis (gallstones), cholangiohepatitis and cholestasis have been diagnosed, often with elements of all three conditions. Gallbladder disease may include inflammation as well as bile stasis. Gallstones may form due to the inflammation and stasis, and may also have an ascending bacterial component (from the duodenum through the bile duct) as a nidus for formation.

Aetiology/pathophysiology

The inflammation in the gallbladder may start with irritation to the mucous membranes probably involving a bacterial component entering from the bile duct. Generalised biliary tree complications during neoplasia or hepatitis/hepatopathy may also be involved. Once gallstones have formed, they may block the duct contributing further to bile stasis. *Helicobacter mustelae* has been found to cause cholangiohepatitis and may be a part of other pathology as well.

Clinical presentation

Non-specific signs of lethargy, anorexia, vomiting and diarrhoea may be seen. Icterus may be present. There may be pain or nausea triggered with palpation of the cranial abdomen.

Differential diagnosis

Hepatitis, hepatic neoplasia.

Diagnostic testing

CBC, serum chemistry. A coagulation panel may also be included. Radiographs and ultrasonography will usually confirm the presence of cholelithiasis and if there is thickening of the gallbladder wall (**Fig. 13.36**). Vitamin K should be administered prior to any biopsy. Fine needle aspirate or biopsy (ultrasound guided) of the liver may show biliary stasis and inflammation. Theoretically you could biopsy the gallbladder although this is rarely done. Exploratory laparotomy may be performed and in some cases cholangectomy is performed. *H. mustelae* PCR can be run as *Helicobacter* may play a role in initiation of inflammation.

Diagnosis

Confirmation of cholangitis, cholelithiasis, cholangiohepatitis and/or cholestasis. There may be elevations of alanine aminotransferase, alkaline phosphatase and/or bilirubin. There may be bilirubinuria.

Management/treatment

If the bile duct is plugged with stones, surgery is indicated and probably a cholangectomy is performed rather than a cholangotomy just to remove the stones. Prior to surgery a coagulation panel should be run. Supportive care includes fluid therapy, and B-complex vitamin supplementation. Antibiotics such as amoxicillin are used. Other liver supportive care may be given including milk thistle, taurine and L-carnitine. Dosages for these are listed in the formulary but are empirical. The author (CAJD) does not use the commercial liver support methionine, inositol, lecithin combination. Famotidine is used to help prevent stress gastric ulceration. If *H. mustelae* is involved, the protocol for treatment should be initiated. Ursodiol may be used to reduce biliary stasis. Prognosis is guarded.

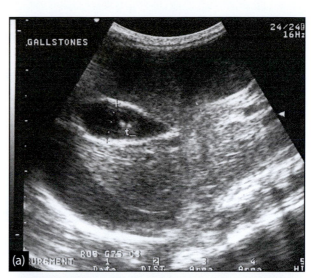

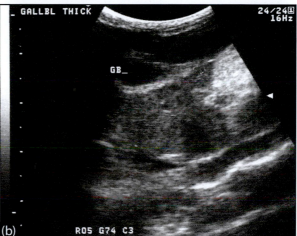

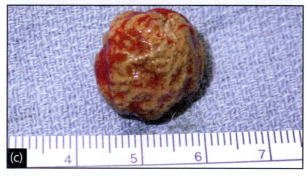

Fig. 13.36 (a) Choleliths and thickened gallbladder wall; (b) thickened gallbladder walls; (c) cholelith.

Hepatic lipidosis

Definition/overview

The liver becomes infiltrated with fat (**Fig. 13.37**).

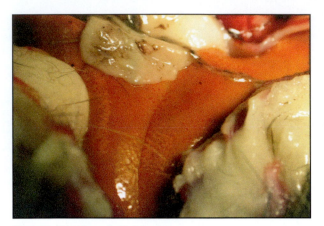

Fig. 13.37 Hepatic lipidosis.

Aetiology/pathophysiology

Anorexia and sudden weight loss predispose the condition. Other factors might play a role in its development: coronavirus enteritis, hepatic lymphocytic hepatitis that compromises hepatic function, steroid usage, endocrine dyscrasias.

Clinical presentation

A ferret that has not been eating for as little as 2 days. Presentation is variable with many cases being subclinical. Presenting signs are related to whatever disease process precipitated the initial weight loss. Severe cases may cause enough hepatomegaly to be palpated. Serum chemistry may be normal or show elevations of alanine aminotransferase, gamma-glutamyl transferase (GGT).

Differential diagnosis

Hepatitis, hepatomegaly due to congestion from heart disease, hepatic neoplasia.

Diagnostic testing

Radiographs, ultrasonography, ultrasound-guided transdermal biopsy. Exploratory surgery and biopsy. Vitamin K should be administered prior to biopsy procedure. CBC and serum chemistry.

Diagnosis

Histopathology showing fat infiltration. Hepatomegaly present on radiographs and/or ultrasound. Grossly the liver appears pale brown to yellow in colour. The lobes tend to be swollen and rounded.

Management/treatment

As with other species, getting nutrition into the ferret is critical. This can be done by the addition of dook soup and a commercial product like Nutrical (Vetoquinol, Fort Worth, TX). Treat underlying disease. Broad-spectrum antibiotics may be used to inhibit GI bacterial overgrowth or low-grade hepatitis. One suggested combination is to use enrofloxacin at 5 mg/kg PO q12h along with amoxicillin at 10 mg/kg PO q12h. Ursodiol (Actigall) can be used to reduce biliary stasis. Dosage is 15 mg/kg PO q24h. Prognosis for reversing hepatic lipidosis is good in most ferrets provided that the underlying cause of the lipidosis is identified and resolved.

Hepatitis

Definition/overview

Inflammation of the liver. Chronic lymphocytic portal hepatitis has been documented on histological examination. It may accompany neoplasia.

Aetiology/pathophysiology

Inflammation may be related to chronic visceral inflammation including IBD. *Helicobacter mustelae* has been found in hepatitis and may be causative. The organism was found in the faeces. Other bacteria may be involved. Often there is concurrent neoplastic disease. Chronic cholangiohepatitis with biliary hyperplasia of variable intensity has been found. Newly identified ferret hepatitis E has been linked with the development of hepatitis (see Chapter 23).

Clinical presentation

May be non-specific signs including anorexia, weight loss, vomiting, diarrhoea. In severe cases there may be icterus (**Fig. 13.38**). Pain may be associated with palpation of the liver and upper abdomen.

Differential diagnosis

Hepatic neoplasia, *Helicobacter* infection, IBD, other causes of vomiting and/or diarrhoea.

Diagnostic testing

Helicobacter may be diagnosed via PCR of the faeces or gastric aspiration. Ultrasonography may show changes in the liver parenchyma, looking more

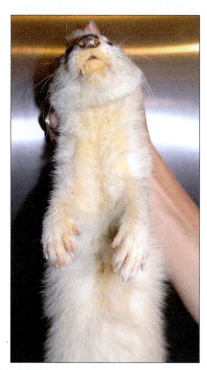

Fig. 13.38 **Icterus.**

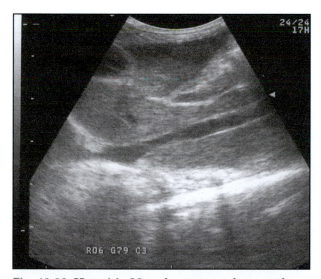

Fig. 13.39 **Hepatitis. Note dense parenchyma and thickened walls of ducts and vasculature.**

dense than normal (**Fig. 13.39**). Radiographs may show hepatomegaly. Vitamin K should be administered prior to any biopsy. Ultrasound-guided biopsy of the liver and histopathology. CBC, serum chemistry to assess liver function primarily. Urinalysis to look for bilirubinuria.

Diagnosis

Histopathology confirmation of a form of hepatitis. Liver enzymes may be elevated particularly alanine transaminase (higher than 275 IU/L) and alkaline phosphatase. If there is bile duct obstructive disease, bilirubin may be elevated. Bilirubinuria may be present. There may be elevated lymphocytes. PCR confirmation of *Helicobacter*. Surgery may be necessary if there is an obstructed bile duct (see on ultrasonography).

Management/treatment

Symptomatic supportive care includes amoxicillin at 20 mg/kg orally q12h, fluids, bismuth subsalicylate at 6 mg/kg orally q12h. If *Helicobacter* confirmed, in addition to those medications metronidazole at 20 mg/kg orally q12h. Dook soup and additional feeding may be necessary if there has been weight loss. If neoplasia is present the prognosis is poor. If there are distinct masses, theoretically the affected lobe of the liver could be excised surgically, but the author does not know of this being done on a routine basis.

NEOPLASIA

Many types of neoplasia have been documented, both benign and malignant. They include lymphoma, haemangiosarcoma, adenocarcinoma, hepatoma, biliary cystadenoma and hepatocellular adenoma. Lymphoma is the most common (**Fig. 13.40**) (see Chapter 16). Pancreatic islet cell tumours may metastasise into the liver. Prognosis is guarded to poor.

Hepatocellular
Definition/overview
Hepatocellular carcinomas significantly outnumber hepatocellular adenomas. Carcinoma is seen with no gender predilection in adult ferrets.

Aetiology/pathophysiology
There is marked hepatomegaly (**Fig. 13.41**). This may be 4 or 5 times the normal weight/size. Grossly there may be white to grey nodules of variable number, shape and size in the parenchyma. There may be ascitic fluid present. Histologically the carcinoma is composed of large cuboidal to pleomorphic

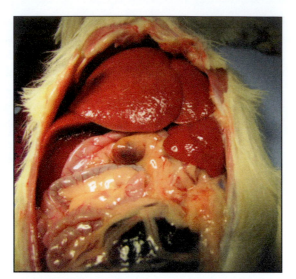

Fig. 13.40 **Hepatic lymphoma. Note concurrent lymphadenopathy.**

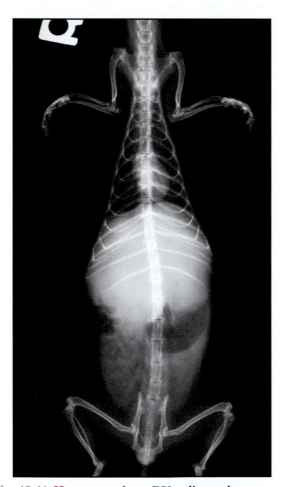

Fig. 13.41 **Hepatomegaly on DV radiograph.**

cells arranged in acini, sheets or cords. There may be metastasis to the spleen and mesenteric lymph nodes. Hepatocellular adenoma was documented as an incidental finding in a 5-year-old male ferret with the tumour mass well circumscribed. It consisted of pleomorphic epithelial cells resembling normal hepatocytes (**Fig. 13.42**).

Clinical presentation
Signs may be non-specific consisting of lethargy, anorexia and weight loss. There may be cranial to mid-abdominal mass or hepatomegaly on palpation. It also may be painful.

Differential diagnosis
Hepatitis, neoplasia including right adrenal, hepatomegaly due to congestive heart failure.

Diagnostic testing
Radiographs and ultrasonography. A coagulation panel prior to any ultrasound-guided fine needle aspirate or biopsy is prudent, particularly if exploratory laparotomy and biopsy are planned. Vitamin K should be administered prior to any biopsy or surgery. Histopathology of samples. Serum chemistry.

Diagnosis
Histopathology confirms hepatocellular carcinoma or adenoma. Serum chemistry of alanine aminotransferase or alkaline phosphatase may be elevated.

Management/treatment
Unfortunately by the time of diagnosis it is often disseminated throughout the liver and individual masses are too many to remove surgically. Many times the diagnosis is made at necropsy. Otherwise, supportive care for the liver may be attempted which includes amoxicillin, fluid therapy, B-complex vitamins, milk thistle, taurine and and L-carnitine. Some practitioners use methionine and inositol as liver supplements. Analgesics should be used if the ferret seems in pain. Famotidine may also be used to try to prevent gastric ulceration from the stress of the neoplasia. Prognosis is poor.

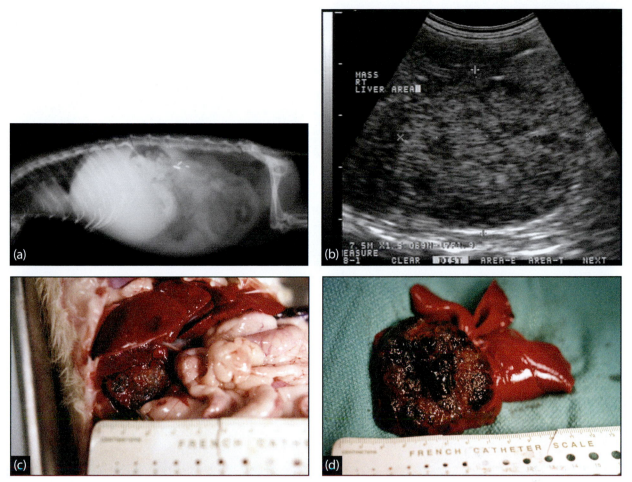

Fig. 13.42 (a) Lateral radiograph showing hepatomegaly and likely mass on the liver, (the haemoclips are from a left adrenalectomy); (b) ultrasonogram of a liver mass; (c) mass in the liver; (d) mass removed with the liver. This was identified on histopathology as a hepatocellular carcinoma.

Biliary

Definition/overview

Neoplasia of the biliary system is a continuum between common benign biliary cysts, benign cyst-adenomas, cystadenocarcinoma and infiltrative chol-angiocellular carcinoma.

Aetiology/pathophysiology

Biliary cysts are common and may be focal or multiple. They are often incidental lesions (**Fig. 13.43**). Biliary cystadenomas are the most common neoplasms of the biliary tract. These cause problems as they are infiltrative and may actually replace one or more lobes of the liver. Grossly the two lesions are easily differentiated. Cystadenomas often arise at the edge of liver lobes. These are composed of interconnected oval to spherical cysts with minimal intervening fibrous stroma. These cysts often have clear intraluminal fluid. Rarely it may be opaque. Histologically these lesions look very similar as both are large empty cystic spaces lined by attenuated epithelium. Differentiating between biliary cysts, cystadenomas, cystadenocarcinoma and cystadenocarcinoma on a limited surgical biopsy, it is important to look closely for the presence of hepatic-specific clinical signs, clinopathologic abnormalities or progressive growth via abdominal palpation or ultrasound (**Fig. 13.44**).

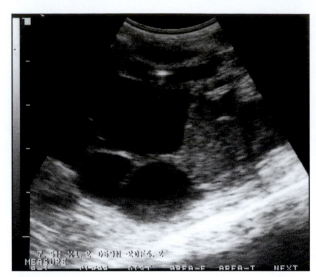

Fig. 13.43 **Ultrasonogram of liver cysts.**

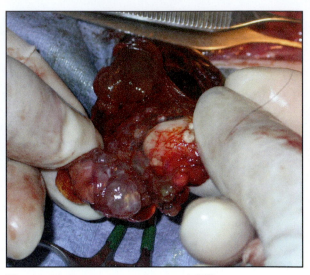

Fig. 13.44 **Surgery exposing cysticbiliary adenocarcinoma.**

Clinical presentation

Signs may be non-specific consisting of lethargy, anorexia and weight loss. There may be cranial to mid-abdominal hepatomegaly. It also may be painful. There may be icterus in advanced stages. There may also be elevations of alanine aminotransferase, alkaline phosphatase and bilirubin.

Differential diagnosis

Hepatic cysts, hepatomegaly, hepatic neoplasia.

Diagnostic testing

Ultrasonography, radiology. CBC, serum chemistry, coagulation panel. Vitamin K should be administered prior to any biopsies or surgery. Exploratory laparotomy with biopsies. Ultrasound-guided biopsy of the liver. PCR for *Helicobacter mustelae.*

Diagnosis

Biliary cysts and cystadenomas may be ruled out if malignant presentation on histopathology is found. Cystadenocarcinoma is diagnosed in cases where there is infiltrative growth and replacement of extensive amounts of liver tissue, even if there are no

cellular features of malignancy. Cholangiocellular carcinoma is easier to diagnose. It is composed of acini-lined cuboidal epithelial cells with large nuclei and a variable mitotic rate. These carcinomas are usually associated with a prominent desmoplastic response. Diagnosis of cholangeiocellular carcinoma may not be made until it is in advanced stages with elevations of alanine aminotransferase, alkaline phosphatase and bilirubin. A positive *Helicobacter* test may validate the disease process.

Management/treatment

General supportive and symptomatic care. Surgical excision of any cystic lesion should be done with wide margins due to the aggressive nature of biliary cystadenoma (a gross pathological stage diagnosis cannot be made). Analgesics, fluid therapy, vitamin B complex, vitamin K, amoxicillin, bismuth subsalicylate (*Helicobacter* treatment regimen), metronidazole, and nutraceuticals (milk thistle, taurine, L-carnitine, coQ10) can be used. Famotidine is used due to likelihood of development of gastric ulcers due to the *Helicobacter* and stress. Prognosis of any hepatic neoplasm involving multiple lobes is poor.

CHAPTER 14

DISORDERS OF THE ENDOCRINE SYSTEM

Nico J. Schoemaker and
Yvonne R.A. van Zeeland

INTRODUCTION

Endocrine diseases are among the most commonly seen conditions in ferrets. Insulinomas (or islet cell tumours) and adrenocortical tumours constitute the majority of the endocrine diseases, seen predominantly in middle-aged to older ferrets, although they may occasionally be seen in younger ferrets as well. Other endocrine disorders that may be encountered in ferrets include persistent oestrus, diabetes mellitus, hypothyroidism and hypoparathyroidism. Of the endocrine diseases described in companion animals, the following have not been documented in ferrets: growth hormone deficiency or growth hormone excess, diabetes insipidus, hyperthyroidism, hyperparathyroidism and spontaneous hypoadrenocorticism (Addison's disease). Despite the lack of reported cases, the above mentioned differentials should not be ruled out, and further diagnostic work-up for such diseases is warranted when confronted with a ferret with clinical signs corresponding to symptoms seen in dogs and/or cats with the aforementioned endocrine diseases.

DISEASES OF THE ADRENAL GLAND

Hyperadrenocorticism/ hyperandrogenism
Definition/overview
The most common form of adrenal disease in ferrets is hyperadrenocorticism, which is characterised by a hyperfunction of the adrenal cortex. The adrenal cortex is built up out of three layers (**Fig. 14.1**). In principle, distinct syndromes may arise from hyperfunctioning of each of these layers: hyperaldosteronism or Conn's syndrome (i.e. increased production of mineralocorticoids by

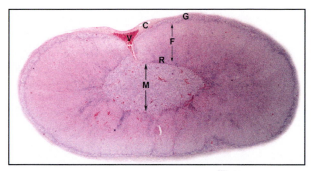

Fig. 14.1 Histological cross-section of a left adrenal gland of a healthy ferret. Key: C, capsule; F, zona fasciculate; G, zona glomerulosa; M, medulla; R, zona reticularis; V, adrenolumbar vein.

the zona glomerulosa), hypercortisolism or Cushing's syndrome (i.e. increased production of glucocorticoids by the zona fasciculata), and hyperandrogenism (i.e. increased production of androgens by the zona reticularis). In pet ferrets, hyperandrogenism is the most common form of hyperadrenocorticism, resulting in increased plasma concentrations of androstenedione, 17-hydroxyprogesterone and oestradiol. In rare instances, hypercortisolism and hyperaldosteronism may also be seen.

Hyperandrogenism is most commonly diagnosed in neutered pet ferrets of 3 years and older. In the USA, however, diagnosis of hyperandrogenism in ferrets may occur as early as 2 years of age. An exact incidence is not known, but it has been reported that up to 95% of ferrets presented for postmortem examination suffered from adrenal pathology. In a recent study, 80% of 125 surgically neutered ferrets developed adrenal cortical disease over a period of 8 years. There appears to be no sex predilection: the disease affects males and females equally.

A unilateral enlargement of the adrenal gland (without atrophy of the contralateral adrenal gland) appears to be most common (present in approximately 85% of ferrets). Bilateral enlargement may be found in the remainder of cases. Adrenal tumours have been histologically classified as (nodular) hyperplasia, adenoma and adenocarcinoma. The histological diagnosis, however, does not provide any prognostic information, nor does it infer information about the functionality of the tumour.

Aetiology and pathogenesis

Different aetiologies have been suggested for the high incidence of hyperadrenocorticism in ferrets. These include (early) neutering of ferrets, housing ferrets indoors and genetic background.

(Early) neutering: In the last two decades, a growing amount of evidence has been gathered supporting the hypothesis that the high incidence of hyperadrenocorticism in pet ferrets is the result of neutering. This evidence has shown that neutering results in increased concentrations of gonadotrophins (due to the loss of negative feedback from the gonads), which stimulate the LH receptors that are present in the adrenal cortex, eventually leading to the development of an adrenocortical neoplasm (**Fig. 14.2**). The prevalence of the disease appears similar in the Netherlands and the USA, where ferrets are neutered at a different age. Based on these findings a significant correlation has been found between the age at neutering and the age at

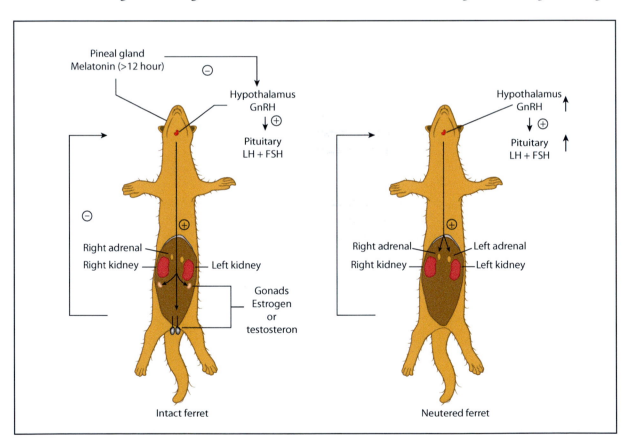

Fig. 14.2 Diagram illustrating the regulation of reproductive endocrinology in intact ferrets, the consequences of neutering on this process and the possible role it plays in the development of hyperadrenocorticism in this species. In short, high melatonin concentrations for more than 12 hours per day suppress the release of gonadotropin-releasing hormone (GnRH). When this suppression is lost, GnRH is released in a pulsatile fashion, resulting in the release of luteinising hormone (LH) and follicle-stimulating hormone (FSH), which in turn stimulate the release of oestrogen and testosterone. This exerts a negative feedback on the hypothalamus and pituitary gland. When ferrets are neutered this negative feedback is lost, resulting in an increased release of the gonadotrophins, which may activate their respective receptors in ferret adrenal glands if they are present.

onset of hyperandrogenism. In addition, they indicate that age of neutering may be of less importance for the development of adrenocortical tumours than neutering itself. Although less common, adrenal disease may also occur in intact ferrets. In these ferrets, diagnosing the disease may be more difficult as the clinical signs with which the ferrets present are difficult to differentiate from the normal hormonally driven physiological changes that occur in healthy intact ferrets.

Housing ferrets indoors: In line with the hypothesis that increased gonadotrophin levels induced by neutering pose an increased risk for developing adrenal gland tumours, indoor housing may also pose as a risk factor for developing increased gonadotrophins and subsequent hyperadrenocorticism. Ferrets that are kept indoors will generally be exposed to more hours of light per day than ferrets that are housed outdoors. As a result, melatonin will be suppressed for longer periods of time, which – as a result of loss of inhibitory action of melatonin – subsequently results in elevated gonadotrophin plasma concentrations and increased risk of developing adrenal gland disease in both neutered and intact ferrets.

Genetic background: As ferrets have a high incidence of both insulinomas and adrenal gland tumours, it has been hypothesised that the hereditary changes causing multiple endocrine neoplasms in humans (MEN1, MEN2a and MEN2b), could also play a role in the aetiology of the formation of adrenal tumours in ferrets. Since many of the ferrets in the USA come from the same breeding facility, thereby sharing a similar genetic background, it is possible that in the USA the limited genetic variation of ferrets poses an explanation for the high incidence of the disease. Thus far, however, no proof for a genetic predisposition has been found. In addition, ferrets in the Netherlands supposedly have a different genetic background from the ferrets in the USA. It therefore remains questionable if a genetic predisposition indeed is involved.

Pituitary adenomas have been detected in ferrets with adrenal tumours. However, these tumours did not seem to secrete any of the pituitary hormones, thereby characterising them as clinically non-functional gonadotrope tumours. Thus, in contrast to dogs with Cushing's disease, pituitary tumours do not seem to be associated with hyperadrenocorticism in ferrets.

Clinical presentation

The most common clinical signs in ferrets with hyperadrenocorticism include symmetrical alopecia (**Fig. 14.3**) and pruritus. Sometimes only a thinning of the hair coat may be seen. Hair loss frequently starts at the base of the tail and back and may gradually progress to a more generalised alopecia. In the first year of symptoms, hair may regrow during the winter after which it will disappear again during the next moult. Skin lesions are usually absent, unless scratching results in excoriations. There may be generalised pruritus. In (neutered) jills, vulvar swelling (**Fig. 14.4**) and occasional mammary gland enlargement may be noted. Bone marrow suppression, resulting in pancytopaenia (anaemia, thrombocytopaenia, leucopaenia) may occur due to hyperoestrogenism, but is considered rare in ferrets with hyperadrenocorticism. In hobs, dysuria, pollakisuria and/or anuria may be encountered due to the androgen-related development of secondary periprostatic or periurethral cysts causing urethral obstruction (**Fig. 14.5**). Hobs (and occasionally jills) may furthermore show recurrence of sexual behaviour. This is often accompanied by an increased skin odour produced by the sebaceous glands. The ferret may also exhibit increased aggression.

Polyuria and polydipsia (PU/PD) have also been documented in ferrets with hyperadrenocorticism. It is not clear whether this clinical sign is resultant from concurrent kidney disease occurring in (elderly) ferrets, or from an increased production of adrenal hormones. In a case of LH-dependent hypercortisolism (Cushing's disease) in a ferret, PU/PD were the predominant clinical sign, with other clinical signs (e.g. alopecia) being minimally present.

Differential diagnoses

The most important differential diagnosis for a female ferret with signs of hyperadrenocorticism is an active ovary, either due to the presence of an ovarian remnant, ovarian neoplasm (granulosa cell tumour) or because the animal has not been ovariectomised (i.e. an intact jill) (**Fig. 14.6**). Other possibilities include a Sertoli cell tumour (in cryptorchid,

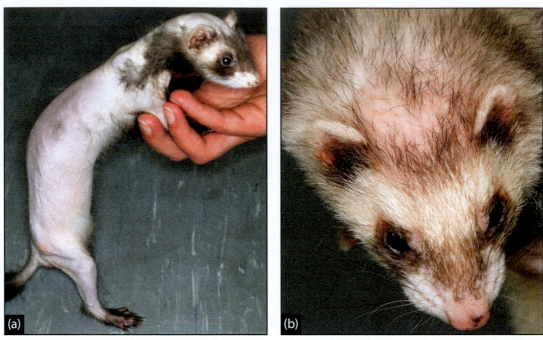

Fig. 14.3 (a) Symmetrical alopecia in a 5-year-old female ferret with hyperadrenocorticism; (b) the alopecia in this female ferret with hyperadrenocorticism was located only on the head.

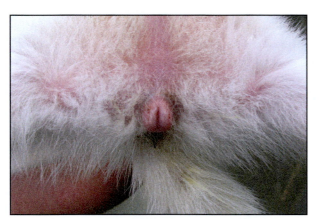

Fig. 14.4 Oestrus can easily be detected in female ferrets as the vulva is greatly enlarged during this period.

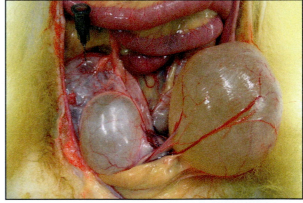

Fig. 14.5 A postmortem view of the abdomen of a 7-year-old male ferret with a periurethral cyst that developed as a result of a right adrenal tumour. The fluid out of the largest cyst has already been collected, after which the needle was kept in place.

intact hobs) and hypothyroidism, although both are considered rare. In addition, hypothyroidism will rarely result in pruritus. If the ferret is showing signs of severe alopecia and pruritus, food intolerance and infectious skin diseases (e.g. dermatophytosis, demodicosis and bacterial dermatitis) should also be considered in the differential diagnoses. In the latter cases, however, skin lesions will often be present, whereas such lesions (other than an incidental superficial scratch mark) will not be present in ferrets with hyperadrenocorticism or food intolerance. Seasonal alopecia, characterised by a seasonal occurrence of

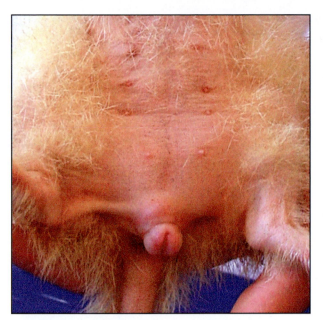

Fig. 14.6 Abdominal alopecia, swollen nipples and an extremely enlarged vulva in a ferret. These signs can be seen during oestrus, but also in cases of hyperadrenocorticism.

alopecia at the base of the tail, is also commonly mentioned as a differential diagnoses. The actual cause for this condition is currently not known, but the authors suspect that it may well be an early sign of hyperadrenocorticism.

Diagnosis

Clinical signs: A tentative diagnosis of hyperadrenocorticism can usually be made based on the presence of the typical clinical signs combined with the exclusion of other differential diagnoses. Aside from the clinical signs mentioned previously, abdominal palpation may reveal presence of a (tiny) firm mass craniomedial to the cranial pole of the kidneys. An enlargement of the left adrenal gland will usually be easier to palpate than a right adrenal gland enlargement as the latter is located more cranial and dorsal to the right caudate process of the caudate liver lobe, thereby obscuring it from palpation unless it is grossly enlarged.

Hormone analysis: This is commonly recommended in the diagnostic work-up of ferrets suspected of hyperadrenocorticism. (Appendix 4 provides normative values). For this purpose, plasma may be collected and submitted to an external laboratory, for analysis of androstenedione, oestradiol and 17-hydroxyprogesterone. Elevation of plasma concentrations of one or more of the aforementioned hormones has been considered as diagnostic for hyperadrenocorticism in ferrets. Plasma androstenedione, oestradiol and 17-hydroxyprogesterone concentrations in intact female ferrets are, however, identical to those in hyperadrenocorticoid ferrets. The authors therefore do not consider the analysis of these hormones useful for differentiating between a ferret with hyperandrogenism and one with an active ovarian remnant. Hormone analysis may, however, be useful to monitor the effect of treatment and progression of the disease (*Table 14.1*).

In contrast to dogs, plasma concentrations of ACTH and α-MSH do not change in ferrets with hyperandrogenism and are therefore not helpful in

Table 14.1 Serum concentrations of adrenal hormones in intact female ferrets and neutered ferrets without and with hyperadrenocorticism

| | | | NEUTERED FERRETS | | |
| | INTACT FEMALE FERRET | | NORMAL FERRETS | | ACD |
STEROID HORMONE	MEAN	REFERENCE	MEAN	REFERENCE	MEAN
Androstenedione (nmol/L)	58	20–96	6.6	<0.1–15	67
Oestradiol (pmol/L)	166	122–210	106	30–108	167
17-OH progesterone (nmol/L)	7.7	2.3–13	0.4	<0.1–0.8	3.2

Key: ACD, adrenal cortical disease.
Adapted from Rosenthal KL, Wyre NR (2012) Endocrine diseases. In Quesenberry KE, Carpenter JW (eds) *Ferrets, Rabbits, and Rodents: Clinical Medicine and Surgery, 3rd edition.* Elsevier, St. Louis. pp 86–102.

establishing a diagnosis. Similarly, plasma cortisol concentrations, ACTH stimulation tests and dexamethasone suppression tests (commonly used to diagnose Cushing's syndrome in dogs) are considered non-diagnostic in ferrets with hyperandrogenism. A stimulation test with human chorionic gonadotrophin (hCG), an LH-receptor agonist, may be performed in those ferrets of which it is certain that their gonads have been completely removed. Blood samples should be collected immediately before and 60 min after an intramuscular injection of 100 IU hCG. In ferrets with hyperadrenocorticism, stimulation with hCG will result in increased androstenedione concentrations, even if baseline androstenedione concentrations were below the detection limit.

Urine analysis: An increased urinary corticoid: creatinine ratio (UCCR) can be found in ferrets with adrenocortical disease ($>2.1 \times 10^{-6}$). The UCCR, however, is considered to be of limited diagnostic value because this ratio is also increased in intact ferrets during the breeding season and in ferrets with an active ovarian remnant. The test is therefore not considered diagnostic, and may only be used as a rough screening tool in case of monitoring a large population of ferrets for the presence of hyperadrenocorticism.

Diagnostic imaging: Radiographs are not ideal for identifying (enlarged) adrenal glands. Adrenal glands will only be visible on radiographs when they are extremely enlarged, or contain mineralisations. Abdominal ultrasonography, on the other hand, is considered by the authors to be a highly useful tool in diagnosing hyperadrenocorticism in ferrets. It should be emphasised, however, that ultrasound only allows evaluation of the size and morphology of the organs and does not provide any information on the functionality of the tumour. It may thus be possible to find only one adrenal gland enlarged, while both adrenal glands contribute to the androgen release, or to find neither gland enlarged in a ferret with clinical signs resulting from hyperandrogenism. Ultrasound is considered particularly useful when surgical intervention is envisaged as it allows identification of the affected adrenal gland(s) and/or a remnant ovary as well as evaluation of other abdominal organs (e.g. prostate, **Figs 14.7, 14.8**). Abdominal lymph nodes

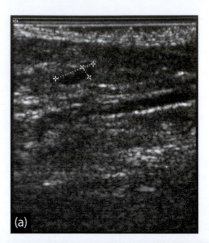

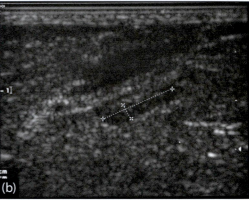

Fig. 14.7 Ultrasound of normal left (a) and right (b) adrenal glands including the normal range of measurements.

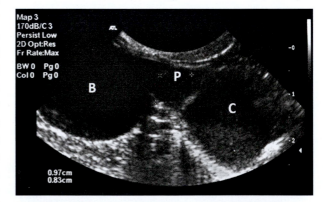

Fig. 14.8 Transverse sonogram of the bladder (B), prostate (P) and a periprostatic cyst (C) in a 4-year-old male ferret with hyperadrenocorticism. This ferret was presented with dysuria that resolved after emptying of the cyst by ultrasound-guided aspiration. The cyst turned out to be a diverticulum of the urethra, filled with turbid urine.

may resemble adrenal glands, thereby requiring the use of specific landmarks to correctly identify the adrenal glands. For the left adrenal gland, which is located lateral to the aorta, the cranial mesenteric and coeliac arteries branch of the aorta may be used as landmarks (**Fig. 14.9**). The right adrenal gland may be located during a transverse scan by first identifying the aorta (most dorsal and pulsating), portal vein (most ventral and widest in diameter) and caudal vena cava in the region of the caudate process of the liver, following which the right adrenal gland may be located at the level of and/or immediately cranial to the origin of the cranial mesenteric artery (**Fig. 14.10**). It is important to realise that the right

adrenal gland is always attached to the dorsolateral wall of the caudal vena cava. This can also be seen during the longitudinal scan, whereby the caudal vena cava can be followed from the liver towards the kidney (**Fig. 14.11**). The ultrasonographic signs suggestive of adrenal gland hyperplasia or neoplasia include increased thickness or echogenicity, rounded appearance, heterogeneous structure and/or the presence of signs of mineralisation in the adrenal gland (**Figs 14.9–14.11**). An extremely large adrenal gland may be suggestive of an adrenal carcinoma, which usually does not respond well to hormone therapy. Ultrasonographic dimensions for adrenal glands are listed in *Table 14.2*.

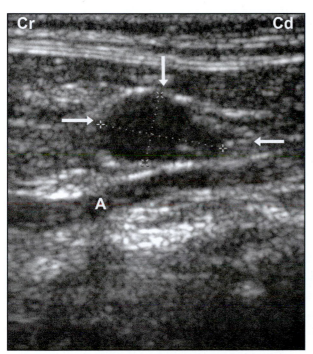

Fig. 14.9 **A longitudinal sonogram of a left adrenal gland (between the arrows) in a 3.5-year-old, spayed female ferret with hyperadrenocorticism. The cranial pole is enlarged. Adrenal length is 10.4 mm, and thickness is 6.4 mm. Histopathological diagnosis was adrenocortical hyperplasia. Note the location of the adrenal gland ventrolateral to the aorta (A). The top of the image is ventral. Cr, cranial; Cd, caudal. (Previously published in: Kuijten AM, Schoemaker NJ, Voorhout G (2007) Ultrasonographic visualisation of the adrenal glands of healthy and hyperadrenocorticoid ferrets.** *J Am Anim Hosp Assoc* **43: 78–84.)**

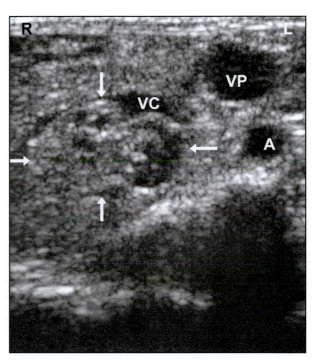

Fig. 14.10 **Transverse sonogram of the right adrenal gland (between the arrows) in a 6.5-year-old, castrated male ferret with hyperadrenocorticism. The adrenal gland length is 15.6 mm, and thickness is 5.5 mm. The right adrenal gland is located dorsolateral to the vena cava (VC). The top of the image is ventral. Key: A, aorta; VP, vena porta; R, right; L, left; Cr, cranial; Cd, caudal. (Previously published in: Kuijten AM, Schoemaker NJ, Voorhout G (2007) Ultrasonographic visualisation of the adrenal glands of healthy and hyperadrenocorticoid ferrets.** *J Am Anim Hosp Assoc* **43: 78–84.)**

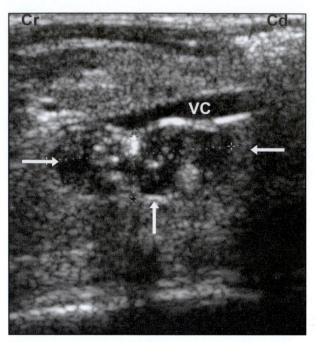

Fig. 14.11 **Longitudinal sonogram of the right adrenal gland (between the arrows) in a 6.5-year-old, castrated male ferret with hyperadrenocorticism. The adrenal gland is hyperechoic, heterogeneous and contains mineralisations (hyperechoic spots). The adrenal gland length is 15.6 mm, and thickness is 5.5 mm. The right adrenal gland is located dorsolateral to the vena cava (VC). The top of the image is ventral. Key: A, aorta; VP, vena porta; R, right; L, left; Cr, cranial; Cd, caudal. (Previously published in: Kuijten AM, Schoemaker NJ, Voorhout G (2007) Ultrasonographic visualisation of the adrenal glands of healthy and hyperadrenocorticoid ferrets.** *J Am Anim Hosp Assoc* **43: 78–84.)**

Table 14.2 **Normal ultrasonographic sizes of adrenal glands**			
	PRESENTED IN MEAN +/– SD, MM		
SEX, GLAND	**LENGTH**	**WIDTH**	**DEPTH**
Female, right	7.5 +/– 1.2	3.7 +/– 0.6	2.8 +/– 0.4
Female, left	7.4 +/– 1.0	3.7 +/– 0.4	2.8 +/– 0.4
Male, right	8.9 +/– 1.6	3.8 +/– 0.6	3.0 +/– 0.8
Male, left	8.6 +/– 1.2	4.2 +/– 0.6	3.0 +/– 0.6

Adapted from Neuwirth L, Collins B, Calderwood-Mays, M, Tran T (1997) Adrenal ultrasonography correlated with histopathology in ferrets. *Veterinary Radiology and Ultrasound* **38(1)**:69–74.

In addition to ultrasonography, CT may be useful when evaluating the adrenal glands in ferrets. When using this technique, intravenous contrast medium will be needed to delineate the adrenal gland better from the caudal vena cava and enable better visualisation of the size of this gland (**Fig. 14.12**).

Preputial cytology: In male ferrets with signs of hyperadrenocorticism, a significantly higher percentage of cornified preputial epithelial cells may be found compared to clinically healthy individuals. Furthermore, this increased percentage in cornified preputial cells was found to correlate strongly with increases in plasma sex hormone concentrations, particularly 17α-hydroxyprogesterone. Preputial cytology has therefore been suggested as a reliable screening test for diagnosing hyperandrogenism in male ferrets. A finding of >70% cornified preputial epithelial cells is considered suggestive of hyperandrogenism.

Management/treatment

Surgery and/or medical intervention using long-acting GnRH analogues are the most commonly used treatment modalities in ferrets with hyperadrenocorticism. The choice of treatment is influenced by many factors. Criteria such as the age of the ferret, presence of concurrent disease (e.g. renal failure, lymphoma and/or cardiomyopathy), risk of surgery (which is higher when the right or both adrenal glands are involved), and/or financial limitations may lead an owner to decline surgery. When surgery (see Chapter 25) is chosen, it is important to realise that gonadotrophin release will persist, thereby resulting in a continued stimulation of the remaining adrenal gland. As a result, this gland may also become hyperplastic or neoplastic at a later stage. The use of hormone therapy (the placement of a long-acting implant containing 4.7 mg deslorelin [Suprelorin-F ®, Virbac]) may therefore be recommended even when the originally affected adrenal gland has been surgically excised. The extra costs for medical treatment may, however, lead an owner to opt for surgery alone.

Surgical treatment: Surgical removal of the left adrenal gland is relatively easy and straightforward and can be accomplished by dissecting the adrenal gland

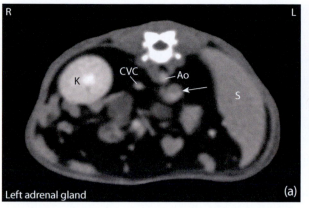
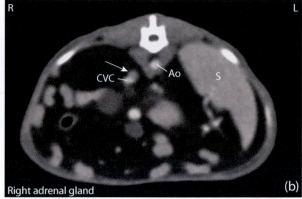

Left adrenal gland (a)

Right adrenal gland (b)

Fig. 14.12 CT images of a 3-year-old female ferret after IV administration of 2 mL contrast medium. The left adrenal gland (a, arrow) is located in close proximity of the aorta (Ao). The right adrenal gland (b, arrow) is located dorsal of the caudal vena cava (CVC), medial to the right kidney (K). The spleen (S) in this ferret is large, which is not uncommon in ferrets.

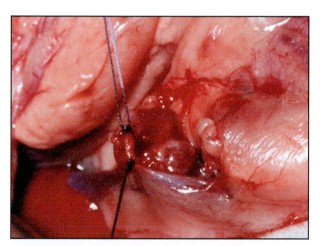
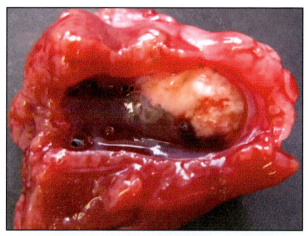

Fig. 14.13 Dissection of the left adrenal gland out of the retroperitoneal fat and ligation of the adrenolumbar vein. The use of haemoclips instead of suture material as shown here allows for a much faster surgery.

Fig. 14.14 View of a right adrenal adenocarcinoma from within the opened caudal vena cava. The adrenal gland is clearly visible together with the venous connections towards this gland.

out of the retroperitoneal fat and ligating the adrenolumbar vein (**Fig. 14.13**; see Chapter 25). Removal of the right adrenal gland is, however, considered more difficult. Its anatomical location (i.e. close proximity to the liver and dorsolateral attachment to the caudal vena cava) hinders its accessibility during a standard ventral abdominal approach. Surgery may furthermore be complicated by the close connection between the right adrenal gland and caudal vena cava (**Fig. 14.14**), thereby rendering it necessary to remove part of the wall of the caudal vena cava to completely remove the adrenal gland. Due to the difficulty of this procedure, however, many surgeons prefer to remove only part of the adrenal gland (**Fig. 14.15**), thereby posing a risk for recurrence of the problems. Some surgeons have ligated the caudal vena cava to allow complete removal of the right adrenal gland. This technique, however, is only possible if this vein is already occluded for a major portion of its diameter and collateral veins have opened up. If this is not the case, there is a serious risk of hypertension distal to ligation that may lead to acute and potentially fatal kidney failure.

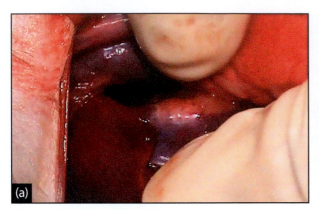 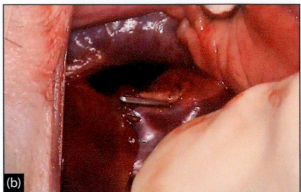

Fig. 14.15 (a, b) Surgery on a right adrenal tumour is complicated by the close connection between this gland and the caudal vena cava. It has therefore been common practice to remove as much of the gland as possible and leave the remaining part attached to this vein. (Courtesy of Angela M. Lennox.)

Removal of both adrenal glands poses a risk of the ferret developing hypoadrenocorticism (Addison's disease). This complication is, however, rarely seen, most likely due to the fact that the right adrenal is seldom removed *in toto*, with the remnant tissue preserving sufficient function, thereby minimising the chance of development of iatrogenic Addison's disease.

Cryosurgery and injection with alcohol have been proposed as alternatives to surgical excision. With cryosurgery, however, it remains uncertain how much of the tumour has actually been destroyed. Alcohol injection in dog testes has been found to be very painful. Because of this finding and the availability of less painful alternatives, the authors are not in favour of injecting alcohol into the adrenal glands of ferrets.

Medical treatment. GnRH agonists: The most effective drugs currently used to treat hyperadrenocorticism in ferrets are the depot GnRH-agonists leuprolide acetate (Lupron Depot®, AbbVie) and deslorelin, which suppress the release of gonadotrophins by continuously releasing GnRH into the circulation, thereby overriding the pulsatile release of GnRH that is needed for the release of gonadotrophins (LH and FSH) (**Fig. 14.16**). The administration of a depot GnRH agonist will initially result in an increased release of GnRH into the circulation, thereby resulting in a (short-lived) release of gonadotrophins. This initial increase in plasma gon-

adotrophin concentrations, which often results in a (temporary, lasting up to 2 weeks) worsening of clinical signs, is soon followed by a drop in gonadotrophin concentrations to baseline levels. Initially, leuprolide acetate, which is registered for use in people and can be administered subcutaneously per injection in a dose of 100 µg IM for ferrets <1 kg and 200 µg IM for ferrets over 1 kg, was the only drug available. In recent years, however, deslorelin implants, which can be placed subcutaneously (**Fig. 14.17**), have become available on the market. Its registration for use in dogs and ferrets renders this drug as the drug of first choice in ferrets with hyperadrenocorticism. In the United States, the implant is licensed for use in ferrets (Suprelorin-F ®, Virbac). Moreover, deslorelin has several other advantages over leuprolide acetate, including: (1) there is no need for reconstitution of the drug; (2) a longer duration of effectiveness (8–30 months for a 4.7 mg-containing deslorelin implant versus 1–3 months for leuprolide injections); and (3) it is much cheaper in use. Deslorelin implants have been found to be very effective for treating hyperandrogenism in ferrets, and are considered a first option over surgical treatment in ferrets diagnosed with adrenal disease, especially in patients considered unacceptable surgical candidates. The implants do not cause any local reaction and may be left in place, even if their activity has worn out (**Fig. 14.18**). Autonomous production of steroids by the adrenal gland may, however, occur over time, resulting in a loss of efficacy of the implant and recurrence of clinical signs.

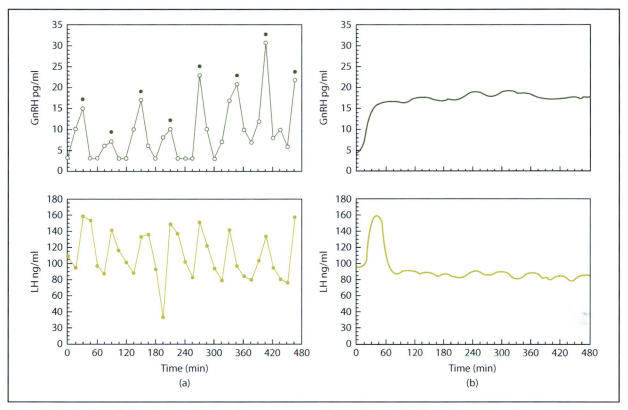

Fig. 14.16 (a) Hypothalamic and pituitary hormones are released in a pulsatile fashion. Gonadotropin release from the pituitary gland is always preceded by the release of GnRH. (b) After deslorelin implant placement the GnRH is constantly high, and now peaks are generated. The initial increase of GnRH results in a single LH peak, after which levels remain at the baseline.

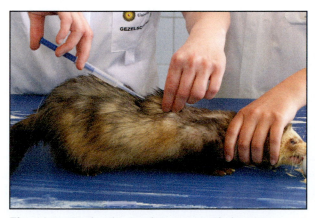

Fig. 14.17 Deslorelin implant can easily be given subcutaneously without anaesthesia as long as ferrets are distracted by giving them food which they like. The skin in the neck is extremely thick. It is therefore recommended to place the implant over the thorax, rather than in the neck.

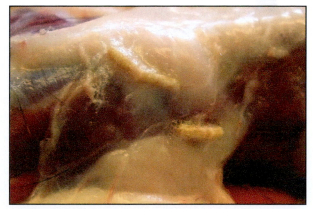

Fig. 14.18 Three years after placement of a deslorelin-containing implant, a 7-year-old ferret died as a result of lymphoma. After removal of the skin, it became clear that the implants were still in place, without showing any local reaction.

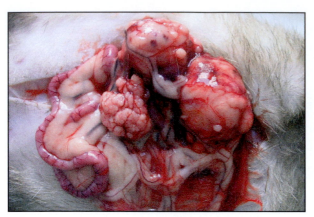

Fig. 14.19 After 2 years of successful treatment with a deslorelin-containing implant of an adrenal adenoma, this ferret was presented with a large mass in its abdomen. This mass turned out to be a huge adrenal adenocarcinoma.

In addition, a study on the use of deslorelin in ferrets with hyperadrenocorticism demonstrated five of fifteen ferrets developing adrenal tumours greater than 2 cm in size within 2 months after the activity of the (3 mg) deslorelin implant had worn off (**Fig. 14.19**). In practice, however, this phenomenon is seldom encountered. It therefore remains unclear why these tumours developed and how high the actual frequency is.

A recent study furthermore demonstrated relief of clinical signs of hyperadrenocorticism following administration of a GnRH vaccine. Currently, the vaccine is available only for research purposes, thereby not rendering it a viable option in practice at this time.

Other medications that have been proposed for the treatment of hyperadrenocorticism in ferrets include flutamide, melatonin, mitotane (o,p′-DDD) combined with ketoconazole, and trilostane.

Flutamide (10 mg/kg PO q12–24h) inhibits androgen uptake and may therefore be beneficial in the first weeks of treating ferrets with a GnRH agonist, when gonadotrophins are increased.

Melatonin (0.5–1 mg/animal PO q24h) has been proposed as a therapeutic option for hyperadrenocorticoid ferrets. It supposedly suppresses the release of GnRH. In the early 1980s, researchers showed that ferrets kept under 8h light:16h darkness (8L:16D),

would come into oestrus only 7 weeks later than ferrets exposed to long photoperiods (14L:10D). It is therefore debatable if melatonin is indeed capable of completely suppressing the release of gonadotrophins. Clinical improvement (e.g. regrowth of fur) is, however, seen in hyperadrenocorticoid ferrets either receiving 0.5 mg melatonin daily PO or an implant containing 5.4 mg melatonin. In general, however, hormone concentrations rose and the tumours continued to grow. Thus, treatment with melatonin poses a risk to the ferret as the disease may progress without the owner noticing it. Especially in the USA, where melatonin can be purchased freely in drugstores, owners may opt for home medication with melatonin which, due to the effective masking of clinical signs, may also delay the time at which ferrets with hyperadrenocorticism will be initially presented to veterinarians.

Mitotane (o,p′-DDD) and *ketoconazole* are well-known drugs for treating hypercortisolism in dogs and humans. These drugs have also been tried in ferrets, but were found to be insufficiently effective, thereby rendering them obsolete for treatment of hyperadrenocorticism in ferrets.

Trilostane, a 3β-hydroxysteroid dehydrogenase (3β-HSD) blocker, is commonly used to treat pituitary-dependent hyperadrenocorticism in dogs, but has been used only incidentally in ferrets. Although the drug theoretically may be effective for treatment of hyperadrenocorticism in ferrets (as 3β-HSD is necessary for the synthesis of androstenedione and 17-hydroxyprogesterone), a pilot study in ferrets with hyperadrenocorticism given 5 mg trilostane PO once daily showed deterioration or no effect rather than improvement of the clinical symptoms. Potentially, this is the result of the decrease in 3β-HSD leading to an activation of 17,20-lyase and thus an activation (rather than deactivation) of the androgen pathway. Higher dosages may potentially overcome this issue, but further research will be necessary to demonstrate whether this is indeed the case and, if so, which dose will be effective and safe for use in ferrets with hyperadrenocorticism.

Management of complicating factors: Ferrets with urinary blockage due to periprostatic or periurethral

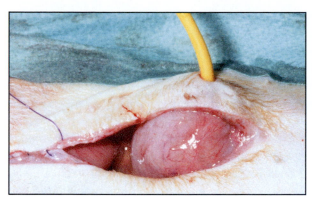

Fig. 14.20 **A prepubic catheter is placed in a periprostatic cyst to allow draining of its content. After placement of a deslorelin-containing implant it will take some time for the cyst to decrease in size. Once this is achieved the catheter may be removed.**

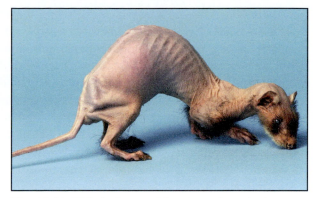

Fig. 14.21 **Elderly ferret with severe alopecia due to hyperadrenocorticism. In this ferret it is also clear to see that hair loss is not the only sign of hyperadrenocorticism, but that emaciation may also occur.**

cysts need immediate medical and/or surgical intervention (cystocentesis, catheterisation and placement of a prepubic catheter) to combat uraemia and/or bladder rupture (**Fig. 14.20**). It will take several weeks before these cysts decrease in size after medical intervention for the hyperadrenocorticism. During this time, close attention should be paid to urinary production.

Prognosis

The prognosis of a ferret with hyperadrenocorticism in general is fair. Ferrets with adrenal pathology may survive for years with this condition, although prognosis may vary depending on factors such as age of the animal, type of tumour, presence of concurrent disease and clinical signs shown by the animal (**Fig. 14.21**). Pruritus will sometimes be unbearable for the animal, and some of these animals appear to be more lethargic as well (**Fig. 14.22**). Anaemia may occur in jills with adrenal tumours due to prolonged hyperoestrogenism but is considered rare. Rupture of the caudal vena cava may also occur incidentally when the right adrenal gland has invaded this vein, thereby resulting in sudden death. In male ferrets, prostate involvement may furthermore result in a life-threatening urinary blockage, thereby influencing chances of survival if not treated promptly. Metastases occur only rarely, thereby hardly influencing the overall prognosis. If metastases are present, however, prognosis will be guarded to poor.

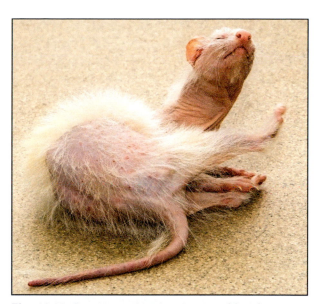

Fig. 14.22 **Severe pruritus in a 7-year-old male ferret with a right adrenal tumour. The pruritus was unresponsive to treatment with corticosteroids.**

Following treatment with a deslorelin-containing implant or surgical intervention, average disease-free periods of 16.5 months and 13.6 months, respectively have been reported. Another study showed 1- and 2-year survival rates of respectively 98% and 88% after surgical intervention. Following surgical removal of a unilateral adrenal tumour, disease commonly recurs due to development of disease in the contralateral adrenal gland.

Prevention

Surgical neutering has been implicated as an aetiological factor in the development of hyperandrogenism in ferrets. Neutering is, however, considered necessary to prevent hyperoestrogenism-related pancytopaenia resulting from persistent oestrus in jills, as well as to reduce intraspecies aggression (enabling ferrets to be kept in groups) and to decrease the intensity of the musky odour in hobs. Chemical neutering using long-acting deslorelin implants may pose a suitable alternative for surgical neutering. In hobs, these implants were found to suppress plasma FSH and testosterone concentrations, decrease testis size, and inhibit spermatogenesis. In addition, the musky odour and sexual behaviour, as well as aggressive behaviour, could be effectively reduced. In jills, deslorelin implants were also found to be effective in preventing oestrus, with duration of effectiveness of a 4.7 mg deslorelin implant varying between 1–3 years in both jills and hobs. Following placement of the implant, minor local side-effects (e.g. scab formation, pruritus) have been noted in less than one out of five ferrets. In the majority of (non-oestrus) females, placement of the implant was reported to induce a temporary oestrus, which in general lasted up to 2 weeks and only incidentally resulted in development of pseudopregnancy that required medical intervention. Based on the results of the aforementioned studies, deslorelin implants are considered a suitable alternative for surgical neutering in ferrets. It does remain uncertain whether these implants will actually reduce the incidence of hyperandrogenism. However, a recent study on a GnRH vaccine in ferrets found that the probability of ferrets developing hyperadrenocorticism was significantly reduced in young (1–3 years old) ferrets following vaccination when compared to untreated, neutered control animals. This finding renders it likely that the GnRH-containing implants will have a similar efficacy in preventing adrenal gland disease in ferrets.

OTHER ANOMALIES RELATED TO THE ADRENAL GLAND

Other forms of adrenal gland neoplasia have been reported in ferrets, but are considered rare.

There is one report of a 6-year-old ferret with an aldosterone-secreting adrenocortical adenoma. The ferret presented with alopecia, pruritus, lethargy and chronic cough. Ancillary tests revealed hypertension, hypokalaemia and increased plasma concentrations of aldosterone, suggestive of Conn's syndrome. Moreover, plasma concentrations of oestradiol, 17α-hydroxyprogesterone and androstenedione were found to be elevated. Despite initial improvement to treatment with leuprolide acetate, potassium gluconate, spironolactone, amlodipine and benazepril, the ferret deteriorated and was euthanased 2 months later. Postmortem examination revealed an 8-cm mass in the left adrenal gland, with immunohistochemistry revealing the neoplastic cells to stain positively for aldosterone.

Hypercortisolism, Iatrogenic hypercortisolism has been found in ferrets. The authors have seen at least two ferrets with iatrogenic hypercortisolism after prolonged treatment of these ferrets with prednisolone for the management of an insulinoma. Once these ferrets were put on a treatment with diazoxide and the administration of prednisolone was gradually decreased, the signs of hypercortisolism disappeared and the ferrets returned to normal. An unusual case of hypercortisolism was also found in a 5-year-old castrated male ferret that presented with PU and polyphagia. Abdominal ultrasonography revealed an enlarged right adrenal gland and atrophy of the left adrenal gland. An hCG stimulation test demonstrated an increase in plasma cortisol and androstenedione concentrations. Based on these findings LH/hCG-dependent hypercortisolism and hyperandrogenism was suspected and treatment was started with a deslorelin-containing implant. Within 3 weeks of placement of the implant all clinical signs had disappeared. Three months later the endocrine parameters had normalised, while abdominal ultrasonography revealed that the right adrenal gland had diminished in size and the left adrenal gland was considered of normal size. No recurrences of clinical signs were seen within 2 years of placement of the deslorelin implant.

Phaeochromocytomas, i.e. tumours of the adrenal medulla, have incidentally been reported in ferrets. Although these tumours are usually much larger than tumours of the adrenal cortex (**Fig. 14.23**), they can

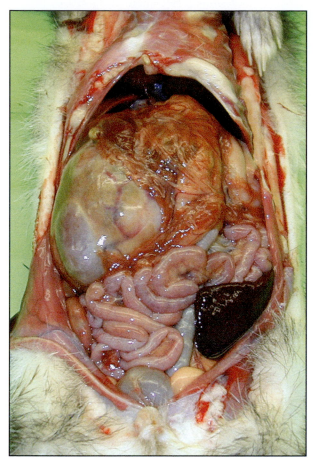

Fig. 14.23 A huge right adrenal gland was found in this ferret. Histology was suggestive of a phaeochromocytoma. Unfortunately, the ferret died before the diagnosis could be confirmed by measuring metanephrines in the urine.

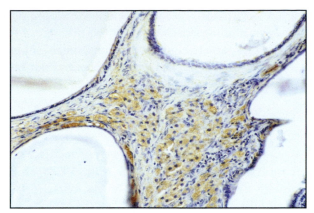

Fig. 14.24 LH-receptor staining of a cystic area located between the right adrenal gland and the liver. The brown coloured cells are LH-receptor positive adrenal cells, while the non-stained cells are hepatocytes. The cysts are dilated biliary ducts. This area is referred to as adrenohepatic fusion and is frequently seen in right adrenal tumours that show cystic alterations.

go unnoticed for a long period of time. Diagnosis has thus far only been made postmortem, without availability of clinical data to indicate whether these ferrets exhibited classical signs of hypertension, arrhythmia, tachycardia, tachypnoea and/or retinal pathology as demonstrated in other species. Some veterinarians have reported clinical signs consistent with cardiovascular collapse, which may be suggestive of phaeochromocytoma. To confirm the diagnosis, measurement of urinary metanephrine would be necessary. To the authors' knowledge, such confirmation has thus far not been reported in ferrets.

Recently, *adrenohepatic fusion*, an anomaly of the right adrenal gland resulting from a union of the adrenal gland with hepatic tissue, has been described in two ferrets. Histologically, a close fusion of the respective parenchymal cells was found, with (partial) absence of an intervening connective tissue septum. Although adrenohepatic fusion has only been reported in these two ferrets without clinical or microscopic evidence of adrenal gland disease, the authors have seen similar fusion in multiple ferrets with right adrenal pathology (**Fig. 14.24**). The most striking finding in these ferrets was the presence of cysts which turned out to be dilated bile ducts. This anatomic anomaly does not seem to have any clinical relevance.

Hypoadrenocorticism

Definition/overview

Hypoadrenocorticism, also referred to as Addison's disease, is a condition characterised by a hypofunction of the adrenal cortex resulting in a decreased secretion of both mineralocorticoids and glucocorticoids.

Aetiology/pathophysiology

Hypoadrenocorticism has been diagnosed in ferrets as a complication of (sub)total bilateral adrenalectomy or following treatment with mitotane in ferrets with hyperadrenocorticism. In a follow-up study concerning long-term outcome following surgery for hyperadrenocorticism, four out of 28 ferrets

(14.3%) with bilateral adrenalectomy developed signs of hypoadrenocorticism within the first weeks following surgery. In contrast to other animals, spontaneous (primary) hypoadrenocorticism has not been diagnosed in ferrets.

Clinical presentation

Clinical signs are similar to those observed in dogs with hypoadrenocorticism and may include lethargy, anorexia, weakness and shock (**Fig. 14.25**). Signs usually develop within days to weeks following (sub) total bilateral adrenalectomy.

Differential diagnosis

The most common differential diagnosis for an animal with hyponatraemia and hyperkalaemia is acute renal failure. Other differential diagnoses for weakness and lethargy include hypoglycaemia, e.g. due to concurrent insulinoma or secondary to prolonged (postsurgical) anorexia, (postsurgical) infection or sepsis, cachexia associated with advanced adrenal disease (including metastases), or other systemic disease that may have been exacerbated following surgery (e.g. cardiac failure, hepatic disease).

Diagnosis

Similar to dogs and cats, evaluation of serum electrolytes may reveal hyponatraemia, hypochloraemia and hyperkalaemia, suggestive of hypoadrenocorticism. An ACTH-stimulation test, during which cortisol is measured at baseline and at t = 60 in a manually restrained ferret following IV injection of 1 µg/kg of a synthetic ACTH, may reveal lack of or diminished response to the injected ACTH, thereby confirming the diagnosis. Previously published cortisol values range from 26–137 nmol/L at baseline. They will increase to 143–309 nmol/L 60 minutes after the administration of ACTH. Instead of administering the ACTH IV, an IM administration of the same dose did not result in significantly different values.

Management/treatment

Treatment consists of supplementation with glucocorticoids and mineralocorticoids. Treatment is often initiated with dexamethasone (0.5 mg/kg SC, IM or IV) followed by prednisone (0.25 mg/kg PO q12–24h). In addition, fludrocortisone acetate (0.05–0.1 mg/kg PO q12–24h) or deoxycorticosterone pivalate (2 mg/kg IM every 3 weeks) may be administered. If shock is present, fluid therapy should be initiated immediately to correct for any fluid deficits and/or electrolyte imbalances (**Fig. 14.26**). Animals generally respond quickly to medical treatment. Once the animal is stable, dosages may be gradually tapered to the lowest dose possible. Careful monitoring of plasma electrolytes is warranted to monitor the effect of the therapy and adjust this accordingly.

Prognosis

Prognosis is considered fair if disease is diagnosed early and treated appropriately. Prognosis may be poor if severe electrolyte abnormalities are present (with hyperkalaemia and hyponatraemia resulting in severe hypotensive shock and life-threatening cardiac arrhythmias).

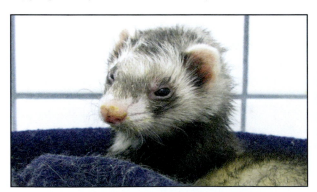

Fig. 14.25 This lethargic ferret was presented with anorexia, hyperthermia, delayed skin tenting and a tachycardia.

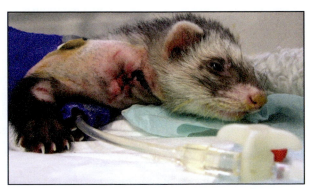

Fig. 14.26 The cephalic vein is an ideal location for administering fluid in dehydrated ferrets, or those in shock.

DISEASES OF THE PANCREAS

Insulinoma

Definition/overview

Insulinomas or islet cell tumours are, usually, small (0.5–2 mm) tumours (**Fig. 14.27**) of the pancreatic beta cells that result in the production of excessive amounts of insulin and subsequent hypoglycaemia. Tumour types may be described as hyperplasia, adenomas or carcinomas (**Fig. 14.28**). Most are well circumscribed, but infiltration in surrounding tissues may occur. In contrast to dogs, insulinomas in ferrets rarely metastasise.

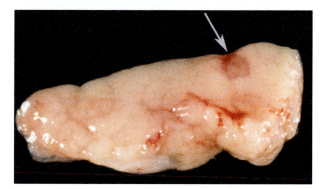

Fig. 14.27 Part of the pancreas which was removed during pancreas surgery in a ferret with hypoglycaemia. On palpation of the pancreas a small firm nodule could be palpated (arrow). Histological evaluation confirmed this to be an islet cell adenoma. The clinical signs in the ferret resolved after the surgery.

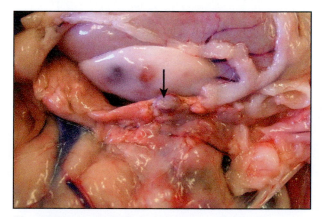

Fig. 14.28 A relatively large tumour within the pancreas (arrow) of a ferret. Histological examination of this tumour proved it to be an adenocarcinoma of islet cell origin.

The distribution of insulinomas is equal among the sexes. With a reported prevalence of 20–25% of the diagnosed neoplasms in ferrets, insulinomas are one of the most commonly diagnosed tumours in middle-aged to older ferrets, with a median age of 5 years (range 2–8 years).

Aetiology/pathophysiology

The aetiology of insulinomas in ferrets is currently unknown. The limited genetic diversity of ferrets, which stem from a limited number of breeder farms, has led to the suggestion that a genetic component may be involved. Another theory suggests that, based on the natural carnivorous diet of mustelids, diets high in carbohydrates may contribute to the development of these tumours. A diet high in protein (42–55%), high in fat (18–30%), low in carbohydrates (8–15%), and low in fibre (1–3%) (percentages on a dry-matter basis) has therefore been advised to reduce the incidence. Alternatively, feeding commercial balanced diets based on entire prey animals has been recommended. No scientific evidence, however, is available to back up any claims on the aetiology of insulinoma, nor has it been proven that the incidence is reduced when ferrets are fed prey-based diets or low-carbohydrate kibble (see Chapter 5).

Clinical presentation

Clinical signs vary from lethargy, slight incoordination (ataxia), stargazing and weakness in the hindlimbs to complete collapse, generalised seizures and coma (**Fig. 14.29**). Progression of clinical signs can extend over a period of days to weeks or months. In humans, an overdose of insulin may result in stimulation of the autonomic nervous system resulting in nausea. The nausea, which is commonly seen in ferrets with an insulinoma, often manifests itself in the form of ptyalism and pawing at the mouth. In addition, owners may notice a glazed look in the eyes of their ferrets. Signs are most evident when the ferret has not eaten for some time, and will often resolve spontaneously after providing the ferret with some food (**Fig. 14.30**) or a calorie-rich beverage. If the waxing and waning of the signs are not seen, other diseases affecting the hindlimbs should also be considered.

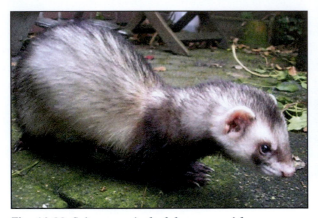

Fig. 14.29 Seizure typical of that seen with hypoglycaemia and insulinoma.

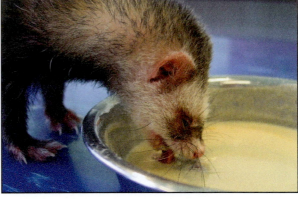

Fig. 14.30 A ferret in a hypoglycaemic crisis may be fed a protein-rich diet to quickly correct the energy balance.

Differential diagnosis

The differential diagnosis of hindlimb weakness consists of: neurological diseases (e.g. trauma, intervertebral disc disease, Aleutian disease), cardiac disease, generalised weakness and metabolic disorders, such as hypoglycaemia. In ferrets, hypoglycaemia is considered the most commonly seen cause of hindlimb weakness.

Within the differential diagnosis of hypoglycaemia, excessive glucose-consuming conditions, such as rapid multiplying neoplastic cells, severe hepatic disease, severe malnutrition or starvation, sepsis or iatrogenic insulin overdose should be considered. These conditions can usually be ruled out based on the results of the history, physical examination and/or diagnostic work-up.

Diagnosis

Blood chemistry: Blood glucose concentrations lower than 3.3 mmol/L (<60 mg/dL; reference range: 5.0–7.0 mmol/L [90–125 mg/dL]), after withholding food for 4 hours, are highly suggestive of an insulinoma when ferrets display the above mentioned signs. In ferrets with blood glucose concentrations between 3.3 and 5.0 mmol/L (60–90 mg/dL), the authors advise to prolong the fast another 2 hours. In many cases, the blood glucose will then drop below 3.3 mmol/L, thereby confirming the tentative diagnosis. Portable blood glucose meters (PBGMs) seem very practical for obtaining quick results (**Fig. 14.31**). They only need one drop of blood that can be collected from any

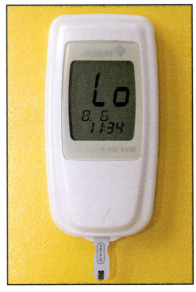

Fig. 14.31 With a glucometer a quick indication of the blood glucose concentration can be obtained. Although glucometers frequently underestimate the actual blood glucose concentration, a reading of 'Lo' can be interpreted as being hypoglycaemic.

vein, but also from a puncture of a footpad. Due to the method of analysis, heparinised blood should not be used. In a comparison study evaluating the agreement between glucose concentrations measured with a laboratory analyser and three different PBGMs it became clear that the human PBGMs severely underestimate the actual glucose concentrations. The veterinary PBGM had two settings in which the canine setting produced the most agreeable values. If one wants to use a PBGM in practice, it is good to realise that underestimation is possible and that accurate values can only be obtained with a laboratory analyser.

Plasma insulin concentrations can also be measured and are usually increased (>108 µU/L or >773 pmol/L), but concentrations within the reference range (4.6–43.4 µU/L; 33–311 pmol/L) may also be seen due to presumed erratic insulin secretion by some insulinomas. The concurrent finding of hypoglycaemia and insulin concentrations within the reference range should therefore be considered abnormal, as insulin plasma concentrations should be low during a hypoglycaemic event.

Diagnostic imaging: In dogs, insulinomas have a high rate of metastasis, which frequently occurs in the liver. These metastases can be visualised on ultrasound. Adenocarcinomas of the ferret pancreas and their metastases have been found on ultrasound. The great majority of insulinomas, however, are benign and do not metastasise. The primary tumour is usually very small in size (0.5–2 mm) as well, rendering these tumours extremely difficult to visualised by ultrasound. In the experience of the authors, insulinomas may occasionally be visualised by ultrasound, but they are frequently missed as well. Diagnostic imaging in the form of radiography or ultrasound examination is therefore not routinely advised.

CT, MRI and nuclear scintigraphy with octreotide or indium-111 have not, to the authors' knowledge, been used in ferrets to diagnose insulinomas. The expense of the nuclear scanning and the lack of sensitivity in finding insulinomas in dogs and humans with CT and MRI make these advanced diagnostic imaging tools less promising for future use in practice.

Management/treatment

Insulinomas may be managed surgically and/or medically. Many factors, such as age of the ferret, desire of the owner to have an instant solution and/or financial restrictions, may play a role in the decision-making process. It is recommended by the authors that a veterinarian presents all facts, in order to allow the owner to make an informed decision based on the pros and cons of each method.

Surgical treatment: To fully eliminate the source of excess insulin production, surgical removal is seemingly the best therapeutic option (see Chapter 25). Due to the limited ability to visualise the tumours, the possibility to excise the insulinoma(s) can only be evaluated upon explorative surgery. Surgical excision may not be successful in alleviating the clinical signs as some tumours may remain undetected during surgery due to their small size. A partial pancreatectomy (**Fig. 14.32**) has therefore been recommended over pancreatic nodulectomy in order to remove as many undetectable islet cell tumours as possible and thus increase the survival time after surgery. In addition, if the neoplasm is located in the body of the pancreas, it is often difficult to remove, as resection of this part of the pancreas is not possible due to the presence of the pancreatic duct. A mean disease-free state after surgery of about 1 year, and survival times of over 3 years, have been reported. Recurrence of clinical signs is mainly due to the occurrence of new insulinomas and not due to metastases of the removed tumour. If too much of the pancreas is removed, complications such as diabetes mellitus may occur. It should be stressed that every effort should be taken to avoid this condition from occurring, since the medical management of insulinoma is far easier than that of diabetes mellitus. It could also be speculated that an exocrine pancreatic insufficiency could occur when too large a portion of the pancreas is removed. Thus far, however, this has not been reported.

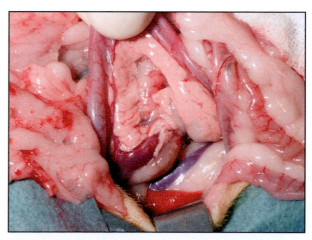

Fig. 14.32 **The pancreas is examined for nodules associated with insulinoma.**

Medical treatment: Prednisone and diazoxide are the most commonly used drugs for treating insulinomas. Octreotide (Sandostatin, Novartis), a synthetic long-acting analogue of somatostatin, which inhibits the synthesis and secretion of insulin by normal and neoplastic beta cells, has also been incidentally used in ferrets in a dose of 1–2 µg/kg q8–12h, but no clear beneficial effects were seen over the other two modes of treatment.

In private practice, prednisone and other glucocorticoids that induce gluconeogenesis, are frequently used as the drug of first choice. Although these drugs commonly induce side-effects in other species, ferrets seem relatively refractory to developing side-effects due to glucocorticoid administration, and generally respond well to the treatment protocol. Weight gain and impaired hair growth (suggestive of iatrogenic Cushing's disease), however, have been reported in ferrets that have received glucocorticoids for prolonged periods in time. In addition, the gluconeogenic mode of action of glucocorticoids results in an increase in glucose, which may be contraindicated in ferrets with insulinomas due to the risk of stimulating the secretion of insulin.

Diazoxide, which is registered for treating human insulinoma patients, inhibits insulin release. The authors therefore prefer this drug over the use of glucocorticoids. The drug, however, is more expensive than prednisone, which may also explain why prednisone is frequently chosen over diazoxide. Although this is a factor to be considered in dogs (especially larger breeds), the ferret's low body-weight limits the daily quantities that are needed of the drug, thereby making diazoxide an affordable alternative for ferrets. Compounding the drug is, however, necessary to allow accurate dosing. Treatment is started at an oral dose of twice daily 5 mg/kg diazoxide. Based on the response to treatment (as judged by disappearance or continuing of clinical signs), the dose may need to be increased gradually. When using plasma glucose concentrations to monitor effect of treatment, blood should always be collected 4 hours after giving the diazoxide. During this period food should be withheld from the ferret. Once the dose of diazoxide has been increased to 15–20 mg/kg q12h and clinical

signs still have not resolved, prednisone may be added to the treatment protocol in a concentration of 0.2–1 mg/kg PO, q24h. For both drugs, doses may be increased further if necessary, with no real upper limits existent. The only limiting factor may therefore be the development of side-effects such as vomiting and anorexia. Medical management based on the aforementioned protocol is usually sufficient to control hypoglycaemia for a period up to 18 months, with some ferrets in the authors' clinic even surviving up to 2 years on medical treatment.

In patients with a hypoglycaemic crisis, emergency treatment may be initiated by intravenously administering a bolus of 50% dextrose diluted 1:1 with saline or lactated Ringer's (0.25–2.0 mL over 1–3 minutes, titrated to effect). Diazepam may be considered in patients that continue seizuring despite the intravenous administration of dextrose (**Fig. 14.29**). Following the initial dextrose bolus, it is recommended to place the ferret on maintenance fluids supplemented with 5% dextrose to prevent rebound hypoglycaemia. In humans, severe hypoglycaemic episodes can often be successfully managed by administering glucagon. Research even suggests that glucagon may be preferable over dextrose for short-term management of hypoglycaemic crises because of the diminished risk for rebound hypoglycaemia and consequent fluctuations in blood glucose concentrations. A recent report, which described the use of constant rate infusion of glucagon as an emergency treatment for a severely hypoglycaemic ferret, suggested a similar effect in this species. Using a dosage of 15–40 ng/kg/min (as extrapolated from data in dogs and cats) the authors were able to increase blood glucose levels and alleviate the clinical signs in an elderly ferret that did not respond sufficiently to other types of therapy.

To prevent rebound release of insulin (which may trigger a hypoglycaemic episode), owners should be instructed to frequently (4–6 times per day) feed their ferrets smaller portions of a low-carbohydrate, high-protein diet and make sure that food is available at all times (i.e. provide food in multiple feeding stations). In addition, owners should be instructed to monitor their ferret closely for signs of hypoglycaemia and feed the ferret immediately if mild signs of hypoglycaemia are noted. In the event of a seizure or comatose condition, the owner should be instructed to drip corn syrup or dextrose (sugar) solution on the mucous membranes (lips, tongue, gingiva). This may help to temporarily relieve the clinical signs so that the ferret can be transported safely to the veterinary clinic.

Prognosis

In ferrets, the prognosis is better compared to dogs, in which metastases are very common. Although metastases are rare in ferrets, multiple tumours and recurrent signs are common. Recurrent signs are probably due to the development of new tumours rather than metastases of the earlier tumour.

OTHER FORMS OF PANCREATIC NEOPLASIA

Pancreatic polypeptidomas are neoplasia that produce and secrete pancreatic polypeptide, a 36-amino-acid polypeptide that exerts various effects on the GI tract, including stimulation of basal gastric acid secretion, promotion of GI motility and gastric emptying and limitation of pancreatic exocrine secretion following a meal. A case report described the finding of multiple endocrine pancreatic tumours in a 4-year-old male ferret with clinical signs of depression, diarrhoea, melena and progressive weight loss. Serum hormone analysis initially revealed elevated basal and postprandial plasma gastrin levels, suggestive of a gastrinoma and concurrent Zollinger–Ellison syndrome. Provocative tests (secretin and calcium challenge tests), however, did not support this diagnosis. Following euthanasia, further testing revealed pancreatic islet tumours, which were found to contain markedly elevated concentrations of pancreatic polypeptide, consistent with pancreatic polypeptidoma.

DIABETES MELLITUS

Definition/overview

Diabetes mellitus (DM) is a metabolic disease characterised by elevated blood glucose concentrations. The disease may result from an absolute or relative insulin deficiency, which impairs the tissues' ability to use carbohydrates, fats and proteins. The impaired use of glucose and ongoing gluconeogenesis subsequently result in persistent hyperglycaemia and glucosuria with concurrent diuresis (**Fig. 14.33**). In most cases, it involves a transient condition that develops following aggressive surgical intervention in ferrets with insulinomas. Spontaneous DM is rare in ferrets, with only sporadic reports found in the literature. No sex, age or breed predispositions have been reported.

Aetiology/pathophysiology

Most cases of DM in ferrets are iatrogenic as a result of aggressive pancreatectomy to debulk insulinomas. Any ferret undergoing (partial) pancreatectomy for treatment of insulinoma should be considered at risk for developing DM.

Reports on spontaneous DM in literature are rare. Causes may include: 1) lack of insulin production (an *absolute* insulin deficiency, e.g. secondary to immune-mediated pancreatitis, i.e. type-I DM); 2) (peripheral)

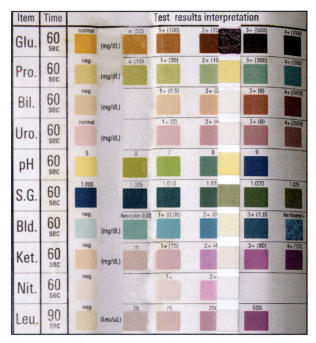

Fig. 14.33 Glucose concentrations in the urine can easily be monitored using urine sticks. In this instance urine was only placed on the glucose area. The result clearly demonstrates the presence of glucose in the urine.

insulin resistance (a *relative* insulin deficiency resulting from diminished response to insulin, i.e. type-I DM); or 3) glucagonoma, resulting in excessive production and release of glucagon in the circulation. In the literature, one case report described pathological findings consistent with a type-I DM. Histologically, the ferret's pancreas not only contained fewer beta cells, but cells also lacked immunoreactivity for insulin. In addition, focal lymphoplasmacytic inflammation was present in the pancreatic tissue, consistent with an immune-mediated pancreatitis, as has been found in dogs with DM. Another report described presence of DM and ketoacidosis in a ferret fed solely on sweet cereals, suggesting that a diet high in glycaemic index may play a role in diabetogenesis in ferrets, similar to other species. Findings in this ferret were thought to be the result of a peripheral insulin resistance brought on by the high-sugar diet, consistent with a type-II DM. Two other ferrets with spontaneous DM were found to have concurrent hyperadrenocorticism. It may be theorised that DM in these ferrets occurred due to peripheral insulin resistance brought on by increased blood cortisol concentrations resulting from adrenal gland disease. Unfortunately, cortisol levels were not reported in either of the two ferrets, thereby rendering it uncertain whether and to what degree adrenal gland disease played a role in DM diagnosed in these ferrets. Alternatively, gonadotrophin-releasing hormone (which had been administered in one of the ferrets to manage its hyperadrenocorticism) may also have played a role in the peripheral insulin resistance, as has been reported in humans.

Clinical presentation

Clinical signs are identical to those in the more common companion animal species and include PU/PD, lethargy and weight loss, despite good appetite. In advanced stages of the disease, anorexia, depression, ataxia, vomiting and/or hepatomegaly may also develop secondary to hepatic lipidosis (**Fig. 14.34**) and ketoacidosis.

Differential diagnosis

Differential diagnoses include other signs of hyperglycaemia and glucosuria such as transient hyperglycaemia resulting from stress or handling,

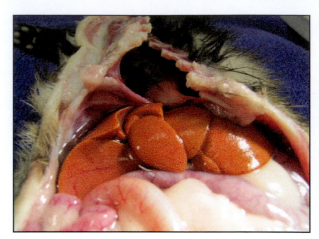

Fig. 14.34 Hepatic lipidosis. (Courtesy of Cathy Johnson-Delaney.)

hyperglycaemia associated with hyperthermia, pregnancy toxaemia, hepatic lipidosis, or renal glucosuria (e.g. occurring in patients with renal disease). These patients will, however, generally not present with PU/PD or weight loss, and have normal blood glucose concentrations (if measured at a time when the animal is not stressed).

Diagnosis

Glucosuria combined with plasma glucose concentrations greater than 21 mmol/L (400 mg/dL) are suggestive of the diagnosis, although repeated measurements are advised. A reference interval has been determined for fructosamine in ferrets (101–202 μmol/L), but to date, no measurements have been performed in cases of (confirmed) DM.

Bloodwork may further reveal low plasma insulin concentrations. Normal to high insulin concentrations accompanied by persistent hyperglycaemia are considered suggestive for peripheral insulin resistance or presence of a glucagonoma. The value of testing insulin is, however, questionable since little is known about regulation of insulin release in ferrets and many laboratories may not offer tests that have been validated for ferrets. Confirmation of glucagonoma requires serum glucagon concentrations or immunohistochemical staining of pancreatic biopsies.

Urinalysis may reveal secondary bacterial cystitis and/or ketonuria (particularly in late stages of the disease). Concurrent diabetic ketoacidosis may be evident by findings of hypokalaemia, hyponatraemia, ketonaemia, hypochloraemia and hypobicarbonaemia. A complete blood cell count and serum biochemistry, radiographs and ultrasound may be performed to rule out concurrent disease (e.g. hepatic lipidosis, atherosclerosis).

Management/treatment

The aim of treatment is to normalise blood glucose concentrations without the animal developing hypoglycaemia. Hyperglycaemia developing as a complication of pancreatectomy is often transient, resolving within 1–2 weeks without further therapeutic intervention. If hyperglycaemia persists and the patient demonstrates signs consistent with DM, treatment with insulin is usually indicated. Treatment often follows the recommendations for diabetic cats, with limited ferret-specific protocols being published.

Treatment of spontaneous DM in ferrets is difficult, as many of the patients appear to have developed concurrent diabetic ketoacidosis at the time of presentation. In this stage of the disease, patients often need to be hospitalised and require intensive care (including aggressive fluid therapy) to correct water and electrolyte balance and reverse the ketonaemia and acidosis. In this stage, the use of regular, crystalline insulin is recommended as this can be given parenterally and has a rapid bioavailability and short duration of action. Despite intensive therapy, however, the prognosis of patients with diabetic ketoacidosis is often poor. For patients that are stable and well-hydrated, SC administration of NPH insulin (0.1–1.0 IU/ferret q12h), which has an intermediate duration of action, may be considered. Similarly, the longer-acting ultralente insulin (1.0 IU/ferret SC q24h) may also be effective for treating DM. Unfortunately this drug is no longer available in most countries. The long-acting glargine insulin – which is the drug of first choice in cats – may pose a suitable alternative: this drug was reported effective for treating DM in an elderly ferret in a dose of 0.5 IU SC q12h.

Patients with spontaneous DM have been reported to respond unpredictably to the administration of insulin. Following the start of insulin therapy, patients therefore need to be monitored closely while gradually increasing insulin dosages until the hyperglycaemia has resolved. For this purpose, it is recommended to hospitalise the patient until the blood glucose levels have stabilised between 6.9–11.1 mmol/L (125–200 mg/dL). Owners should furthermore be instructed to monitor their ferret's urine closely for glucosuria and ketonuria and offer a low-carbohydrate, protein-rich diet in smaller portions throughout the day (i.e. divided into four portions that are fed concurrently with each insulin injection and 4–6 h following the injection). Since it is unsure which type of DM occurs in ferrets, the use of oral hypoglycaemic drugs, such as glipizide, is questionable.

Prognosis

The prognosis of ferrets with DM following partial pancreatectomy is usually good, with most patients becoming euglycaemic within 1–2 weeks postsurgery. In patients with spontaneous DM or those that continue to be hyperglycaemic for more than 2 weeks following surgery or develop ketoacidosis, prognosis is usually guarded to poor as these patients often prove difficult to regulate.

DISEASES OF THE THYROID GLAND

Hypothyroidism
Definition/overview
Hypothyroidism is characterised by impaired production or secretion of thyroid hormones by the thyroid gland, resulting in a decreased concentration of circulating thyroid hormone and associated clinical signs. Although the disease is one of the most common endocrine diseases seen in dogs, hypothyroidism has only rarely been described in ferrets.

Aetiology/pathophysiology
The aetiology and pathogenesis of hypothyroidism in ferrets is currently not known. In dogs, primary hypothyroidism, resulting from either immune-mediated lymphocytic thyroiditis or idiopathic thyroid atrophy, is most common. On rare occasions, primary or metastatic neoplasia may also cause hypothyroidism. In cats, hypothyroidism is most commonly iatrogenic, resulting from treatment for hyperthyroidism.

Clinical presentation
Clinical signs observed in ferrets may include obesity and lethargy, as indicated by decreased activity

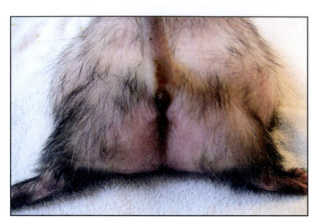

Fig. 14.35 **Morbid obesity is seen in this 5-year-old female ferret. Plasma T4 concentrations did not increase during a TSH stimulation test. (Courtesy of Angela M. Lennox.)**

and excessive sleeping (**Fig. 14.35**). Hindlimb weakness has also been noted in some ferrets with hypothyroidism. Of the clinical signs commonly noted in dogs, hair loss, hypercholesterolaemia and hypoglycaemia have not been consistently noted in the ferrets diagnosed with hypothyroidism.

Differential diagnosis

The vague, non-specific clinical signs such as lethargy and decreased activity may be encountered in most diseases seen in ferrets. Owners may occasionally also incorrectly assume that the decreased activity is the result of normal aging. Obesity may also be seen in ferrets that are on long-term steroid therapy (e.g. for management of insulinoma). Weakness in the hindlimbs may be associated with hypoglycaemia, myasthenia gravis, thromboembolism, cardiac disease or generalised weakness.

Diagnosis

After finding low thyroid hormone levels (<10 ng/mL*), hypothyroidism may be suspected (Appendix 4). Similar to dogs and cats, a thyroid-stimulating hormone (TSH) stimulation test is needed to confirm the diagnosis and eliminate the possibility of sick euthyroid syndrome. Experimentally, an IM injection

---

* Normal baseline values in ferrets for (neutered) male and female pet ferrets were determined as 29.9 ± 5.8 ng/mL and 21.8 ± 3.3 ng/mL, respectively.

of 100 µg of human recombinant TSH (thyrogen) resulted in successful stimulation of the thyroid gland, with poststimulation levels increasing to 1.4 times prestimulatory levels after 4 hours in euthyroid ferrets. In contrast, this stimulation was not seen in ferrets with true hypothyroidism.

Management/treatment

Oral treatment with levothyroxine (50–100 µg q12h) was found effective to resolve the clinical signs and normalise serum T4 concentrations. Ferrets with sick euthyroid syndrome do not appear responsive to T4 supplementation.

Prognosis

In the hypothyroid ferrets that thus far have been treated with levothyroxine, prognosis has been excellent. Prognosis in the long term is, however, uncertain as the underlying cause for the hypothyroidism as well as efficacy of the therapy in the long term are currently unknown.

Thyroid neoplasia

Although thyroid adenomas and adenocarcinomas have been reported in ferrets, their incidence appears low. Since most thyroid neoplasms were reported in large retrospective studies on neoplasms in ferrets, little is known about the clinical signs, diagnosis and treatment of these tumours.

One case report listed the clinical signs and postmortem findings in an adult neutered male ferret diagnosed with a C-cell carcinoma (medullary thyroid carcinoma). According to this report, the ferret exhibited vague signs of reduced appetite, weight loss, lethargy, decreased activity and thinning of the hair coat. Physical examination revealed a firm, infiltrative soft tissue mass in the region of the thyroid gland. Diagnostic work-up included radiographs, serum biochemistry and a fine needle aspirate of the mass, based on which the tentative diagnosis of thyroid neoplasia was made. Efforts to surgically excise the tumour were unsuccessful, following which the animal was euthanased. In addition to the C-cell carcinoma, a postmortem examination revealed presence of multiple other endocrine neoplasms, including adrenocortical adenoma, phaeochromocytoma and islet cell adenoma, consistent with MEN syndrome in humans. Unfortunately, immunohistochemical staining for calcitonin was unsuccessful, thereby preventing confirmation of functionality of the tumour.

DISEASES OF THE PARATHYROID GLAND

Hypoparathyroidism
Definition/overview
Hypoparathyroidism is characterised by a decreased function of the parathyroid glands with decreased production of parathyroid hormone. This may subsequently result in hypocalcaemia and associated clinical signs. The disease is considered rare in ferrets, with only a single case report of suspected primary hypoparathyroidism in a ferret found in literature.

Aetiology/pathophysiology
Primary hypoparathyroidism is a state of inadequate parathyroid hormone (PTH) activity, resulting in concomitant hypocalcaemia. The condition may be inherited, but has also been reported following thyroid or parathyroid gland surgery or immune-mediated parathyroid disease. In the ferret from the case report, primary hypoparathyroidism was suspected based on the inability to identify the parathyroid glands upon necropsy.

Besides primary hypoparathyroidism, pseudohypoparathyroidism (characterised by elevated serum PTH concentrations resulting from peripheral PTH resistance) and secondary hypoparathyroidism (characterised by decreased serum PTH concentrations in response to a primary process that causes hypercalcaemia) may also be distinguished.

Clinical presentation
Clinical signs in the ferret included intermittent seizures and depression. Other clinical signs that may result from the hypoparathyroidism-associated hypocalcaemia and hyperphosphataemia include cramping and twitching of muscles or tetany (involuntary muscle contraction) and cardiac arrhythmias.

Differential diagnosis
Differential diagnoses for hypocalcaemia include hypoparathyroidism, pseudohypoparathyroidism, hypomagnesaemia, (chronic) renal disease (renal secondary hyperparathyroidism), nutritional secondary hyperparathyroidism, hypoalbuminaemia and tumour lysis syndrome. Of the aforementioned diseases, only hypoparathyroidism results in a combination of low serum calcium concentrations, high serum phosphorus concentrations, and normal renal function in the face of low PTH concentrations.

Diagnosis
Diagnosis is usually made using blood analysis. Plasma biochemistry will reveal concurrent hypocalcaemia and hyperphosphataemia. Serum PTH concentrations are low to low–normal.

Management/treatment
The treatment of hypoparathyroidism is limited by the fact that there is no artificial form of the hormone that can be administered as replacement; calcium replacement therapy (e.g. calcium gluconate or calcium carbonate) and/or vitamin D supplementation can ameliorate the symptoms but can increase the risk of kidney stones and chronic kidney disease. In the ferret suspected of primary hypoparathyroidism, treatment was initiated with calcium gluconate (2.0 mg/kg/h IV) followed by a treatment with calcium carbonate (53 mg/kg PO q12h) and dihydrotachysterol, a vitamin D analogue (0.02 mg/kg PO q24h). The animal responded well to both emergency and long-term treatment and lived for approximately 2 years after the initial time of presentation.

Pseudohypoparathyroidism
Pseudohypoparathyroidism is a hereditary condition that clinically resembles hypoparathyroidism but is caused by a lack of response to high circulating concentrations of PTH, rather than a deficiency of this hormone. It is characterised by low serum calcium, high serum phosphorus, and high serum PTH concentrations.

One report described the clinical findings and diagnostic work-up in a ferret suspected of pseudohypoparathyroidism. The animal, a 1.5-year-old neutered male ferret, presented with intermittent seizures, muscle fasciculations, disorientation and lethargy. Blood biochemistry revealed low serum calcium, high serum phosphorus and high serum

PTH concentrations, consistent with pseudohypo-parathyroidism. Unfortunately no PTH (Ellsworth-Howard) challenge test or diagnostic imaging were performed to confirm the diagnosis. Clinical improvement was seen following treatment with calcium carbonate (100 mg PO q12h) and dihydrota-chysterol (0.01 mg/kg PO twice per week).

REPRODUCTIVE ENDOCRINE DISEASES

Persistent oestrus and hyperoestrogenism
Definition/overview
Persistent oestrus is a well-known endocrine con-dition that affects sexually mature, non-neutered female ferrets. It is characterised by elevated con-centrations of feminising sex hormones such as oestradiol, oestriol and oestrone that may result in pancytopaenia. Hyperoestrogenism due to pro-longed oestrus is relatively rare in the USA as most ferrets are surgically neutered at the breeding farm when they are 5–6 weeks of age.

Aetiology/pathophysiology
Female ferrets are seasonally polyoestrous (breed-ing season lasts from March to August) and induced ovulators. As a result, they remain in oestrus until they are mated, or for as long as daylight lasts lon-ger than 12 hours. The prolonged oestrus and asso-ciated hyperoestrogenism may subsequently result in an oestrogen-induced bone marrow suppression of the erythroid, myeloid and megakaryocytic cell lines, and thus pancytopaenia. As a result, females are at risk of developing life-threatening anaemia and blood loss due to thrombocytopaenia if oestrus persists over longer periods of time (**Figs 14.36, 14.37**).

On occasion, hyperoestrogenism may also be encountered in neutered ferrets of both genders as a result of hyperandrogenism, or in females with rem-nant ovaries or ovarian tumours. The bone marrow suppression associated with hyperandrogenism is generally mild.

Clinical presentation
Clinical signs that may be noted include bilateral symmetrical alopecia (usually starting at the base

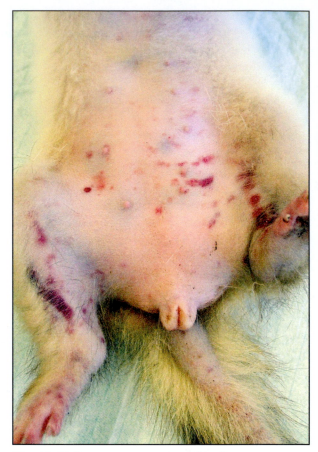

Fig. 14.36 Bone marrow suppression due to hyperoestrogenism has led to a pancytopaenia in this ferret. The petechiae that can be seen in this ferret were due to the thrombocytopaenia.

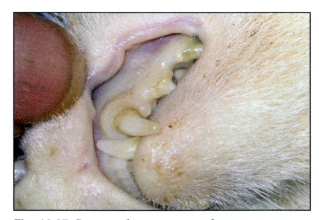

Fig. 14.37 Severe pale mucous membranes are seen in this female ferret with persistent oestrus and associated pancytopaenia. (Courtesy of Cathy Johnson-Delaney.)

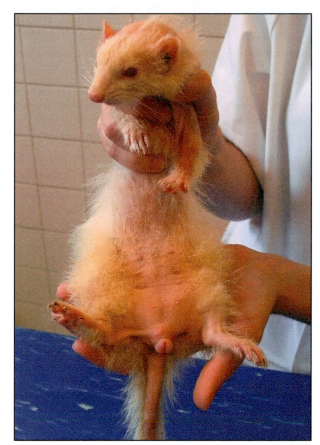

Fig. 14.38 An 18-month-old ferret was presented with a swollen vulva and generalised alopecia consistent with hyperoestrogenism due to persistent oestrus.

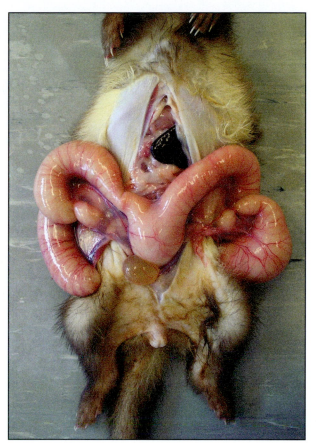

Fig. 14.39 This 3-year-old ferret was never mated with and had been in oestrus for 6 months per year, prior to being presented with a distended abdomen, which proved to be a mucometra.

of the tail and progressing cranially) and vulvar swelling (**Fig. 14.38**). Pale mucous membranes may indicate anaemia resulting from bone marrow suppression (**Fig. 14.37**). In addition, melena, haematuria, petechiae, ecchymosis and other signs of haemorrhage may be present (**Fig. 14.36**). Ferrets may also display anorexia, weakness, lethargy and depression, as well as signs associated with pneumonia, sepsis or muco-/pyometra (**Fig. 14.39**) that may result from the neutropaenia associated with bone marrow suppression. Galactorrhea and gynaecomastia may be seen on rare occasions.

Differential diagnosis

The most important differential diagnoses include hyperadrenocorticism (which is usually seen in ferrets over 3 years of age, and associated with milder disease that is slower in onset), ovarian remnant and granulosa cell tumours in neutered females. Rule-outs for anaemia include blood loss (e.g. due to trauma, gastric ulcers), rodenticide toxicity, hepatic disease, neoplasia, anaemia of chronic disease, renal failure, and haemolysis. Differential diagnosis for alopecia includes hyperadrenocorticism, seasonal alopecia, ectoparasites, mast cell tumours, food allergy and dermatophytosis.

Diagnosis

Diagnosis is usually based on the finding of classical clinical signs combined with the results of a haematological profile that reveals non-regenerative anaemia, thrombocytopaenia and leucopaenia. Bone marrow aspirates may reveal hypoplasia of the erythroid, myeloid and megakaryocytic cell lines.

Increased plasma oestradiol concentrations may help confirm a suspected diagnosis, although it should be noted that elevated plasma oestradiol levels may also be seen in ferrets with hyperadrenocorticism or an ovarian remnant or neoplasia. In spayed females with a swollen vulva, an abdominal ultrasound is extremely useful in distinguishing hyperadrenocorticism from the presence of an (altered) ovary. Additionally, an hCG challenge test may be performed. If the vulvar swelling disappears following administration of hCG (100 IU IM, repeat after 14 days), an ovarian remnant becomes likely.

Management/treatment

Treatment may be initiated with either hCG (100 IU/ferret IM), GnRH (20 µg/kg) or a deslorelin implant to induce ovulation and terminate oestrus. Alternatively, surgical intervention (ovariectomy or ovariohysterectomy, see Chapter 25) may be considered if the ferret is stable with a PCV >30%. In ferrets with PCVs <30%, blood transfusions may be considered prior to surgery. Patients that are severely anaemic, thrombocytopaenic and/or have secondary infections due to neutropaenia need to be stabilised first, if possible.

To prevent hyperoestrogenism-associated pancytopaenia, (surgical or chemical) neutering is recommended in any female ferret that is not bred. Alternatively, intact females that are not bred should not be allowed to remain in heat for more than 2 weeks. In these animals, ovulation may be induced by administering hCG (100 IU/ferret IM) or GnRH (20 µg/kg). In the UK it is also common practice to place the female with a vasectomised male, which will result in mating-induced ovulation.

Prognosis

Prognosis is good in case of timely intervention. Oestrus will generally be terminated within 7 days following administration of hCG in 95% of jills. Similarly, signs of oestrus will usually resolve within the first week following surgery (i.e. ovario[hyster]ectomy, adrenalectomy). Ferrets with a PCV of >25% are generally reported to carry a good prognosis and respond well to treatment with hCG; ferrets with a PCV of <25% carry a fair to guarded prognosis, dependent on the severity of the clinical signs and presence of concurrent disease.

CHAPTER 15

DISORDERS OF THE EARS AND EYES

Cathy A. Johnson-Delaney

EARS

The pinnae and external ear canals in ferrets are fairly small. Many breeders tattoo the ears of the ferrets. In the USA, one major breeder puts two dots in the right pinna signifying neuter/spay and demusking (**Fig. 15.1**). A breeder in Canada does a stripe in the right ear. Laboratory animal sources tend to put in small metal clip ear tags with individual numbers (**Fig. 15.2**). The pinna sometimes becomes infected or traumatised around these clips. Ferrets may tear them out; resulting in damage to the pinna.

The author promotes the use of an ear cleaner formula developed by Dr. Robert Wagner DVM, Dipl. ABVP-ECM. *Box 15.1* lists the 'recipe'.

AURAL HAEMATOMA

Definition/overview
Haematoma on the pinna, fluid pocket either on the cranial or caudal pinna (**Fig. 15.3**).

Aetiology/pathophysiology
Usually starts from trauma to the pinna. Haemorrhage trapped between the skin and cartilage. The most common scenario for this development is rough play, although the author knows of one case where the ferret's head was slammed in a cupboard door.

Clinical presentation
Fluctuant swelling on either the cranial or caudal pinna. May be discoloured (deep red to purple/bluish).

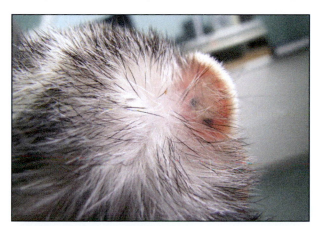

Fig. 15.1 **Two dots tattoo in the right ear signifying neutering and demusking.**

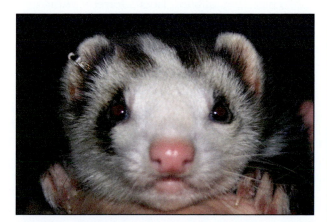

Fig. 15.2 **Metal ear tag used frequently in laboratories.**

Box 15.1 **Ferret ear cleaner formula**

- 1 and $^1/_3$ cups white vinegar.
- 2 and $^2/_3$ cups water.
- 2 tablespoons boric acid powder (Note: do not get powder in eyes or on wet skin while you are making this).
- 2 aspirin (325 mg ea).
- Mix ingredients well.
- It mixes faster if you use hot water.
- Store in a tightly sealed, plastic container.
- Makes about 1 litre of ear cleaner.

Developed by Dr Robert A. Wagner.

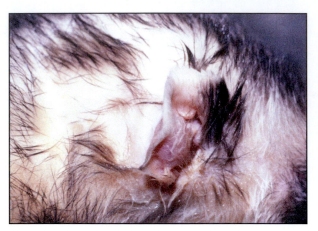

Fig. 15.3 **Aural haematoma.**

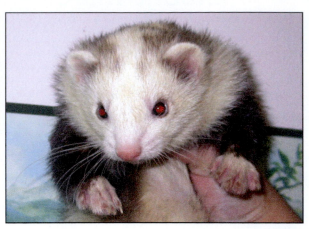

Fig. 15.4 **Blaze coat pattern associated with deafness.**

It may be painful on palpation. There may be accompanying bite marks or small scabs in the area around the ear.

Differential diagnosis
Abscess, neoplasia.

Diagnostic testing
After application of a topical anaesthetic, 22–23 gauge needle and syringe used to aspirate, evaluation of fluid with cytology.

Diagnosis
Fluid aspirated appears to be whole blood.

Management/treatment
Drainage of haematoma is usually sufficient although it may return requiring subsequent draining. In severe cases, a through-and-through suturing to compress the skin against the cartilage can be done, similar to how the haematoma would be corrected in a dog.

DEAFNESS

Definition/overview
Deafness linked with coat colour is the most common form. This is congenital sensorineural deafness (CSD). It can also be acquired following severe otitis or trauma.

Aetiology/pathophysiology
The most common form of deafness is CSD. A European study was recently published examining the association with coat colour. Seven per cent of ferrets out of 152 examined were unilaterally deaf; 22% were bilaterally deaf. The trait was not sex-linked and it was not found in Angora ferrets. White patterned ferrets or those exhibiting premature greying (ferret has sable or silver coat initially but as it ages it turns white) had an 87% prevalence of deafness. The dark-eyed white (DEW) exhibited a 4% deafness rate. Silver ferrets had a 4% deafness rate. Mitt ferrets (white paws) without other white markings had a 31% deafness rate. Mitt ferrets with other white markings had a 2% incidence of deafness. Panda (entirely white head, silver body, white feet), American Panda (large white areas anywhere on trunk, white feet) and Blaze (white stripe on the head that begins on the muzzle and extends to at least the level of the ears) were 100% bilaterally deaf (**Fig. 15.4**).

The lay public label ferret deafness as Waardenburg's syndrome. It is defined as an inherited form of deafness accompanied by characteristic markings and eye colouring. It is inherited as an autosomal dominant disease, although severity is variable. Confirmation of the genetics of heritable coat and eye colour is not possible in most cases of pet ferrets as they are not traceable back to the jill and hob. Waardenburg's syndrome is named for the Dutch ophthalmologist Petrus Johannes Waardenburg (1886–1979) who identified it in humans in 1951.

Differential diagnosis
Deafness acquired through otitis, neoplasia or trauma.

Diagnosis

History and coat colour. Greying ferrets' coat change may begin as early as 1 year of age with subsequent moults becoming whiter so that the ferret ends up being white.

Clinical signs

Coat colour and pattern. Usually the ferret acts totally normally and often the owner is unaware except they may have noted the ferret sleeps excessively soundly, squeals loudly during play, and otherwise ignores sounds and vocal commands. Some ferrets are startled easily and may nip.

Management/treatment

There is no treatment for coat colour. If otitis, neoplasia or trauma are the cause, treat the conditions as listed in this chapter. Once deaf, it will not resolve. It does not affect the ferret's quality of life. Owners need to be aware of this and alter their behaviour (do not startle the ferret) around the ferret to prevent nipping.

EAR MITES

Definition/overview

Infestation with *Otodectes cynotis*. The mite is transmitted by direct contact with other infested animals (**Figs 15.5, 15.6**).

Aetiology/pathophysiology

Otodectes cynotis is usually contracted from other ferrets but it is possible to be contracted from dogs or cats in the household, so these pets should be checked and treated accordingly if infested. The mite does not typically cause pruritis in the ferret, but some ferrets do rub at their ears during head grooming, although the frequency of this may be normal and not attributed directly to mite infestation. Long-standing infestation is sometimes noted by pigmentation of the pinnae.

Clinical signs

Ear wax with visible white mites or microscopically visible mites and eggs. There may be pigmentation to the pinnae and ear canal if chronic (**Fig. 15.7**). There may be deformities of the pinnae if there has been concurrent trauma from rubbing.

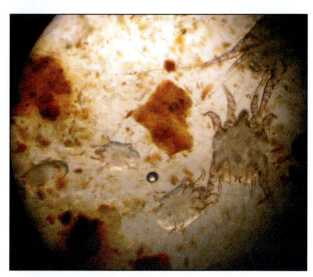

Fig. 15.5 *Otodectes cynotis.*

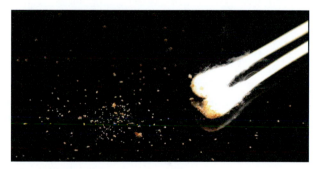

Fig. 15.6 *Otodectes cynotis* **visible macroscopically. (Courtesy of Vondelle McLaughlin.)**

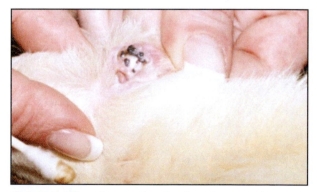

Fig. 15.7 **Chronic ear mites lead to pigmentation spots in the ear canal.**

Generally ear mites are non-pruritic but some ferrets do seem to include rubbing in head grooming.

Differential diagnosis

Excessive wax formation.

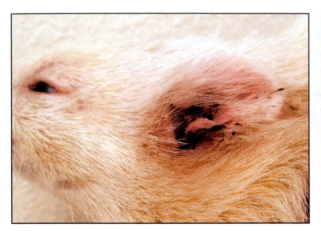

Fig. 15.8 Ear mite infestation with typical excess cerumen.

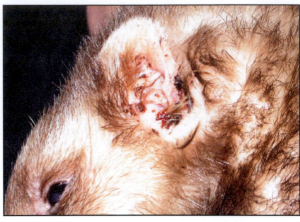

Fig. 15.9 Ear mite infestation contributing to otitis externa.

Diagnosis

Visible mites (white on dark wax) and/or microscopic examination of ear wax for mites and eggs (**Fig. 15.8**).

Management/treatment

Ivermectin at 0.5–1 mg/kg applied topically (mixed with propylene glycol to a volume of about 0.1–0.2 mL) or given orally or subcutaneously at 0.4 mg/kg repeated in 14–28 days or selamectin at 15 mg/kg topically every 30 days. Frequent ear cleaning and changing of bedding should accompany the parasiticide treatment regimen. All ferrets in the household should be treated as well. It does take persistence to eliminate a mite infestation. Imidaclopid plus moxidectin (Advantage Multi™ US, Advocate™ UK, BayerDVM, www.bayerdvm.com) has also proved effective in controlling ear mites.

OTITIS EXTERNA, MEDIA, INTERNA

Definition/overview

Otitis can be classified by segment of the ear infected or inflamed.

Aetiology/pathophysiology

Otitis externa is the most common, often due to infestation by ear mites and subsequent damage by the ferret rubbing at the ear (**Figs 15.9, 15.10**). Media is usually seen on otoscopic examination. Interna can be secondary to externa and media, but

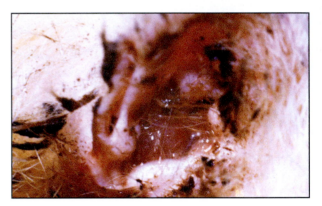

Fig. 15.10 Otitis media and externa.

may also be from ascending infection through the Eustachian tubes. Otitis can be unilateral or bilateral. In the author's experience media and interna are most frequently unilateral. Otitis generally is due to bacterial infection, but yeasts have been found, particularly in chronic cases that have been treated repeatedly with otic antimicrobial preparations. Wax in ferrets is normally pigmented, so using it as a measure of otitis cannot be done (**Fig. 15.11**). The tympanic bullae may be intact or ruptured. In some cases there may be bullae osteitis visible on radiograph (**Fig. 15.12**).

Clinical signs

May present with a head tilt (**Fig. 15.13**), excessive shaking of the head and pawing at the ear(s), exudate-filled ear canal(s), excessive wax formation and/or inflammation of the pinnae (**Fig. 15.13**).

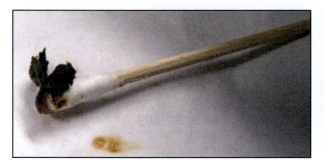

Fig. 15.11 **Excessive pigmented cerumen.**

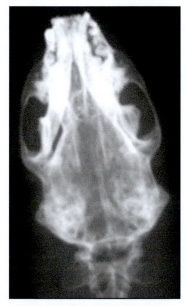

Fig. 15.12 **Bilateral bullae osteitis.**

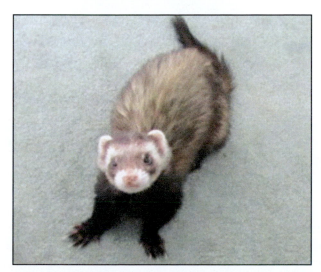

Fig. 15.13 **Head tilt due to otitis interna.**

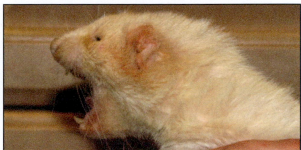

Fig. 15.14 **'Cauliflower' ear from trauma secondary to otitis.**

The pinnae may exhibit changes frequently called 'cauliflower ear' if there has been trauma to the pinnae from shaking, rubbing and chronic inflammation (**Fig. 15.14**). Pigmentation of the pinnae may be seen with the chronic inflammation.

Differential diagnosis
Heavy ear mite infestation. Neoplasia of the inner or outer ear.

Diagnosis
Cytology of the exudate. Culture of the exudates. Radiographs to examine the canal and bullae. Direct otoscopic examination of the ear canal and tympanic bullae.

Management/treatment
After cleaning the ear canal, and determining the integrity of the tympanic bullae, topical treatment of the ear canal with ophthalmic antimicrobial drops should be initiated (**Fig. 15.15**). The author prefers using ophthalmic preparations as they are mild on the ear canal and can be used with rupture of the tympanic bullae. Choice of antimicrobial should be based on culture results. If otitis interna is present, the use of systemic antimicrobials should be undertaken as well as administration with an analgesic and/or non-steroidal anti-inflammatory drug (NSAID). When using an NSAID use a stomach protectant as well, such as famotidine.

NEOPLASIA

Definition/overview
There are few reports of neoplasia involving the inner ear, but neoplasia is found involving the canal

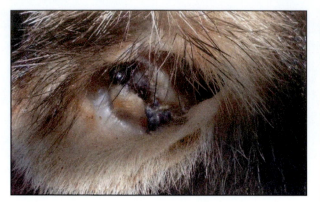

Fig. 15.15 **Chronic otitis externa. (Courtesy of Vondelle McLaughlin.)**

and pinna. Various types of tumours have been found including squamous cell carcinoma.

Aetiology/pathophysiology

Neoplasia involving the ear is not uncommon. Several types of tumours have been found associated most frequently with the pinna including squamous cell carcinoma. Neoplastic changes are unilateral (**Figs 15.16, 15.17**).

Clinical signs

There may be swelling, ulceration, and exudates from the ear canal and/or pinna. The area is usually painful with the ferret exhibiting shaking of the head or rubbing of the ear area. The area surrounding the ear may be swollen.

Differential diagnosis

Otitis media or externa, with involvement of the pinna and skin surrounding the ear.

Diagnosis

After cleaning out the ear canal to fully visualise the ear with direct otoscopy, biopsy the lesion for histopathology. As there is often secondary microbial infection of the tissue, cytology and culture of the lesion may direct otic antimicrobial therapy.

Treatment

Excisional surgery may be possible depending on the location of the mass. Treatment of the secondary otitis should be done. The author prefers to use ophthalmic preparations for the ear including the use of

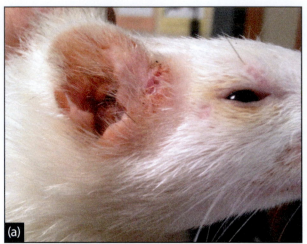

(a)

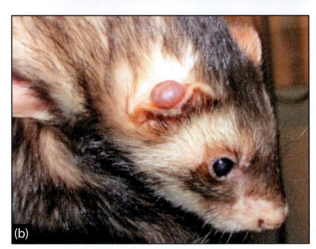

(b)

Fig. 15.16 **(a) Neoplasia of the pinna; (b) fibroma on the pinna.**

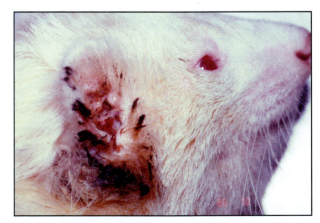

Fig. 15.17 **Squamous cell carcinoma involving the pinna.**

a topical NSAID such as flurbiprofen to help control inflammation and pain. Prognosis depends on the type of neoplasia plus the effectiveness of the surgery to debulk or completely remove the mass. Systemic antimicrobials along with an NSAID or analgesic may also treat the accompanying otitis externa and skin, particularly if there is ulceration. Depending on the type of neoplasia, appropriate chemotherapy and/or radiation therapy may be tried.

TRAUMA TO PINNAE

Definition/overview
Ferrets play roughly and often grab each other by the ear and drag each other across the floor. Puncture wounds are not uncommon. Laboratory ferrets may tear the ear tag out, leaving a lacerated pinna. Other trauma may occur from constant rubbing of the pinnae when there is otitis or neoplasia.

Aetiology/pathophysiology
Trauma to the pinnae occurs during play, removal of the ear tag or secondary to rubbing with otitis, or rarely severe ear mite infestation.

Clinical signs
The pinna may be lacerated, have puncture wounds or scabs and may be swollen. Chronic changes may occur with the skin of the pinnae becoming pigmented as seen with chronic ear mite infestation. The ferret may exhibit pain on palpation of the pinna. Signs are usually unilateral, although wounds acquired during play may be bilateral. Pinnae pigmentation is usually bilateral.

Differential diagnosis
Swelling and ulceration due to neoplasia, otitis.

Diagnosis
History. If accompanying exudates in the lesions, cytology and culture of the wounds may be warranted. If thickening or mass-like presentation, biopsy may be warranted.

Management/treatment
If infected, treatment can be initiated prior to culture results with a broad-spectrum ophthalmic preparation.

Systemic antimicrobial and NSAID may be used adjunctive to topical therapy. Consider changing playmates if this infected ear is due to bite wounds. Laceration from ear tag is usually treated with just the topical antimicrobial. If otitis is present, treat as outlined in 'Otitis'. If neoplastic, surgical excision and subsequent therapy per histopathology results may be warranted.

EYES (SEE CHAPTER 3)

The ferret globe is small at 7.0 ± 0.24 mm with a relatively large lens at 3.4 ± 0.15 mm. It has a wide cornea for optimal light gathering in low light conditions. The pupil is horizontally ovoid. The nictitating membrane is well developed. It has lymphoid tissue that can be a site of infection and lymphoma.

CATARACTS

Definition/overview
Lens opacification in one or both lenses. Most occur in ferrets older than 5 years of age. Nuclear sclerosis of the lens often precedes development of the cataract (**Fig. 15.18**).

Aetiology/pathophysiology
Opacity of the lens may start with focal spots before it becomes more diffuse. Some are seen as a diffuse haze or more profound opacity similar to what is seen in other species. These changes are considered age related. The author has seen cataracts in very young ferrets so there may be a congenital condition. It has been considered that all ferrets by 7 years of age have some degree of age-related cataract formation.

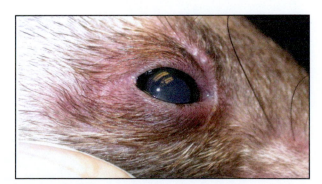

Fig. 15.18 **Cataract.**

Clinical presentation
Uni- or bilateral lens opacity (**Fig. 15.19**).

Differential diagnosis
Rule out nuclear sclerosis, focal opacities versus mature or hypermature cataracts.

Diagnosis
Using direct or indirect ophthalmic examination.

Management/treatment
Removal of the lens is difficult because of the small size of the globe. Irrigation–aspiration has been successful. Most ferrets adapt to blindness well so treatment may not be necessary.

CONGENITAL OCULAR DEFECTS

Definition/overview
There are a number of congenital defects found in ferrets, including microphthalmos, corneal dermoids, primary hyperplastic vitreous and cataracts (see above). Most congenital ocular defects do not require treatment.

CORNEAL DERMOIDS

Definition/aetiology/pathophysiology
Dermoid tissue growing on the cornea. May be inherited or a sporadic defect.

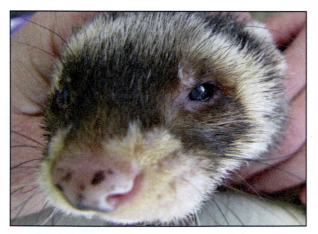

Fig. 15.19 Bilateral cataracts.

Clinical presentation
These are aberrant islands of dermal tissue appearing within the conjunctiva or cornea.

Differential diagnosis
These are distinctive.

Diagnosis
Ophthalmological examination including slit-lamp.

Management/treatment
Superficial keratectomy.

MICROPHTHALMIA

Definition/aetiology/pathophysiology
Probably a genetic heritable finding. In one closed colony it was found to have a simple dominant inheritance. It may be uni- or bilateral and does not behaviourally appear to cause any vision problems. In a few cases, a persistent conjunctival sac infection may occur due to the over-large conjunctival sac relative to the small size of the eye.

Clinical presentation
Unilateral or bilateral small eye with normal lids. If unilateral it is more noticeable as that side of the face may also seem small compared to the normal side. Conjunctivitis may be present due to excess conjunctival sac tissue (**Fig. 15.20**).

Differential diagnosis
Infection of the globe causing phthsical eye.

Diagnosis
Visualising globe and face.

Management/treatment
None needed unless there is persistent conjunctivitis. This requires regular management with topical ophthalmological agents.

CONJUNCTIVITIS

Definition
Inflammation of the conjunctiva, usually with epiphora or discharge. The lids may also be swollen.

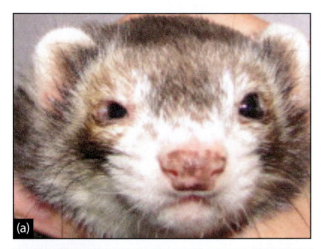

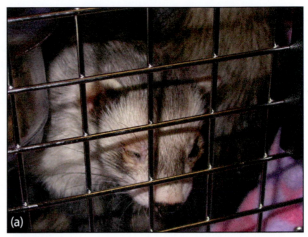

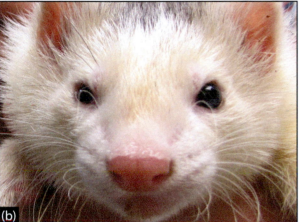

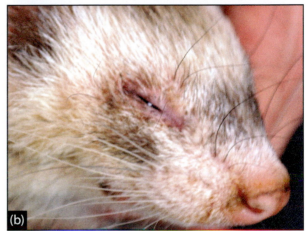

Fig. 15.20 (a, b) Microphthalmia right eye.

Fig. 15.21 (a) Nonspecific conjunctivitis; (b) canine distemper conjunctivitis. (Courtesy of Vondelle McLaughlin.)

Aetiology/pathophysiology

Local irritants such as dusty bedding, conjunctival foreign body or a corneal lesion may contribute although the latter two are usually unilateral in signs. Conjunctivitis is also seen with canine distemper or influenza (see Chapter 20). *Mycobacterium genovense* has been reported with proliferative or a chemotic conjunctivitis. Conjunctivitis has been associated with *Salmonella* infection although a minor clinical sign.

Clinical presentation

Appearance of conjunctival hyperaemia, oedema, and an obvious mucoid to mucopurulent ocular discharge. There may be fur wetness or loss around the eye if discharge has been lengthy or the ferret shows signs of rubbing the eyes. Because of the swelling the ferret may appear to be squinting. Blepharospasm may also be present (**Fig. 15.21**).

Differential diagnosis

Rule out local causes versus systemic such as canine distemper, influenza, *Mycobacterium*, *Salmonella*.

Diagnosis

History of exposure to distemper and influenza, along with thorough physical examination of the ferret and consideration of its environment. An ophthalmological examination for presence of foreign body. PCR of conjunctival swabs or biopsies has been used for distemper, influenza, and mycobacterial infections. *Salmonella* infections are usually diagnosed from the GI symptoms and sampling.

Management/treatment

Remove foreign body if present. Change environment if dusts are suspected. If canine distemper, see Chapter 20. If influenza, topical antimicrobials and NSAIDs may be used to decrease physical signs. Mycobacteria (see Chapter 20), *Salmonella* (see Chapter 20).

DISTICHIASIS

Definition/aetiology/pathophysiology

Abnormal eyelashes growing within the conjunctival sac or meibomian glands rubbing against the cornea or sclera.

Clinical presentation

Chronic blepharospasm, epiphora and conjunctivitis from one or both eyes.

Differential diagnosis

Topical irritants, entropion with trichiasis (rare), if unilateral, particularly foreign body, corneal trauma.

Diagnosis

Ophthalmic examination including thorough examination of the conjunctival sac for visualisation of the hairs.

Management/treatment

Transconjunctival unipolar electrocautery and/or full thickness wedge excision.

ENTROPION

Definition/aetiology/pathophysiology

This is rare in the ferret. It is due to lid inturning that causes ocular discomfort. In severe cases there may be corneal ulceration due to the trichiasis with skin hair abrading onto the cornea. While anatomical abnormalities may be present, another cause can be ocular foreign body, which may be responsible for the initial blepharospasm that later turns into a more long-lasting defect.

Clinical presentation

Blepharospasm and epiphora are usually present. The cornea may be ulcerated or abraded. The ferret is in pain.

Differential diagnosis

Foreign body corneal lesions, blepharospasms, conjunctivitis.

Diagnosis

Careful direct ophthalmic examination to look for foreign body, direct and indirect ophthalmoscopy, fluoroscein dye to assess cornea.

Management/treatment

Remove foreign body and treat ocular pain and corneal lesions as with other species (topical NSAID such as flurbiprofen ophthalmic drops, and a broad-spectrum antibiotic ophthalmic drop or ointment). If an anatomical defect is the cause, a standard Hotz-Celsus excision of a small strip of lid skin can resolve the problem. This surgery is usually done under an operating microscope due to the small size and delicate tissue of the ferret.

EXOPHTHALMOS

Definition

Protrusion of the globe. Unilateral or bilateral. Usually there is protrusion of the third eyelid in association with the proptosed eye.

Aetiology

Pressure behind the globe. Trauma to the head, usually results in bilateral but not always. May be a sign of retrobulbar space-occupying lesion.

Pathophysiology

Retrobulbar mass effect. This can be soft-tissue neoplasia, boney neoplasia of the orbit, or retrobulbar abscess. An infraorbital salivary mucocele from the zygomatic salivary gland may develop, particularly following head trauma (**Fig. 15.22**).

Clinical presentation

Globe appears to be protruding. It may be partially or fully outside the bony orbit. Globe may appear injected, cornea may be clouded depending on length of time condition has existed. The third eyelid is usually also proptosed and may be swollen, injected.

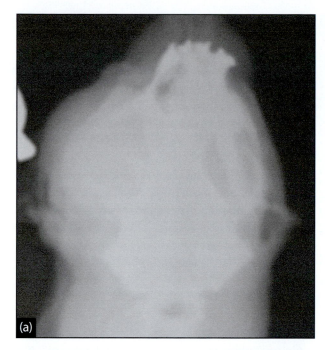

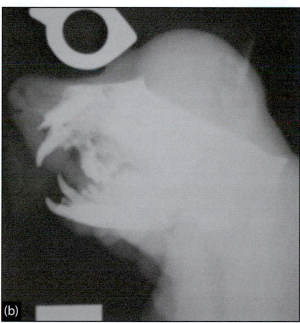

Fig. 15.22 (a) DV radiograph of mass effect proptosing the right eye; (b) lateral radiograph mass effect with proptosed globe.

Diagnostic testing

Skull films. Ophthalmic examination. Fine needle aspirate or biopsy of the retrobulbar tissue. Ultrasonography of the globe and retrobulbar tissue. In extreme cases CT scan.

Diagnosis

Abnormal placement of the globe.

Management/treatment

Depending on the length of time the globe has protruded, this will determine if the globe itself has been damaged. If globe is exophthalmic due to retrobulbar mass effect, it will need to be reduced if the globe is to be replaced. If glaucomatous or injected globe, treatment may need to include a topical NSAIDs (flurbiprofen), topical antibiotics, topical antiglaucoma ophthalmics. In severe cases the globe may need to be enucleated. The ferret has a sizeable retrobulbar venous plexus which can complicate surgical intervention. Prognosis is guarded for the health of the globe, particularly if the retrobulbar mass effect cannot be easily treated.

GLAUCOMA

Definition

Intraocular hypertension of the eyes.

Aetiology/pathophysiology

Glaucoma in the ferret is usually secondary to trauma or luxation of cataractous lenses. Primary glaucoma has not been reported. In the laboratory, glaucoma is induced in ferrets used as models for human disease.

Clinical presentation

The eye may be grossly swollen (**Fig. 15.23**). This may include episcleral injection, mydriasis and blindness as in other species. If due to lens luxation, the lens may appear as a half moon (**Fig. 15.24**).

Differential diagnosis

Globe disease including glaucoma, neoplasia. Abscessation or neoplasia of the retrobulbar tissue.

Differential diagnosis

Trauma to the globe and adnexa. Uveitis with secondary development of glaucoma.

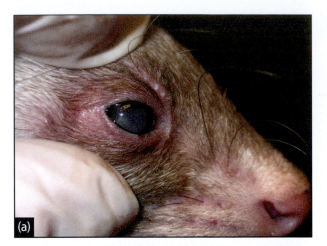

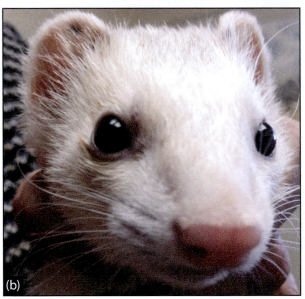

Fig. 15.23 (a) Glaucoma causing swelling of the globe; (b) there may be tearing of the glaucomatous eye.

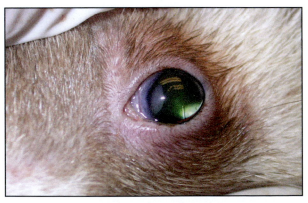

Fig. 15.24 Luxated lens.

Diagnosis

Full ophthalmic examination including use of an applanation tonometer to measure intraocular pressure. Normal intraocular pressure has been published as 13.1 ± 1.1 mmHg, although it also has been published using a different type of tonometer as 22.8 ± 5.5 mmHg as well as 14.5 ±3.2 mmHg.

Management/treatment

As primary glaucoma is rare in ferrets, responses to treatments of dorzolamide, pilocarpine or the prostaglandin analogue latanoprost used in other animals have not been reported. One article successfully used trans-scleral diode laser cytophotocoagulation to control raised intraocular pressure in one ferret.

KERATITIS

Definition

Corneal ulceration or non-ulcerative keratitis. Non-ulcerative keratitis if characterised by vascularisation and cellular infiltrate.

Aetiology/pathophysiology

Corneal ulceration can be due to trauma, tear deficiency or exposure keratitis. Older ferrets may have delayed epithelial healing, which could be associated with epithelial basement membrane dystrophy. There may be decreased tear production. Non-ulcerative keratitis may be immune mediated as seen in canine chronic superficial keratitis. However, it has been reported as an early sign of multicentric lymphoma.

Clinical presentation

The ferret may have ocular pain, corneal abrasion or ulceration, conjunctivitis and blepharospasm (**Fig. 15.25**).

Differential diagnosis

Corneal trauma, dry eye due to exposure (exophthalmos).

Diagnosis

The Schirmer tear test strop works in ferrets to see when tear deficiency is involved in the corneal defect. Tear production in ferrets has been documented at

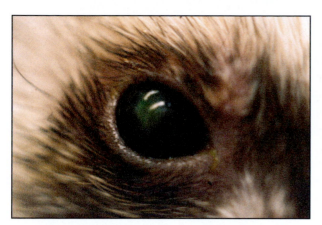

Fig. 15.25 **Keratitis with fluorescein dye showing corneal lesion.**

5.3 ±1.3 mm/min. Fluoroscein dye is used to assess the cornea.

Management/treatment

Corneal ulceration is managed using topical antibiotics and NSAIDS. If ulceration is due to lack of tears, a topical ciclosporin ointment and tear replacement should be used like treating keratoconjunctivitis sicca. If exposure keratitis is the cause, amelioration of the cause of the globe protrusion is necessary. If that is not possible, lateral canthoplasty will reduce the degree of exposure of the cornea.

LYMPHOMA OF GLANS NICTITANS, ADNEXA, CONJUNCTIVAL TISSUE

Definition

Lymphoma of the tissues surrounding the eye; may be diffuse or more definitive mass (**Fig. 15.26**).

Aetiology/pathophysiology

Common finding in the older ferret and may or may not be associated with lymphomas in other organs. The eye itself is not the site of the lymphoma. There may be enlargement on the bulbar surface of the glans nictitans. One or both of the eyes may be affected. If the mass enlarges, it may proptose the globe and cause blindness.

Clinical presentation

The tissue around the eye may appear swollen and hyperaemic. The glans nictitans may be swollen

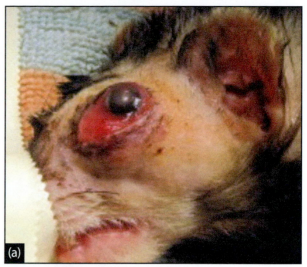

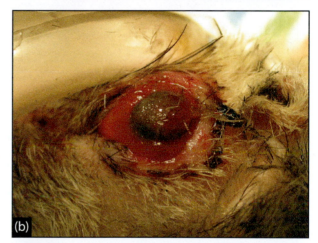

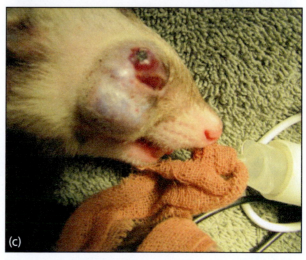

Fig. 15.26 **(a) Mass effect proptosing eye (the globe is compromised); (b) lymphoma involving the globe; (c) mass involving the globe.**

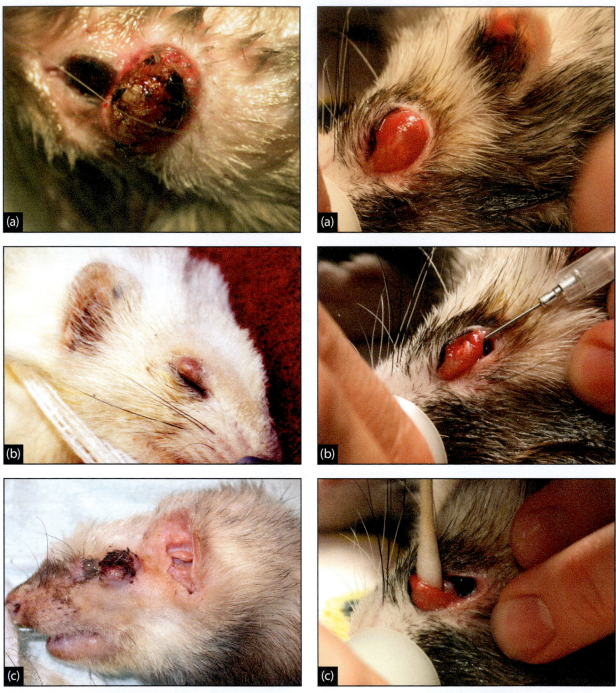

Fig. 15.27 (a) Lymphoma mass at the canthi of the eye; (b) lymphoma of the eyelid; (c) lymphoma of the skin adjacent to the eye.

Fig. 15.28 (a) Lymphoma in the glans nictitans; (b) aspiration of the tissue (submit for cytology) to decrease the mass; (c) replacement of the glans within the canthi.   *(Continued)*

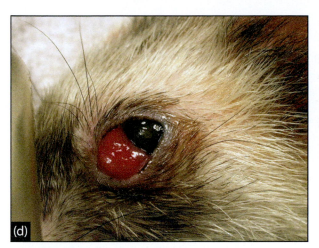

Fig. 15.28 (continued) (d) another example of glans nictitans involvement.

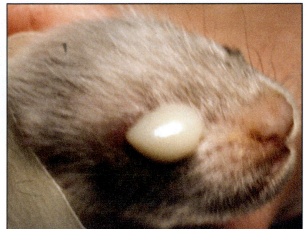

Fig. 15.29 Ophthalmia neonatorum in a 3-week-old kit.

and protruding from the eyelids, often covering the cornea (**Figs 15.27, 15.28**).

Differential diagnosis

Conjunctivitis and severe swelling of the adnexal tissue. A foreign body on the cornea may elicit a lymphoid response by the glans nictitans. Retrobulbar abscess.

Diagnosis

Examination under sedation to elevate the glans nictitans and biopsy. Adnexal tissue exhibiting swelling may also be biopsied.

Management/treatment including prognosis

If lymphoma, the tissue may be excised (debulked). In some cases the glans nictitans if involved may be removed to prevent corneal damage. Topical prednisolone ophthalmic drops may be tried, along with an antibiotic drop. Prognosis for continued lymphoma is poor, as the growth of the lymphatic tissue may have an impact on vision and may cause progressive pain to the ferret.

OPHTHALMIA NEONATORUM (SEE CHAPTER 26)

Definition

Infection of the conjunctival sac in the newborn kit before the eyelids open.

Aetiology/pathophysiology

Ocular infection may occur at birth, but more commonly it is seen when kits suckle a jill with mastitis. There may even be development of panophthalmitis and septicaemia resulting in death if untreated.

Clinical presentation

There may be swelling of lids and/or discharge from between the opening lids. Affected kits may be anorexic and dehydrated. This may be due to pain involved, but also due to systemic infection spreading from the ocular region (**Fig. 15.29,** see **26.10**).

Differential diagnosis

Only what species of bacteria involved and the extent of the lesion(s).

Diagnostic testing

Culture of the eye may be taken from between the lids. An antibiogram should also be run.

Diagnosis

Confirmation of bacterial involvement determined from the culture.

Management/treatment

The eyelids should be coaxed apart using cotton buds wetted with saline. In younger kits the lids may need to be surgically opened. A topical broad-spectrum ophthalmic antibiotic ointment should be applied at least 3–4 times a day. If the kit is listless, pyrexic, anorexic, dehydrated or if the jill has mastitis, systemic antibiotics should be used, based on the culture and sensitivity. Supportive care including systemic fluids and analgesics may be given. Antibiotics started may be adjusted pending the bacterial sensitivity. Prognosis is generally good with response to treatment.

PYOGRANULOMATOUS PANOPHTHALMITIS DUE TO CORONAVIRUS

Definition
Panophthalmitis with pyogranulomatous lesions.

Aetiology/pathophysiology
Case of systemic coronavirus with multi-systemic necrotising granulomas in the lung, spleen, kidneys, mesenteric lymph nodes and serosa of the duodenum. This is consistent with ferret systemic coronavirus (FRSCV). The case reported was unilateral. In cats with systemic coronavirus (FIP) anterior uveitis, chorioretinitis, optic neuritis and retinal detachment have been documented.

Clinical presentation
Focal area of opacity on the cornea. The ferret in this case had poor body condition, lethargic and dehydrated. Other signs included azotaemia, hyperproteinaemia, hypoalbuminaemia, mild hyperphosphataemia and hyperchloraemia. On radiographs showed multifocal thoracic nodular disease, splenomegaly and renomegaly. Abdominal ultrasound showed bilateral enlarged kidneys, hypoechoic liver and spleen and a caudal abdominal hypoechoic mobile nodule.

Differential diagnosis
For the eye, trauma to the cornea; panophthalmitis due to infection, abscess. Neoplasia.

Diagnosis
Immunohistochemistry of the eye confirmatory for FRSCV. Granulomatous lesions may be tested with reverse transcriptase polymerase chain reaction (RT-PCR). Formalin-fixed paraffin embedded tissue from lung, spleen and kidneys has been found to be negative for FRSCV but positive for ferret enteric coronavirus (FRECV) (Chapter 13).

Management/treatment
There is no treatment for FRSCV. FRECV treatment is largely symptomatic and supportive. Prognosis is generally poor.

RETINAL DISEASE

Definition
Abnormalities of the retina including hyper-reflectivity and vascular attenuation similar to that in the dog or cat, with inherited degeneration as seen in progressive retinal atrophy.

Aetiology/pathophysiology
Because ferrets are obligate carnivores like cats, taurine deficiency may play a role in retinal atrophy. However, unlike cats that have changes in the area centralis, there are no reports of this in the ferret. Experimental intrauterine infection with feline panleucopaenia virus has caused widespread devastating retinopathy with subsequent blindness. This infection has not been reported to occur naturally.

Clinical presentation
The ferret may be blind. The tapetum may have hyper-reflectivity, vascular attenuation.

Differential diagnosis
Retinitis, retinal atrophy.

Diagnosis
Direct and indirect ophthalmoscopic examination.

Management/treatment
Taurine supplementation may slow the progression as is seen in cats. Dosage of taurine is empirical at 10 mg per day. The ferret may be blind but adapts well to this condition.

TRAUMA

Definition
Injury to the eye (**Fig. 15.30**).

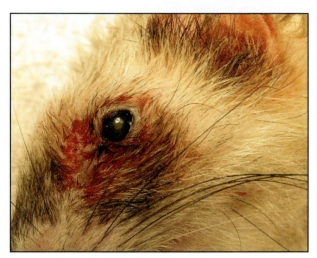

Fig. 15.30 Trauma to the eye may involve swelling of the glans nictitans, conjunctiva, cornea and globe.

Aetiology/pathophysiology

Ferrets may run into things during play. They also get foreign objects in their eyes, often while digging or burrowing in substrate. Lacerations occur to the cornea and occasionally the sclera. Ferrets can also exhibit retinal detachment or lens luxation from a blow to the head, often accidental from being hit with a door or other trauma.

Clinical presentation

The cornea may be opaque, there may be conjunctivitis, blepharospasm, ophthalmic pain and vision compromise. Epiphora and swelling of the glans nictitans is seen fairly commonly, especially with corneal abrasion/laceration. On ophthalmic examination, lens luxation and retinal detachment may be seen.

Differential diagnosis

Glaucoma, uveitis, foreign body in conjunctiva, neoplasia of adnexa or other ophthalmic manifestations.

Diagnosis

Direct and indirect ophthalmoscopy. If cornea is severely opaque, examination of the lens and retina may be difficult. Fluoroscein dye to the cornea will show abrasion/laceration. Full examination of the conjunctiva and glans nictitans needs to be done to rule out foreign body.

Management/treatment

For corneal abrasion/laceration treatment depends on depth of the lesion. It may be necessary to suture the cornea and eyelids to provide healing as in other species and indications. Corneal lesions may be treated with a broad-spectrum antibiotic ophthalmic gel or solution, and in some cases a topical NSAID for the pain. A systemic analgesic is also recommended as the eye is usually painful. Rest and quiet is recommended for retinal detachment but that is difficult in the ferret and it is likely to be/become blind. A luxated lens might be removable but due to the small size of the eye, it may be extremely difficult. A luxated lens may cause glaucoma (see above). Usually these are just left alone. Rechecks of the eye, particularly monitoring intraocular pressure, should be done with the lens luxation as the dynamics of the inner eye have been changed. Most ferrets have no problems with lens luxation.

UVEITIS

Definition

Inflammation of the iris and ciliary body.

Aetiology/pathophysiology

Uveitis is not common. It may involve the breakdown of the blood–aqueous barrier secondary to trauma or corneal ulceration. Aleutian disease, a systemic parvoviral immune complex disease (see Chapter 16), has been shown to cause uveitis in mink and otters, so may also do so in ferrets. The disease causes vasculitis and inflammation of uveal vasculature causes a breakdown in the blood–aqueous barrier and subsequent uveitis. Due to the small size of the ferret eye this may be difficult to visualise, particularly if there is corneal opacity.

Clinical signs

Miosis, episcleral hyperaemia and signs of intraocular inflammation such as keratic precipates, hypopyon, pain and photophobia. Corneal oedema is the most common sign.

Differential diagnosis

Glaucoma, corneal/eye trauma.

Diagnosis

Rule out Aleutian disease (see Chapter 16) or other systemic diseases that can cause uveitis including toxoplasmosis (see Chapter 18), blastomycosis, cryptococcosis (see Chapter 20). Rule out glaucoma with tonometry. Fluoroscein dye to check corneal integrity. Direct and indirect ophthalmoscopy.

Management/treatment

Atropine (topical mydriatic, cycloplegic) is used with caution due to the small size of the ferret eye and small blood volume. This is a parasympatholytic that if overused may cause systemic toxicity. As uveitis is often seen with other disease, a full physical examination and clinical work-up is warranted.

DISORDERS OF THE HAEMIC, IMMUNOLOGICAL AND LYMPHATIC SYSTEMS

*Samantha Swisher and
Angela M. Lennox*

INTRODUCTION

The normal ferret haemogram is similar to other mammals (see Appendices 2, 3 for normal values). Anaemia is a common finding in ferrets, and morphological changes associated with a regenerative response are similar to other mammals (**Fig. 16.1**). As in other mammals, heterophils are typically the predominant cell type, followed by lymphocytes, monocytes, eosinophils and basophils.

It should be noted that ferrets may experience marked splenic sequestration of blood cells during inhalent anaesthesia, resulting in artifactual reduction in cell counts in samples collected under anaesthesia. The effects of injectable sedation on the haemogram have not been investigated.

Maternal transfer of immunoglobulins to neonates is primarily via passive transfer from milk, and studies have demonstrated transmucosal uptake of immunoglobulin (Ig) G across the intestinal mucosa for the first 30 days of life.

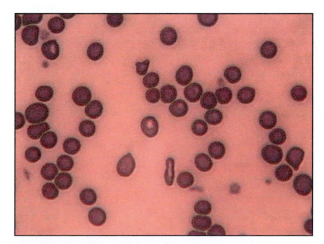

Fig. 16.1 **Peripheral blood film demonstrating polychromasia, consistent with a regenerative response to anaemia.**

Disorders of the haemolymphatic system in ferrets are very common. Many haemolymphatic diseases are secondary to another primary disease process (often infectious) that affects the function of the bone marrow or the immune system, but primary haemolymphatic diseases, such as lymphoma, are also commonly reported.

ALEUTIAN DISEASE

Definition/overview
Aleutian disease (ADV) is a viral disease of mustelids. This disease was initially documented in mink and is referred to as Aleutian disease because mink with the Aleutian coat pattern have a genetic mutation that makes them more susceptible. Because ADV is relatively uncommon in pet ferrets, much of the information available in the literature is from mink, and may not always be applicable to ferrets with the disease. While seroprevalence in ferrets has been reported to be as high as 10% in some populations, only a few clinical cases of ADV have been documented in recent years, and it is believed to be relatively rare in the pet ferret population. The authors have seen two confirmed cases in 20 years of practice.

Aetiology/pathophysiology
Aleutian disease is caused by a parvovirus that was first reported in mink farms in the USA in the 1940s. There have been three strains of parvovirus documented in ferrets with clinical signs of ADV, all of which are believed to be mutations of the mink virus. Ferrets may also be infected with mink strains of the virus, though it is generally believed that each species is more severely affected by its own strains of the virus.

Virus transmission is by aerosol or contact with infected bodily secretions, including blood, urine, faeces and saliva. Parvoviruses are very stable in the environment, so direct contact with an infected animal is not required. Vertical transmission has not been documented in ferrets, but is known to occur in mink. It is possible for an infected animal to be asymptomatic and still actively shedding the virus.

Once infected, ferrets typically mount a marked humoral immune response. The resulting hyper-gammaglobulinaemia leads to the immune-complex deposition that is responsible for many of the clinical signs of this disease, including glomerulonephritis, biliary hyperplasia and pneumonitis. Because of the marked immune response focused on the virus, affected animals often have poor immune responses to other pathogens, leaving them vulnerable to bacterial and other viral infections.

Clinical presentation

Most clinically affected ferrets present with progressive weight loss, muscle wasting and weakness (**Fig. 16.2a**). Some animals present with neurological signs, including ataxia, paresis, muscle fasciculations, tremors and seizure activity. Ferrets with liver involvement may appear icteric (**Fig. 16.2b**), and those with renal compromise may present with dehydration, nausea or oral ulcers. Respiratory signs have occasionally been reported, primarily in juvenile ferrets. In contrast with other parvoviruses, ferret parvoviruses typically do not cause GI signs, except in cases that develop *Helicobacter mustelae* gastritis as a result of immune alteration.

Asymptomatic carrier states have been reported and are thought to be most common in animals that are exposed as adults. These animals may remain persistently infected for years and develop clinical signs (including sudden death) at any time. Infected animals can shed the virus in the absence of clinical signs. Persistently infected breeding animals may have decreased fertility or increased incidence of abortion.

Differential diagnosis

Many of the clinical signs of ADV are non-specific. Weight loss, ataxia, and posterior paresis occur in ferrets with a wide variety of diseases, including insulinoma, lymphoma and chronic inflammatory

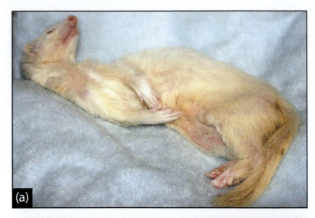

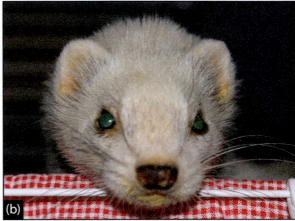

Fig. 16.2 Ferrets with Aleutian disease demonstrating (a) severe emaciation and (b) icterus. (Courtesy of Vondelle McLaughlin.)

GI diseases. Differential diagnoses for neurological signs include insulinoma, exposure to toxins and distemper virus. Differentials for haematological signs include lymphoma, bone marrow suppression, chronic GI blood loss and a wide variety of other chronic diseases. Respiratory signs in young ferrets may be caused by mediastinal lymphoma or pneumonia. The most common differential for hyperglobulinaemia is ferret systemic coronavirus (FRSCV), though marked hyperglobulinaemia has also been reported in ferrets with lymphoma.

Diagnostic testing

Because many of the clinical signs of ADV can be caused by other, more common diseases, initial diagnostics should include a CBC, biochemistry, and imaging (radiographs and/or abdominal ultrasound). The most common abnormality on biochemistry is a marked hyperglobulinaemia, with an inverted albumin:globulin ratio. Further characterisation by protein electrophoresis typically reveals marked increases in gamma globulins. Other findings on blood work vary depending on the organ system(s) affected, but may include azotaemia, elevated liver values and anaemia. White blood cell abnormalities described with parvovirus infections in other species are uncommon in ferrets.

With the exception of splenomegaly and rare cases of pneumonitis, there are rarely any radiographic changes associated with ADV, but radiographs may still be indicated to rule out other disease processes. Abdominal ultrasound may reveal renal, hepatic, or splenic changes.

Specific testing for viral pathogens can be by direct detection of the virus or by serology. For ferret parvovirus, serology by counterimmunoelectrophoresis (CEP) is currently the most commonly employed screening test, and a negative CEP result is required for entrance into shows sponsored by the American Ferret Association (AFA). A positive CEP test, while evidence of exposure, does not necessarily imply active disease; serological surveys have demonstrated a seroprevalence of 8.5–10% in ferrets without clinical signs.

As of this writing, CEP testing is available through Blue Cross Animal Hospital (208-678-5553, submission instructions available at www.ferret.org/read/CEP_testing.html). Michigan State University (www.ferrethealth.msu.edu/Diagnostics.php) and University of Georgia (www.uga.eud/idl/test) offer PCR testing on faecal material, tissue samples or blood (University of Georgia only). A positive result on any of these tests is suggestive of active shedding.

Diagnosis

A diagnosis of active ADV should be based on a combination of positive serology, PCR and compatible clinical signs. Positive results in an asymptomatic animal may still be helpful in guiding colony management.

Management/treatment

Parvoviruses are highly infectious and are included in core vaccination protocols for dogs and cats.

Unfortunately, there is no vaccine available for ferret parvovirus, and it is unclear whether vaccination would be beneficial, given the immune-mediated nature of the disease.

In mink, serology-based test-and-cull strategies have allowed the eradication of the disease from individual facilities. While this may not be practical in pet ferrets, it should be considered in breeding or shelter situations. In companion animals, all animals with evidence of active shedding should be quarantined and segregation of seropositive animals should be considered.

There is no specific treatment for animals with ADV. As with most viral diseases, good supportive care is critical and may consist of fluid and nutritional support, antibiotics for secondary infection and GI protectants as indicated. Due to the immune-mediated nature of the disease, treatment with immunosuppressive agents may be beneficial. A study in mink found that intraperitoneal administration of cyclophosphamide controlled clinical signs, but virus levels were unaffected. Another study documented decreased mortality in mink kits treated with ADV antibody, but this is probably impractical for clinical use. In pet ferrets, immunosuppressive therapy with prednisolone, cyclophosphamide or other drugs may be considered, but the risks should be carefully considered and the patient should be closely monitored for secondary infection.

Unfortunately, most existing studies of treatment and prognosis for ADV have been conducted in farmed or laboratory mink, so information about prognosis for individual patients that receive intensive care is unknown, but probably guarded.

ANAEMIA

Definition/overview

Anaemia is a decreased number of red blood cells in the systemic circulation. Depending on the source, ferrets are considered anaemic when packed cell volume (PCV) drops below 35–40%. Anaemia is commonly reported in ferrets with a wide variety of disease processes and determining the underlying cause can sometimes be challenging.

Aetiology/pathophysiology

All causes of anaemia fall into three major categories: decreased red blood cell production, increased destruction and haemorrhage. Decreased production can result from bone marrow disease (neoplasia, hyperoestrogenaemia, pure red cell aplasia), iron deficiency, renal disease or anaemia of chronic disease. Increased destruction has not been commonly reported in ferrets, but in other species, haemolytic anaemia can be associated with infectious diseases (especially tick-borne disease), neoplasia, heavy metal toxicosis, drugs and vaccine administration. One of the most common causes of haemorrhage seen in pet ferrets is GI blood loss secondary to *Helicobacter* gastritis, but haemorrhage into body cavities secondary to trauma, coagulopathy or neoplasia should also be considered. In 2008, an outbreak of unexplained haemorrhage was reported in juvenile ferrets as the result of a coagulation disorder of unknown aetiology (see below, Haemorrhagic syndrome).

Clinical presentation

Common findings on physical examination may include pale mucous membranes (**Fig. 16.3**), weakness, tachycardia, and increased respiratory rate and effort. Animals with very severe anaemia may develop neurological signs as a result of poor oxygen delivery. The severity of clinical signs depends both on the degree of anaemia and on the chronicity; patients that have become anaemic gradually generally tolerate much more severe anaemia than patients with acute blood loss. The authors have encountered ferrets apparently tolerating haematocrits as low as 8–10%. In ferrets, the spleen plays an important role in haematopoiesis (especially if the bone marrow is compromised) and splenomegaly is a common finding in anaemic ferrets.

Differential diagnosis

The primary differential for patients that present pale, weak, tachypnoeic and tachycardic is shock (hypovolaemic, septic, etc.). Basic diagnostic testing and response to treatment will help to determine whether the patient's clinical signs can be attributed to anaemia.

Diagnostic testing

A diagnosis of anaemia can often be achieved with a simple PCV and total solids (**Fig. 16.4**). In the case of acute anaemia, PCV may be relatively normal in the face of marked blood loss. Further diagnostics are required to determine the underlying cause of the anaemia.

- Complete blood count with blood smear evaluation – the results of a CBC can help to classify anaemia as regenerative or non-regenerative, based on RBC indices and the presence of increased numbers of reticulocytes (**Fig. 16.1**). In rare cases, there may also be morphological changes suggestive of iron deficiency or haemolysis.

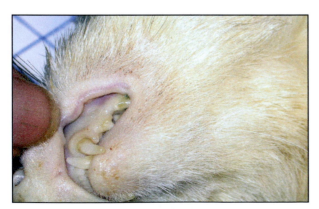

Fig. 16.3 Ferret with pale mucous membranes as a result of severe anaemia. (Courtesy of Cathy Johnson-Delaney.)

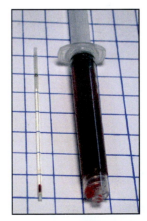

Fig. 16.4 Haematocrit tube from an anaemic ferret. (Courtesy of Cathy Johnson-Delaney.)

- Chemistry – renal disease can produce anaemia as a result of decreased production of erythropoietin. BUN can also be elevated in patients with GI bleeding. Chemistry results may also help to detect other underlying conditions that might produce anaemia of chronic disease.
- Imaging – imaging should be performed as indicated based on clinical signs and physical examination findings. Radiographs, ultrasound and endoscopy may all be helpful, depending on the case.
- Faecal occult blood (**Fig. 16.5**) – use of faecal occult blood testing in obligate carnivores is controversial due to concerns about cross-reaction with dietary components, though more recent studies have suggested that changes in the manufacturing of these tests may have reduced the likelihood of cross-reaction. Both false positives and false negatives are possible, and results should be interpreted with caution, since these tests have not been validated in ferrets.
- Bone marrow aspirate/biopsy (**Fig. 16.6**) – if anaemia is believed to be non-regenerative, a bone marrow biopsy can be helpful to determine the underlying aetiology. See Chapter 10 for more information on performing bone marrow biopsies in ferrets.

Diagnosis

Anaemia is diagnosed with a PCV/TS. Further testing is required to determine underlying aetiology.

Management/treatment

Treatment for anaemia should be directed at resolving the underlying cause. For patients experiencing haemorrhage, the source of bleeding should be addressed as soon as possible. Aplastic anaemia has been successfully managed with immunosuppressive drugs (after appropriate diagnostics to rule out underlying infectious aetiologies). Outcomes for females with anemia secondary to hyperoestrogenemia have not been well-documented, but some may resolve with surgical or chemical neutering.

While the ultimate goal of therapy for anaemic animals should be to resolve the underlying disease process, patients that are experiencing severe clinical signs as a result of anaemia (tachycardia, respiratory effort, etc) may require a blood transfusion to ensure adequate oxygen delivery until the underlying cause of the anaemia can be addressed. Ideally, this should be achieved using packed red blood cells for euvolaemic patients and whole blood for patients that are volume-contracted. However, most patients that are free of underlying heart disease can tolerate a whole blood transfusion if given slowly with careful monitoring. The goal of treatment should be to achieve resolution of clinical signs, rather than restoration of a specific PCV. See Chapter 10 for more detail about blood transfusion in ferrets. Depending on cause and severity, administration of iron dextran (10–20 mg/kg IM once, repeat weekly as needed) and/or erythropoietin (50–150 U/kg IM q48h) should also be considered.

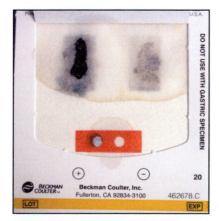

Fig. 16.5 **Faecal occult blood test demonstrating a positive (left) and negative sample.**

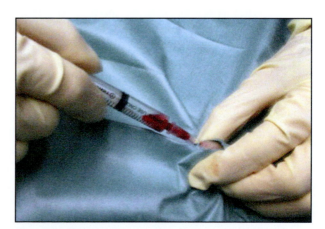

Fig. 16.6 **Bone marrow aspiration from the femur.**

Prognosis for anaemic patients is highly variable, depending on the underlying disease process.

FERRET HAEMORRHAGIC SYNDROME

Definition/overview
This syndrome was first reported in 2006 and 2007. There were at least 35 reported cases in kits roughly 8–24 weeks of age, which had all been recently shipped from the same commercial breeder. Often the only sign was haemorrhage and acute death. The disease is now rarely reported.

Aetiology/pathophysiology
Studies in ferrets have shown that ferret coagulation pathways do not differ significantly from those of other mammals. While the clinical signs exhibited by affected ferrets are consistent with defects in both primary and secondary haemostasis, the primary clinico-pathological finding was prolonged prothrombin time (PT)/partial thromboplastin time (PTT), suggesting a defect in secondary haemostasis. The few affected ferrets that had coagulation panels available all had prolonged coagulation time compared to age-matched ferrets, but the number tested was not statistically significant. No aetiological agent was discovered.

Clinical presentation
Most ferrets present due to the presence of large amounts of blood in the cage or for unexplained epistaxis. Bleeding may stop and spontaneously recur at any time. Some ferrets may have bleeding from other mucosal surfaces, such as the mouth (**Fig. 16.7a**) or rectum. Severe cases may develop petechiation/ecchymosis or internal haemorrhage (**Figs 16.7 b, c**). Ferrets may be presented for acute death due to severe haemorrhage.

Differential diagnosis
Differentials for unexplained bleeding include hereditary coagulopathies, anticoagulant rodenticide toxicity and disseminated intravascular coagulation (DIC).

Diagnostic testing
Ferrets with compatible clinical signs should have a blood sample submitted for a coagulation profile, including a platelet count, PT and PTT (normal values

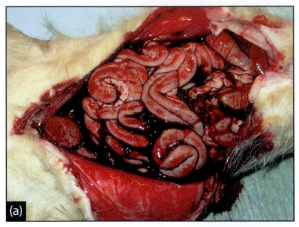

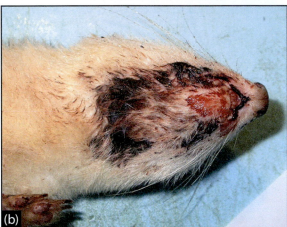

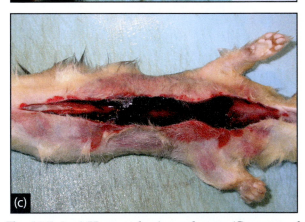

Fig. 16.7 (a–c) Haemorrhagic syndrome. (Courtesy of Drury Reavill, Zoo/Exotic Pathology Service.)

provided in Appendix 2). The classical finding for this disease is prolonged PT/PTT, but platelet counts may be decreased in severe cases due to consumptive losses. Other specialised clotting tests are available for small animals, but reference ranges have not been established for ferrets. It is prudent to check with the laboratory before submitting samples, as many clotting tests have specific sample handling requirements.

Diagnosis

Antemortem diagnosis is based on prolonged PT/PTT in the absence of known toxin exposure. On necropsy, affected ferrets (n = 35) had subacute to non-suppurative cholangitis, mild vacuolar hepatopathy, mild interstitial pneumonia and haemorrhage of the mucosa and wall of the urinary bladder and thymus, but these histological findings were not considered specific for any disease entity.

Management/treatment

The mainstay of therapy is oral vitamin K1 (1.5–2.5 mg/kg PO q12h, given with a fatty meal). Since the underlying aetiology has not been determined, there are no specific recommendations for duration of therapy. Consider treating for 1 month, then rechecking PT/PTT 48–72 hours after discontinuing therapy. With good supportive care, animals caught in the earlier stages of disease may recover, but once severe haemorrhage occurs, the disease is typically fatal. Ferrets that recover may relapse at any time.

FERRET SYSTEMIC CORONAVIRUS

Definition/overview

Ferret systemic coronavirus (FRSCV; also referred to as granulomatous inflammatory syndrome or ferret FIP in earlier literature) is an emerging disease syndrome in ferrets, characterised by granulomatous lesions induced by a coronavirus. It closely resembles the 'dry form' of feline infectious peritonitis (FIP), and most management recommendations are derived from protocols used in cats.

Aetiology/pathophysiology

FRSCV is caused by a coronavirus that may be a mutated form of the virus that causes ferret epizootic catarrhal enteritis, or ferret enteric coronavirus (FRECV). In cats, the mutation (that allows the virus to invade and replicate in macrophages) is generally believed to occur individually in each affected animal. It is unknown if the same is true in ferrets.

Most clinical signs are caused not by the virus itself, but by the marked immune response that it elicits. Many affected animals are febrile on presentation, and histopathology generally reveals multifocal pyogranulomatous inflammation affecting multiple organ systems.

Clinical presentation

Affected ferrets are generally young (<18 months) and most commonly present for weight loss, lethargy and GI signs, though neurological and respiratory signs have also been reported. Abnormal findings on physical examination often include a mid-abdominal mass effect and elevated body temperature.

Differential diagnosis

When taken individually, many of the clinical signs associated with FRSCV are non-specific. However, suspicion for the disease should be high when presented with a young ferret with weight loss, GI signs, abdominal mass(es) and hyperglobulinaemia. The primary differentials for this combination of findings include juvenile lymphoma (or other neoplasia), infectious/inflammatory GI disease, chronic gastric foreign body or ADV.

Diagnostic testing

Blood work: The classical finding on serum biochemistry is hyperglobulinaemia, characterised by a large, polyclonal gamma-globulin fraction. Anaemia and lymphopaenia have also been reported. Other abnormalities may be seen, depending on the organ system(s) affected.

Imaging: Radiographic findings commonly reported in ferrets with confirmed FRSCV include severe muscle wasting, loss of serosal detail, renomegaly, splenomegaly and a mid-abdominal mass effect. Abdominal ultrasound may be a more helpful modality in many cases. Common ultrasound findings include peritonitis, a heterogenous abdominal mass surrounded by hyperechoic fat or abnormal lymph nodes (more commonly a change in echotexture, rather than enlargement) (**Fig. 16.8**). Ultrasound-guided fine needle aspirates (FNAs) of masses or abnormal lymph nodes may reveal pyogranulomatous inflammation.

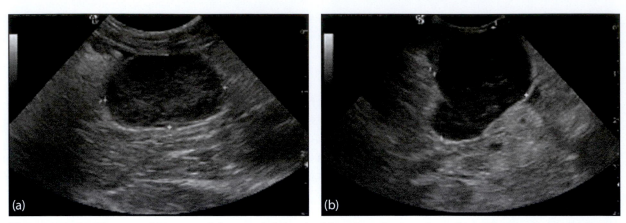

Fig. 16.8 (a, b) Ultrasound images of abnormal abdominal lymph nodes in a ferret later diagnosed with ferret systemic coronavirus.

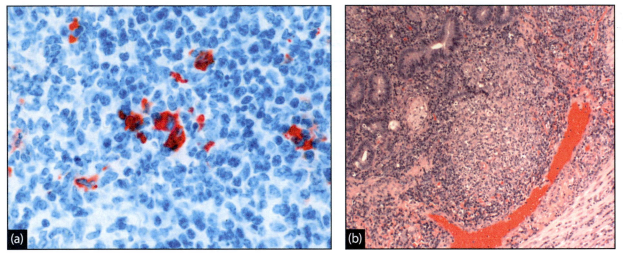

Fig. 16.9 (a) Ferret coronavirus-associated lymphadenitis. Note intracytoplasmic immunoreactivity for corona virus antigen (red) within macrophages. Streptavin-biotin, hematoxylin counterstain. (Courtesy of Dr. Timothy Baszler, Washington Animal Disease Diagnostic Laboratory, Washington State University, Pullman, WA.) (b) Pyogranulomatous inflammation extending across the muscular tunics of the small intestine. A few mucosal glands are in the upper left and the smooth muscle tunics are in the lower right. The central region (in the submucosa) is a mixture of lymphocytes, plasma cells, macrophages and neutrophils. H&E stain. (Courtesy of Dr. Drury Reavill, Zoo/Exotic Pathology Service.)

Histopathology: While FNAs can be helpful in some cases, definitive diagnosis requires a biopsy of affected tissue demonstrating characteristic pyogranulomatous inflammation and confirming presence of coronavirus on immunohistochemistry (**Fig. 16.9**). A real-time PCR test is also available for samples that have not been fixed in formalin (Michigan State University, Diagnostic Center for Population and Animal Health, www.ferrethealth.msu.edu/Diagnostics.php).

Diagnosis

Definitive diagnosis is by histopathology of affected lymph nodes or granulomas. Unfortunately, diagnosis may be made at necropsy (**Fig. 16.10**).

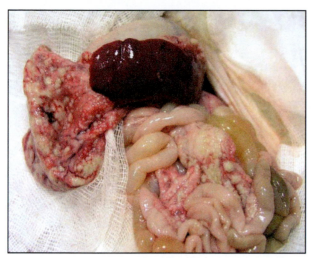

Fig. 16.10 Necropsy of a ferret with ferret systemic coronavirus demonstrating granulomas throughout the abdominal organs. (Courtesy of Jordi Jimenéz, Clinica Veterinária Els Altres, Barcelona.)

Management/treatment

As for FIP in cats, there is no cure for FRSCV, but palliative care can be attempted. Management of FRSCV is typically modelled after feline FIP treatment protocols. However, it is important to remember that even in cats, there are limited data on the efficacy of various treatments. In many cases, treatments that anecdotally improve quality of life have not proven to have statistically significant effects on outcome. Since waxing and waning clinical signs are a common feature of this disease, objectively determining whether a given treatment was helpful can be challenging.

There are three basic approaches to the management of viral diseases like FRSCV: (1) treatment with antiviral drugs; (2) immunosuppression to reduce negative sequelae associated with a dramatic immune response; and (3) non-specific immune stimulation in hopes of clearing or better controlling the virus. In human medicine, the primary focus for most viral diseases is on identifying appropriate antiviral drugs, but there are no data on the use of these drugs in FRSCV, and they have generally proven ineffective against feline FIP.

Immunosuppressive drugs used in management of FIP include steroids, cyclophosphamide and pentoxyfilline (a tumour necrosis factor inhibitor). While there are anecdotal reports of the benefits of these drugs, controlled studies have failed to demonstrate any effect on survival, quality of life, or other measures of disease progression in cats. The immunosuppressive drug most commonly reported in the ferret FRSCV literature is prednisolone (at doses ranging from 1–2 mg/kg/day), which anecdotally seems to help to decrease the size of abdominal masses and improve quality of life in many cases. However, this should be interpreted with caution, due to the highly variable course of the disease and the lack of controls that did not receive steroids.

A wide variety of immune stimulants have been used in cats with FIP, including ImmunoRegulin™ (Neogen, Lexington, KY) (Staph A protein), acemannan and polyprenyl immunostimulant. These drugs are typically very expensive and there is very little evidence to support their efficacy.

Regardless of the primary treatment modality, good supportive care is required to assure appropriate hydration and nutritional support as the disease progresses. Since immunosuppression is a common feature of the disease, prophylactic antibiotics may be indicated. Survival times reported in the literature vary widely, from a few days to over a year. The authors have had at least one ferret with a histopathologically confirmed diagnosis survive over 2 years after diagnosis.

It still unknown whether the mutated form of the virus is communicable or if the mutation occurs individually in each affected animal. For this reason, it is prudent to isolate affected animals. No vaccine is available.

LYMPHOMA/LYMPHOSARCOMA

Definition/overview

Lymphoma is a group of cancers arising from lymphoreticular cells. In lymphoma, the malignant transformation occurs in the lymphatic system, in comparison with leukaemia, where the neoplastic transformation occurs in the bone marrow. There are a number of subclassifications based on the cell type (T vs. B cell), organ system(s) affected, and degree of malignancy. Lymphoma is the third most common neoplasm in ferrets and accounts for 10–15% of all neoplasms reported in ferrets.

Aetiology/pathophysiology

While most cases of lymphoma in ferrets appear to develop spontaneously, in some cases infectious or chronic inflammatory disease may play a role. In humans, an association has been demonstrated between chronic *Helicobacter* gastritis and development of gastric mucosa-associated lymphoid tissue (GALT) lymphoma. The high rate of inflammatory GI disease in ferrets may also predispose them to the development of GI lymphoma, but this potential association has not yet been investigated. There have been several reports of clusters of lymphoma in high-density ferret populations, suggesting a potential infectious aetiology for some cases. One study documented development of lymphoma in ferrets inoculated with cells or cell-free medium from a ferret diagnosed with lymphoma, and retrovirus-like particles were isolated from the inoculum. Potential associations with feline leukaemia virus and/or Aleutian disease virus have been investigated and determined to be unlikely.

Clinical presentation

Clinical presentation varies dramatically, depending on the organ system affected.

- Multi-centric – generalised lymphadenopathy (**Fig. 16.11a**), splenomegaly, hepatomegaly.
- Gastrointestinal – clinical signs may include diarrhoea, weight loss, palpable thickening of the stomach or intestines or mesenteric lymphadenopathy (**Figs 16.11b, c**).
- Mediastinal – enlargement of mediastinal lymph nodes with secondary respiratory distress is the most common presentation of lymphoma in young ferrets (**Fig. 16.11d**).
- Cutaneous – erythema and oedema of affected skin, most commonly affecting feet and extremities (**Fig. 16.11e**).
- Other sites (liver, kidneys, CNS, eyes, bone, muscle) – signs vary, depending on organ system affected (**Figs 16.11f–m**).

Differential diagnosis

- Multi-centric – in other species, peripheral lymphadenopathy is reported with fungal or tick-borne disease, although these diseases have not been commonly reported in ferrets. Localised lymphadenopathy may occur with severe local infection. Obese ferrets may also have heavy fat deposition around lymph nodes, and care should be taken to distinguish this from true lymphadenopathy. Splenomegaly can occur with extramedullary haematopoiesis or other neoplasia.
- Gastrointestinal – early GI lymphoma can easily be mistaken for chronic inflammatory GI disease, which is also common in ferrets. Gastric lymphoma (pyloric thickening, ulceration, local lymphadenopathy) manifests similarly to *Helicobacter* gastritis, which may in some cases play a role in its pathogenesis.
- Mediastinal – differentials for a cranial mediastinal mass include thymoma and mediastinal abscess, though neither of these are commonly reported in ferrets.
- Cutaneous – differentials include bacterial, fungal, parasitic and autoimmune/inflammatory skin disease.

Diagnostic testing

Lymphoma in ferrets can affect a variety of body systems and present with a wide range of clinical signs. For this reason, a thorough diagnostic work-up should include full blood work and imaging.

- Complete blood count – mild to moderate anaemia is common. In advanced cases, evidence of bone marrow suppression may be evident. While presence of lymphocytosis or atypical lymphocytes in the blood is relatively rare, evaluation of a blood smear should always be included in the diagnostic work-up.
- Biochemistry – paraneoplastic hypercalcaemia has been reported with T-cell lymphoma, and hyperglobulinaemia may be seen with either T-cell or B-cell lymphoma. Other abnormalities (azotaemia, elevated liver enzymes, albuminaemia) may be present as well, depending on the organ systems affected.

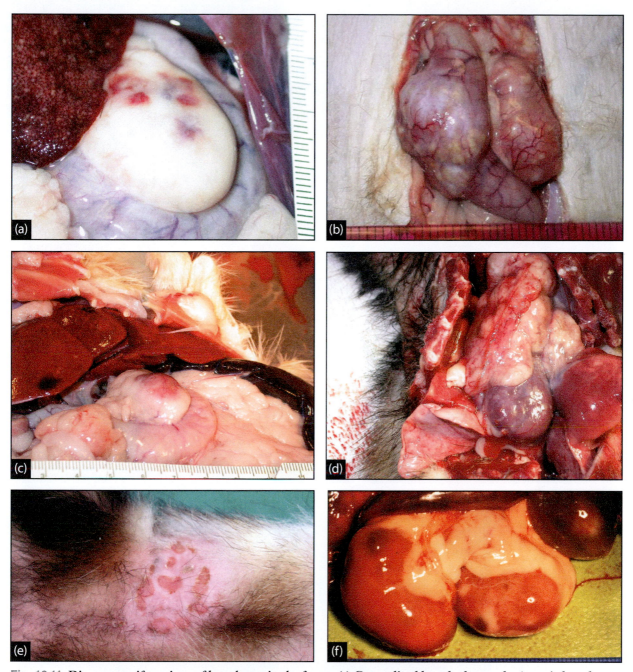

Fig. 16.11 Diverse manifestations of lymphoma in the ferret. (a) Generalised lymphadenopathy (gastric lymph nodes); (b) intestinal lymphoma; (c) pyloric node lymphadenopathy; (d) mediastinal lymphoma; (a–d courtesy of Cathy Johnson-Delaney); (e) cutaneous lymphoma (courtesy of Vittorio Capello); (f) renal lymphoma. *(Continued)*

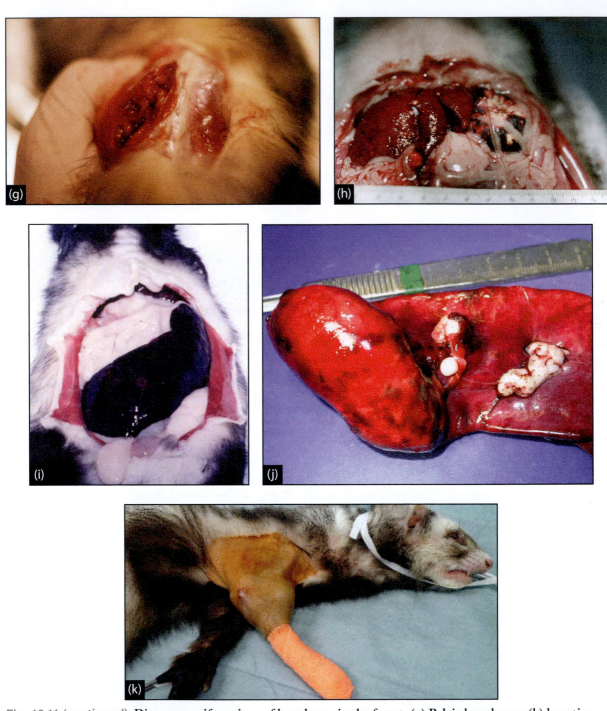

Fig. 16.11 (continued) Diverse manifestations of lymphoma in the ferret. (g) Pelvic lymphoma; (h) hepatic lymphoma; (i, j) splenic lymphoma; (g–j courtesy of Cathy Johnson-Delaney); (k) forelimb lymphoma (courtesy of Vittorio Capello).

(Continued)

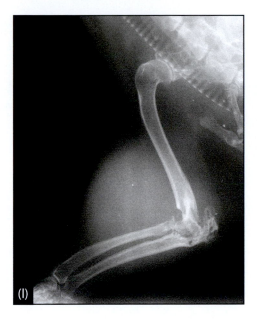

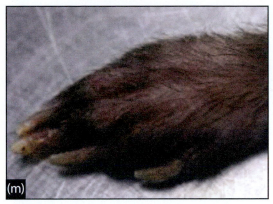

Fig. 16.11 (continued) Diverse manifestations of lymphoma in the ferret. (l) Radiograph of (k), also showing arthropathy (courtesy of Vittorio Capello); (m) lymphoma of skin and paw.

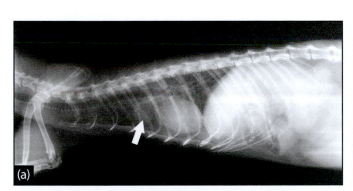

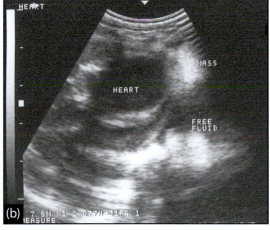

Fig. 16.12 (a) Radiographic (arrow; courtesy of Vittorio Capello) and (b) ultrasound images of mediastinal lymphoma in a ferret (courtesy of Cathy Johnson-Delaney).

- Thoracic radiographs – the involvement of mediastinal lymph nodes is common, especially in young ferrets (**Fig. 16.12a**).
- Thoracic ultrasound (**Fig. 16.12b**).
- Abdominal ultrasound – abdominal ultrasound should be performed to identify visceral lymphadenopathy and abnormalities of liver, spleen, kidneys and GI tract. It is recommended that the ultrasound be performed by a radiologist who is familiar with ferrets, as their normal lymph node appearance is slightly different from dogs and cats and may be mistaken for pathology (**Fig. 16.13**).
- Fine needle aspirate/biopsy of lesions – while FNAs may be suggestive of lymphoma, a biopsy of the affected tissue is usually required for a definitive diagnosis (**Fig. 16.14**). This can be relatively straightforward in cases with peripheral lymphadenopathy or cutaneous lymphoma, but may require more invasive procedures for other types.

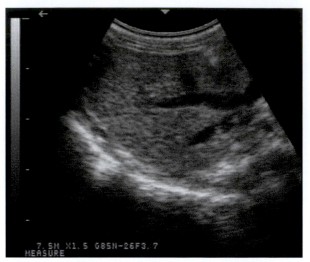

Fig. 16.13 Ultrasound image of a ferret with hepatic lymphoma. (Courtesy of Cathy Johnson-Delaney.)

Diagnosis

Once a patient has been diagnosed with lymphoma, the disease should be graded, staged and ideally immunophenotyped in order to provide the owners with the most accurate prognosis possible. While detailed prognostic data have not been collected for ferrets with different classifications of lymphoma, some information may be extrapolated from other species.

Grading/classification: Grading is an assessment of malignancy made by a pathologist based on cell size, mitotic index and other morphological characteristics. While grading can be performed on cytology or histopathology samples, human studies show poor agreement of grading results between cytology and histopathology, and biopsy samples are preferred. There are a number of different grading schemes in use in veterinary medicine, and there is currently no accepted standard. The World Health Organisation Revised European-American Lymphoma (WHO-REAL) classification system has been proposed as a standard for future lymphoma research in ferrets. Immunophenotyping may also be helpful, although data regarding the effect of phenotype on outcome in ferrets are limited. Current literature suggests that malignant lymphomas of T-cell origin are most common.

Staging: In dogs and cats, staging is considered an important tool for predicting prognosis and

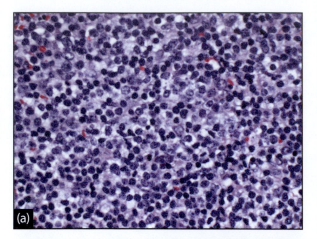

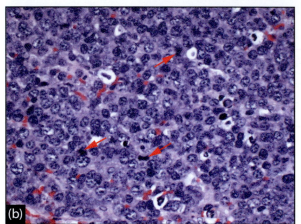

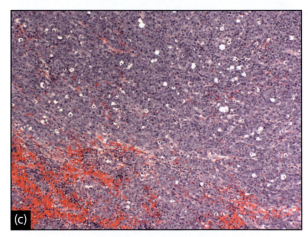

Fig. 16.14 (a) A sheet of closely packed neoplastic lymphocytes (H&E stain, 40×); (b) a sheet of closely packed neoplastic lymphocytes – the arrows are indicating mitotic figures (H&E stain, 40×); (c) a sheet of closely packed neoplastic lymphocytes effacing a lymph node (H&E stain, 10×). (Courtesy of Dr. Drury Reavill, Zoo/Exotic Pathology Services.)

monitoring response to therapy. Staging is often based on the WHO lymphoma staging scheme:

Stage 1: Single site.
Stage 2: Single site with spread to regional lymph nodes, all on one side of the diaphragm.
Stage 3: Generalised lymph node involvement.
Stage 4: Visceral involvement.
Stage 5: Blood/bone marrow involvement.

An alternative staging scheme that may be more relevant for some species involves staging primarily by body system affected:

Multi-centric: Affecting multiple peripheral lymph nodes, liver, spleen, and/or bone marrow.

Gastrointestinal: Affecting GI tract and/or associated lymph nodes.

Mediastinal: Affecting mediastinal lymph nodes (and potentially thymus).

Cutaneous: Affecting the skin.

Extranodal: Affecting organ systems other than those listed above (kidneys, CNS, eyes, bone).

Management/treatment

In most cases, lymphoma is considered a systemic disease that is most appropriately managed with chemotherapy. Exceptions include cutaneous lymphoma and other localised tumour manifestations, which may be controlled with local excision. In cases where a single large mass requires rapid size reduction for palliative purposes (e.g. mediastinal lymphomas), radiation therapy may also be helpful.

A variety of canine/feline chemotherapeutic protocols have been adapted for use in ferrets (*Tables 16.1, 16.2*). Unfortunately, no studies exist to determine the relative efficacies of these protocols. Many of the drugs used in canine/feline protocols require repeated, reliable venous access, which can sometimes be achieved with peripheral catheters, but often requires placement of a venous access port. For patients in which this is not feasible, there exist published protocols that involve only oral and

Table 16.1 Tufts No-IV Protocol for the treatment of lymphoma

WEEK	TREATMENT	MONITORING
Week 1	L-asparaginase Cyclophosphamide Prednisolone	
Week 2	L-asparaginase	CBC
Week 3	L-asparaginase Cytarabine	
Week 4	--------------	CBC
Week 5	Cyclophosphamide	
Week 7	Methotrexate	CBC
Week 8	--------------	CBC
Week 9	Cyclophosphamide	
Week 11	Cytarabine Chlorambucil	
Week 12	--------------	CBC
Week 13	Cyclophosphamide	
Week 15	Procarbazine	
Week 16	--------------	CBC
Week 17	--------------	CBC
Week 18	Cyclophosphamide	
Week 20	Chlorambucil Cytarabine	
Week 23	Cyclophosphamide	
Week 26	Procarbazine	
Week 27	--------------	CBC, Chemistry
If not in remission:	Repeat weeks 20–26 for three cycles	

Cytarabine (Cytosar) 300 mg/m² SC × 2 days (dilute 100 mg in 1 mL sterile water)
Cyclophosphamide (Cytoxan) 250 mg/m² PO with SQ fluids
L-asparaginase (Elspar) 10,000 IU/m² SC once, premedicate with diphenhydramine
Methotrexate 0.8 mg/kg IM once
Chlorambucil (Leukeran): 2 mg (1 tablet) PO once or 1 mg PO SID x 2 days
Prednisolone 2 mg/kg PO q24h for 1 week, then q48h
Procarbazine 50 mg/m² PO q24h × 14 days
Dose reduction: If marked myelosuppression is noted on complete blood count (CBC), decrease next dose by 25%
Ferret body surface area = (weight in kg)²ᐟ³
Adapted from Mayer J, Erdman SE, Fox JG (2014) Diseases of the haematopoietic system. In: Fox JG, Marini RP (eds). *Biology and Diseases of the Ferret, 3rd Edition*. Wiley-Blackwell, Hoboken, NY. pp. 311–334.

Table 16.2 **Gulf Coast Veterinary Specialists Protocol for the treatment of lymphoma**

WEEK	L-ASPARGINASE	VINCRISTINE	CYCLOPHOSPHAMIDE	PREDNISOLONE
– 3 days	X			
Week 1		X	X	q 12
Week 2		X		q 12
Week 3		X		q 24
Week 4		X	X	q 24
Week 7		X	X	q 24
Week 10		X	X	q 24
Week 13		X	X	q 24–48
Week 16		X	X	q 24–48
Week 19		X	X	q 24–48
Week 22		X	X	q 24–48
Week 25		X	X	q 24–48
Week 28		X	X	q 24–48
Week 31		X	X	q 24–48
Week 34		X	X	q 24–48
Week 37		X	X	q 24–48
Week 40		X	X	q 24–48
Week 43		X	X	q 24–48
Week 46		X	X	q 24–48
Week 49		X	X	q 24–48
Week 52		X	X	q 24–48

L-asparaginase (Elspar): 400 IU/kg IM, premedicate with diphenhydramine
Prednisolone 1 mg/kg PO
Vincristine 0.12 mg/kg IV
Cyclophosphamide (Cytoxan) 10 mg/kg PO or SC
Complete blood count (CBC) should be performed at every treatment. If neutrophil count <1,000, delay
   treatment 5–7 days and repeat CBC
Adapted from Antinoff N, Williams B (2012) Neoplasia. In: Quesenberry KE, Carpenter JW (eds). *Ferrets,
   Rabbits, and Rodents: Clinical Medicine and Surgery, 3rd Edition*. Saunders, Philadelphia, PA. pp. 103–121.

subcutaneous chemotherapeutic agents. These protocols have not undergone rigorous testing, but are anecdotally effective in prolonging survival. Frequent monitoring of CBC is required to detect possible immunosuppression.

If chemotherapy is declined, palliative therapy with oral prednisolone (2 mg/kg PO q24h) may provide temporary control of clinical signs. It is important to warn owners that prior exposure to high doses of steroids may promote resistance to chemotherapeutic drugs, if more aggressive therapy is elected in the future.

Regardless of the protocol selected, the primary goal is to prolong survival and provide a good quality of life; the vast majority of cases of lymphoma are ultimately fatal.

Survival data for specific forms of lymphoma and modes of treatment are not available. It has generally been thought that younger ferrets were more prone to a more aggressive lymphoblastic form, whereas older ferrets typically developed a more slowly progressive small-cell form, similar to that reported in cats. In recent years, this has become more controversial, and it is unclear what impact (if any) the age of the ferret has on prognosis. One study reported survival times ranging from a few weeks to 19 months, with B-cell lymphomas tending to be associated with longer survival times, but the sample size was relatively small and included ferrets with a wide variety of forms of lymphoma and different treatment protocols. Another informal study found a mean survival time of 8 months, with a range of 0–40 months. Ferrets receiving chemotherapy (specific protocols not specified) had a longer mean survival time of 14 months.

DISORDERS OF THE SPLEEN

Introduction
Enlargement of the spleen (**Fig. 16.15**) is common in ferrets. Pathological causes of splenomegaly include extramedullary haematopoiesis (EMH), neoplasia, heart failure (as a result of splenic congestion), splenitis, splenosis and hypersplenism. The ferret spleen has also been reported to enlarge significantly with inhalant anaesthesia, and the size of the spleen should always be carefully evaluated in the awake ferret before anaesthetised imaging or surgery. Diagnostic investigation of splenomegaly can be frustrating, and it not uncommon for no underlying cause to be identified.

Aetiology/pathophysiology
Extramedullary haematopoiesis: EMH is the most common histopathological diagnosis for ferrets with splenomegaly. EMH represents a compensatory reaction in response to either inadequate bone marrow function or increased blood cell needs. It may be a result of chronic antigen stimulation or anaemia. In many cases, the exact disease process resulting in EMH is undetermined. Anaemia is assumed to be a potential cause; however the author and others have noted apparently normal-sized spleens in ferrets with chronic anaemia and enlarged spleens in ferrets with normal blood counts and bone marrow analyses. Enlarged spleen size and weight can be induced in laboratory rats after injection of substances noted to produce marked inflammation, lending credibility to the theory that EMH is produced by chronic inflammation in the ferret. Chronic subclinical *Helicobacter* gastritis and other inflammatory GI disease are commonly suggested as a possible cause. EMH is

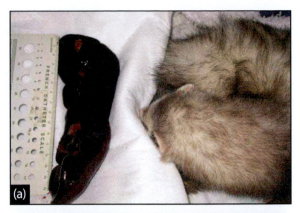
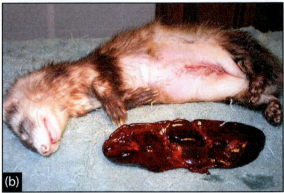
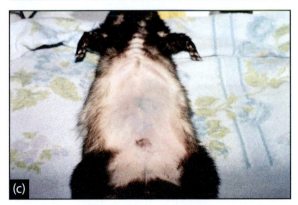

Fig. 16.15 **(a, b) Postsplenectomy demonstrating marked splenomegaly in a ferret; (c) note that splenomegaly can be so severe at times that it is visible externally on physical examination. (Courtesy of Cathy Johnson-Delaney.)**

also believed to be responsible for the splenomegaly commonly reported in ferrets with disseminated idiopathic myofasciitis (DIM).

Splenic cysts: Cystic structures may be found on palpation or on ultrasound. These are typically

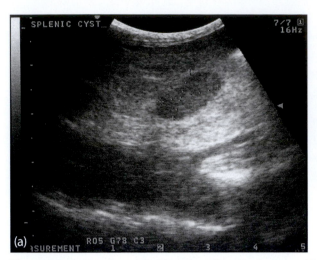
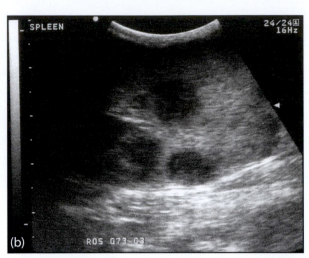

Fig. 16.16 (a, b) Ultrasound images of a splenic cysts. (Courtesy of Cathy Johnson-Delaney.)

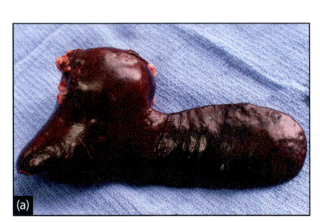
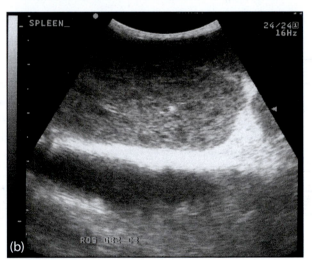

Fig. 16.17 (a) Neoplasia of the spleen; (b) abnormal ultrasound indicative of neoplasia. (Courtesy of Cathy Johnson-Delaney.)

blood filled. It is unknown if they correspond to trauma or neoplastic processes (**Fig. 16.16**).

Splenic neoplasia: Lymphoma is the most common neoplasia of the ferret spleen, but other cancers, including haemangiosarcoma, should be considered. Histopathology is recommended to help determine appropriate follow-up treatment and long-term prognosis (**Fig. 16.17**).

Splenic nodules: These may be found upon ultrasound or palpation. The nodules may be fibrotic, congested tissue or neoplastic (**Fig. 16.18**).

Splenitis: Inflammation of the spleen has been reported in association with ferret systemic coronavirus, *Mycobacterium*, or fungal organisms. While many infectious processes can cause enlargement of the spleen due to EMH, cases of true splenitis require the infectious agent to directly infect the spleen.

Ectopic splenic tissue (Fig. 16.19): Accessory foci of splenic tissue are occasionally reported in humans and other species. Splenic tissue that is found separate from the body of the spleen can either be the result of failure of two sections to fuse during fetal development (accessory spleens) or traumatic/surgical splenic

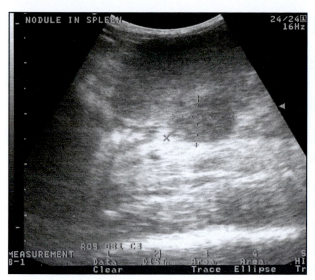

Fig. 16.18 **Ultrasound of splenic nodule. (Courtesy of Cathy Johnson-Delaney.)**

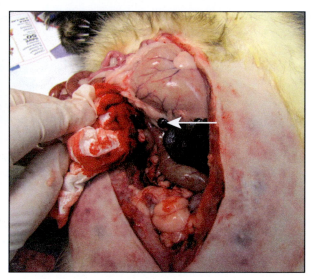

Fig. 16.19 **Ectopic splenic tissue in a ferret (white arrow). (Courtesy of Cathy Johnson-Delaney.)**

fracture (splenosis). These can be distinguished histopathologically, but usually not by gross appearance. They are usually asymptomatic, but their anatomical position may sometimes predispose them to torsion, rupture or other complications that result in clinical signs. There is one report of splenosis in a domestic ferret.

Hypersplenism: While it is part of the normal function of the spleen to removed damaged or senescent blood cells, in some cases the spleen may perform this function excessively or prematurely. This condition is referred to as hypersplenism and results in an enlarged spleen with anaemia and/or leucopaenia that resolves with splenectomy. There are several anecdotal reports of this disease in ferrets, but no published case studies.

Clinical presentation

The normal ferret spleen can measure up to 5–7 cm long and 2 cm wide, making it proportionately much larger than spleens in other species. An enlarged spleen should be palpated for masses and other irregularities, but the absence of a discrete mass does not rule out neoplasia. Palpation should be performed carefully, as certain types of splenic pathology can predispose the spleen to rupture. Many ferrets with splenomegaly are asymptomatic, but animals with profound splenomegaly may

exhibit decreased activity or gait abnormalities due to the weight and size of the spleen itself. Ferrets whose splenomegaly is a secondary disease process may also have clinical signs associated with their primary disease.

Differential diagnosis

As previously discussed, the normal ferret spleen is proportionately larger than most other species', and clinicians inexperienced with ferret palpation may mistake a normal spleen for an enlarged one. Masses at the head of the spleen are similar in location to the adrenal glands and kidney and may be mistaken for enlargement of these structures. Primary differentials for true splenomegaly include EMH, neoplasia and splenic congestion secondary to anaesthesia. Less common causes include splenitis, splenosis and hypersplenism.

Diagnostic testing

Complete blood count: Since the spleen is an important haematopoietic organ in the ferret, a CBC is a critical diagnostic step for any patient presenting for splenomegaly. In cases of EMH, red and white blood cell counts may be low, normal or elevated, depending on how effectively the spleen is compensating for the primary disease process. In cases of anaesthesia-induced splenomegaly, blood cell counts may be artificially decreased. With hypersplenism, counts will be decreased due to inappropriate destruction of blood cells. Lymphoma is rarely detectable in peripheral blood, but a blood smear should always be evaluated to assure that morphological changes are not missed.

Chemistry: While there are no changes on the chemistry panel specific to splenic disease, evidence of other organ dysfunction may help to identify underlying disease processes that contributed to the development of splenomegaly.

Radiology (Figs 16.20a, b): Splenomegaly and splenic masses are often readily apparent on radiographs, though these abnormalities can typically be identified on physical examination without the use of radiography. Radiographs should still be considered, however, as they may reveal other underlying disease processes.

Ultrasound (Fig. 16.20c): In some cases, ultrasound may reveal changes in echogenicity or the contour of the splenic capsule suggestive of neoplasia. Nodules and cystic structures may be identified (**Figs 16.16, 16.18**). However, in dogs and cats, ultrasound is generally not considered helpful to distinguish between benign and malignant splenic abnormalities, except when peritoneal effusion or other abnormalities help to raise the suspicion for a neoplastic process. The same is probably true for the ferret.

FNA/biopsy: FNAs of abnormalities identified on ultrasound may be helpful in some cases; however in many cases pathology may be focal and not easily identified on ultrasound, leading to false negatives. Percutaneous biopsy of the spleen is generally not recommended due to risk of bleeding. Surgical biopsy may be considered, but the benefits of preserving a potentially normal spleen should be weighed carefully against the risk of bleeding and the need for a second surgery, should the biopsy results reflect malignant neoplasia.

Management/treatment

If splenomegaly is believed to be the result of a systemic disease process, such as lymphoma, chronic inflammation or an infectious disease, management

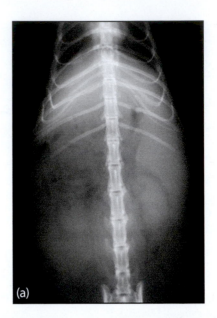
(a)

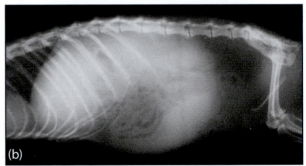
(b)

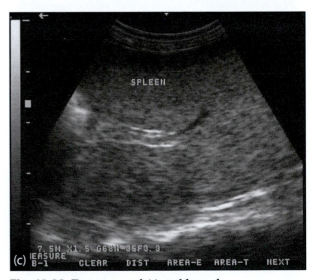
(c)

Fig. 16.20 Dorsoventral (a) and lateral (b) radiographs, and (c) ultrasound of a ferret with an enlarged spleen. (Courtesy of Cathy Johnson-Delaney.)

should be focused on addressing the underlying disease. However, clinical experience shows that attempted treatment of an underlying aetiology often does not result in reduction of the size of the spleen.

If splenomegaly is determined to be the result of a primary splenic disease process or if the aetiology cannot be determined, splenectomy may be considered.

Splenectomy is technically straightforward in the ferret (see Chapter 25) but the decision about when to remove an abnormal spleen can be more challenging. Most cases of mild to moderate splenomegaly do not require splenectomy. However, there is a concern that severely enlarged spleens and those with focal abnormalities may be more prone to rupture, resulting in a potentially fatal haemoabdomen. Some ferrets with severe splenic enlargement may experience impaired mobility, and splenectomy often dramatically improves their quality of life. Splenectomy may be beneficial for certain types of splenic neoplasia; for instance, splenectomy has been shown to prolong survival in dogs with splenic haemangiosarcoma, and splenectomy may be curative for certain types of primary splenic neoplasia. Splenectomy may also be indicated to prevent blood cell destruction in cases of hypersplenism or haemorrhage in cases of splenic trauma.

Prior to splenectomy, bone marrow analysis is important to ensure that the bone marrow is functioning appropriately; there have been a number of anecdotal reports of ferrets developing refractory anaemia after splenectomy, presumably because their bone marrow function was inadequate and they were relying on the spleen as a major source of erythrocytes.

CHAPTER 17

DISORDERS OF THE MUSCULOSKELETAL SYSTEM

Cathy A. Johnson-Delaney

INTRODUCTION

The muscles of the ferret differ little from those of other carnivores. Intact hobs have well-developed cervical muscles and appear 'thick necked'. Many ferrets 'bulk up' for the winter by putting on additional body fat. The vertebral formula is C7, T14–15, L5–7, S3–4; varying coccygeal number (usually >15) (see Chapter 3). Ferrets do have 5 digits on each foot, which differs from dogs and cats. The compact body is extremely flexible and the ferret can turn in the diameter of its body by compressing the chest and abdomen (**Fig. 17.1**).

ATAXIA, POSTERIOR PARESIS

Definition/overview
Incoordination. It is most often presented as posterior paresis and unsteady movements. (see posterior paresis) (**Fig. 17.2**).

Aetiology/pathophysiology
Ataxia can be characterised as either cerebellar, vestibular or proprioceptive. Cerebellar is due to a disruption of transmission of sensory impulses from the vestibular system, cerebral cortex and spinal cord through the cerebellum. Cerebella-affected patients will demonstrate abnormal rate, range or force of movement with normal strength. Paresis is not present with cerebellar dysfunction. Vestibular ataxia occurs when there is damage or disease affecting the vestibular system within the inner ear. It may be seen with otitis interna (see Chapter 15).

Dysfunction manifests with a loss of balance. The ferret may list or fall or one side. There may be head tilt. Proprioceptive ataxia is due to spinal disease. Deficits are localised to the affected region of the spinal corn. Trauma, intervertebral disc disease and tumours within or compressing the spinal cord or nerves may cause the ataxia (**Fig. 17.3**).

Clinical presentation
The ferret cannot ambulate normally. It wobbles in the hindquarters, and may drag itself by the front legs. The forelimbs may also be affected making crawling difficult. The ferret may tire easily and stop trying to ambulate. There may be muscle spasms over any area that is painful. Head tilt may be present. If vestibular, there may be nystagmus. There may be normal or abnormal peripheral reflexes.

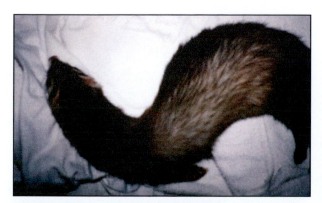

Fig. 17.1 **Ferrets are extremely flexible.**

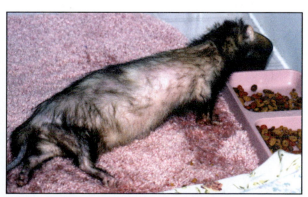

Fig. 17.2 **Posterior paresis in an aged ferret.**

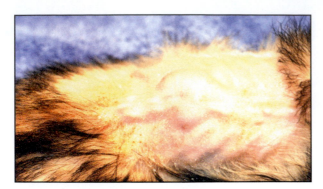

Fig. 17.3 Spinal tumour.

There may be pain exhibited and localised to a specific joint or limb. If generalised, there may be arrhythmias. If presented for acute ataxia, there may be hypoglycaemia as found with islet cell disease (see Chapter 14).

Differential diagnosis

Posterior paresis, otitis interna, spinal cord compression (trauma, neoplasia, etc.), generalised muscle weakness as seen with systemic disease including cardiomyopathy (severe arrhythmias), myasthenia gravis, hypoglycaemia, fractures, luxations in legs or hips, degenerative disc disease with subsequent nerve impingement, any systemic disease that may be causing pain, generalised weakness. While toxicosis is not common in ferrets, lead and other heavy metals could possibly cause signs relating to central neurological disease.

Diagnostic testing

Physical and neurological examinations, otic examination, radiographs, CT scans (head, spinal column), haematology, serum chemistry. Ultrasonography including echocardiography. A history of which toys may be chewed on or environment might be relevant if toxicosis is suspected.

Diagnosis

The definitive cause of the ataxia is discerned. Posterior paresis may be a part of the symptomatology.

Management/treatment

Depending on the causative aetiology, treatment should be geared to eliminating pain and discomfort first and addressing individual diseases. In many cases with ataxia and posterior paresis, supportive care (fluids, food, analgesics) may accompany definitive disease treatment. If there is muscle weakness, some ferrets respond to supplements such as L-carnitine and B-complex vitamin supplementation. The L-carnitine may be delivered in an omega 3–6 oil and is listed as Cardiac Formula in Appendix 10.

CHONDROSARCOMA

Definition/overview

A tumour that may form anywhere in the appendicular skeleton, comprised of neoplastic chondrocytes that invade normal bone.

Aetiology/pathophysiology

A malignant bone tumour that produces a cartilaginous matrix. There may be new bone formation due to some endochondral ossification of tumour cartilage, but generally there is a lack of direct bone formation. Most reported arise from within the medullary cavity. They are considered slow to metastasise. Chondrosarcomas are considered less malignant than osteosarcomas. Without removal, they grow slowly to large sizes. Metastasis can occur to the lungs, although other organs may be affected. They do not evoke the same periosteal response as seen with osteosarcomas. Histopathology yields inconsistently sized lacunae within the matrix of hyaline cartilage. There are nests of pleomorphic chondrocytes with indistinct nucleoli. There are clusters of chondrocytes that invade normal bone. The mitotic index in the reported cases was low at 0–1 per high-power field.

Clinical presentation

Firm, immobile, and non-alopecic swelling arising from any bone. In the literature this tumour was found in the distal tibia and one in the right scapula. Initially no lameness was associated with the mass until it became so large as to inhibit joint movement. Normal range of motion was found when the ferrets were first presented.

Differential diagnosis

Abscess, lymphoma, chondroma, osteoma, osteosarcoma, fibroma or bone cyst.

Diagnosis

Radiographs first step, then CT scan to determine bone involvement and structure of the mass. Fine needle aspirate may rule out abscess, but wedge biopsy and histopathology are necessary for the diagnosis. Radiographs should also be taken of the chest and abdomen to rule out metastasis. Lymph node biopsy in the area of the mass should be obtained.

Management/treatment

Surgical excision with wide margins including bone attachments can be tried. Limb amputation may be necessary. Prognosis is good if total excision; however, that may be difficult depending on how the tumour is situated. Recurrence is expected if there is incomplete excision. In dogs chemotherapy and radiation have been used where surgical excision is not possible. There are no reports of therapy in ferrets other than amputation resulting in full surgical excision.

CONGENITAL MALFORMATIONS

Definition/overview

A number of skeletal deformities have been noted in ferrets including elbow luxation (uni- or bilateral), hemivertebrae, hemiribs, differing number of vertebrae and missing digits (**Fig. 17.4**). Spina bifida aperta (also known as spina bifida manifest) has been documented in a stillborn kit. Other rare conditions that have been reported include agenesis of limbs, anencephaly, scoliosis, cranioschisis, cleft lip, cleft palate, kinked tail and shortened tail.

The vertebral column has differing numbers of thoracic vertebrae, lumbar vertebrae and sacral vertebrae. The majority of ferrets are C7/T14/L6/S3. However in screening 161 radiographs that only looked at T/L, 13.7% of ferrets had differing numbers than the 'standard' formula. Three had T15/L7; 8 had T15/L6; 2 had T15/L5; 1 had T14/L5; 7 had T14/L7. Overall 16 males had abnormalities, and 6 females. Several with T15 had corresponding ribs or partial ribs either uni- or bilateral (**Fig. 17.5**).

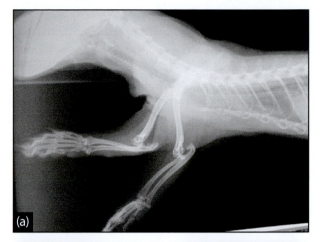
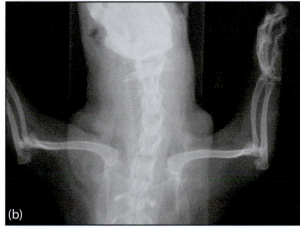

Fig. 17.4 (a) Lateral radiograph of congenital bilateral elbow luxation; (b) DV of luxated elbows.

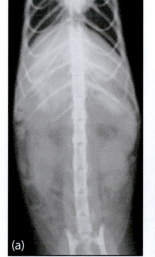
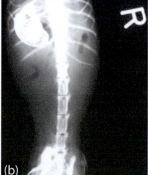

Fig. 17.5 (a) Hemirib (transitional) left; (b) hemirib (transitional) right.

Aetiology/pathophysiology
Likely to be inheritable defects that present as kits.

Clinical presentation
Elbow luxation: abnormal ambulation, elbows usually held out to the side. Frequent stumbling. Does not seem painful. On palpation, elbows are lax and can be moved abnormally, including rotation. Hemivertebrae may present with kyphosis and/or scoliosis. Hemiribs are often found on palpation or on radiographs and do not seem to pose a clinical problem. Missing digits is an anomaly but does not seem to cause problems in ambulation.

Differential diagnosis
Trauma for elbow luxation. Others, no differentials.

Diagnostic testing
Radiographs.

Diagnosis
Presence on radiographs and by palpation.

Management/treatment
Theoretically elbow luxation could be surgically corrected. However this is rarely done. Instead, splinting the legs with the elbows in extension seems to allow improvement in ambulation with the formation of false joints. The splinting seems to allow for stabilisation of the luxated joint (**Fig. 17.6**). There is no treatment for vertebral or rib deformities or missing digits.

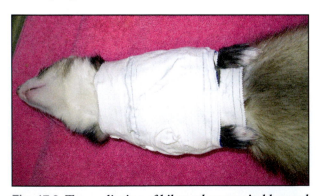

Fig. 17.6 Tape splinting of bilateral congenital luxated elbows. When the splint was removed, seemingly false joints were formed as the ferret was able to ambulate with only a slight limp.

CRUCIATE LIGAMENT RUPTURE

Definition/overview
The ferret has the same cruciate ligament anatomy as in other mammals.

Aetiology/pathophysiology
Trauma usually from jumping or falling can cause rupture of any of the cruciate ligaments.

Clinical presentation
Usually acute lameness of one leg. The knee may be swollen and painful.

Differential diagnosis
Rupture of one or more of the cruciate ligaments. Fractures of the distal femur, patella or tibia.

Diagnostic testing
Radiographs of the leg: the positioning of the knee should be in flexion. Under sedation with analgesic, manipulation of the knee to test for drawer signs and rotational instability. The technique to do this is described by placing a finger and thumb of one hand on the patella and lateral fabella proximal to the knee joint. Place the finger and thumb of the other hand on the fibular head and tibial crest distal to the knee joint. A positive drawer sign can be determined by moving the tibia cranial relative to the femur.

Diagnosis
Positive drawer signs.

Management/treatment
Surgery to repair the knee joint, technique as in the dog.

DISSEMINATED IDIOPATHIC MYOFASCIITIS

Definition/overview
Disseminated idiopathic myofasciitis (DIM) is described as a pyogranulomatous inflammatory involvement of cardiac and skeletal muscles. It affects young adults (average age 10 months, range of 11 weeks to 4 years). It does not appear to have a sex predilection (**Fig. 17.7**).

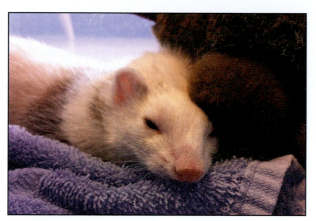

Fig. 17.7 Febrile ferret with severe lethargy associated with DIMS. (Courtesy of Vondelle McLaughlin.)

Aetiology/pathophysiology

The common denominator may have been vaccination with at least one dose of a distemper vaccine (Fervac-D), which is no longer on the market. Recently ferrets have been presented with DIM that have been vaccinated with Purevax (Merial, Athens, GA) and/or Nobivac® Puppy-DPv (Merck & Co. Inc., Whitehouse Station, NJ) or Galaxy-D (Schering Plough, Omaha, NE). It is unknown if vaccination history is linked at all with development.

There is diffuse infiltration of inflammatory cells in affected muscles, with progressive atrophy rather than necrosis of muscle fibres. On necropsy, gross lesions may have white mottling and dilation of the oesophagus. There may be white streaks on the heart, diaphragm and intercostal muscles. There may be moderate to severe atrophy of limb and lumbar muscles. There may be atrophy of the tongue. The diaphragm may be thin and semi-transparent. Splenomegaly is usually seen. Histologically there is moderate to severe, suppurative to pyogranulomatous inflammation in skeletal muscle of the limbs, lumbar region, head muscles, sternum and abdominal wall. The oesophagus muscle is affected with inflammation extending into the submucosa and serosal tunics. The inflammation primarily affects the perimysium and endomysium, with extension into the fascia and adipose tissue. Myeloid hyperplasia of the spleen and bone marrow has also been found. No aetiological agent has been found. Histological lesions point to an autoimmune inflammatory process, which is the working hypothesis for this disease at this time.

Clinical presentation

A rapid onset of clinical signs of fever, lethargy, depression, inappetance, recumbency with apparent pain in the rear legs. The fever may be marked at 39.5–40°C or higher. There is a reluctance to walk, ataxia and posterior paresis. Bruxism and difficulty swallowing may be contributing to the inappetance. There may be tachycardia, tachypnoea and heart murmurs. The ferret seems to be in pain. There may be mild to moderate neutrophilia along with mild to moderate non-regenerative anaemia. Serum alanine aminotransferase is elevated in some ferrets. There is no elevation of creatine kinase or aspartate aminotransferase that would be markers of muscle damage.

Differential diagnosis

Systemic disease including ferret systemic coronavirus, cryptococcosis or systemic bacterial disease causing fever.

Diagnostic testing

Haematology, serum chemistry, radiographs, muscle biopsy with histology.

Diagnosis

Existence of neutrophilia, anaemia, fever and positive inflammatory infiltration of muscles on histopathology.

Management/treatment

Supportive care first including fluids and opioid analgesics. NSAIDs may help with the inflammation. Multiple antibiotics are usually used and glucocorticoids, cyclophosphamide and interferon have been tried. Prognosis is poor. A newer treatment modality has been shown to be of use in treatment. Cyclophosphanide (10 mg/kg on day 1, day 14, then monthly for 3 months or until recovered), prednisolone (1 mg/kg PO q12h for 3 months, then q24h until recovered, taper off dosage at end of treatment), and chloramphenicol palmitate (50 mg/kg PO q12h for 6–8 weeks) together have resulted in remission in a number of ferrets. Cyclophosphamide has immunosuppressive effects. Success using this combination may indicate that DIM is an acquired immune-mediated disease.

FRACTURES

Definition/overview
Fractured bones. Surprisingly, ferrets seem fairly resistant to limb fractures despite the number of times ferrets fall from climbing.

Aetiology/pathophysiology
Trauma – usually from falling. Ferrets also may be stepped on or caught in furnishings such as recliner chairs.

Clinical presentation
Depending on location of fracture, favouring of the limb and reluctance to bear weight if it is a limb. If vertebral, there may be paresis or paralysis. Skull fractures (non-lethal) may show signs of head tilt, nystagmus, pain on touching the head. Jaw fractures usually present with degree of open mouth, lolling of tongue to one side and ptalysm.

Differential diagnosis
Severe haematoma due to soft tissue crushing. Luxation of joints rather than fracture. Soft tissue trauma especially to head, neck, jaws.

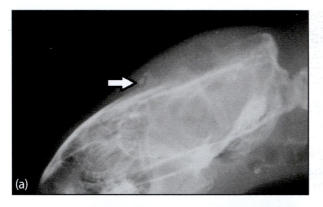
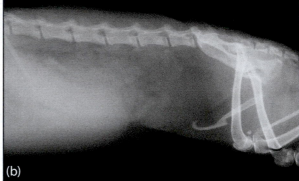
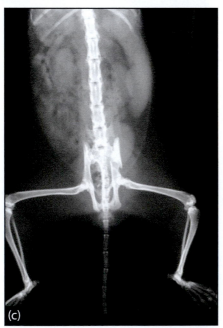
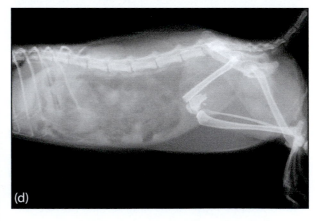

Fig. 17.8 (a) Fracture fragments of anterior sagittal crest (arrow); (b) fractured os penis; (c) fractured wing of ileum; (d) fractured distal femur. *(Continued)*

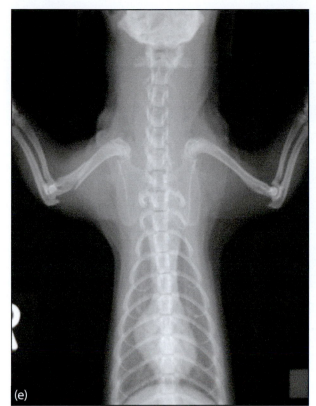

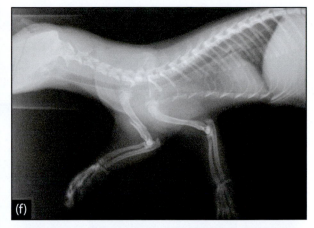

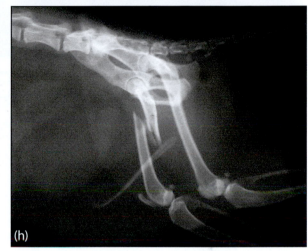

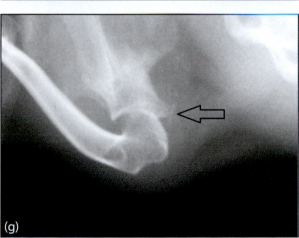

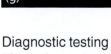

Fig. 17.8 (continued) (e) DV of fracture right humerus; (f) lateral view of same fracture as (e); (g) fracture of distal scapula (arrow); (h) facture of femur.

Diagnostic testing

Physical examination, radiographs. Dental examination in cases of jaw fractures. Neurological examination may be necessary if there have been skull or vertebral fractures.

Diagnosis

Presence of fracture(s) (**Fig. 17.8**).

Management/treatment

For fractures, management is the same as in other mammals using internal or external fixation (**Fig. 17.9**). Skull fractures that are non-displaced will be allowed to heal by themselves. Jaw fracture fixation may require some tooth extraction if roots are damaged and/or teeth are fractured. A soup diet may be needed in cases of jaw fractures. Fractures may develop large calluses if unstable during the healing process (**Fig. 17.10**).

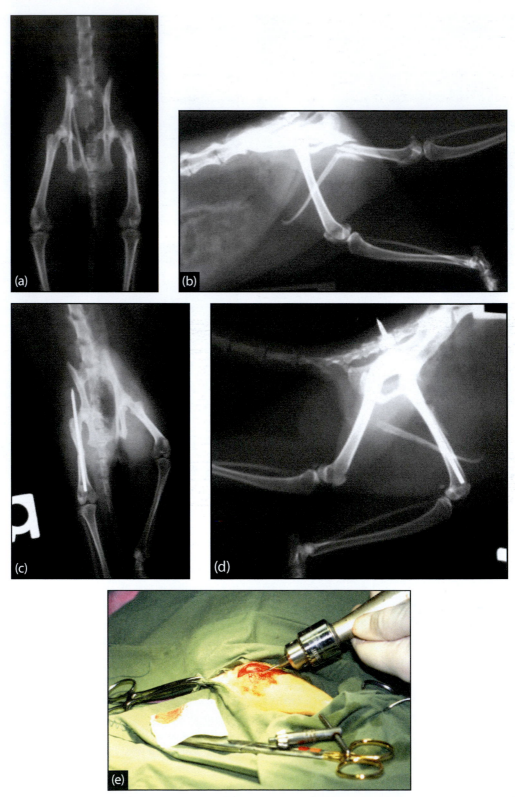

Fig. 17.9 (a) VD radiograph of fractured femur; (b) lateral radiograph of fractured femur; (c) lateral view; (d) VD view intramedullary pin placed; (e) surgery showing pin placement.

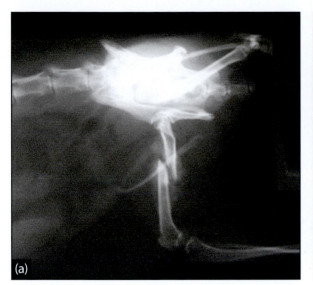
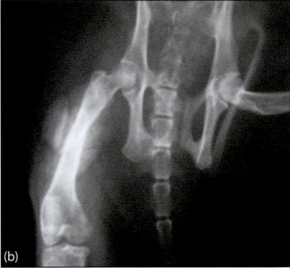

Fig. 17.10 (a) Lateral view of callus formation around the femoral fracture; (b) VD of callus formation.

INTERVERTEBRAL DISC DISEASE (SEE ALSO CHAPTER 18)

Definition/overview

Compression of vertebral discs most commonly T14–L1 but also found in other locations, particularly lumbar intervertebral spaces. Intervertebral discs are the shock absorbers between the vertebral bodies and can partially or completely herniate, compressing the spinal cord. This compression alters the function of the spinal cord, and the symptoms that result depend on the site along the spinal cord and the degree of compression. Pain, weakness or paralysis may occur from the mechanical compression or from secondary vascular or other changes of the tissue around the site.

Aetiology/pathophysiology

Discs may become compressed as a function of trauma or age. The exact cause of herniation of the intervertebral disc is unknown. This condition may be caused by trauma or other causes including genetics, neoplasia and infection. The intervertebral discs consist of the nucleus pulposus that offers flexibility to the vertebral column and it is surrounded by the annulus fibrosus, a tough fibrous structure. Degeneration of the disc leads to calcification of the nucleus with weakening of the annulus, leading to rupture. Trauma can also result in rupture of the disc. Compression or alteration of the

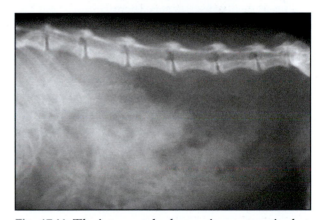

Fig. 17.11 The intervertebral space is compromised at L2–L3, L3–L4, L4–L5. Spondylosis is present at L2–L3, L3–L4. Physical signs included hindlimb paresis.

structure by tumour cells or infectious agents can weaken and cause rupture of the disc. Spondylosis may be noted that may contribute to nerve pinching (**Fig. 17.11**).

Clinical presentation

Usually manifests with posterior ataxia or paresis. There may also be incontinence or problems urinating/defaecating depending on which discs are affected. There may be pain in the back and hindquarters. The presentation will depend on the location of the herniation of the disc. In a recent report of intervertebral disc prolapse, the ferret presented with hindlimb lameness. There was paresis of both hindlimbs with absent proprioception and lack of muscle tone. Deep pain was present. In this case, there was protrusion between the second and third lumbar vertebrae.

Differential diagnosis
Neoplasia, trauma, botulism, spinal abscess.

Diagnostic testing
Radiographs, myelogram, MRI.

Diagnosis
Evidence of decreased space between vertebral bodies and/or protrusion of disc seen on myelogram, MRI.

Management/treatment
Theoretically disc surgery (hemilaminectomy) with decompression at the site. Could be performed as in dogs. However, ferrets due to their size are problematic. Initially corticosteroids may be tried to minimise inflammation associated with the rupture. Analgesics will help alleviate the pain involved. Physical therapy may help to keep the muscles from atrophy. Prognosis is generally poor for recovery if the ferret cannot walk. Lack of deep pain is indicative of a very poor prognosis.

L-CARNITINE DEFICIENCY WEAKNESS

Definition/overview
This is a recently characterised genetic problem.

Aetiology/pathophysiology
The Animal Genetics Center at the University of California at Davis has identified this as a genetic disorder resulting in L-carnitine metabolism defect.

Clinical presentation
Overall muscle weakness but particularly hindquarters paresis. There may also be dilated cardiomyopathy.

Differential diagnosis
Ataxia and/or posterior paresis from other causes (see above).

Diagnostic testing
At this time none is commercially available. Radiographs may rule out vertebral problems. Echocardiography of the heart is warranted.

Diagnosis
Generally based on treatment response.

Management/treatment
Supplementation with L-carnitine and decreased clinical signs. The heart muscle will improve. The author has used the Cardiac Formula with increased L-carnitine to 2000 mg in 1 ounce of the omega 3–6 solution (Appendix 10).

LYMPHOMA, MYELOMA AND LEUKAEMIA OF THE BONE

Definition/overview
Lymphosarcoma may invade the skeleton. Lymphoma may metastasise particularly to the vertebra. The invading tumour causes osteolytic lesions (**Fig. 17.12**).

Aetiology/pathophysiology
Lymphosarcoma may be found as a disseminated disease. In the literature there has been a lobulated, firm, light tan mass occupying the body of the lumbar vertebra. The mass had invaded the bone marrow, adjacent bone, muscles and vertebral canal.

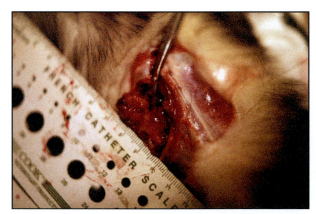

Fig. 17.12 Lymphoma invaded the ilium and surrounding muscle.

The bone was fractured. It was a poorly demarcated and unencapsulated mass of neoplastic plasma cells. The adjacent bone was necrotic and in some areas replaced by fibrous connective tissue. There was also reported a cystic bone lesion in the proximal humerus with a non-supporting lameness of the foreleg. Lytic masses have been noted in various bones.

Clinical presentation
There may be generalised lymphadenopathy, weakness, lethargy, posterior ataxia and paresis, anorexia, weight and condition loss and splenomegaly.

Differential diagnosis
Multiple myeloma.

Diagnostic testing
Haematology, serum chemistry. Radiographs. Biopsy can be done of spleen, rarely done *ante mortem*. If peripheral lymph nodes are involved, biopsy and histopathology may confirm.

Diagnosis
Presence of lesions and lymphadenopathy.

Management/treatment
Poor prognosis if lymphoma has caused skeletal lesions. In some cases of distal limb lytic lesions, amputation has been tried to control the spread. Histopathology should be done to determine systemic disease.

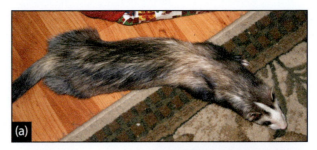

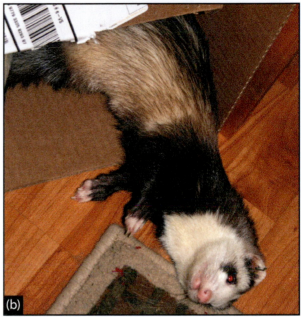

Fig. 17.13 **(a, b) Weakness associated with myasthenia gravis. Note the blaze: this ferret is deaf. (Courtesy of Vondelle McLaughlin.)**

MYASTHENIA GRAVIS

Definition/overview
An autoimmune disease of the muscles including the oesophagus.

Aetiology/pathophysiology
It is due to antiacetylcholine receptor antibodies.

Clinical presentation
Episodic hindlimb weakness, flaccid paraparesis progressing to tetraparesis. There may be megaoesophagus of varying degrees which is accompanied by projectile vomiting and weight loss (**Fig. 17.13**).

Differential diagnosis
Posterior paresis, ataxia due to disc disease, L-carnitine metabolic disorder, neoplasia of spine, spinal cord compression. Gastrointestinal disease if megaoesophagus is present (see Chapter 13).

Diagnosis
Nerve conduction velocity testing, serology positive for antiacetylcholine receptor antibodies. A test using neostigmine methylsulphate positive response. Dosage for the test: 40 µg/kg IM or 20 µg/kg IV. Muscle biopsy and histopathology. Radiographs for megaoesophagus.

Management/treatment

Published case used 1 mg/kg PO q8h of pyridostigmine bromide, which aided in remission of symptoms. The published dog dosage is 0.5–3 mg/kg q8h so higher doses may be needed to control the condition. Concurrent administration of prednisolone may help decrease the autoimmune response. The condition may be put in remission with medications but it is usually progressive. If megaoesophagus is present, small meals, preferably dook soup (Appendix 6), frequently may aid in peristalsis and decrease the vomiting. Famotidine is recommended as there may be stomach irritation and ulceration from the stress as well as likelihood of *Helicobacter* ulcers. Metoclopramide has been used as an antiemetic but response is questionable.

NEOPLASIA (SPINAL TUMOURS, BONE TUMOURS) OTHER THAN LYMPHOMA

Definition/overview

Many different tumours have been described involving the musculoskeletal system. This includes osteoma, osteosarcoma, chordoma (see Chapter 18), chondrosarcoma, and fibrosarcoma.

Aetiology/pathophysiology

The types of neoplasia derive from the tissue of origin. Chordomas arise from remnants of the notochord. Osteomas arise from the skull, zygomatic arch, parietal bone or occipital bone. Chondrosarcomas have been described appearing on the tail. Morphological description is similar to chordomas but can be differentiated with immunohistochemistry. Fibrosarcomas arise from the periosteal tissue of the perivertebral connective tissue.

Clinical presentation

Usually there is a mass that the owner has noted. If cervical chordoma, ferret may have posterior paresis and ataxia (see above). Chordomas most frequently involve the last vertebrae at the end of the tail. They also can be located anywhere on the tail (**Fig. 17.14**). Osteomas are found most frequently on the skull. The mass may become quite large. It is firm to hard and may put pressure on the

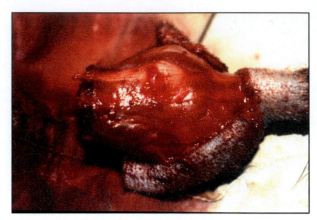

Fig. 17.14 Chordoma of the tail. Amputation was curative.

eye or ear (**Fig. 17.15**). The report that describes the fibrosarcoma had posterior paresis with the tumour being on the spine. It did metastasise to the lungs.

Differential diagnosis

Types of neoplasia.

Diagnostic testing

Radiographs. For suspected tumour impinging on the spinal cord, a myelography can be done. CT scan. Biopsy with histopathology, immunohistochemistry (to determine chondrosarcoma vs. chordoma).

Diagnosis

Presence of neoplasia on testing modality.

Management/treatment

Any tumour surgically removed should be submitted for histopathology to aid in prognosis. Surgical amputation of the tail several vertebrae anterior to suspected chordoma or chondrosarcoma. Surgical excision of the osteoma. If full excision it should not recur at the site. The report on the fibrosarcoma indicated that despite surgical intervention, the tumour recurred at the site and metastasized.

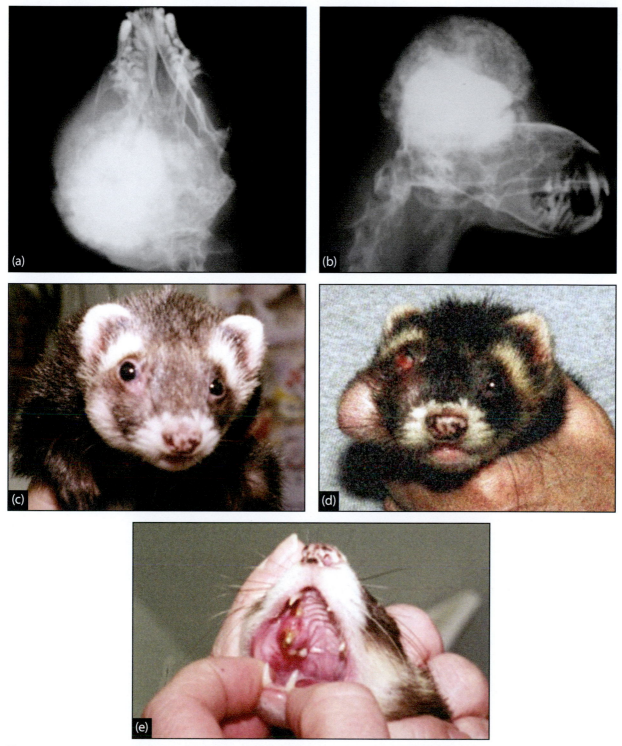

Fig. 17.15 (a) DV of skull osteoma; (b) lateral view of osteoma; (c) osteoma beginning to impinge on eye;
(d) large osteoma involving the maxilla and orbit; (e) oral cavity penetration and involvement with the osteoma.

CHAPTER 18

DISORDERS OF THE NERVOUS SYSTEM

Susan E. Orosz and
Cathy A. Johnson-Delaney

INTRODUCTION

There are few primary diseases that affect the nervous system of ferrets but secondary problems need to be addressed, particularly as systemic illness has an impact on the nervous system. Historical questions should be similar to those for other mammals and include, but are not limited to: rabies and/ or distemper vaccination history, onset of clinical signs, exposure to potential toxins such as lead or insecticides, treatment for concurrent illness and if other pets in the household are affected.

After taking a history, the ferret should have a thorough physical examination as there are diseases of ferrets that mimic neurological diseases but are systemic or involve the liver and/or pancreas. Systemic diseases that cause weakness can mimic neurological disease. The physical examination is best done first, including heart rate and auscultation of the heart and lungs, rectal temperature, abdominal and peripheral lymph node palpation, abdominal palpation and inspection of the mucous membranes and the teeth, ears and eyes and the body surface including the fur coat, before performing the neurological examination.

NEUROLOGICAL EXAMINATION

The purpose of the neurological examination is to rule in or out a neurological problem and to determine if a single lesion can be localised to explain those findings.

The neurological examination is divided into the following components:

* Mentation.
* Posture and gait.
* Postural reactions.
* Cranial nerves.

* Spinal reflexes.
* Palpation and pain perception.

Mentation

While taking the history, you can put the ferret on the floor of the examination room and watch its behaviour and movement. It is important to observe the patient for the level of consciousness (alertness) and the content of consciousness (awareness). The categories for mentation are as follows:

* Normal – bright and alert and responsive.
* Lethargic – decreased activity but normal mental status.
* Depressed – slow responses and will sleep while undisturbed.
* Obtunded – slow responses with a decreased level of consciousness; will sleep in unfamiliar locations but is easily aroused.
* Stuporous – decreased consciousness but responds to noxious stimuli.
* Comatose – unable to arouse and unconscious.

Lethargy and depression are associated with metabolic conditions while patients that are obtunded, stuporous or comatose have a condition that affects the brainstem or cerebrum.

Posture and gait

Posture is the position of the animal at rest and there can be a number of alterations from normal. These can include:

* Kyphosis – dorsal curvature of the spine.
* Lordosis – ventral curvature of the spine.
* Head tilt – tipping of the head down; describe the direction of the head on the examination form.

- Curvature of the head and neck – note the direction the head and neck are turned; the body often follows this direction.
- Wide-based stance – the legs appear splayed from the body.

There are conditions that are rare but the postures can help in localisation of the lesion:

- Decerebrate rigidity – extension of all four limbs.
- Decerebellar rigidity – extension of the thoracic limbs and flexion of the pelvic limbs.
- Opisthotonus – dorsiflexion of the head and neck.
- Schiff–Sherrington posture – increased tone of the thoracic limbs with paralysis of the pelvic limbs.

Gait is the assessment of movement of the limbs and is evaluated as the patient moves about the examination room. The patient can be:

- Ambulatory – able to walk and support the body weight with all four limbs and advance without assistance.
- Non-ambulatory – the patient is not able to support its weight or walk. It may refer to all limbs affected or may be only the hindlimbs.

One common abnormality of gait is ataxia or the alteration of coordinated voluntary muscle movement. There are a number of types of ataxia. These include:

- Proprioceptive ataxia – lack of awareness of the muscles and joints in 3-dimensional space so that there is a stomping type of gait that worsens when the visual system is impaired.
- Vestibular ataxia – the lack of vestibular input so that the body tends to fall or drift to one side of the midline.
- Cerebellar ataxia – is often symmetrical and is hypermetric, which results in a bouncy gait.

Postural changes may occur with vestibular or cerebellar disease or asymmetrical lesions of the cervical spinal cord. Purposeful coordinated movement requires an intact extrapyramidal system. Paresis is a weakness of voluntary muscle movement. This is usually associated with stumbling or knuckling of the patient. It can be caused by reduced or absent sensory pathways to the brain or by upper motor neuron disease. Lesions from the brainstem caudally result in gait disturbances characterised by ataxia, paresis or even paralysis. Paralysis is a loss of voluntary movement to the muscles.

Postural reactions

These tests evaluate complex actions that require integration of the proprioceptive sensory systems for initiation of movement and the motor systems for follow-up. In mammals, these reactions require intact sensory systems, the cerebral cortex for integration and the motor systems for a response. Deficits in postural reactions cannot localise a lesion by themselves but may help in context with other tests. For example, a lesion in the cerebral cortex may result in changes in postural reactions without any changes in gait. These reaction tests are not easy to perform, require good technique and require cooperation on the part of the patient. The most common tests performed are the paw placement and the hopping tests, which are more challenging in ferrets.

Paw placement test

The patient is typically supported under the chest to prevent loss of balance when placing the paw in dorsiflexion. With the short legs of ferrets, a thin surgical towel can be wrapped around the chest to provide this support.

Place a finger over the top or dorsal surface of the limb and then gently flex the paw so that the tops of the toes are touching the ground but not supporting the weight of the body on that limb.

For the hindlimb, the towel can be used to support the pelvis as well. The finger(s) supports the limb while flexing the paw.

Normally, the patient replaces the paw into its normal position with weight bearing on the ventral metacarpal or tarsal pads.

It is important to use a non-slip surface and support the patient to determine subtle changes.

Visual and tactile placing of the paw (Figs 18.1, 18.2)

This is much easier to do in ferrets due to their anatomy. For this test, the ferret is supported in your arm and the paw away from your arm and body is exposed to a slow approach of the examination table or other smooth surface. Let the dorsum of the paw touch the surface of the table.

This test should be done slowly to not evoke a vestibular response and should be done both with the animal sighted and with your hand covering the face. In visual placing the patient is allowed to see the table and in the tactile portion of the test it is not.

The patient, when the dorsum of the paw is 'aware' of the table, will then attempt to place the paw correctly on the surface.

Hopping reaction (Figs 18.3, 18.4)

This should be done with both the fore- and hindlimbs. It can be challenging due to the short legs and long torso of ferrets.

For the forelimb, place a hand under the torso and lift the hindlimbs from the ground while holding one of the forelimbs up off the ground as well. You may use a towel to fold one of the forelimbs toward the chest. Push the patient over towards the foot that is remaining on the ground.

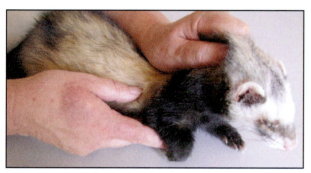

Fig. 18.1 Paw placement reflex, forelimb. The ferret is either scruffed or supported under the chest and held just over the table. Repeat for the other side.

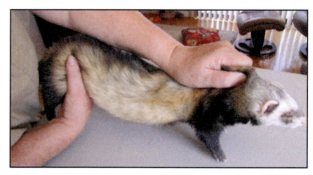

Fig. 18.3 Hopping, forelimb. Gently scruff holding the opposite leg elevated or against the body; place one hand under the abdomen to lift the hindlimbs from the surface. Push the ferret towards the standing limb. Repeat with the other limb.

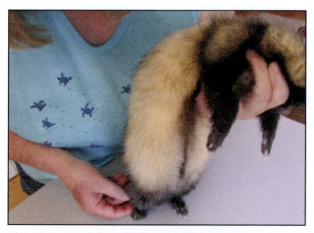

Fig. 18.2 Hindlimb placement reflex. The ferret is either scruffed or supported under the pelvis or caudal abdomen. The hand is placed above the paw and it is knuckled over. Repeat for the other side.

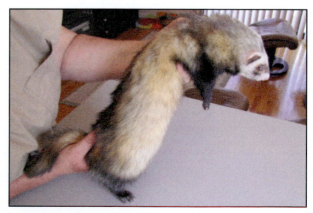

Fig. 18.4 Hopping, hindlimb. One hand placed under the chest lifts the forelimbs off the ground. The other hand is placed by the femur; lift one hindlimb off the surface. Push the ferret towards the standing limb. Repeat for the other limb.

Poor initiation of the hopping reaction suggests that there are proprioceptive deficits, while poor follow-through suggests a motor system problem or motor paresis.

Cranial nerve examination (*Table 18.1*)

CN I (olfactory nerve)

The olfactory nerve; not routinely tested as most ferrets are easily observed to sniff the table, the handler, and the veterinarian(!); Can use a noxious substance such as alcohol on a swab placed near the nose; causes response from CN V. A piece of normal food can be placed at the nose and then normal sniffing reaction can be observed.

CN II (optic nerve)

For the optic nerve, check for normal pupillary size and for anisocoria; there should be a direct and consensual light reflex for the pupils of both eyes.

Menace test: Move your hand toward the eye in a menacing manner and the patient should blink as a response. Covering one eye and testing the other both at the temporal and the nasal fields, further localisation can be determined. Many normal ferrets lack a menace response.

Visual following: Drop cotton balls or roll a ball to see if the patient follows with both eyes.

CN III (oculomotor nerve), CN IV (trochlear nerve), CN VI (abducent nerve)

These are considered together as they control eye movements. The parasympathetic supply to the eye is from CN III that causes pupillary constriction. Move the head and watch the movement of the eyes as they should move in concert. This can be difficult to determine in ferrets due to their small eyes.

Corneal reflex: The corneal surface is touched lightly with a cotton bud and the globe will retract

Table 18.1 **Cranial nerve assessment**	
CRANIAL NERVE (CN)	**ASSESSMENT**
I	Place a cotton bud soaked in alcohol under the nose, or a bit of food
II and III	Pupillary light reflex
II and VI	Menace reflex. Some ferrets do not have this normally
III, IV, VI	Symmetry of eyes, pupils
V ophthalmic branch	Touch medial canthus of eye
V maxillary branch	Touch lateral canthus of eye
III, IV, VI	Move head from side to side, observe vestibular eye movements
V	Paralysis: bilateral dropped jaw; unilateral decreased jaw tone
VI	Retractor bulbi muscle with the palpebral and corneal reflex
V and VII	Touch, pinch nose and lower jaw
VII	Symmetry of face
VIII	Cochlear part: test with response to loud noise (ascertain whether ferret is genetically deaf). Vestibular lesions: unilateral ataxia, nystagmus, head tilt to the side of the lesion
IX and X	Stimulate back of the pharynx to induce gag reflex
XI	Palpate the trapezius muscle, parts of the sternocephalicus and brachiocephalicus for symmetry
XII	Put dab of treat on nose, evaluate the ability of the tongue to extend forward

Adapted from Lewis W (2009) Ferrets: nervous and musculoskeletal disorders. In: Keeble E, Meredith A (eds). *BSAVA Manual of Rodents and Ferrets*. BSAVA, Quedgeley, UK. pp. 303–310.

due the normal function of CN VI. The sensory component to the corneal surface is from CN V (trigeminal nerve).

CN V (trigeminal nerve)

The *motor component* supplies the masseter and temporalis muscles that close the jaw. Jaw tone will test the integrity of these muscles along with palpation of the muscle mass above the globe.

The sensory components are:

- *Lingual nerve: principal sensory nerve to rostral three-fourths of the tongue ophthalmic division (V1):* this division provides sensory supply to the cornea and the upper portion of the face; the corneal reflex has the sensory portion from V1 and the motor component from VI. When the medial canthus is touched lightly, the eyelids blink. The sensory component is V1 and the motor is CN VII and/or the facial nucleus.
- *Maxillary division (V2):* this division supplies the sensory component to the upper lip. Pinching the upper lip lateral to the canine tooth results in a wrinkling of the skin and a blink. This response is from CN VII and/or the nucleus.
- *Mandibular division (V3):* this division supplies the sensory component to the lower lip. Pinching will cause the animal to pull away, which involves the forebrain.

CN VII (facial nerve)

This nerve supplies the muscles of facial expression; note blinking of the eyelid; symmetry of the face including the lips. It also innervates the taste buds and secretory motor fibres to the lingual gland. This nerve mediates tearing from the lacrimal gland.

CN VIII (vestibulocochlear nerve)

This nerve is divided into the cochlear portion that sends information on hearing to the brainstem from the inner ear. The vestibular portion brings information regarding the head and neck in 3-dimensional space from the semicircular canals to the vestibular nucleus.

- *Cochlear portion:* this can be tested with a squeaky toy or other noises and the ferret should direct

its attention to the source of the sound. Ferrets with a blaze as well as panda markings are deaf (see Chapter 15).

- *Vestibular portion:* physiological nystagmus will result when the head is turned from the midline in a horizontal plane both to the right and the left. The fast phase for the eye movement will be directed towards the side the head is rotated. Signs of vestibular disease include head tilt, circling, ataxia with a broad-based gait and abnormal nystagmus. It may be difficult to observe nystagmus due to the dark iris and the lack of the white sclera for contrast as the lid margins in ferrets are next to the corneal surface.

CN IX (glossopharyngeal nerve) and CN X (vagus nerve)

These nerves have both the sensory and motor components to the oral cavity for swallowing. Clients may report that the ferret may have trouble swallowing, may regurgitate or may have dysphagia. The sensory component of this test is to lightly touch the right or left side of the back of the oral cavity and the ferret should gag.

CN XI (spinal accessory nerve)

This nerve supplies the trapezius and the sternocephalicus muscles over the dorsal shoulders and is difficult to assess clinically.

CN XII (hypoglossal nerve)

This nerve supplies the intrinsic tongue muscles. There may be atrophy of these muscles and the nerve can be assessed by watching the ferret lick some soft food. The tongue will move to the side of the lesion.

Spinal reflex examination

Spinal reflexes are used in conjunction with postural reactions to help localise lesions to either the central nervous system (CNS) or the peripheral nervous system (PNS). The reflex response helps to define whether the lesion represents a deficit of the upper (UMN) or lower motor neuron (LMN) of the PNS. An LMN deficit results from a problem with the final common pathway or the ventral grey horn of the spinal cord. This pathway includes the motor root and spinal nerve, the motor endplate and the

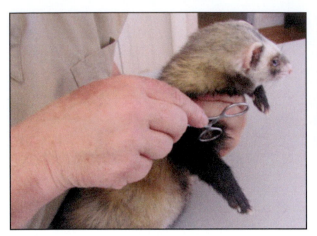

Fig. 18.5 **Biceps reflex. While pulling the limb slightly caudally, place a finger over the tendon and tap the finger with the handle of a haemostat or just tap the tendon with the haemostat handle. The limb can be just suspended as shown in the picture.**

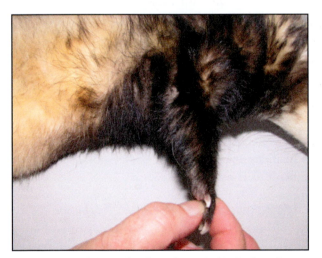

Fig. 18.7 **Withdrawal reflex, thoracic limb. Gently pinch a toe. Watch for flexion of all joints. A reduced reflex is often best seen in the shoulder joint.**

muscle fibres of the particular reflex being tested. LMN paresis or paralysis is characterised by hyporeflexia or areflexia, decreased motor tone and neurogenic atrophy that is often marked and rapid.

UMN pathways represent long descending tracts from the brain and brainstem that affect motor tone and direct wilful movement. For example, the rubrospinal tract increases flexor muscle tone, whereas the vestibulospinal tracts increase extensor muscle tone.

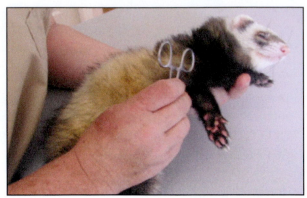

Fig. 18.6 **Triceps reflex. Hold the ferret so that the limb is suspended and elbow slightly bent. Tap the triceps tendon with a finger or the handle of a forceps.**

Dysfunction of these UMN pathways results in either a normal reflex or hyperreflexia with mild disuse atrophy of the muscles affected and either decreased, normal or increased muscle tone, depending on the tracts affected.

When performing spinal reflexes, it is important to use the percussion or reflex hammer or handle of a haemostat appropriately for interpretation of test results. It is important to keep the muscle and tendon slightly stretched before hitting the tendon of the muscle. In ferrets due to their small size and short limbs, it can be difficult to perform the spinal reflex examinations appropriately for interpretation.

Forelimb reflexes:

- Biceps reflex – this test evaluates spinal nerves from C6 to C8 and the musculocutaneous nerve. Pull the forelimb slightly caudally and place a finger over the tendon near the elbow and tap the tendon (**Fig. 18.5**).
- Triceps reflex – this test evaluates spinal nerves C7 to T1 and the radial nerve peripherally. Flex and abduct the elbow. Tap the tendon just proximal to the tip of the elbow with the reflex hammer (**Fig. 18.6**).
- Withdrawal reflex engages all of the cervical/thoracic nerves of the forelimb. The skin of the paw is pinched. The response is for the flexion of the joints of the thoracic limb. A reduction in tone is more often observed in the shoulder joint (**Fig. 18.7**).

Hindlimb reflexes:

- Patellar reflex – this test evaluates L4 to L6 spinal nerves and the femoral nerve. Slightly flex the stifle and place your hand under the limb for support. Tap the tendon just proximal to the point of the tibia and the patella. The tibia should extend forward and the stifle be extended (**Fig. 18.8**).
- Gastrocnemius reflex – this test evaluates L4 to L6 spinal nerves and the tibial branch of the sciatic or ischiatic nerve. The hock should be flexed keeping the tendon tensed and abducted while holding the metatarsal region of the leg (**Fig. 18.9**).
- Withdrawal reflex – this engages all of the lumbar and sacral intumescence when the skin of the paw is pinched from the hindlimb. The response is flexion of all of the joints of the hindlimb. A reduction in tone is more commonly observed in the hock joint. This is just to test the reflex at the spinal cord level, not for detection of conscious perception of pain (**Fig. 18.10**).
- Perineal (anal) reflex – this evaluates the sacral nerves and the branches of the pudendal nerve. The perineal/anal region is stroked lightly with the tip of the haemostat or a cotton bud on each side. The response is contraction of the sphincter and flexion of the tail (**Fig. 18.11**).
- Cutaneous trunci (panniculus) reflex – the patient should be laying in lateral recumbency and the skin just ventral to the vertebral column is pinched with a forceps starting near the

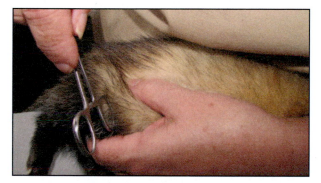

Fig. 18.8 Patellar reflex. Slightly flex the stifle and tap the patellar tendon with a handle of a forceps.

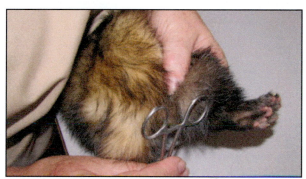

Fig. 18.9 Gastrocnemius reflex. Flex and adduct the hock by holding the limb. Keep the hock flexed, which keeps the tendon tense. Tap the tendon with the handle of a forceps.

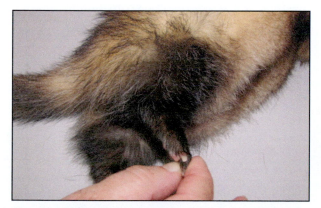

Fig. 18.10 Withdrawal reflex, hindlimb. Gently pinch a toe. Watch for flexion of all joints. The reduced reflex is often best seen in the hock.

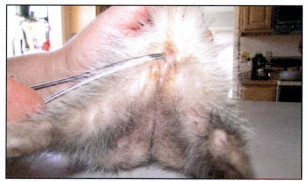

Fig. 18.11 Perineal (anal) reflex. This evaluates the sacral nerves and branches of the pudendal nerve. The perineal/anal region is stroked lightly with the tip of a forceps or a cotton swab on each side. The response is contraction of the sphincter.

lumbosacral region and proceeding cranially trying to do one vertebral body segment at a time. The response is for the cutaneous trunci muscles to contract, making the skin twitch where pinched (**Fig. 18.12**).

Palpation and pain perception

During the neurological examination, careful palpation of the entire body should be done. While doing so, the animal may respond to pain over any muscle mass, bone or joint. The responses may vary

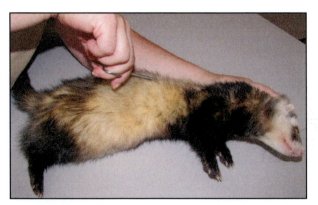

Fig. 18.12 Cutaneous trunci (panniculus) reflex. The ferret should be laying in lateral recumbency (you can gently scruff if the ferret will not lay on its side willingly). The skin just ventral to the vertebral column is pinched with a forceps starting near the lumbosacral region and proceeding cranially trying to do one vertebral body segment at a time. The response is for the cutaneous trunci muscles to contract making the skin twitch where pinched.

depending on severity of the pain in the area. The ferret may close its eyes, tremble, vocalize, jerk the body part away or try to get away from the examiner. The ferret may snap at the affected area or try to bite the examiner. If pain is perceived, an attempt should be made to determine if it is superficial (one test can be using a 25 gauge hypodermic needle and gentle pricking the skin) or deep (deeper palpation or joint manipulation). Knowledge of the innervation to the area can pinpoint the site of the pain.

Muscle tone

Muscle tone of each of the thoracic and pelvic limbs should be examined after the spinal reflexes are performed. Each limb should be manipulated passively, and each of the muscle masses of the long bones palpated in order to detect atrophy. The limbs should be flexed and extended to help determine differences in muscle tone (**Fig. 18.13**). Rarely will the examiner be able to observe muscle fasciculations, but these abnormalities are important findings if present. Differences in muscle tone are graded as increased, normal or decreased for each limb.

There may be an increased resistance to manipulation of the limb. This can occur with lesions of the UMN system, increased facilitation of the efferent pathway and alterations in muscle movement. It may be difficult to separate increased muscle tone from restriction of muscle movement from some mechanical cause. In addition to UMN disease causing increased tone, tone may be increased with muscle irritation or decreased inhibition of the

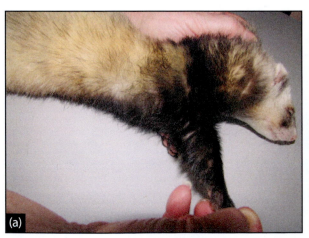
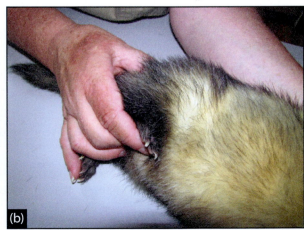

Fig. 18.13 (a) Forelimb; (b) hindlimb. To test muscle tone, the limbs should be flexed and fully extended.

intact LMN pathways. A perceived increase in tone may result with chronic LMN disease and muscle replacement with connective tissue. An example of a disease problem that results in increased muscle rigidity not of UMN origin is tetanus.

Muscle tone can be decreased with both upper and lower motor neuron disease. However, decreased muscle tone is associated more commonly with LMN problems. Deep palpation of the limbs is used to determine pain of the limb or joints. It is also important to check range of motion of the joints.

NEUROLOGICAL DISEASES

The standard tests that are used for a diagnostic work-up of neurological disease in dogs and cats can be used for ferrets as well. Blood work consisting of a CBC and chemistry panel are important. Of these, the blood glucose is important in distinguishing an insulinoma from other true neurological diseases that affect mentation and/or posterior or caudal paresis (see Chapter 14). Use of radiographs along with CT and MRI images is helpful in distinguishing changes in the vertebral column and skull, particularly with traumatic, lytic, proliferative and/or neoplastic lesions. Common neurological diseases that affect the ferret are discussed below.

INFECTIOUS DISEASE: BACTERIAL

Botulism
Definition/overview
Clostridium botulinum produces endotoxins. Ferrets are moderately susceptible to *C. botulinum* types A and B. They are highly susceptible to type C which is usually lethal.

Aetiology/pathophysiology
This is often related to eating contaminated food; symptoms of dysphagia, ataxia and hindlimb paresis occur about 12–96 hours after ingestion.

Clinical presentation
Symptoms usually include paralysis, which starts with the hindlimbs and progressively extends forwards for some days. Sensation remains. There is usually no temperature rise. Respirations become shallow and slow due to partial paralysis of the intercostals and diaphragm. There may be protrusion of the third eyelid and then death from respiratory failure.

Differential diagnosis
Neoplasia of the nervous system, otitis media/interna, spinal trauma/abscess, toxicosis (lead, chocolate, nicotine, bromethalin, liquid potpourri etc.), botulism, infectious disease (distemper, rabies, Aleutian disease, listeriosis, toxoplasmosis, cryptococcosis, other bacterial meningitis/encephalitis).

Diagnostic testing
Bacterial identification from vomitus, faeces or stomach contents at necropsy.

Diagnosis
Presence of the bacteria. Theoretically presence of the toxins in the blood would be diagnostic, but the authors are not aware of any commercial testing of these for ferrets.

Listeriosis
Definition/overview
Listeria monocytogenes is a saprophyte and is common in soils. It appears to be mildly infectious to ferrets.

Aetiology/pathophysiology
Infection may result from ingestion of contaminated food or inhalation. It may be secondary to debilitating disease such as TB and salmonella. The incubation period between ingestion of infected food and disease onset can be 1–90 days, making tracking of source difficult. Recently a number of raw food diets sold for dogs and cats but fed to ferrets have been recalled due to *Listeria* contamination.

Clinical presentation
Ataxia, paresis, paralysis and other CNS signs.

Differential diagnosis
Neoplasia of the nervous system, otitis media/interna, spinal trauma/abscess, botulism, toxicosis (lead, chocolate, nicotine, bromethalin, liquid potpourri, etc.), botulism, infectious disease (distemper, rabies, Aleutian disease, toxoplasmosis, cryptococcosis, other bacterial meningitis/encephalitis).

Diagnostic testing

Regular haematology and serum chemistry should be performed. A CSF tap and culture may be definitive. Radiographs may be needed to rule out skeletal differentials.

Diagnosis

A positive culture of *Listeria*.

Management/treatment

The ferret should be started on a broad-spectrum antibiotic that can penetrate the CNS such as penicillins and chloramphenicol, to which *Listeria* is usually sensitive.

INFECTIOUS DISEASE: FUNGAL

Blastomycosis

Definition/overview

The organism *Blastomyces dermatitidis* has been reported in ferrets. While this is more often classified as a respiratory disease or skin disease, it can result in multifocal granulomatous mengoencephalitis (see Chapter 20).

Aetiology/pathophysiology

The disease incidence is sporadic. It is in soil, and route of infection is probably inhalation of conidia. There is apparently no animal/animal or animal/human transmission. It has been reported in the USA, Canada, Africa and Central America. Ferrets housed outdoors may be at higher risk.

Clinical presentation

Most often ferrets develop chronic granulomatous mycosis in the lungs, with cough and sneezing. A cutaneous form has ulcerative swellings which spread closely over the skin. The footpads can have ulcerative swellings. Ataxia, paresis and paralysis and other CNS signs are seen when meningoencephalitis has developed.

Differential diagnosis

For the nervous system signs: neoplasia of the nervous system, otitis media/interna, spinal trauma/abscess, botulism, toxicosis (lead, chocolate, nicotine, bromethalin, liquid potpourri, etc.), botulism, infectious disease (distemper, rabies, Aleutian disease, listeriosis, toxoplasmosis, cryptococcosis, other bacterial meningitis/encephalitis).

Diagnostic testing

Organisms can be extracted from skin lesion or lung aspirates. Tissue imprints may show budding yeasts. Circulating antibody titre to the organism can be shown by agar immunodiffusion test.

Diagnosis

Presence of the organism. Subsequent changes seen at necropsy may include a reticulonodular interstitial pneumonia. The lung may have focal consolidation and pleural fluid. There may be a bilateral diffuse granulomatous pneumonia and pleuritis, a meningoencephalitis and an enlarged spleen.

Management/treatment

IV amphotericin B has been used in ferrets at 0.4–0.8 mg/kg with some regression of signs; however, side-effects may cause anorexia, pyrexia and azotaemia. Ketoconazole has been given at 5 mg/kg orally SC every other day. Prognosis is poor.

Cryptococcosis

Definition/overview

A rare disease in ferrets caused by *Cryptococcus neoformans* (see Chapter 20).

Aetiology/pathophysiology

Reported infrequently for producing subacute or chronic meningoencephalitis. It is an inhaled organism that spreads to the lungs, brain and abdomen.

Clinical presentation

Initially it may be serous or purulent unilateral or bilateral nasal discharge that may have small amounts of blood. The ferret may have neck stiffness, incoordination, ataxia then death.

Differential diagnosis

Neoplasia of the nervous system, otitis media/interna, spinal trauma/abscess, botulism, toxicosis (lead, chocolate, nicotine, bromethalin, liquid potpourri, etc.), botulism, infectious disease (distemper, rabies, Aleutian disease, listeriosis, toxoplasmosis, other bacterial meningitis/encephalitis).

Diagnostic testing

CSF tap for culture, cytology. Often histopathology at death.

Diagnosis

Positive for the organism in the CSF. Often unfortunately the diagnosis is made at necropsy.

Management/treatment

None at this time. Prevention may be to eliminate contact with soil.

INFECTIOUS DISEASE: PARASITIC

Toxoplasmosis

Definition/overview

Ferrets are susceptible to *Toxoplasma gondii* infection through ingesting raw meat and from cat faeces infected with the parasite.

Aetiology/pathophysiology

Ferrets may become infected or possibly may act as intermediate hosts. One study showed that *Toxoplasma* isolated from ferrets was morphologically, biologically and serologically indistinguishable from that found in rabbits in England. In one case report on a fur farm in New Zealand, 30% of 750 neonatal ferrets died without clinical signs. Multifocal necrosis was observed in lung, heart and liver.

Clinical presentation

Signs depend on the organs involved and may include: anorexia, lethargy, corneal oedema, retinitis, iritis, blindness, ataxia, fever, anaemia, hepatitis, CNS signs, respiratory disease and diarhhoea.

Differential diagnosis

For neurological signs: neoplasia of the nervous system, otitis media/interna, spinal trauma/abscess, botulism, toxicosis (lead, chocolate, nicotine, bromethalin, liquid potpourri, etc.), botulism, infectious disease (distemper, rabies, Aleutian disease, listeriosis, cryptococcosis, other bacterial meningitis/encephalitis).

Diagnostic testing

ELISA tests for IgG and IgM as well as *T. gondii*-specific antigens in the serum.

Diagnosis

Positive test results as well as response to treatment.

Management/treatment

Sulphonamides continued for at least 2 weeks and a short time after cessation of clinical signs. A regimen may include pyrimethamine at 0.5–1 mg/kg PO q12–24h along with sulfadiazine at 60 mg/100 mL of drinking water.

INFECTIOUS DISEASE: VIRAL

Aleutian disease

Definition/overview (see Chapter 16)

A chronic wasting disease with hypergammaglobulinaemia.

Aetiology/pathophysiology

Aleutian disease virus (ADV) is a parvovirus that causes a persistent infection in mink and in ferrets.

Clinical presentation

Splenic enlargement with lymphadenopathy. Nervous system signs include posterior paresis and ataxia with paraplegia or hemiplegia. There may be faecal and/or urinary incontinence with paraplegia.

Differential diagnosis

Neoplasia of the nervous system, otitis media/interna, spinal trauma/abscess, botulism, toxicosis (lead, chocolate, nicotine, bromethalin, liquid potpourri, etc.), botulism, infectious disease (distemper, rabies, listeriosis, toxoplasmosis, cryptococcosis, other bacterial meningitis/encephalitis).

Diagnostic testing

ELISA test serology is available, but may be confusing as clinically normal ferrets may have a positive titre but do not develop disease. A very high titre might point to clinical disease. Paired sera 2 weeks apart may be more definitive.

Diagnosis

Ferrets with clinical signs have disseminated non-suppurative encephalomyelitis. This is usually confirmed on necropsy.

Management/treatment

For those with signs, there is no specific treatment and they can be provided supportive care or euthanased (see Chapter 16). Supportive care may include fluid and nutritional support, antibiotics for secondary infections and gastrointestinal protectants. Due to the immune-mediated nature of the disease, treatment with immunosuppressive agents may be beneficial. A study in mink found that intraperitoneal administration of cyclophosphamide controlled clinical signs, but virus levels were unaffected. Another study documented decreased mortality in mink kits treated with ADV antibody, but this is probably impractical for clinical use. In pet ferrets, immunosuppressive therapy with prednisolone (0.25–1 mg/kg PO q12–24h), cyclophosphamide (10 mg/kg PO, SC q24h), or other drugs may be considered, but the risks should be carefully considered and the patient should be closely monitored for secondary infection. There is no vaccine that cross-protects even though this is a parvovirus.

Unfortunately, most existing studies of treatment and prognosis for ADV have been conducted in farmed or laboratory mink, so information about prognosis for individual patients that receive intensive care is unknown, but probably guarded.

Canine distemper virus
Definition/overview (see Chapters 20, 21)
This is a devastating disease in ferrets, and was first described by use of ferrets in characterising the disease and designing vaccines for dogs.

Aetiology/pathophysiology
Canine distemper virus (CDV) is an RNA virus from the genus *Morbillivirus* in the family Paramyxoviridae. It affects mustelids and other carnivores including some Felidae. The severity of the disease depends on the viral strain and immunocompetence of the host. Some strains produce neurological disease with high mortality rates while others only produce pneumonia with lower death rates

Clinical presentation
The disease manifests first with conjunctivitis, rash, anorexia, fever, and respiratory signs ranging from catarrhal rhinitis to fulminating pneumonia, GI signs including diarrhoea and melena, followed by CNS signs that include myoclonus or paresis along with muscle tremors and hyperexcitability.

Differential diagnosis
Differential diagnoses for neurological signs include ADV, rabies, ferret systemic coronavirus infection, botulism, brain tumours, toxicoses, fungal infections of the brain (cryptococcosis, blastomycosis) and toxoplasmosis.

Diagnostic testing
PCR techniques can be used for detection in the blood. ELISA testing is also available.

Diagnosis
Positive results on PCR, ELISA, postmortem histopathology.

Management/treatment
See *Table 20.1* for treatment regimens. By the time CNS signs are observed, treatment usually fails and euthanasia is the only option. Commonly used disinfectants will kill the virus in the environment. Vaccination of exposed ferrets in the face of an outbreak in a multiple ferret household or shelter is recommended. A two-vaccine series may be necessary.

Rabies virus
Definition/overview
Uncommon but of public health concern in the USA. The virus occurs worldwide except in Australia, New Zealand, UK, Hawaii, Japan and parts of Scandinavia. May be transmitted to ferrets from dogs, cats, raccoons, foxes, polecats, other land mammals and bats. Ferrets housed outdoors may be at risk of exposure.

Aetiology/pathophysiology
The most common exposure is from a bite as the virus is primarily transmitted by saliva. It has been shown experimentally to have an incubation period of 28–33 days with death ensuing in 4–5 days in ferrets.

Clinical signs
Signs relating to infection of the CNS range from posterior paresis or paralysis and paresthesia to anxiety and behavioural changes.

Differential diagnosis

Neoplasia of the nervous system, otitis media/interna, spinal trauma/abscess, botulism, toxicosis (lead, chocolate, nicotine, bromethalin, liquid potpourri, etc.), botulism, infectious disease (distemper, rabies, ADV, listeriosis, toxoplasmosis, cryptococcosis, other bacterial meningitis/encephalitis).

Diagnostic testing

Necropsy: virus is detected in the salivary glands and the CNS.

Diagnosis

Confirmed at necropsy with immunohistochemistry and histopathological changes.

Management/treatment

Killed rabies vaccine is available. Imrab vaccine (Merial, Duluth, GA USA) SC for 1 year protection starting at 12 weeks of age. Current vaccination may help if the ferret bites a human by allowing a quarantine period instead of euthanasia. The veterinarian must consult local and state laws. For example, in the state of Washington, USA, it is law that all dogs, cats and ferrets be vaccinated for rabies.

INTERVERTEBRAL DISC DISEASE (SEE CHAPTER 17)

Definition/overview

Intervertebral discs are the shock absorbers between the vertebral bodies and can partially or completely herniate, compressing the spinal cord. This compression alters the function of the spinal cord and the symptoms that result are dependent on the site along the spinal cord and the degree of compression. Pain, weakness or paralysis may occur from the mechanical compression or from secondary vascular or other changes of the tissue around the site.

Aetiology/pathophysiology

The exact cause of herniation of the intervertebral disc is unknown. This condition may be caused from trauma or other causes including genetic, neoplasia and infection.

The intervertebral discs consist of the nucleus pulposus that offers flexibility to the vertebral column and it is surrounded by the annulus fibrosus, a tough fibrous structure. Degeneration of the disc leads to calcification of the nucleus with weakening of the annulus leading to rupture. Trauma can also result in rupture of the disc. Compression or alteration of the structure by tumour cells or infectious agents can weaken and cause rupture of the disc.

Clinical presentation

The presentation will depend on the location of the herniation of the disc. In a recent report of intervertebral disc prolapse, the ferret presented with hindlimb lameness. There was paresis of both hindlimbs with absent proprioception and lack of muscle tone. Deep pain was present. In this case, there was protrusion between the second and third lumbar vertebrae.

Differential diagnosis

Neoplasia of the nervous system, spinal abscess, botulism, trauma.

Diagnostic testing

In the reported case, a myelogram was able to be used to demonstrate the herniation at L2–3. MRI may prove beneficial in diagnosing disc disease as well.

Diagnosis

Evidence of decreased space between vertebral bodies and/or protrusion of disc seen on radiograph, myelogram, MRI.

Management/treatment

Treatment is best with a hemilaminectomy with decompression at the site. Some patients may improve with the use of steroids based on the degree of compression of the spinal cord. Those that cannot walk have reduced prognosis with medical management alone. Lack of deep pain is indicative of a very poor prognosis.

NEOPLASIA

While neoplasia is common in ferrets, lesions localised to the CNS are uncommon. As with other animals, the signs are related to the part of the CNS affected by the tumour. The most common are lymphomas that often spread to the CNS, and chordomas (see Chapters 16, 17).

Chordoma (Fig. 18.14)

Definition/overview

These localised tumours of the spinal cord are rare in most mammals except ferrets.

Aetiology/pathophysiology

They are considered to be of embryonic origin of the notochord and tend to affect the tail of the ferret. These tumours are slow growing, firm masses that may be lobulated in the tail of adult ferrets.

Clinical presentation

A mass usually on the end of the tail, although they may occur elsewhere associated with the spinal cord. Neurological signs associated with spinal cord suppression may be seen with cervical or thoracic chordomas.

Differential diagnosis

Other types of neoplasia, abscess.

Diagnosis

A biopsy and histopathology can confirm chordoma.

Management/treatment

Tumours should be removed by amputation of the tail proximal to the tumour with wide surgical margins (**Fig. 18.15**). Prognosis is good when the tumour is distal on the tail. Metastasis is slow but leaving the tumour reduces the prognosis.

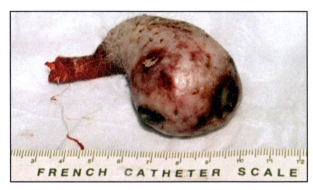

Fig. 18.15 **Amputated chordoma. Note the ulcerated surface.**

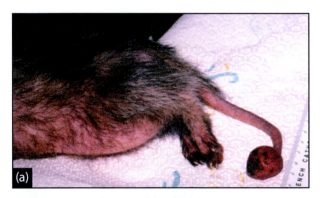

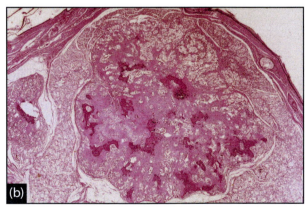

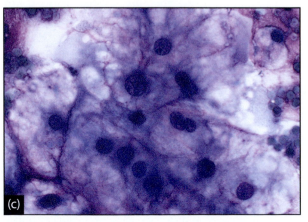

Fig. 18.14 **(a) Chordoma; (b) aspiration cytology of a neck mass with clusters of large vacuolated polygonal cells (physaliferous cells) (May-Grunwald Giemsa stain, 40×); (c) from tail, multinodular mass comprised of variably concentrically arranged aggregates of bone, cartilage and lobules of physaliferous cells (H&E stain, 40×). (Courtesy of Dr. Drury Reavill, Zoo/Exotic Pathology Service.)**

Cervical or thoracic chordomas can rarely be excised and clinical signs will be progressive, with euthanasia the only option.

T-cell lymphoma

Definition/overview
It has been described in a case report in a 22-month-old ferret. The tumour was of T-cell lymphocyte origin.

Aetiology/pathophysiology
A form of lymphoma (see Chapter 16).

Clinical presentation
The ferret had acute paraparesis of the hindlimbs. This progressed rapidly to plegia with incontinence.

Differential diagnosis
Spinal trauma/abscess, botulism, toxicosis (lead, chocolate, nicotine, bromethalin, liquid potpourri, etc.), botulism, infectious disease (distemper, rabies, ADV, listeriosis, toxoplasmosis, cryptococcosis), other bacterial meningitis/encephalitis).

Diagnostic testing
Radiographs showed bony lysis of the lumbar spine in this case. If the tumour is elsewhere in the nervous system, MRI or CT scan may be needed.

Diagnosis
The tumour was located and histopathology and immunohistochemistry were used to demonstrate cell of origin of the mass. Adjacent tissue may be invaded. In the reported case there was bony lysis of the lumbar spine.

Management/treatment
Predisolone may be attempted but is probably ineffective. Treatment regimens for lymphoma are listed in Chapter 16. Euthanasia is the option if signs progress.

TOXICOSIS (SEE CHAPTER 29)

Definition/overview
A number of substances are potentially toxic to ferrets.

Aetiology/pathophysiology
Ibuprofen toxicosis has been documented in ferrets causing severe lethargy progressing to coma, apnoea and death. Other toxicoses potentially include lead, chocolate, nicotine, bromethalin, narcotics, liquid potpourri, insecticides, etc. Nervous system symptomatology would be similar to other animals.

Clinical presentation
Nervous system signs may include lethargy, ataxia, paresis, tremors and seizures (**Fig. 18.16**). Other systems may be affected as well with clinical signs of apnoea, respiratory depression, vomiting and diarrhoea. History of exposure to chemicals listed above would be suspect.

Differential diagnosis
For nervous system signs: neoplasia of the nervous system, otitis media/interna, spinal trauma/abscess, botulism, infectious disease (distemper, rabies, ADV, listeriosis, toxoplasmosis, cryptococcosis, other bacterial meningitis/encephalitis).

Diagnosis
Serum testing is possible for a number of toxins, including ibuprofen, although testing may not be practical as the quantity of serum needed for some tests may be prohibitive. Test results may be definitive but may take time, which in an acute case is problematic. Unfortunately, necropsy with histopathology may be needed for the final diagnosis.

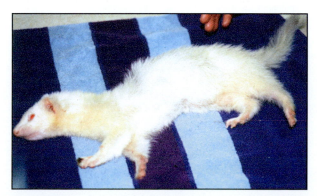

Fig. 18.16 **Generalised seizure.**

Management/treatment

Ascertaining the toxin involved in acute cases may point to specific antidotes such as naloxone for narcotics toxicosis or calcium EDTA for lead, but for most cases supportive care is all that can be done. This includes fluids, stomach protectants and symptomatic treatment for seizures, vomiting and diarrhoea.

TRAUMA

Definition/overview

Trauma is often from falling as ferrets like to climb. Occasionally they are dropped as they often squirm when held. Head injury can also occur from being slammed in a door as they try to pop through.

Aetiology/pathophysiology

Trauma to the head or spine may cause symptoms as in other animals.

Clinical presentation

CNS signs, ataxia, incoordination, paresis, paralysis, seizures, head tilt, anisocoria, nystagmus.

Differential diagnosis

Neoplasia of the nervous system, otitis media/interna, spinal abscess, botulism, toxicosis (lead, chocolate, nicotine, bromethalin, liquid potpourri, etc.),

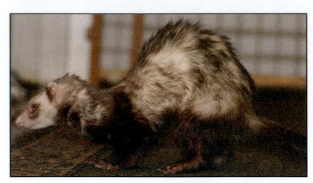

Fig. 18.17 **Pain posture associated with trauma. (Courtesy of Vondelle McLaughlin.)**

botulism, infectious disease (distemper, rabies, ADV, listeriosis, toxoplasmosis, cryptococcosis, other bacterial meningitis/encephalitis).

Diagnostic testing

Radiographs may show fractures. MRI or CT scans may be necessary to determine trauma to the CNS.

Diagnosis

Often by response to supportive care, or by positive lesion findings on imaging.

Management/treatment

Symptomatic supportive care including analgesics for pain (**Fig. 18.17**).

CHAPTER 19

DISORDERS OF THE ORAL CAVITY AND TEETH

Cathy A. Johnson-Delaney

INTRODUCTION

The domestic ferret has 28–30 deciduous teeth (di3-4/3: dc1/1: dm3/3). Eruption of the canines begins at 8 weeks of age (**Fig. 19.1**). The permanent dental formula is I3/3: C1/1: PM3/3: M1/2 = 34. The mandibular second molar is congenitally missing in some ferrets. There may also be supernumerary teeth, most commonly found between the first and second maxillary incisors (**Fig. 19.2**). Periodontal and gingival tissues and structures are similar to that of other carnivores. Using dog and cat dentistry as guidelines for home and veterinary care appears to be relevant. Oral microflora of the gingival sulcus and related mucosa was cultured at the mid-buccal surface of the right upper P4. In this study nearly 100% of the total cultivable flora were composed of facultative anaerobic gram-negative and gram-positive rods. *Pasteurella* spp., *Corynebacterium* spp., and *Rothia* spp. were the major components. No anaerobic bacteria

were detected. Detailed anatomy and physiology are in Chapter 3. Prognathism is found occasionally as a congenital defect (**Fig. 19.3**).

Dental instruments used in ferrets include the 'Nazzy' ferret mouth gag (Universal Surgical Instruments, Glen Clove, NY), scalers such as the McColl's scaler, pictured, double-ended elevator, small feline elevator, dental probe, and regular dental drill and polisher (**Fig. 19.4**). Dental surgery follows the same guidelines as those used in dog and cat practice. Infraorbital anaesthesia block is routinely used for canine extractions or root canal (**Figs 19.5, 19.6**). The most common dental surgery is extraction. Deciduous teeth can be removed without surgically closing the gingiva (**Fig. 19.7**). For adult teeth, after local blocking, gingivectomy is performed, the periodontal ligaments severed and the tooth extracted. The gingiva is then sutured (**Fig. 19.8**). The remaining teeth should be probed, scaled and polished (**Fig. 19.9**).

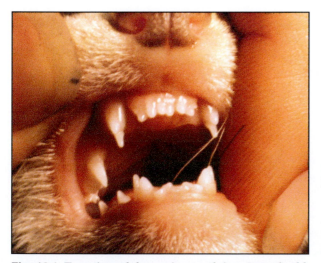

Fig. 19.1 Eruption of the canine teeth in a 9-week-old ferret.

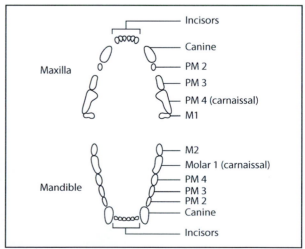

Fig. 19.2 Dental diagram. Key: M, molar; PM, premolar.

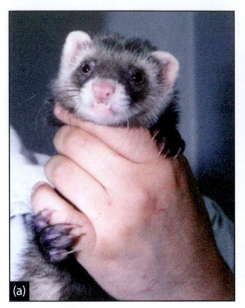

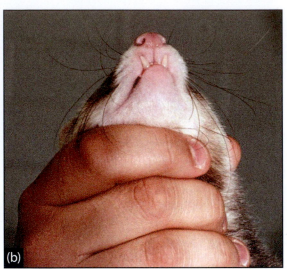

Fig. 19.3 (a, b) Prognathism.

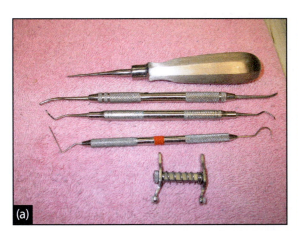

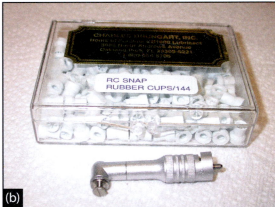

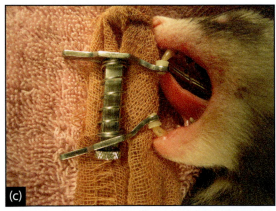

Fig. 19.4 (a) Instruments useful for ferret dental work; (b) prophy head and cups for polishing following scaling; (c) the 'Nazzy' ferret mouth gag in position.

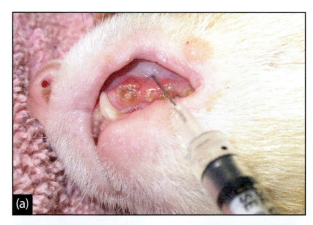

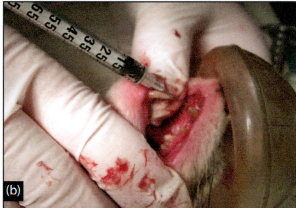

Fig. 19.5 (a) Infraorbital local anaesthesia block; **(b)** anaesthetic injected into pulp cavity.

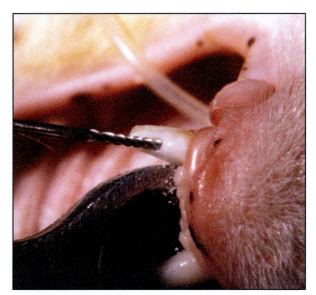

Fig. 19.6 Drill bit placed for root canal.

DENTAL PROPHYLAXIS

Cleaning of ferret teeth should be done at least annually under anaesthesia. The 'Nazzy' ferret mouth gag was designed by the author (Universal Surgical Instruments, Glen Clove, NY) for ferrets' mouths to hold them open. The Nazzy ferret mouth gag got its name from the oral measurements taken from the author's ferret, Nazzy. Deep planing of the teeth and removal of calculi can be done using a McColl's scaler that will fit under normal ferret gingivae. After gingival recess planing has been done, further removal of plaque can be achieved using an ultrasonic dental cleaning system or by further hand scaling (**Fig. 19.9**). Polishing of the teeth can be done using a prophy cup on a low-speed hand-piece with a mild abrasive polish (Zircon-F, Henry Schein, Melville, NY). After rinsing and removal of

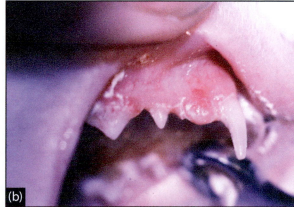

Fig. 19.7 (a, b) Extraction of retained deciduous canine tooth.

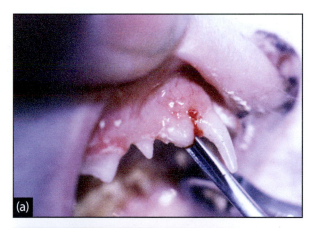

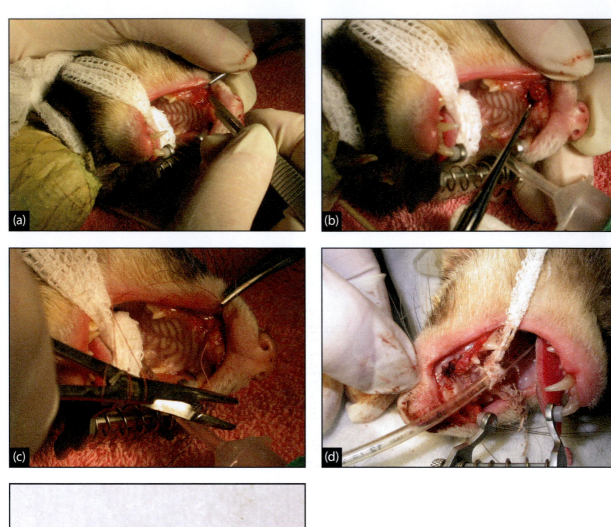

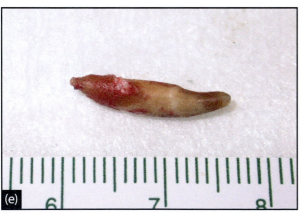

Fig. 19.8 (a) Gingivectomy; (b) the periodontal ligaments are severed and the tooth root is elevated; (c) the gingiva are sutured; (d) the mouth at the conclusion of the surgery; (e) extracted necrotic canine tooth.

debris, the teeth can be dried thoroughly and either a fluoride paste or varnish (several brands as used in dogs, Henry Schein, Melville, NY) can be applied or a sealant (Oravet, Merial, Duluth, GA) can be used.

Home dental prophylaxis

Home dental care should include the continued application of Oravet (if that was used) on a weekly basis. If teeth are not sealed, then owners should be instructed on how to brush their ferret's teeth.

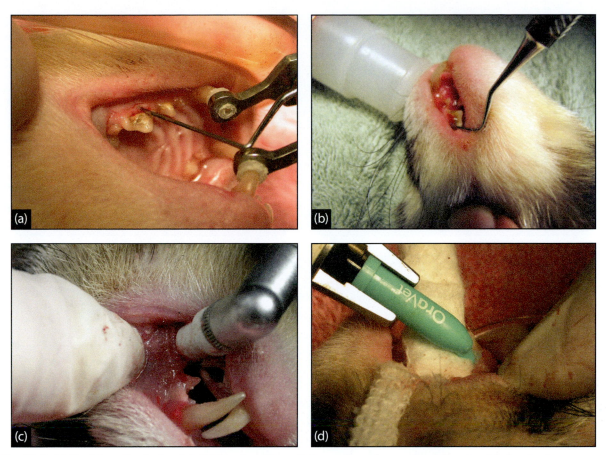

Fig. 19.9 (a) Probing gingival sulci; (b) hand scaling of the teeth – ultrasonic scaling could also be done; (c) prophy polish using a polish containing fluoride; (d) a sealant being applied to the teeth.

The author uses cotton buds and an enzymatic toothpaste (CET, Virbac, Fort Worth, TX) in either malt or poultry flavour. Most pet ferrets do not mind tooth brushing as they like the taste of the toothpaste. Following brushing, the teeth and gingiva can be 'painted' with a children's non-alcohol mouthwash on a cotton bud. Follow-up examinations should be done on a regular basis (**Fig. 19.10**).

THE DENTAL EXAMINATION

Examination of the ferret mouth is an essential part of any physical examination. If the ferret is prone to bite, a sedative may be necessary for full examination. Most pet ferrets will readily open their mouths for the examination. Teeth and gingiva can be examined using a cotton bud to elevate the lips (**Fig. 19.11**). The author photographs the teeth

before and after the procedure to give the pictures to the owner. These are a good practice builder (**Fig. 19.12**).

The author has developed a grading system to assist in determining a dental programme for each ferret. A healthy mouth is one with no gingivitis, although there may be a small amount of calculi if the ferret is over 1 year of age. No oral ulcers should be present (**Fig. 19.13**).

Stage 1: gingivitis, with inflammation of the gingiva due to plaque. Some of the plaque may be mineralised (calculus), although build-up is usually fairly minimal. The gingiva will be erythematous, and may be slightly swollen along the edge abutting the teeth. These usually do not bleed when the pockets are probed (**Fig. 19.14**).

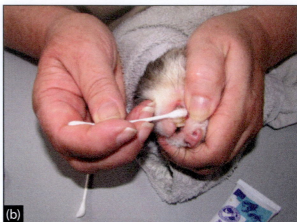

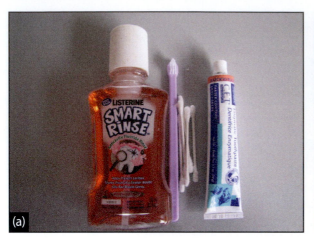

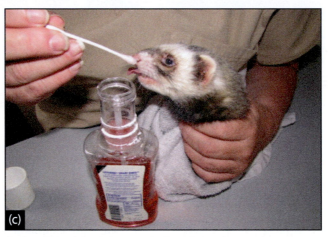

Fig. 19.10 (a) Products for home dental healthcare; (b) brushing the teeth using a cotton bud; (c) using a cotton bud dipped in the children's mouthwash for painting the teeth and gingiva.

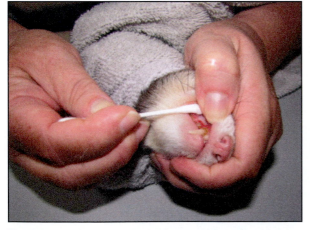

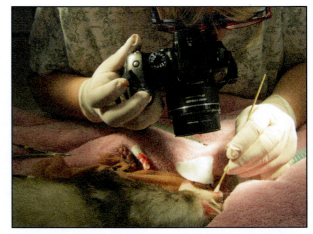

Fig. 19.11 Using a cotton bud to examine the teeth and gingiva.

Fig. 19.12 The author photographing the mouth for the dental record. (Courtesy of Vondelle McLaughlin.)

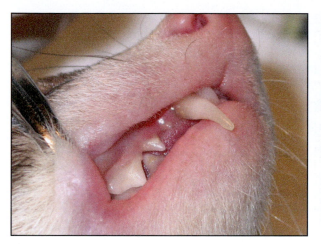

Fig. 19.13 **Normal teeth and gingiva.**

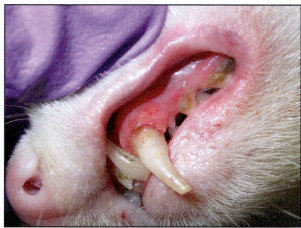

Fig. 19.14 **Stage 1 gingivitis and some calculus.**

Stage 2: early periodontitis. The gingivitis has progressed to actual infection of the gingiva, periodontal tissues and even the bone, although the teeth are still firmly attached, and on radiographs roots are still viable. There may be gingival abscesses at this point and there may be some gingival recession or periodontal pocket formation. Up to 25% of the dental attachments may have been lost. For oral examination and probing in the awake ferret at this stage, the author first applies an oral lidocaine 2% gel (lidocaine gel, Henry Schein, Melville, NY) to the gingival areas (**Fig. 19.15**).

Stage 3: moderate periodontitis. Bleeding usually occurs during dental probing and affected teeth may have up to 50% loss of attachments. There may be root exposure. Some teeth may be slightly loosened. Abscesses are frequently found around the roots and accumulations of food and debris encountered in the periodontal/gingival pockets. Most ferrets require light sedation, parenteral analgesia and topical dental anaesthetics for a full oral examination at this stage (**Fig. 19.16**).

Stage 4: advanced periodontitis. There is greater than 50% loss of attachments, and tooth roots are usually exposed due to gingival and bone recession. On radiographs, tooth roots will show the lack of attachment and often a degree of abscessation or destruction (lysis), and loss of viability. There is often blood and pus surrounding the tooth. The tooth may also

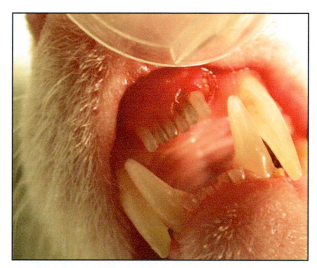

Fig. 19.15 **Stage 2 has early periodontitis and possible gingival abscesses.**

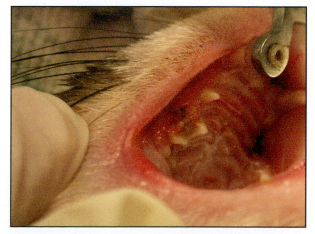

Fig. 19.16 **Stage 3 has moderate periodontitis.**

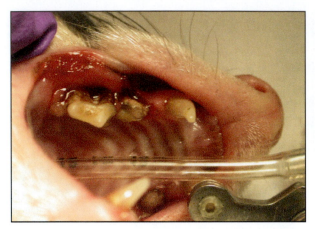

Fig. 19.17 **Stage 4 has severe periodontitis often with tooth roots exposed.**

be loose. This condition is painful and further examination requires heavy sedation, analgesia or anaesthesia. Teeth may be lost at this stage even if periodontal treatment is initiated using protocols used in dogs (including resection of gingiva, packing with an antibiotic gel, parenteral/oral antibiotics and brushing of the teeth) (**Fig. 19.17**).

DENTAL SURGERY

Endodontic procedures

Superficial pulpotomy can be done in the canine tooth presented with the tip broken off if the tooth is not discoloured (**Fig. 19.18**). This involves using a high-speed burr into the pulp a few millimetres below the exposed surface, drying and sterilising the pulp chamber with calcium hydroxide and filling with a composite as is done in other species. Local anaesthetic block is given using lidocaine 2%.

Root canal treatment is difficult in the ferret owing to their small size and the canine tooth curvature. The procedure is as in other species (**Fig. 19.6**).

Extraction

If extraction of teeth is necessary, the author advocates first locally blocking the area with lidocaine 2% (volume dependent on size of the dental area and weight of the ferret – for most teeth 0.05–0.1 mL is adequate), then gingivectomy. Incise the periodontal tissues. In some cases, it may be necessary to remove

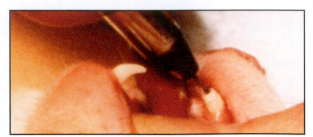

Fig. 19.18 **Drilling performing a pulpotomy.**

some alveolar bone. Once the ligamentous tissues have been severed, the tooth can be easily elevated using a fine-tipped elevator or 18 gauge needle (for the smaller teeth), and extracted often with just haemostats. If there is an open alveolus (as with the canine teeth), the cavity may be packed with a hydrostatic gel or synthetic bone matrix material (Consil Bioglass, Nutramax, Baltimore, MD). The gingiva can be sutured with 4- or 5-0 absorbable suture on a fine swaged-on taper-point needle. Suturing the gingiva encourages healing and decreases the risk of debris being introduced (**Fig. 19.19**). Analgesics, NSAIDs, and often antibiotics will be used postextraction. Owners are usually instructed on how to apply a mild chlorhexidine rinse to the sutured area twice daily for up to a 1 week as well.

DENTAL DISEASES

Dental diseases include dental abscesses, calculus, periodontal disease associated with tooth infection and/or gingival infection or inflammation, fractured teeth and teeth lost or necrotic teeth, due to a variety of disease processes including malnutrition, renal disease and neoplasia, and wear from diets or toys. While tooth resorption, caries, stomatitis and tumours are possible, these seem to be uncommon.

Abscess

Definition/overview

Abscess of a tooth may come from diseased gingiva, periodontal tissues or underlying bone. Infection may also enter the tooth from the pulp cavity if it becomes exposed due to fracture or caries (rarely seen in ferrets). Generally the tooth root is involved.

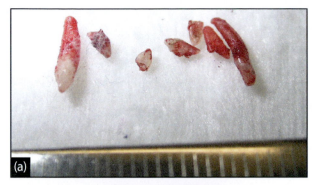

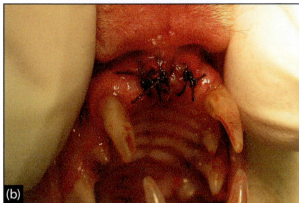

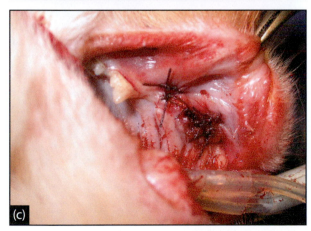

Fig. 19.19 (a) extracted teeth; (b, c) sutured gingiva following extractions.

Aetiology/pathophysiology

Abscesses may get started with trauma to an individual tooth or gingival area, or with calculus formation typically in the gingival sulcus. In many cases by the time the abscess is discovered, the tooth is no longer viable, and there is enough periodontal disease and bone loss to make root canal and tooth retention not an option. Secondary anorexia,

dehydration and weight loss may be seen if the condition is causing oral pain.

Clinical presentation

There will be exudate and swelling from the affected site. The tooth may be fractured, discoloured or loose. In many cases there will be a fistula where the root is (**Fig. 19.20**). The gingiva itself may be discoloured and regressed over the abscessed tooth. There is pain associated with this. There may be odour from the site. The ferret may also be anorexic and in some cases dehydrated and may have lost weight because of this.

Differential diagnosis

Infection may/may not be in the root, and may/may not be affecting periodontal tissue and underlying bone. Foreign body to gingival sulcus.

Diagnostic testing

Dental radiographs particularly to look at tooth roots and surrounding bone. Full probing under anaesthesia to determine extent of the abscess.

Diagnosis

Confirmation of abscess involving tooth, gingival sulcus, periodontal tissues and/or bone.

Management/treatment

If there is a tooth root abscess, theoretically a root canal could be performed but due to the size and curvature of the tooth (canine) it may not be feasible. If tooth is loose, extraction is necessary. The abscess should be drained. The tissue involved should be irrigated and flushed usually with a dilute chlorhexidine oral solution (2%). If there is a sizeable gap when the tooth is removed, it is possible to do a gingivectomy, packing of the gap with antibiotic impregnated matrix material (Gelfoam, Pfizer, NY, NY) and gingiva sutured to loosely cover the gap. This is to hold the gel in place but also to prevent food material becoming impacted in the pocket. If there is a fistula, flushing can also be through it. Parenteral broad-spectrum oral antibiotics along with an NSAID and possibly an opioid analgesic should be given. Oral swabbing with a dental rinse can be done daily to cleanse the mouth.

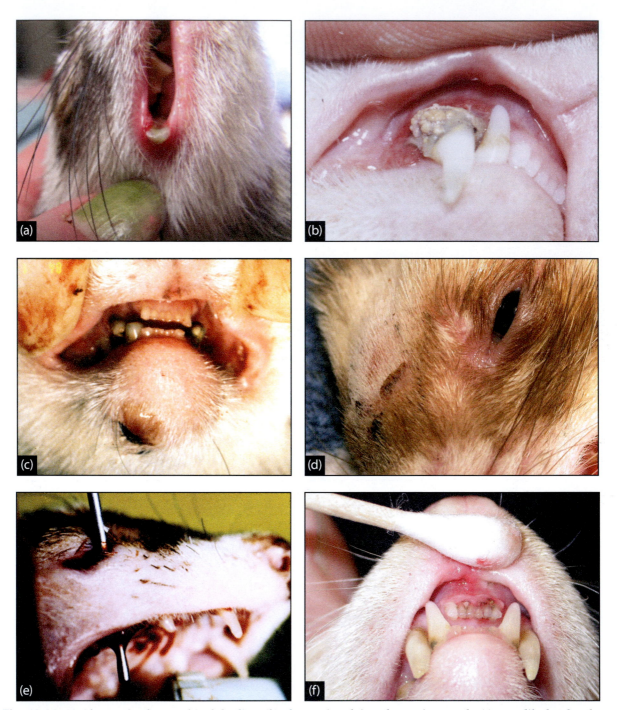

Fig. 19.20 (a) Abscess in the canthi of the lips; (b) abscess involving the canine tooth; (c) mandibular fistula from the canine tooth; (d) swelling of the face below the eye is associated with canine root abscess; (e) fistula from premolar abscess; (f) apical abscesses of the incisors. *(Continued)*

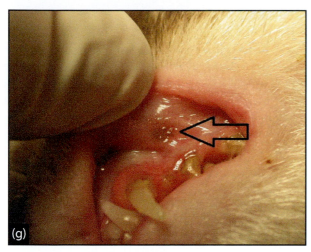

Fig. 19.20 (continued) **(g) Root abscess with fistula (arrow).**

This can be done using a cotton swab. Prognosis is good for healing of the mouth.

Calculus
Definition/overview
Calculus is defined as the mineralised build-up of plaque on tooth surfaces. It is often referred to as 'tartar'.

Aetiology/pathophysiology
Plaque is a build-up of saliva, bacteria, cellular and food debris, epithelial cells and bacterial by-products. The pH and enzyme content of the saliva and enzyme release from bacteria, as well as content of the diet and consistency of the diet, influence the degree of plaque build-up. However, plaque appears in pet ferrets whether fed kibble, canned diet or dook soup. The domestic ferret fed a processed diet appears to lack some of the dietary components that inhibit plaque build-up in wild mustelids. The conformation of the mouth itself may influence the build-up as the bite may allow pocketing of material. The author has not found studies done on the pH (particularly in periodontal and gingival sulci), and enzyme characterisation and levels. These, in combination with diet content, would aid in development of effective prophylaxis treatments.

Clinical presentation
Calculus and plaque left on tooth surfaces. It may extend into the gingival pockets where it accumulates

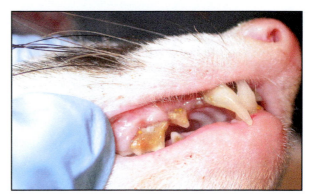

Fig. 19.21 **Build-up of calculus.**

causing gingivitis. There may be periodontitis as well, and even abscess. There may be oral odour. The gingiva and teeth may be painful. The ferret may be anorexic, dehydrated and losing weight (**Fig. 19.21**).

Differential diagnosis
Gingivitis, periodontal disease, osteomyelitis accompanying the calculus. Anorexia from other causes.

Diagnostic testing
Dental radiographs to determine health of tooth roots and gingivae. Probing gingival sulci and teeth under anaesthesia to determine degree of gingivitis. Probing may also find abscesses of the gingiva and teeth.

Diagnosis
Presence of calculus (and plaque) on the teeth.

Management/treatment
Calculus should be removed by scaling, by hand and ultrasonically. Remove necrotic or loose teeth. Fractured teeth (canines in particular) should be assessed for pulp exposure. If pulp is not exposed in a canine tooth, nothing needs to be done. If the pulp is exposed, a superficial pulpectomy ('drill and fill') can be done. All scaled teeth should be polished using a polish with fluoride. A fluoride rinse can be 'painted' onto the teeth following the polish. Prophylactic tooth brushing at home is encouraged using an enzymatic toothpaste. Twice-yearly dental cleaning under anaesthesia is recommended.

Extrusion of canine teeth

Definition/overview
As the ferret ages, the canine teeth extrude accompanied by gingival recession. There may also be bulging of the gingiva around the crown. In one study 93.7% of ferrets had this.

Aetiology/pathophysiology
This appears to be a very common occurrence and accompanies aging.

Clinical presentation
Canine tooth appears elongated with thickened area at crown. The gingiva above appears erythematous and sometimes swollen (**Fig. 19.22**). It is not painful to probing.

Differential diagnosis
Abscess, gingivitis, periodontal disease.

Diagnostic testing
Dental radiographs to look at health of the root and rule out underlying disease.

Management/treatment
Just normal dental prophylaxis. Regular home oral hygiene.

Fractured teeth

Definition/overview
The canine teeth are usually fractured, particularly at the tip. Other teeth may be fractured following extensive oral trauma.

Aetiology/pathophysiology
In one study, tooth fractures were exclusively associated with canine teeth and were found in 31.7% of all ferrets examined. Pulp exposure was confirmed in 60.0% of these canine teeth. The author feels that the maxillary canine is most affected. Pet ferrets frequently bite and pull at their cage bars when they want to get out (**Fig. 19.23**). They also fracture teeth during falls and during play when they hit walls and other obstacles.

Clinical presentation
The teeth are fractured. The pulp may/may not be exposed. The tooth may be sensitive to touch or cold (cotton bud wetted then frozen works well to touch teeth). If sensitive, the tooth may be dying. Many owners are not aware that the teeth are fractured. The tooth (teeth) may be discoloured, necrotic, and/or loose. Unless the pulp is exposed and the ferret is in pain and/or has associated dental disease with the tooth, the finding may be incidental (**Fig. 19.24**).

Differential diagnosis
None.

Diagnostic testing
Dental radiographs to assess health of the tooth root, viability of the tooth. Visual examination and probing under anaesthesia to determine if pulp is exposed.

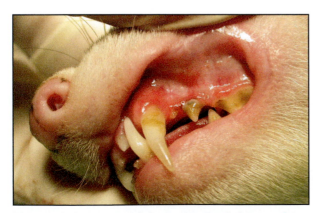

Fig. 19.22 **Extrusion of the canine teeth frequently seen in older ferrets.**

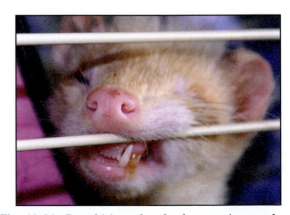

Fig. 19.23 **Cage biting often leads to canine tooth fractures. (Courtesy Vondelle McLaughlin.)**

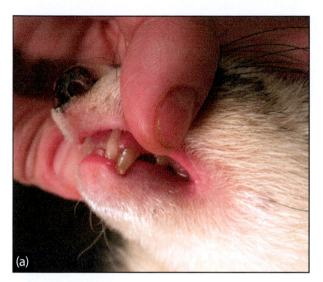

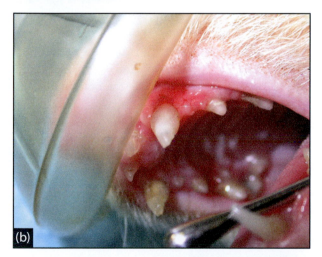

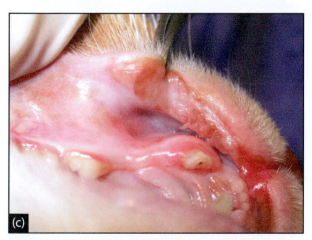

Fig. 19.24 (a) Tip fractured off, tooth is necrotic (courtesy of Vondelle McLaughlin); (b) bilateral fractured canines; (c) pulp exposed in fractured canine.

Diagnosis
Confirmation of the fracture.

Management/treatment
If presented immediately after the fracture and the pulp cavity is exposed and the tooth is still viable, a superficial pulpectomy can be done in the canine tooth. This involves using a high-speed burr into the pulp a few millimetres below the exposed surface, drying and sterilising the pulp chamber, and filling with a composite as is done in other species. The danger is in overheating the pulp cavity and destroying the pulp in the process, which will lead to eventual necrosis. The author prefers to try to preserve canine teeth if possible, particularly in young ferrets, but despite 'drilling and filling' many teeth proceed to fracture again or progress to necrosis. Parenteral antibiotics should be instigated as well as oral rinses when doing endodontic procedures. Prognosis is good if the pulp is not exposed. If the pulp is exposed, the prognosis for the long term is that the ferret will probably have to have the canine removed at some point if it becomes abscessed or necrotic.

Gingival hyperplasia
Definition/overview
Hyperplasia of the gingiva. This occurs with administration of phenytoin. It may also be associated with gingivitis.

Aetiology/pathophysiology
Phenytoin administered at therapeutic oral dosing of 40 mg/kg induces this change. This is similar to what happens in humans. It is due to a drug-induced folic acid deficiency.

Clinical presentation
Hyperplastic gingiva (**Fig. 19.25**). Ferret was being treated for seizures with phenytoin and not supplemented with folic acid in the literature report. Hyperplastic gingiva may also be seen with gingivitis that proliferates over the teeth, causing deep gingival pockets.

Differential diagnosis
Gingivitis, severe, proliferative.

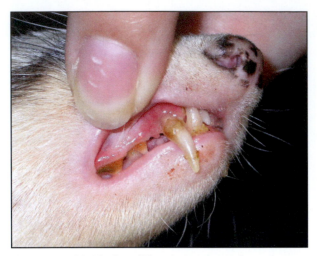

Fig. 19.25 Gingival proliferation over teeth.

Diagnostic testing
History, biopsy.

Diagnosis
History, biopsy.

Management/treatment
It is suggested that supplementation with folic acid may decrease the condition. Dosage is unknown. Oral hygiene is warranted to avoid complications of gingivitis, calculus and periodontal disease.

Gingivitis
Definition/overview
Inflammation of the gingiva. As the inflammation increases, the depth of the sulcus increases, which leads to periodontal disease. In one study, the normal gingival sulcus depth measured <0.5 mm in 87.8 % of anaesthetised ferrets being screened for dental disease. Gingivitis was defined as probing depths of >0.5 mm but <2 mm, which is also evidence of periodontal disease. Clinical evidence of periodontal disease was present in 65.3% of anaesthetised ferrets (gingivitis or probing depths >0.5 mm). Advanced periodontal disease (i.e. periodontal pockets >2 mm or stage 3 furcation exposure) was not found upon clinical examination. There is also considerable pain with both the gingivitis and the act of probing.

Aetiology/pathophysiology
Calculus and plaque left on tooth surfaces extends into the gingival pockets and accumulates, causing gingivitis. Gingivitis left unchecked, along with calculus and time, contributes to periodontal disease where the tissue destruction extends into the periodontal ligaments and the bone itself. As this process continues, infection and inflammation can involve the tooth root and abscess, with permanent damage occurring to the tooth. This is a painful process. Many ferrets become anorexic due to oral pain.

Clinical presentation
The ferret may be anorexic, losing weight or gags when eating or drinking. On oral examination, the gingiva is erythematous and swollen (**Fig. 19.26**). The gingiva may extend over the tooth surface. Calculus is present, sometimes very large amounts. There may be halitosis. Tonsils are usually swollen. There may be excess salivation, and gagging upon opening the mouth and doing the examination.

Differential diagnosis
Abscess, neoplasia. Periodontitis. Tonsillitis due to systemic disease.

Diagnostic testing
Dental radiographs to check root health, periodontal disease with bone changes.

Diagnosis
Oral examination positive for gingival inflammation.

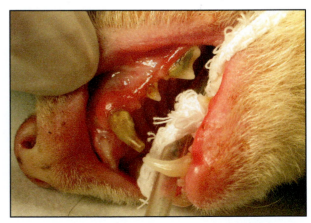

Fig. 19.26 Severe gingivitis. Note canine tooth is discoloured and presumed necrotic.

Management/treatment

Analgesic for the pain. Anaesthesia for tooth probing sulci, scaling and dental prophy polishing. Oral rinse can be used applied with a cotton bud to gingiva and teeth routinely (Listerine® Smart Rinse Berry Flavour, McNeill-PPC, Inc., Fort Washington, PA). Home brushing using an enzymatic pet toothpaste is recommended.

Malocclusion

Definition/overview

Mismatched bite. This may be due to congenital changes (such as prognathism), traumatic changes (fracture of jaw, teeth loss), or supernumerary teeth. It is most commonly seen with the mandibular second incisor teeth being caudal to the other incisors.

Aetiology/pathophysiology

Mandibular second incisor teeth being caudal to the other incisors may be a congenital change to the eruption of the teeth. Unknown aetiology. Prognathism is probably congenital and possibly hereditary (**Fig. 19.27**). Trauma to the jaw and mouth may result in a malocclusive bite pattern. It is also possible that loss of a tooth (teeth) may result in malocclusion as well.

Clinical presentation

The malocclusive incisors are an incidental finding and are very common (**Fig. 19.28**). Prognathism is distinctive. Other changes are found on oral/dental examination and are probably asymptomatic or incidental unless there is trauma such as jaw fracture. Acute trauma will result in pain and possible haemorrhage from the mouth and/or individual teeth.

Differential diagnosis

Chronic changes from previous trauma.

Diagnostic testing

Radiographs including dental films, oral examination.

Diagnosis

Confirmation via visual and radiograph examination.

Management/treatment

Jaw fractures should be treated as they are in other species. If teeth are loose or haemorrhaging, extraction needs to be done. Analgesics for the pain. Prognathism and mandibular second incisor malocclusion do not need treatment. Additional dental disease should be addressed, particularly if the malocclusion has resulted in abnormal positioning of the teeth and lips, with accompanying abscessation (**Fig. 19.28**).

Periodontal disease

Definition/overview

The periodontal ligament is compromised and inflammation/infection usually extends into the periodontal tissues and deeper to the bone, causing

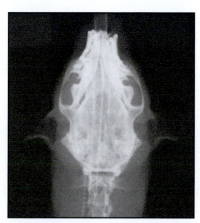

Fig. 19.27 **DV radiograph of ferret with congenital malformation of the mandible and maxilla resulting in an abnormal dental arcade.**

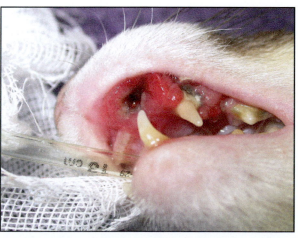

Fig. 19.28 **Malocclusion resulting in abnormal tooth positioning into gingiva and lips, resulting in abscesses.**

an osteomyelitis. The periodontal pocket will be >2 mm. Periodontitis is present. The author uses the grading system as listed above.

Aetiology/pathophysiology

Usually the condition starts with calculus build-up on the tooth surface. Gingivitis progresses and the inflammation/infection extends into the sulcus, then deepens into the periodontal tissues. If the ligament is compromised, the tooth will become loose. The tooth root itself may become exposed (**Fig. 19.29**). Osteomyelitis develops. It may involve more than one tooth. This is a painful condition.

Clinical presentation

There will usually be calculus and gingivitis present. The pockets will be deep when probed under anaesthesia. The tooth (teeth) may be loose. The ferret may be anorexic due to oral pain. The ferret may gag and have excess salivation. Tonsillitis may be present.

Differential diagnosis

Abscess, neoplasia. Tonsillitis due to systemic disease.

Diagnostic testing

Probing under anaesthesia. Dental radiographs to look at the periodontal tissue and bone.

Diagnosis

Presence of periodontal lesions. Osteomyelitis is frequently present as well.

Management/treatment

Scaling of teeth. If gingival tissue is covering teeth, laser or incise the excess tissue back to normal sulci depth. The sulci can be treated directly with instillation of a dental antibiotic as used in dogs and cats. If roots of a tooth are exposed and the tooth is loose, extraction is usually necessary. Gingivectomy for extraction; pack the gap with gelfoam impregnated with a broad-spectrum antibiotic and suture gingiva. Loose teeth unfortunately usually are extracted; however, just a very minor movement may tighten back up with treatment of the periodontal disease. Parenteral antibiotics such as amoxicillin and NSAIDs such as meloxicam are used. Daily swabbing of the mouth with an oral rinse (Listerine® Smart Rinse Berry

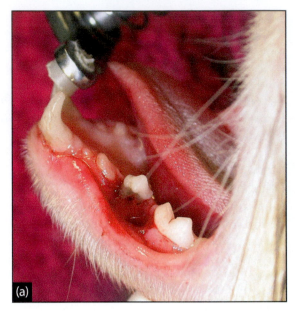

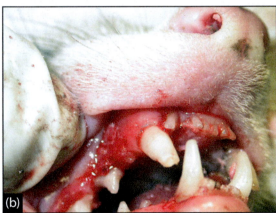

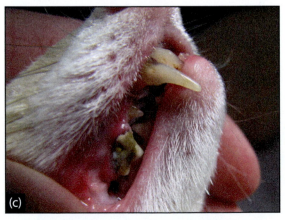

Fig. 19.29 **(a) Exposure of mandibular PM3 roots; (b) exposure of maxillary PM3 roots; (c) heavy calculus and abscess, retraction of gingiva with root exposure of maxillary PM4.**

Flavour, McNeill-PPC, Inc., Fort Washington, PA) will also aid healing. Gingival massage with the cotton bud helps to heal the gingiva. Ferrets should routinely have dental cleaning, which will help prevent further disease.

Tooth loss

Definition/overview
Absence of a tooth.

Aetiology/pathophysiology
A tooth may never have erupted such as when mandibular M2 is missing, congenitally. There may be a history of trauma or dental disease. It may be due to a variety of disease processes including malnutrition, renal disease or neoplasia.

Clinical presentation
There are missing teeth. There may be concurrent dental and/or systemic disease. It may be an incidental finding at the examination (**Fig. 19.30**).

Differential diagnosis
Oral or systemic disease involved with tooth loss.

Diagnostic testing
Thorough oral examination, dental radiographs (will determine if tooth root is still present for example), blood work, work-up for systemic disease.

Diagnosis
Lack of the tooth.

Management/treatment
If there is a retained root, the root should be extracted as it may become a nidus for infection/osteomyelitis. Presence of dental disease should be addressed as listed above. Systemic disease should be addressed per aetiology.

Tooth necrosis

Definition/overview
Necrotic 'dead' tooth. The nerve and pulp are no longer viable. The tooth is usually discoloured brown or is translucent.

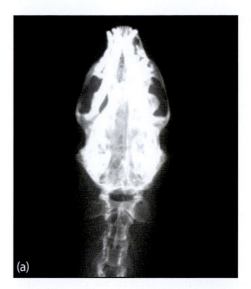

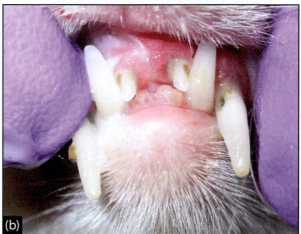

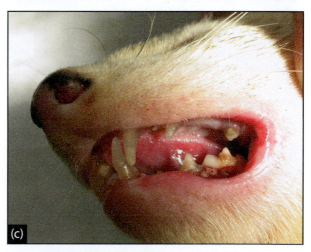

Fig. 19.30 (a) DV radiograph showing missing left mandibular canine; (b) missing incisors; (c) missing maxillary premolars.

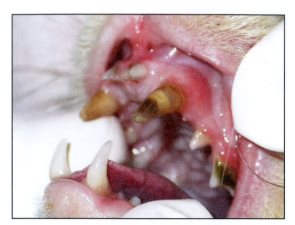

Fig. 19.31 **Necrotic maxillary canine teeth.**

Aetiology/pathophysiology
This is frequently seen in the canine tooth that has had a fractured tip or trauma. Tooth death can also be from abscess or periodontitis, or itself may be a nidus for infection and periodontitis. History of trauma to the teeth is the usual case.

Clinical presentation
Usually incidental finding on examination. Tooth is discoloured (**Fig. 19.31**). Owner may not have even noticed. Usually is not painful. There may be other dental disease present.

Differential diagnosis
None.

Diagnostic testing
Dental radiographs to look at viability of root.

Management/treatment
Concurrent dental disease should be addressed. If the tooth is loose it should be extracted. If the tooth is quiescent, not loose, not painful and there is no abscess associated with it, extraction may not be necessary. Frequent dental examinations should be done to ensure the status does not change.

ORAL DISORDERS

Cleft palate, cleft lip
Definition
Palate and lip malformation – did not fuse in development.

Aetiology/pathophysiology
Congenital defect. Unknown if it may be hereditary.

Clinical presentation
Open lip area and palate appears split. There may be secondary abscessation due to food entering the cleft. Severe cleft palate makes nursing difficult – there may be milk in the nasal cavity.

Differential diagnosis
None.

Diagnostic testing
Radiographs may show the extent of the bone deformation and if there is interference with the maxillary teeth roots.

Diagnosis
Presence of the split.

Management/treatment
Surgery to close the tissues as in other animals.

Oral neoplasia
Definition/overview
Primary tumours of the oral cavity or secondary to tumours of the head such as osteoma.

Aetiology/pathophysiology
Tissue source may be any dental tissue including gingiva, periodontal structures, bone, tooth. Squamous cell carcinoma, osteoma and lymphoma are the most common. Tumours can be benign such as an epulis, or malignant.

Clinical presentation
Various swellings and proliferations involving the oral cavity (**Fig. 19.32**). Secondary abscessation may be present along with compromised dental structures. The teeth may be loose.

Differential diagnosis
Abscess.

Diagnostic testing
Biopsy, radiographs.

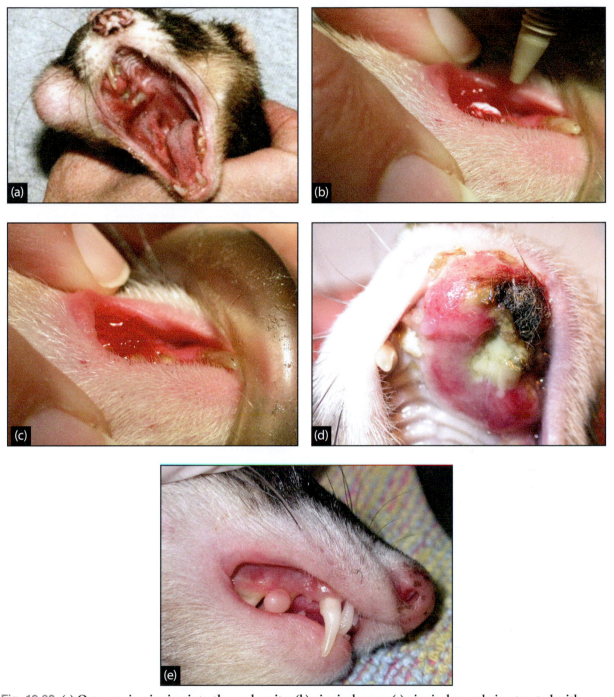

Fig. 19.32 (a) Osteoma impinging into the oral cavity; (b) gingival mass; (c) gingival mass being treated with cryosurgery; (d) mass, determined to be squamous cell carcinoma; (e) small mass not histologically typed, removed with radiosurgery. *(Continued)*

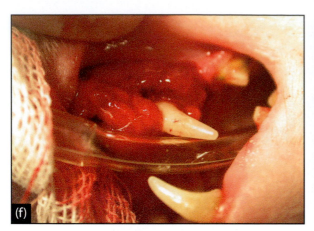
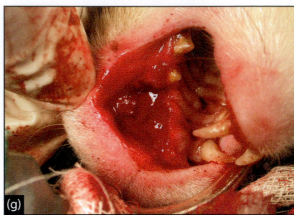

Fig. 19.32 (continued) **(f)** Large gingival mass; **(g)** surgical excision of mass; this required removal of the canine tooth. It did not reoccur. No histopathology was done.

Diagnosis
Confirmation of neoplasia on histopathology, radiographs

Management/treatment
If the mass is resectable, surgery is indicated. Underlying dental structures and teeth may be removed along with the mass if possible. Depending on the type of neoplasia, prognosis is varied.

Oral ulcers
Definition/overview
Ulcers of the mucosa anywhere in the mouth but most commonly on the buccal mucosa or hard palate (**Fig. 19.33**).

Aetiology/pathophysiology
There is usually a history of stress or systemic disease such as renal disease or lymphoma. They may also be present with dental disease. Although they resemble herpesviral ulcers in other species, no virus as yet been found. Oral ulceration has been seen with electrocution. The ulcers are usually painful. There may be concurrent tonsillitis.

Clinical presentation
Visible ulceration within the oral category (**Fig. 19.33**). Often there is anorexia, gagging, hypersalivation and bruxism, probably due to pain. Dental disease may be seen. Systemic disease such as renal disease, lymphoma or other neoplasia may be present.

Differential diagnosis
Ulceration due to a disease process rather than strictly an oral cause. History of stress.

Diagnostic testing
Full work-up including blood work, urinalysis, radiographs, dental examination.

Diagnosis
Presence of the ulcer.

Management/treatment
Direct soothing of the oral ulcer can be done by using sucralfate liquid and administration of an analgesic. Treatment should address the underlying cause of the ulcer whether local (dental) or systemic. A broad-spectrum oral antibiotic may help to prevent secondary bacterial infection.

Salivary microliths
Definition/overview
Salivary microliths are small concretions of mineral usually in the parotid salivary gland.

Aetiology/pathophysiology
The parotid gland produces secretions rich in calcium. The glands contain pockets of inefficient secretion that may lead to microlithiasis. They may be incidental but can reduce flow and allow ascending bacteria to infect the gland, leading to inflammation. Uncomplicated microliths

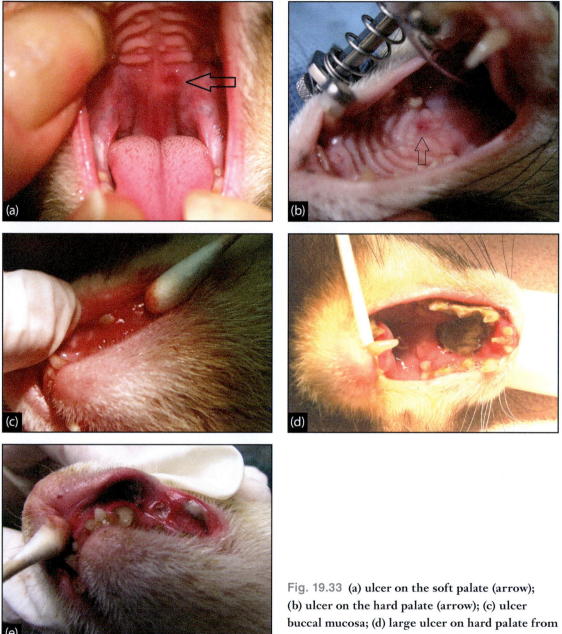

Fig. 19.33 (a) ulcer on the soft palate (arrow); (b) ulcer on the hard palate (arrow); (c) ulcer buccal mucosa; (d) large ulcer on hard palate from a burn; (e) multiple ulcers and abscessation.

are found fairly frequently. One study showed 5 out of 7 ferrets had them with no problems. It is not clear if they contribute to mucocele development.

Clinical presentation

Usually are asymptomatic and can be unilateral or bilateral. May just be found on radiographs.

Differential diagnosis

Neoplasia with small areas of calcification.

Diagnostic testing

Radiographs.

Diagnosis

Presence in the parotid gland.

Management/treatment

As these rarely cause a problem, they do not need treatment unless the gland becomes infected or forms a mucocele. Then treat as below. Infection without mucocele may clear with broad-spectrum antibiotic therapy.

Salivary mucocele

Definition/overview

Damage to one of the five paired salivary glands leads to leakage of saliva into surrounding tissue. There will be swelling in the affected area.

Aetiology/pathophysiology

Swelling is the first indication of the problem. Damage can be due to trauma to the duct openings by other oral pathology or trauma to the glands themselves.

Clinical presentation

Swelling in the jaw area and neck. On palpation the swelling may be mildly fluctuant.

Differential diagnosis

Neoplasia, lymphadenopathy, abscess.

Diagnostic testing

Aspiration with cytology, radiographs, contrast agent into the mass to show its extent.

Diagnosis

Fluid is acellular with debris and occasional red blood cells. The fluid resembles thickened saliva. Radiographs with contrast media determine which salivary gland is causing the mucocele.

Management/treatment

Surgery is required to make a linear or large circular incision in the medial aspect of the mucocele. The gland is then marsupialised into the oral cavity. If the incision is too small, the mucocele will probably reoccur. In many cases it requires removal of the gland itself.

Tonsillitis

Definition/overview

Inflammation of the tonsils.

Aetiology/pathophysiology

Infection or inflammation in the oral cavity. This includes *Streptococcus B* infection, which can be zoonotic. Tonsillitis has also been noted with upper respiratory disease such as influenza. Systemic lymphoma may also involve the tonsils, which will then be enlarged rather than truly inflamed, although on oral visual examination the difference is difficult to discern.

Clinical presentation

Swelling and erythema of tonsils beyond their crypts. There may be excessive salivation, gagging and difficulty swallowing in severe cases.

Differential diagnosis

Lymphoma, upper respiratory infection, bacterial infection.

Diagnostic testing

Throat swab for *Streptococcus*. Blood work, dental radiographs, scout radiographs, urinalysis to rule out systemic disease. If warranted, ultrasonography of abdomen and heart may be added to the work-up.

Diagnosis

Presence of tonsil inflammation, with tonsils protruding from their crypts.

Management/treatment

Treat the source of the inflammation. If infection including bacterial upper respiratory infection, broad-spectrum oral antibiotics may resolve it. Treat dental disease if present. If lymphoma, parenteral lymphoma protocols may be tried (see Chapter 16). If influenza, symptomatic treatment only to alleviate discomfort such as an NSAID along with sucralfate orally.

DISORDERS OF THE RESPIRATORY SYSTEM

*Jenna Richardson and
David Perpiñán*

ANATOMY AND PHYSIOLOGY REVIEW

Refer to Chapter 3. Ferrets have a relatively short nasal cavity that leads to the nasopharyngeal opening at the nasopharynx. The trachea consists of 60–70 C-shaped cartilages and extends proximally from the larynx to the bifurcation of the bronchi distally.

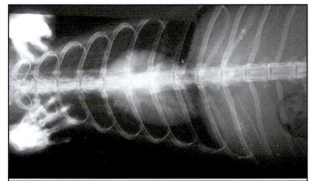
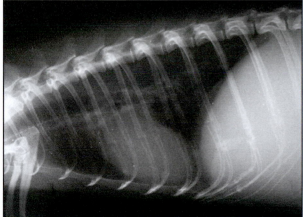

Fig. 20.1 Ventrodorsal (top) and lateral (bottom) radiographs of a healthy ferret showing long thoracic cavity in proportion to body size.

The mediastinal inlet is naturally very narrow due to the reduced length of the first ribs.

The lung field in ferrets extends as far caudal as the 10th/11th intercostal space. The lung volume is relatively large in relation to bodyweight, exceeding the predicted lung volume by 297% (**Fig. 20.1**). This high total lung capacity has made ferrets the subject of research into human respiratory conditions. Anatomically, ferret and human lungs share similarities, both containing excess submucosal glands in the bronchial wall and lacking sialic acid.

The left lung contains cranial and caudal lobes, while the right one is divided into four lobes (cranial, middle, caudal and accessory). The lungs are orientated laterally and dorsally around the heart. The normal respiration rate in a healthy ferret is 33–36 breaths per minute.

EVALUATION OF THE RESPIRATORY SYSTEM

A respiratory rate should ideally be obtained before the physical examination begins. The auscultation of the chest should be performed in quadrants, with dorsal and ventral sections on each side. The auscultation of the trachea may help to differentiate between upper and lower respiratory tract disease. Abnormal findings include wheezes, crackles and absent sounds. The location of respiratory sounds should also be noted. Percussion of the chest is useful with solid lung audibly duller. This, along with reduced chest compliance, can be suggestive of neoplasia, abscess formation or consolidation. A checklist for respiration evaluation is shown in *Box 20.1*.

<table>
</table>

Box 20.1 **Evaluating respiratory rate and pattern**

- Is the breathing excessively noisy? If so, can it be differentiated between the upper or lower respiratory tract?
- Is there increased effort for inspiration or expiration?
- Is there an abdominal component to the breathing?
- Is there any nasal discharge present?
- Has any coughing been noted?

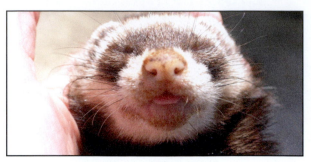

Fig. 20.2 **Conjunctivitis and photophobia in a ferret with canine distemper. (Courtesy of Vondelle McLaughlin.)**

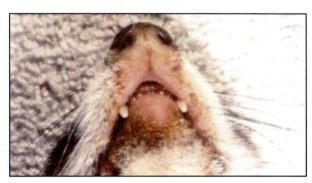

Fig. 20.3 **Chin rash in a ferret with canine distemper.**

CANINE DISTEMPER

Definition/overview

Acute viral disease affecting mainly respiratory system, nervous system and skin. It produces severe symptomatology with high mortality.

Aetiology/pathophysiology

Canine distemper virus (CDV) is an RNA virus from the genus *Morbillivirus* in the family Paramyxoviridae. The severity of the disease depends on the viral strain and immunocompetence of the host. Some strains produce neurological disease with high mortality rates while others only produce pneumonia with lower death rates. Transmission occurs by aerosol or contact with fluids and exudates containing the virus. Close contact between affected and susceptible animals is necessary due to the relative fragility of CDV in the environment. The virus replicates rapidly in multiple organs and viraemia persists until the virus is neutralised by antibodies or the ferret dies. There may be subclinically infected ferrets that shed virus for a period of time.

Clinical presentation

Initial clinical signs include anorexia, inability to gain weight in growing animals, pyrexia, photophobia (semiclosed eyes) (**Fig. 20.2**), lethargy (increase in sleeping times), and respiratory signs (serous nasal discharge, sneezing, coughing, dyspnoea). An erythematous, pruritic rash appears on the chin and eventually spreads to the inguinal area (**Figs 20.3, 20.4**). Generalised pruritus, particularly in the dorsal cervical and interscapular areas, and generalised desquamation with progression to foci of hyperkeratosis (small

scabs) occur inconsistently and usually in the mid–late course of the disease. There may be 'segmenting' of the fur (**Fig. 20.5**). Pasty faeces and soiled perineal area can be seen occasionally (**Fig. 20.6**). There may be a slight distention of the rectum and pigmentation around the anus resembling a 'ring' (**Fig. 20.7**). The oculonasal exudate becomes mucopurulent and develops into brown, encrusted material surrounding the lips, nose, chin and eye (**Fig. 20.8**); the eyelids usually stick shut. Hyperkeratosis of the footpads occurs inconsistently (**Fig. 20.9**). Pneumonia (complicated sometimes with bacterial infections) and/ or neurological signs (myoclonus, paresis, muscular tremors, convulsions and coma prior to death) can be seen with some strains. Even in ferrets infected with neurotropic strains, neurological signs may not be seen if death occurs early in the course of the disease (see Chapter 18).

Variability in clinical signs, as well as other characteristics of the disease (incubation period, duration of disease, etc.), are due to the type of strain, infective dose, route of infection and immune status

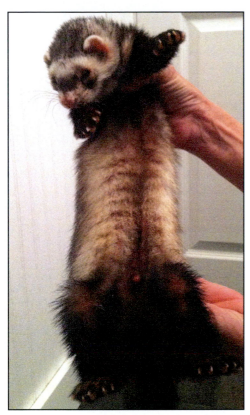

Fig. 20.4 Rash extending on trunk with canine distemper. (Courtesy of Vondelle McLaughlin.)

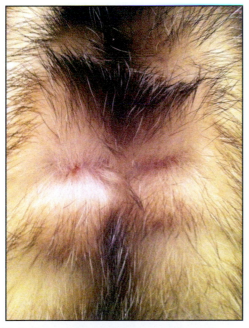

Fig. 20.5 'Segmenting' of the fur with canine distemper. (Courtesy of Vondelle McLaughlin.)

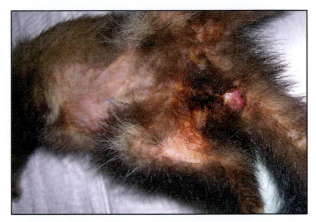

Fig. 20.6 Soiled perineal area with canine distemper. (Courtesy of Vondelle McLaughlin.)

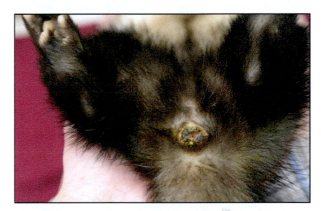

Fig. 20.7 Distention of rectum with pigmentation around the anus with canine distemper. (Courtesy of Vondelle McLaughlin.)

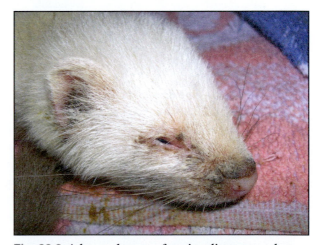

Fig. 20.8 Advanced stage of canine distemper where the initial inflammation around eyes, nose and mouth progresses into encrusted material.

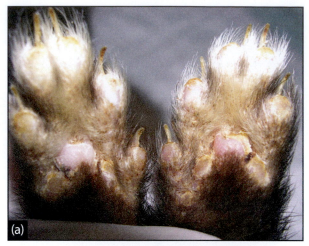

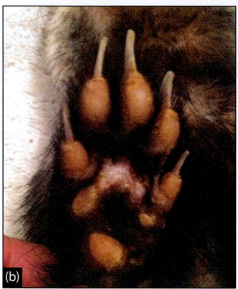

Fig. 20.9 (a, b) Hyperkeratosis of footpads.
(b, courtesy of Vondelle McLaughlin.)

periods and duration of disease than experimental infections with very pathogenic strains.

Disease outcome is also affected by factors such as age and immune status of the ferret, strain of virus etc. The mortality of ferrets with clinical signs of CD may be high, approaching 100% in some outbreaks, but some animals can recover from the disease, particularly those infected with low pathogenic strains and treated early in the course of the disease. Once clinical signs are severe, recovery is not usually possible. Ferrets may die or be euthanased based on severe neurological, respiratory and/or dermatological problems. It is unknown whether it is possible for ferrets to get infected with CDV and not develop disease.

Differential diagnosis

Clinical signs and findings in ferrets with CD are very characteristic (particularly when neurological, respiratory and/or dermatological signs are combined), but the clinician may occasionally be puzzled by observing a disease that does not follow exactly the characteristics described in many articles and books. This is due to the huge body of information available on experimental infections with very pathogenic strains and the fact that naturally occurring distemper in ferrets (generally caused by less pathogenic strains) are uncommonly reported in the literature.

Influenza is common in ferrets and can cause respiratory disease that initially resembles the respiratory signs of CD, but CD progresses faster and the ferret quickly develops more severe clinical signs. Sarcoptic and demodectic mange are rare conditions in ferrets, but could produce pruritic and crusting dermatitis, although the distribution of lesions in ferrets with CD (mainly face, perineal area and paws) is very characteristic. Differential diagnoses for neurological signs include Aleutian disease, rabies, ferret systemic coronavirus infection, botulism, brain tumours, toxicoses, fungal infections of the brain (cryptococcosis, blastomycosis) and toxoplasmosis.

Diagnostic testing

Clinical examination of ferrets with CD may show tachypnoea and increased lung sounds, splenomegaly on palpation (an unspecific indicator of disease in

of the ferret. As a general rule, experimental infections published in scientific articles cause more acute death with neurological signs, while common cases seen in practice may not be as severe and may develop a stronger respiratory component. Atypical cases of canine distemper (CD) have also been described in ferrets with only dermatological problems or in ferrets with disease induced by vaccination. Incubation periods range from 4 to 56 days, and duration of the disease can range from 5 to 35 days or even longer in atypical cases. As a general rule, clinical cases tend to have longer incubation ferrets) and an inconsistent rise in rectal temperature up to 41°C (more common in the early stages of disease). Lung changes compatible with pneumonia can be observed on radiography, and mild non-regenerative anaemia can be seen on blood analysis. Serology can be used to identify CD in an outbreak, and can be used to diagnose recovery and clearance. Detection of antigen on conjunctival, tonsillar or respiratory samples may be performed using immunofluorescent antibody or RT-PCR; immunochemistry, *in situ* hybridisation or viral isolation are less commonly used. Postmortem diagnosis can be performed using histopathology (ideal samples are lung, skin, brain, bladder) to detect characteristic lesions and inclusion bodies, although additional detection of antigen can also be performed on histological samples.

Diagnosis

Diagnosis should be based on clinical history, vaccination status, clinical signs and findings and fluorescent antibody labelling (or RT-PCR) of conjunctival smears or respiratory secretions.

Management/treatment

Treatment may be successful in some situations, particularly in ferrets infected with low pathogenicity strains and when treatment is applied very early in the course of disease. However, animals with severe clinical signs are unlikely to recover. Even with treatment, prognosis should be considered poor in most cases, and any treatment should only be started after a thorough discussion with owners. Therapy is listed in *Box 20.2*.

Therapy should include antibiotics as secondary bacterial pneumonias are common. The use of vitamins A and C may be beneficial to treat ferrets with distemper, although there is more scientific evidence supporting the use of vitamin A over the use of vitamin C. Hyperimmune serum against CD can also be useful, but it is not easily available commercially; alternatively, serum from a healthy and appropriately vaccinated ferret can be used. Nutritional and symptomatic treatment may include the use of easily digestible diets, fluid therapy, antipruritic drugs, anti-inflammatory drugs, bronchodilators, etc. Vaccination can be used as a treatment, but is required to be given a few hours after infection in order to be

Box 20.2 Treatments for canine distemper

- Broad-spectrum antibiotics, ideally based on culture and sensitivity of discharges, in general use: amoxicillin/clavulanate (12.5 mg/kg PO q12h).
- Vitamin A: 50,000 IU (15 mg) of retinol palmitate IM q24h (SID) × 2 days.
- Vitamin C: 250 mg IV q24h × 3 days.
- Hyperimmune serum against CDV: 1 mL IV.
- Vaccination (only effective if done early after infection).
- Interferon (60–120 units SC q24h).
- Meloxicam (0.2 mg/kg PO q24h).
- Famotidine (2.5 mg/ferret SC q24h).
- Diphenhydramine (0.5–2 mg/kg IM, IV, PO q8–12 prn).
- Buprenorphine (0.01–0.5 mg/kg IV, IM, SC q8–12h) if painful.
- Supportive and symptomatic treatment (nutritional support, fluid therapy, bronchodilators).

Key: IM, intramuscular; IV, intravenous; PO, per os; SC, subcutaneous; SID, once daily.

effective. As a general rule, large doses of vaccinal virus are necessary and this treatment is not effective once more than 48 hours have elapsed between infection and vaccination.

Prevention is achieved by vaccination (see Chapter 9) and avoidance of contact with potential carriers of the disease (dogs, other ferrets, wildlife).

INFLUENZA

Definition/overview

Viral infection frequently causing mild respiratory disease in ferrets. It is a zoonotic disease.

Aetiology/pathophysiology

Influenza viruses are RNA viruses in the family Orthomyxoviridae. Influenza viruses have a significant global importance as they can cause serious disease in poultry and humans. Influenza can be transmitted from humans to ferrets and from ferrets to humans, and clinical history may reveal contact with an infected person a few days before illness was noted in the ferret. Transmission usually occurs by aerosol droplets. Ferrets are very susceptible to human influenza owing to a lack of sialic acid in lung mucus.

Clinical presentation

The characteristics of the disease depend on factors such as age of the ferret, virus strains and presence of secondary infections. Clinical signs appear within 48 hours of exposure and include sneezing and serous oculonasal secretion for 3–5 days. Ferrets recover after that period if there are no complications. Morbidity is high but mortality is low. Complicated cases may occur in young or immunocompromised ferrets, or when the strain involved is highly pathogenic. Strains that are highly pathogenic for humans tend to be highly pathogenic for ferrets. Severe and complicated cases may develop disease of the lower respiratory system and show lethargy, dyspnoea, conjunctivitis, photophobia, otitis, periocular and perinasal dermatitis and neurological symptoms such as ataxia, hindlimb paresis and torticollis.

Differential diagnosis

Differential diagnoses should include conditions causing pneumonias such as canine distemper or bacterial pneumonias.

Diagnostic testing

Physical examination of affected ferrets may show temporal fever and signs of mild upper respiratory tract infection. Serology is usually unrewarding as antibody production starts at the time the ferret is recovering from infection. Detection of antigen can be done by RT-PCR or virus isolation, and tests are easily available in many laboratories due to the importance of the disease in humans. Histopathology and immunohistochemistry are tools available for the postmortem diagnosis of influenza in ferrets.

Diagnosis

Diagnosis is based on clinical history, clinical signs and findings and a positive result on antigen detection.

Management/treatment

The disease is generally mild and animals may recover with or without treatment. Treatment may include antibiotics, supportive feeding or symptomatic treatment with decongestants, bronchodilators, etc. Highly pathogenic strains may need more aggressive treatment. Several antiviral drugs against influenza infection have been tested in ferrets, including oseltamivir (Tamiflu®), zanamivir (Relenza®), cianovirin N and others. As a general rule, in order to see a positive effect from these drugs they should be administered at the time of (or soon after) infection (i.e. before the ferret starts showing clinical signs), and therefore their utility in clinical practice is limited.

Contact with infected humans or ferrets should be avoided in order to prevent the disease. Ferrets are also susceptible to influenza viruses of birds and pigs, but contact with these species is less common. The virus is easily inactivated by thorough cleaning and removal of organic matter, followed by the application of common disinfectants, such as bleach, quaternary ammonium compounds, etc. Heat, ultraviolet light and drying also reduce the amount of virus in the environment. Vaccines used for humans are considered safe and effective in ferrets, but vaccination is generally unwarranted as the disease is mild and there is great antigenic variation. It is recommended that owners and others working with ferrets be immunised against influenza to decrease the potential of transmission to the ferret.

BACTERIAL PNEUMONIA

Definition/overview

Bacterial pneumonia is relatively uncommon in ferrets, usually occurring secondary to an underlying disease or process (e.g. viral infection, aspiration pneumonia, etc). It can be characterised by a suppurative inflammation affecting the bronchial tree and/or lung lobes.

Aetiology/pathophysiology

Bacterial infection can occur via inhalation, aspiration or by haematogenous spread. Severity of disease depends on the pathogen implicated and its rate of multiplication. Immunocompromised animals are at greatest risk of developing a bacterial pneumonia. Primary respiratory pathogens affecting ferrets include *Streptococcus zooepidemicus*, *Mycobacterium* spp. and gram-negative bacteria such as *Klebsiella pneumonia*, *Listeria monocytogenes*, *Bordetella bronchiseptica* and *Escherichia coli*.

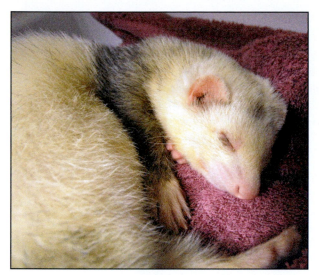

Fig. 20.10 Initial signs of bacterial pneumonia can often be non-specific, with patients presenting subdued.

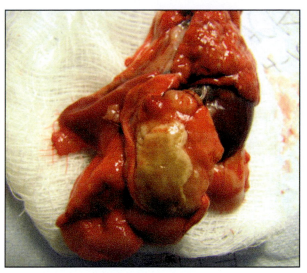

Fig. 20.11 Bacterial pulmonary abscess. (Courtesy of Cathy Johnson-Delaney.)

Clinical presentation

Initially, patients may present with non-specific signs such as lethargy, weight loss, weakness, anorexia and pyrexia (**Fig. 20.10**). In severe cases, clinical signs of respiratory distress can occur and the ferret can show nasal discharge, tachypnoea, dyspnoea, cough and increased respiratory effort. In severe cases cyanotic mucous membranes may be observed and death can result.

Differential diagnosis

Viral pneumonia, e.g. canine distemper virus and influenza virus; fungal pneumonia, e.g. coccidiodomycosis, blastomycosis, histoplasmosis, cryptococcosis; neoplasia, e.g. mediastinal lymphoma, lung metastasis from a primary neoplasia; pleural effusion; congestive heart failure; pulmonary abscessation (**Fig. 20.11**).

Diagnostic testing

The possibility of contact with other ferrets or with humans infected with influenza should be investigated. Thoracic auscultation is always a useful diagnostic aid for the detection of some respiratory diseases. Thoracic radiography can show increase in the alveolar/interstitial pattern and the presence of air bronchograms. Lateral and ventrodorsal views can be performed under manual restraint, sedation or anaesthesia. When the patient may be too compromised for restraint or anaesthesia, sternal recumbency may produce dorsoventral (vertical beam) and lateral (horizontal beam) views of the thorax. When availability and cost are not a problem, a CT scan can provide a superior form of imaging the respiratory tract.

Bronchoalveolar lavage (BAL) performed under general anaesthesia is extremely useful to obtain samples for cytological and microbiological analyses (see *Table 20.4* for procedure). Due to the rare occurrence of primary bacterial pneumonias in ferrets, BAL may be a good starting point when lung pathology is suspected; in addition, it is also indicated in cases that fail to respond to medical therapy or in those situations where multiple ferrets are displaying clinical signs. Alternatively, when an area of consolidation is identified on imaging, a fine needle aspirate of the lung (under ultrasound guidance) can be performed; care should be taken to avoid inducing a pneumothorax.

Diagnosis

Diagnosis is made based on clinical signs and findings and the isolation of pathogenic bacteria from BAL. Underlying causes of pneumonia (such as distemper or influenza) should always be investigated.

Management/treatment

The primary aim of treatment is to stabilise the patient while providing appropriate antibiotic therapy.

Table 20.1	**Medications used for nebulisation**	
	NEBULISED DRUG	**DILUTION**
Antibiotics	Doxycycline	200 mg in 15 mL saline
	F10 solution	5 mL of F10 solution (1:250 dilution in water)
	Enrofloxacin	100 mg in 10 mL saline
	Gentamicin	50 mg in 10 mL saline
	Tylosin	100 mg in 10 mL saline
Mucolytics	Acetylcysteine	200 mg in 10 mL sterile water
	Bromhexine	1.5 mg in 10 mL saline

Broad-spectrum antibiotics including anaerobic coverage are recommended, such as a combination of amoxicillin/clavulanic acid and enrofloxacin. Supportive care should include fluid therapy and nutritional supplements.

Oxygen therapy should be provided to patients displaying signs of respiratory distress or hypoxia. Nebulisation with antibiotics and/or mucolytics for 10–15 minutes (q24h [SID] or q12h [BID]) can be a useful adjunct to medical therapy (*Table 20.1*). The drugs are diluted in saline and dispersed into small-sized particles that are delivered into the upper and lower airways. This can result in high concentrations of the nebulised agent to the targeted area, with less systemic absorption and fewer side-effects. The smaller the particle, the better the distribution (the best nebulisers will produce particles <0.5 μm). Nebulising just with saline may help to rehydrate the natural mucociliary escalator, therefore assisting the ferret to remove bacteria from the lungs. Mucolytics and bronchodilators may also be administered parenterally or orally if indicated. Massage of the thorax and exercise, particularly after nebulisation, can encourage evacuation of mucus from the airway.

MYCOPLASMOSIS

Definition/overview
Novel *Mycoplasma* species have recently been identified in ferrets causing respiratory disease. This was initially seen on a very large scale with over 8,000 ferrets affected from one breeding facility.

Aetiology/pathophysiology
Mycoplasma pulmonis is a significant cause of respiratory disease in rodent species, but the species of *Mycoplasma* affecting ferrets have been more problematic to identify, although they appear most similar to *M. molare* and *M. lagogenitalium*.

Most *Mycoplasma* species are host specific and spread between animals occurs via aerosol transmission. In the respiratory system, *Mycoplasma* attaches to ciliated epithelial cells, causing damage and disruption to their normal function.

Clinical presentation
Clinical signs are varied depending on the severity of the disease and the presence of concurrent illness. *Mycoplasma* should be considered for any ferret presenting with a chronic non-productive cough. Other clinical signs include haemoptysis, sneezing, laboured breathing and conjunctivitis. While morbidity levels may be high, mortality rates are low.

Differential diagnosis
Similar as for bacterial pneumonia.

Diagnostic testing
Samples obtained from a BAL (see *Table 20.4* for procedure) can be used for cytology, bacterial culture and sensitivity and PCR. Ocular swabs for standard microbiological technique (bacteria + *Mycoplasma*) have proven non-diagnostic in affected patients.

If a large group is affected, a diagnostic postmortem examination may be necessary and will allow collection of samples directly from affected lung tissue. Grossly, multi-focal nodules may be visible throughout the airways and lung tissue (**Fig. 20.12**). Histopathology of lung tissue can reveal lymphoplasmacytic perivascular

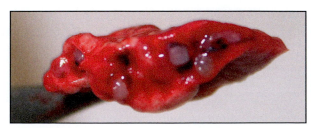

Fig. 20.12 Multifocal nodules present in the lung of a ferret infected with *Mycoplasma* sp. (Courtesy of Cathy Johnson-Delaney.)

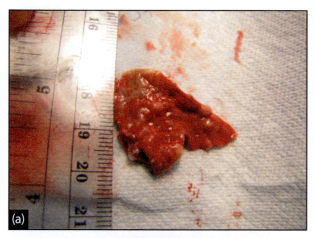

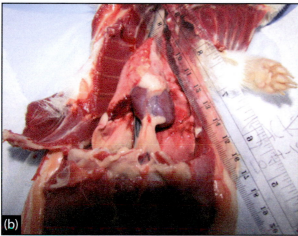

Fig. 20.13 (a, b) Gross pathology of the lungs typically seen with *Mycoplasma* sp. infection. (Courtesy of Cathy Johnson-Delaney.)

cuffing and extensive bronchiole-associated lymphoid tissue (BALT) hyperplasia (**Fig. 20.13**).

Diagnosis
Positive culture or PCR for *Mycoplasma* in a BAL or postmortem sample is conclusive of mycoplasmosis.

Management/treatment
Specific treatment should include antibiotics that are effective against *Mycoplasma*, such as doxycycline, enrofloxacin or azithromycin. Additional and supportive treatment has been described in the section of bacterial pneumonias. Infection may be lifelong in some cases, with coughing symptoms recurring in times of stress. It is unknown if this sets up a carrier state as it may in rodents.

CRYPTOCOCCOSIS

Definition/overview
Cryptococcus is a dimorphic fungus that can cause localised and systemic disease in ferrets. It has a worldwide distribution with reports of infected ferrets in the USA, Canada, UK, Spain and Australia.

Aetiology/pathophysiology
Cryptococcosis can be caused by both *Cryptococcus bacillisporus* and *Cryptococcus neoformans* var. *grubii*. The organism can infect many hosts including humans and wild and domestic mammals. The infection is acquired from the environment, and therefore cryptococcosis is not believed to be a contagious disease. However, infected ferrets and other pets act as sentinel species for humans, which is particularly important in immunocompromised people. Digging and soil excavation can increase exposure to spores. *C. neoformans* var. *grubii* has been associated with avian faeces, particularly contaminated pigeon excrement.

Clinical presentation
The clinical presentation of cryptococcosis is varied and largely depends on both the location and the severity of the disease. When localised to the respiratory system, both upper and lower respiratory disease can occur. Nasal cryptococcosis can present initially with a nasal discharge leading to the development of a chronic rhinitis. One or both nostrils can be affected, and discharge can range from serous to mucopurulent. Upper respiratory stertor, nasal mucosa ulceration and erosion can be seen. Lower respiratory clinical signs, if present, include coughing, dyspnoea and tachypnoea.

The disease can be disseminated in immunocompromised ferrets, affecting multiple organs and producing lymphadenopathy, chorioretinitis, central nervous system signs and swollen limbs (see Chapter 18).

Differential diagnosis
The list of differential diagnoses will depend on the organ or organs affected by the disease. For nasal cryptococcosis, differentials include bacterial rhinitis, other fungal rhinitis, nasal tumour and nasal

foreign body. For other respiratory signs, the differentials listed under the section of bacterial pneumonias should apply.

Diagnostic testing

Diagnosis can be readily achieved using cytological examination of fine needle aspirates or impression smears from affected areas (**Fig. 20.14**). Routine stains such as Diff-Quik will show the organism in encapsulated or budding forms. Biopsy of lesions followed by histopathology examination can also be used for a diagnosis.

Fungal culture on Sabourard's dextrose agar at 28°C can also confirm the diagnosis. Additional tests include latex antigen agglutination test and slide agglutination assay to determine serotype and mating type of the *Cryptococcus* isolate. Further imaging such as radiography, CT, MRI or rhinoscopy will help to collect samples and to assess the degree of invasion (particularly important as a previous step in surgery).

Diagnosis

Any positive test described under the previous section (cytology, histopathology, culture, etc.) will confirm the diagnosis. Nasal cryptococcosis is often more promptly diagnosed than lesions within the lower respiratory tract due to owner awareness, as nasal discharge is readily noticed.

Management/treatment

Early detection and treatment provide the best prognostic outcome. Antifungal medication is required as

Table 20.2 **Antifungal therapy**			
DRUG	**DOSE RATE**	**ROUTE**	**FREQUENCY**
Amphotericin B	0.4–0.8 mg/kg	IV	q24h for 7 days
Fluconazole	10 mg/kg	PO	q24h
Itraconazole	25–33 mg/kg	PO	q24h
Ketoconazole	10–30 mg/kg	PO	q24h–q12h

Key: IV, intravenous; PO, per os.

the main form of therapeutic treatment, with itraconazole being the drug of choice. Treatments are often lengthy; one reported case required a 10-month course of itraconazole, which was endured without adverse effects. Monitoring of biochemistry parameters is advised during prolonged antifungal treatment to avoid induced hepatopathies or azotaemia. Other treatment possibilities include ketoconazole, fluconazole, voriconazole and amphotericin B (*Table 20.2*).

Surgical debulking of masses caused by the aggregations of fungal-infected tissue is recommended. This can be achieved by rhinoscopy in cases of nasal cryptococcosis. More invasive surgical intervention may be needed in cases of chronic rhinitis, including rhinotomy or rhinostomy to debulk lesions in the nasal cavity and leave an indwelling catheter in place for a number of weeks to facilitate flushing and the application of topical treatment to an affected area.

OTHER FUNGAL PNEUMONIAS

Other than cryptococcosis, infection by *Blastomyces dermatitidis* and *Coccidioides immitis* can produce disease in endemic areas. Fungal spores are found in the soil, and therefore animals with access outdoors are more likely to get infected. *B. dermatitidis* is endemic in southeastern USA, the Ohio River Valley and the Mississippi River valley, while *C. immitis* is endemic in southwestern USA and areas Central and South America.

RESPIRATORY DISEASE SECONDARY TO CARDIAC DISEASE

Primary cardiac disease is more common in ferrets than primary respiratory disease; therefore, thorough cardiac auscultation should be performed with

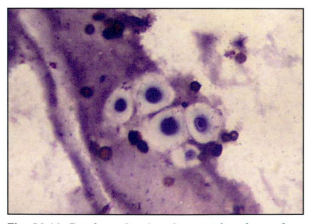

Fig. 20.14 **Cytology showing the capsulate form of** *Cryptococcus.* **(Courtesy of Peter Forsythe.)**

any ferret presenting in respiratory distress to rule out cardiac origin. Ferrets that develop congestive heart failure (CHF) can present with lethargy, weakness, ascites, increased respiratory effort or exercise intolerance. Diagnosis is aided with radiography, electrocardiography (ECG) and echocardiography. Radiographic findings of CHF include pulmonary oedema and pleural effusion. Treatment is based on ECG abnormalities (see Chapter 12).

HEARTWORM (SEE CHAPTER 12)

Definition/overview

Heartworm disease caused by the parasitic nematode *Dirofilaria immitis* has been reported in ferrets, dogs and cats and is endemic in areas of the USA, South America, southern Europe, Asia and Australia. The parasite can cause significant disease and even death in ferrets.

Aetiology/pathophysiology

The heartworm is a small thread-like worm. Due to the relative small size of the ferret, even the presence of one worm in a blood vessel can result in clinical disease. Although referred to as 'heartworm', the parasite is often found in the pulmonary arterial system, as well as in the heart.

Heartworm infections are spread between hosts by mosquito vectors. Naïve vectors become infected when feeding from a contaminated host. Mosquitoes can also be considered as true intermediate hosts, as the parasite larvae (microfilariae) require a period of time for maturation within the insect. After maturing from L1 to L3 larvae, the parasite is then ready to infect a new host. During a blood meal, the microfilariae leave the mosquito and move on to ferret's skin through the bite wound created by the mosquito. The parasite infects the subcutaneous tissues, matures, and then the young adult worms migrate to the cardiopulmonary vessels where they become adults. Sexual reproduction between worms occurs within the bloodstream, after which the female worms release L1 microfilariae into the bloodstream.

Clinical presentation

Ferrets may present with lethargy, dyspnoea, coughing, cyanosis and, in some cases, sudden death. If the worms are present in the right side of the heart, clinical signs associated with right-sided CHF may be noted, which include ascites and pleural effusion; this is due to the parasites causing a mechanical obstruction.

Differential diagnosis

CHF, pleural effusion; viral, fungal or bacterial pneumonia; neoplasia, e.g. mediastinal lymphoma, lung metastasis from a primary neoplasia; other causes of pleural effusion, e.g. endogenous lipid pneumonia, infection by *Pseudomonas luteola*.

Diagnostic testing

Thoracic ultrasonography can visualise worms within blood vessels and associated changes to the heart. The worms are usually visible in the right atrium, right ventricle or pulmonary artery. Structural changes detected with ECG include enlargement of the right side of the heart and triscuspid regurgitation. False negatives can be obtained in ultrasound when the infection is caused only by a small number of worms.

An ELISA antigen test can be performed; however, to get a positively testing result, at least two adult female worms must be present within the bloodstream. False-negative results can occur if only one female or several male worms are present.

Diagnosis

Diagnosis is made by a positive result on ultrasound and/or ELISA.

Management/treatment

Prevention is the proactive approach to heartworm. Ferrets at risk should be treated on a regular basis to prevent the development of the infection. Treatment of a positively testing ferret should begin with an adulticide drug, along with concurrent systemic steroid therapy. Due to the possibility of false negatives, when there is a history of potential exposure and compatible clinical signs, treatment should be started.

Two drugs are used to kill the adult worms: melarsamine and ivermectin. Melarsomine kills the adult worms faster than ivermectin, but it has been associated with a greater risk of adverse reaction. Anaphylaxis is a possibility with any drug choice and ferrets should be observed closely when starting

Table 20.3 **Heartworm therapy**

PREVENTION	DRUG(S)	DOSAGE	ROUTE	FREQUENCY
	Imidacloprid/moxidectin	1.9–3.3 µg/kg	Topically	Once monthly
	Milbemycin oxime	1.15–2.33 mg/kg	PO	Once monthly
	Ivermectin	0.5 mg/kg	PO	Once monthly
	Selamectin	18 mg/kg	Topically	Once monthly
TREATMENT	Ivermectin	0.05 mg/kg	PO	Once monthly until negative ELISA
	Melarsomine with	2.5 mg/kg	IM	One injection followed by two injections 24 hours apart on days 30 and 31
	Prednisolone with	1 mg/kg	PO	Once daily for the duration of treatment course
	Ivermectin	50 µg/kg	PO	Microfilariae dose once monthly until thought heartworm free
	Moxidectin	0.17 mg	SC	Once

Key: ELISA; enzyme-linked immunosorbent assay; IM, intramuscular; PO, per os; SC, subcutaneous.

a new treatment. Antithrombotic drugs can be used concurrently with adulticide treatment, and strict rest is advised at time of treatment. *Table 20.3* summarises treatments for heartworm.

OTHER RESPIRATORY CONDITIONS

Endogenous lipid pneumonia
This is a pulmonary disease characterised by the accumulation of foamy macrophages in the pulmonary parenchyma. It is an idiopathic and endogenous condition that presents as a minor and common incidental histological finding for many conditions (e.g. FRSCV). There has been one report of a ferret with lethargy, tachypnoea and pleural effusion where severe endogenous lipid pneumonia was the only relevant finding at necropsy and histopathology (**Fig. 20.15**). This rare clinical condition can be diagnosed using radiographs to demonstrate lung consolidation and BAL to demonstrate foamy macrophages. Treatment involves the use of steroids, but the only reported case did not respond to treatment.

Pleuropneumonia caused by *Pseudomonas luteola* infection
Infection by *Pseudomonas luteola* in ferrets can produce pyothorax, mediastinal lymphadenopathy

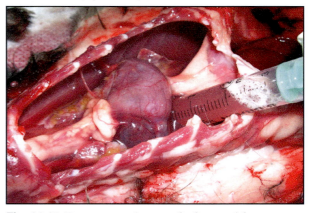

Fig. 20.15 **Postmortem image of a ferret with endogenous lipid pneumonia and pleural effusion. Note golden areas of the lung indicative of lipid deposits.**

and multiple white nodules (1–2 mm) in the lungs (**Fig. 20.16**). Affected animals present with acute onset of dyspnoea and can also show cough, lethargy, anorexia and fever. Bloodwork may reveal anaemia, severe neutrophilic leucocytosis with toxic neutrophils, hyperglycaemia, hyperglobulinaemia and hypoalbuminaemia. Pleural effusion can be visualised using radiography or ultrasound (**Fig. 20.17**). Diagnosis is confirmed based on culture or cytology of the purulent fluid found in the thorax. Cytology demonstrates a severe purulent inflammation with

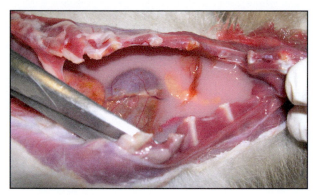

Fig. 20.16 **Pyothorax is common in cases of infection with *Pseudomonas luteola*.**

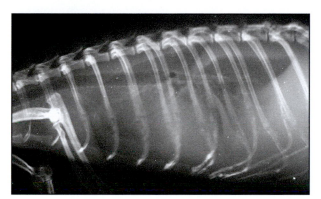

Fig. 20.17 **Pleural effusion can occur in cases of infection with *Pseudomonas luteola*, endogenous lipid pneumonia and bite-related pyothorax, among other causes.**

abundant clusters of rod-shaped microorganisms with a clear surrounding halo. Treatment involves drainage of the thoracic exudates, antibiotic treatment based on culture and sensitivity and supportive and symptomatic treatment. Prognosis is poor, and sensitivity testing of this gram-negative aerobic rod is mandatory.

Other respiration conditions

Dyspnoea can occasionally be seen with anaphylactic reactions after vaccination against distemper or rabies; other important signs of an anaphylactic reaction will also be observed (see Chapter 11). Acetaminophen (paracetamol) toxicity can also produce tachypnoea as part of an acute disease with other clinical signs such as depression, salivation, vomiting, cyanosis and haematuria (see Chapter 29). Megaoesophagus produces a loss of muscle tone in the

oesophagus and facilitates regurgitation and aspiration pneumonia (see Chapter 13). Nausea, a common clinical sign in ferrets seen in cases of gastritis, may be confused by some owners with respiratory disease. Hyperoestrogenism in female ferrets induces aplastic anaemia, which can lead to tachypnoea when the haematocrit value decreases significantly. Other signs would be expected with this condition including a swollen vulva, alopecia and pale mucous membranes. Increased respiratory effort can be observed with mediastinal lymphoma (**Fig. 20.18**). Pregnancy toxaemia can also produce dyspnoea together with weight loss, anorexia, dehydration and other symptoms. Traumatic injuries such as falls from significant heights or bites into the thorax can produce respiratory symptoms due to pneumothorax or pyothorax. Dyspnoea can also be seen if there is neoplastic metastasis to the lungs and thorax (**Fig. 20.19**).

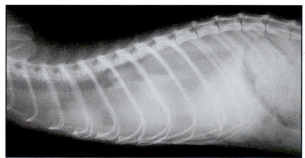

Fig. 20.18 **Thoracic lymphoma demonstrated on radiograph. (Courtesy of Cathy Johnson-Delaney.)**

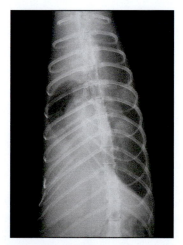

Fig. 20.19 **Metastasis of fibrosarcoma on radiograph. (Courtesy of Cathy Johnson-Delaney.)**

Table 20.4 Bronchoalveolar lavage and thoracentesis techniques

DIAGNOSTIC PROCEDURES	USE	METHOD	PRACTICAL TIP
Bronchoalveolar lavage (BAL)	Collection of fluid for microbiology and cytology from the lower airways	1. The ferret should be anesthetised and intubated with a sterile endotracheal tube (ET) 2. Positioning in lateral recumbency is required. If unilateral lung disease is present, the affected lung should be downwards 3. A sterile urinary catheter should be placed through the ET tube, and gently advanced to the distal trachea 4. Sterile saline (1 mL/kg) is instilled through the ET and immediately suctioned using a syringe to collect fluid. Approximately half the total fluid volume instilled should be aspirated back 5. Samples should be collected in sterile tubes and EDTA for analysis	Premeasure the catheter alongside the ET tube prior to use to judge the length of insertion
Thoracocentesis	To remove excessive accumulations of fluid (pleural effusions) or air (pneumothorax) within the pleural space. This procedure involves the surgical puncture and drainage of the pleural space. Analysis of aspirated fluids helps aid diagnosis (culture, cytology, fluid analysis and specific gravity)	1. The ferret is positioned in sternal recumbency with supportive oxygen therapy provided 2. The fur over the 6th to 10th ribs on both sides is clipped and prepared aseptically. Thoracocentesis is usually performed on the right side of the thorax 3. The procedure can either be performed under light sedation or conscious with the use of local anaesthetic infiltrated in the chosen intercostal space 4. Ultrasound should be used to identify the correct site and for monitoring drainage 5. A 21 g butterfly catheter needle or intravenous cannula with stylet can be used. The needle is inserted at an oblique angle, with the bevel end pointed downwards. To avoid traumatising vessels and nerves, the needle should be introduced at the cranial border of the ribs 6. The needle should be slowly advanced through the skin, into the pleural space. In some cases an audible 'pop' is heard once the needle is in the pleural space 7. The needle should then be positioned parallel to the body wall to reduce the risk of trauma to the lungs 8. Suction is applied using a three-way valve and a 10 mL syringe 9. Continue aspiration until negative pressure is reached or the fluid or gas pocket on ultrasound has significantly reduced	1. This is usually a three person procedure. One person is required to restrain the patient, another to hold the needle and ultrasound probe, while the final person aspirates fluid or air using a three way valve 2. Insert the butterfly catheter needle 1/3rd of the way up the thorax from the ventrum in cases with pleural effusion and mid-thorax in cases with pneumothorax

CHAPTER 21

DISORDERS OF THE SKIN

Cathy A. Johnson-Delaney

INTRODUCTION

The skin of the ferret is similar to that of other carnivores, although it is thicker in the shoulder area. There are two well-developed anal glands that secrete a pungent musk common in the Mustelids. The coat has fine underfur, with longer, coarser guard hairs. It provides dense insulation and is a durable fur that makes it useful for the fur industry, where it is called 'fitch'. The coat can change dramatically seasonally. The winter coat is thicker and softer than the summer coat, and even colour and markings may change (**Fig. 21.1**). The tail is densely furred and aids in swimming. Guard hairs and sensory hairs on the muzzle are grouped as a mystacial pad. Sensory hairs, innervated by three types of nerves, arise from the infraorbital branch of the trigeminal nerve. Deep and superficial vibrissal nerves innervate nearly exclusive targets in large follicle–sinus complexes at the base of each tactile vibrissa. Dermal plexus nerves innervate the fur between the vibrissae.

ABSCESS/WOUNDS

Definition/overview
An infection of the skin, often started with a wound acquired during rough play. Abscesses also may form at any place of skin puncture or damage. There may be accompanying pyoderma or cellulitis. The area is usually fluctuant, swollen and may be painful to touch.

Aetiology/pathophysiology
Bacterial infection may set in where there is skin damage. As the body walls it off an abscess forms. Bacteria isolated from ferret abscesses are most frequently *Staphylococcus aureus* or *Streptococcus* spp. Infection

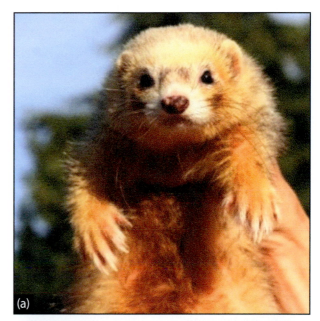

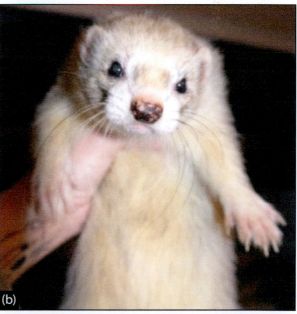

Fig. 21.1 The winter (a) and summer coat (b). Intact male. (Courtesy of Vondelle McLaughlin.)

can also be caused by *Corynebacterium* spp., *Pasteurella* spp., *Actinomyces* spp., and *Escherichia coli*. Frequently small punctures and lacerations occur primarily in the ear and neck area where ferrets tend to bite each other, usually during play.

Clinical presentation
Swellings, sometimes ulcerated or draining, and usually freely movable from deep tissue can be found anywhere on the body. Punctures and lacerations are more probably found in the neck and ear area from rough play, but can be found anywhere on the body (**Fig. 21.2**).

Differential diagnosis
Neoplasia, which is fairly common in ferret skin and dermal/subdermal tissues.

Diagnostic testing
If suspicious for neoplasia, excisional biopsy and histopathology may be in order (**Fig. 21.3**). Otherwise, a culture can be taken from the tissue to determine bacterial infection.

Diagnosis
Negative for neoplastic process on histology. Positive for bacterial infection.

Management/treatment
If abscess, lancing and draining can be done, followed with systemic antimicrobials and NSAIDs for discomfort. Topical antimicrobial cream may also be applied to the skin area if small lacerations and puncture are not fully abscessed, in addition to the systemic antimicrobials.

ALOPECIA

Adrenal disease/hyperoestrogenism
Definition/overview
Loss of hair starting from tail and rump, following on body and usually fairly symmetrically patterned. Eventually spreads to entire body. There may also be an eczema-like scabbiness in some areas.

Aetiology/pathophysiology
Hyperoestrogenism and alopecia are one of the major signs of adrenal disease (see Chapter 14).

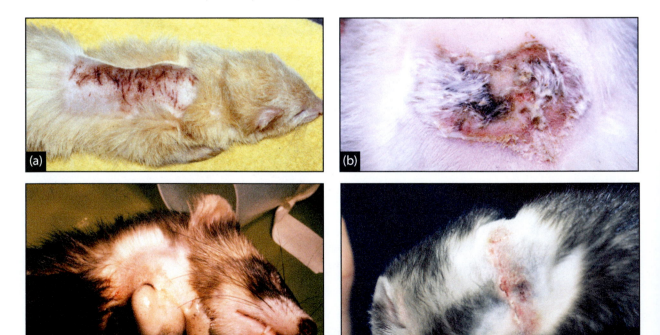

Fig. 21.2 (a) Lacerations; (b) infected wound; (c) abscess; (d) lacerations from a too tight collar.

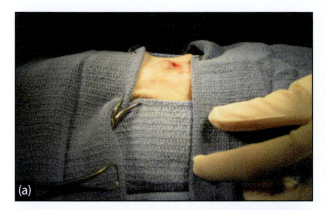

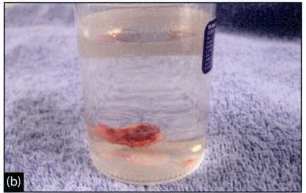

Fig. 21.3 (a) Lump draped for aseptic surgical excision; (b) submit tissues for histopathology.

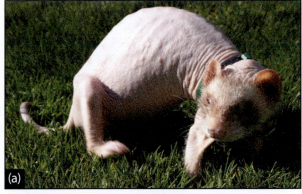

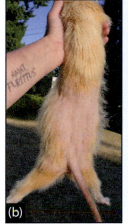

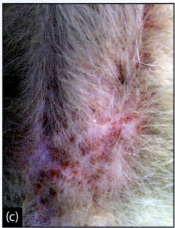

Fig. 21.4 (a, b) Alopecia of the trunk is typical of adrenal disease (courtesy of Vondelle McLaughlin); (c) dermatitis is frequently seen with adrenal disease.

There may also be an imbalance between the oestrogens and androgens, which also contributes to the pattern of hair loss and the timetable for development of the disease. The eczema-like rash may be in part due to altered sebaceous and skin metabolism due to the hormone imbalance. The rash does not seem to respond to topical therapies but does resolve with treatment for adrenal disease.

Clinical presentation

Ferret usually presents with hair loss on the tail, 'rat tail', complete with comedones. There may be sparse hair over the rump or total alopecia spreading from the hindquarters cranially. In severe cases the ferret may be totally hairless. The ferret often acts pruritic and may have traumatised the skin in areas from scratching. There may be eczema-like patches that have some sebaceous scurf (**Fig. 21.4**). Widespread petechiation has been seen in adrenal disease due to thrombocytopaenia (**Fig. 21.5**).

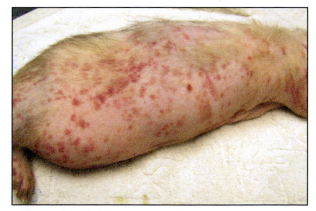

Fig. 21.5 Petechiation seen with thrombocytopaenia.

Differential diagnosis

Hair loss due to seasonal coat changes as frequently it starts with hair loss on the tail and rump. Usually there is corresponding shedding that the owner has noted. Seasonal coat change is especially prominent in the autumn. A poor hair coat can also be seen with hypothyroidism (see Chapter 14), and in cases of starvation/malnutrition.

Diagnostic testing
Testing for adrenal disease includes serum hormone levels, ultrasonography, adrenalectomy with histopathology and/or response to sex steroid hormone suppression using a GnRH agonist analogue (see Chapter 14). History and full physical examination will rule out nutritional status. A thyroid hormone level may be taken but the tests from most laboratories have not been validated in ferrets.

Diagnosis
If the above is positive for adrenal disease, signs usually regress with appropriate therapy (see Chapter 14).

Management/treatment
Usually alopecia resolves in all or part following adrenalectomy with concurrent GnRH agonist treatment (see Chapter 14). Note: it is not uncommon for the abdominal skin following adrenalectomy to have bruising, which may be quite severe (**Fig. 21.6**). This is in part due to the high oestradiol levels that may suppress clotting. In some ferrets with adrenal disease there may be thrombocytopaenia as well, which may contribute to postsurgery bruising. Some adrenal disease ferrets also show petechiation and small bruises on the skin that will resolve with adrenal disease treatment.

Hypothyroidism
Definition/overview
Lowered levels of thyroid hormone. This has been deduced in cases where there appear to be skin and coat changes consistent with hypothyroidism in other species. Validation of the disease has largely been anecdotal as there has not been a commercially validated test for ferrets (see Chapter 14).

Aetiology/pathophysiology
Dysfunction of the thyroid gland. Histopathology reports for this have been lacking. The thyroid gland may exhibit imbalances in cases of adrenal disease (see Chapter 14).

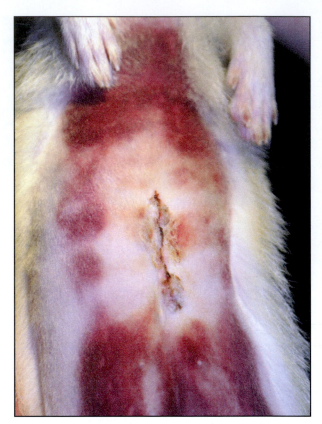

Fig. 21.6 Bruising following adrenalectomy due to thrombocytopaenia.

Clinical presentation
Obesity, generalised poor hair coat (**Fig. 21.7**).

Differential diagnosis
Obesity, often seasonal. Adrenal disease alopecia.

Diagnostic testing
T3 and T4 levels. Ideally a TSH could be run. Levels of these hormones have not been validated in pet ferrets.

Diagnosis
Validated low T3, T4. A TSH stimulation test would have a poor response.

Management/treatment
Supplementation with thyroxine, dosage based on dog dosages. If concurrent adrenal disease, hypothyroid-like clinical signs may resolve with treatment of the adrenal disease (see Chapter 14).

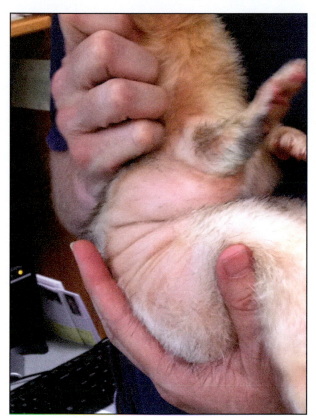

Fig. 21.7 Trunkal alopecia associated with presumed hypothyroidism.

Seasonal alopecia

Definition/overview

Ferrets change hair coats twice yearly, with changes happening in the autumn and spring. The lay term for this is 'blowing their coats'. It often starts with shedding of the tail hair which gives them a 'rat tail' look although new hair begins to grow in conjunction with the rest of the body growth, unlike with adrenal disease. The winter coat has a dense undercoating. The spring moult is the most dramatic as the undercoat is shed. The ferret may actually change coat patterns and colours from one season to the next. Owners are encouraged to take photographs of their ferrets in each season to see the changes over time.

Aetiology/pathophysiology

Ferrets are seasonal animals and undergo the coat changes in conjunction with ancestral climate changes. They are similar in this regard to other members of the Mustelid family, in particular to mink. Seasonal weight changes usually accompany the coat change; ferrets bulk up for the winter and slim down for the summer.

Clinical presentation

There may be rat tail and generalised poor hair coat. The owners usually report a lot of hair being present in the bedding. This is particularly true during the spring moult of the winter coat.

Differential diagnosis

Adrenal disease.

Diagnostic testing

Hormone levels in the adrenal panel, ultrasonography of the glands (see Chapter 14).

Diagnosis

Adrenal disease has been ruled out. History and time of year correlate to coat change.

Management/treatment

Use of a ferret laxative or cat laxative regularly during the change is recommended to prevent trichobezoar formation. Otherwise there is no treatment needed.

Starvation/malnutrition

Definition/overview

Poor nutrition and/or emaciation presents with a poor hair coat.

Aetiology/pathophysiology

Ferrets require a high-protein, high-fat, low-fibre diet. They are obligate carnivores (see Chapter 5). A diet that does not meet their requirements or a lack of food results in a dry hair coat, sparse with areas of alopecia. Concurrent with this is usually poor body condition.

Clinical presentation

Poor hair coat and generalised poor body condition. This may include loss of muscle mass. Body score 1–2 of 5 (**Fig. 21.8**).

Differential diagnosis

Adrenal disease, other causes of alopecia.

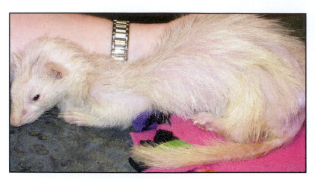

Fig. 21.8 Poor hair coat due to emaciation, malnutrition and possibly adrenal disease.

Diagnostic testing
History is usually all that is needed. Ruling out concurrent adrenal disease is by hormone level testing and/or ultrasonography, or response to GnRH agonist treatment.

Diagnosis
History of diet, lack of food, body condition.

Management/treatment
Usually switching to an appropriate diet will correct the hair coat with time. The coat may change at the usual moult time. For emaciation/starvation, a supplementary meal(s) of dook soup may aid in weight and condition gain (see Chapter 5).

Telogen defluxion
Definition/overview
The hairs move through the telogen (resting phase of growth) and are subsequently lost.

Aetiology/pathophysiology
This form of alopecia occurs 2–3 months after a stressful event. Stressors include pregnancy, suckling of young or a debilitating systemic disease.

Clinical presentation
The ferret undergoes a very heavy moult. In some cases overt alopecia is not seen; only a generalised thinning of the coat will be present.

Differential diagnosis
Other causes of alopecia including adrenal disease (Chapter 14).

Diagnostic testing
History; biopsy, histopathology.

Diagnosis
Confirmation about history, and histopathology results.

Management/treatment
None. With next moult it usually corrects itself. Ovariohysterectomy to prevent further pregnancies may be warranted.

ATOPY

Definition/overview
Atopy is an allergic reaction to environmental allergens. It has been presumptively diagnosed in the ferret.

Aetiology/pathophysiology
The ferret may exhibit generalised inflammation of the skin with pruritis due to systemic and skin release of histamines.

Clinical presentation
Symmetrical, non-lesional pruritus over the trunk, rump and paws. Pruritis may be intensified at flexural surfaces and the perianal area.

Differential diagnosis
Rule out other causes of generalised pruritis including adrenal disease.

Diagnostic testing
History with diet and environment should be noted. Skin biopsies may show an allergic dermatitis.

Diagnosis
Result of the histopathology. Rule out potential allergens including diet related.

Management/treatment
Antihistamines, corticosteroids, omega 3–6 fatty acid supplementation and diet change may help with clinical signs. In severe cases, hyposensitisation programme using allergen preparations may be needed.

BLUE FERRET SYNDROME

Definition/overview
Blue discolouration of the abdominal skin.

Aetiology/pathophysiology
Idiopathic syndrome affecting ferrets of either sex, neutered or intact. It is seen primarily in ferrets clipped for surgery during catagen – the intermediate phase of the hair growth cycle.

Clinical presentation
A blueish discolouration of the abdominal skin but no other symptoms. The clipped skin area remains hairless then turns blue and it appears that the hair follicles are producing melanine to be incorporated into growing hairs. Usually discolouration disappears within a few weeks.

Differential diagnosis
Hyperadrenocorticism.

Diagnostic testing
History, skin biopsy may verify cause.

Diagnosis
Clinical signs.

Management/treatment
None necessary.

BURNS

Definition/overview
First, second or third degree burns as occur in other species. The most common cause in ferrets is spilled boiling water for thermal burns and contact chemical burns usually due to application of ectoparasite products designed for other species.

Aetiology/pathophysiology
Burns to the skin may penetrate all layers.

Clinical presentation
Skin may be reddened, blistered, sloughing (**Fig. 21.9**). Extremely painful (first, second degree. Author considers third degree also painful although not listed as such in other species).

Differential diagnosis
Severe pyoderma.

Diagnostic testing
None needed. Visual examination sufficient.

Diagnosis
History and clinical signs.

Management/treatment
Analgesics should be administered first. First-degree burns may be handled with just cold water application.

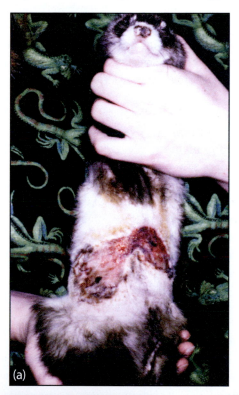

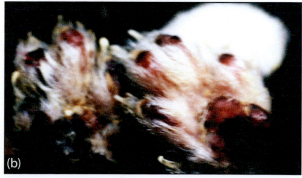

Fig. 21.9 (a) Burned abdomen from a boiling water spill; (b) burned feet.

Second- and third-degree burns should be handled as in other species: protection bandaging if possible to localised areas and systemic antimicrobials. Fluid therapy may also be necessary as burn wounds seep fluids. Prognosis is guarded with second- and third-degree burns covering most of the body.

DERMATOPHYTOSIS

Definition/overview
Fungal infection of the skin. Commonly called 'ringworm'. Report in one ferret with pneumonia and an ulcerated foot pad attributed to *Blastomyces dermatitidis*. Histoplasmosis and coccidiomycosis have also been diagnosed as causing subcutaneous nodules. For this section, the discussion is limited to primary dermatomycosis as listed below.

Aetiology/pathophysiology
Dermatomycosis is not a common disease in ferrets but is seen in highly stressed, immunosuppressed, young, or malnourished ferrets and those in an animal shelter. It is caused by either *Microsporum canis* or *Trichophyton mentagrophytes*. It is transmitted by direct contact. It is potentially zoonotic. It is thought that cohabiting with cats may be a source. It is also possible that the ferret contracted it from contact with an infected human, particularly a child. Spontaneous remission of lesions has been reported but in the author's experience does not seem to happen. It is a zoonotic disease.

Clinical presentation
The lesions may present in several ways but are non-pruritic. There may be areas of annular alopecia, broken hairs, erythema, diffuse scaling and crusting (**Fig. 21.10**).

Differential diagnosis
Early neoplastic lesion such as mast cell tumour, bacterial dermatitis.

Diagnostic testing
Microscopic examination of the hairs from the edge of the lesion may show fungal elements. A skin scraping and hairs plucked from the edges can be used for fungal culture. Some isolates of *Microsporum canis* fluoresce and use of the black light to screen is recommended.

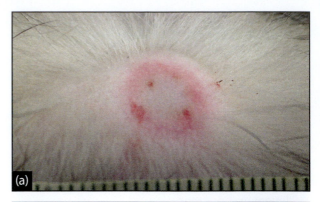

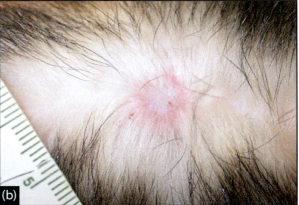

Fig. 21.10 (a, b) Dermatomycosis with the typical 'ring' pattern.

Diagnosis
Fungal elements seen on microscopic examination. Positive fungal culture.

Management/treatment
Topical treatment of the lesions is usually effective using microconazole cream 1% or terbinafine cream 1% 2–3 times a day until the lesion(s) are resolved. In severe cases systemic oral griseofulvin may be used at 25 mg/kg q24h × 21–30 days. The environment also needs to be disinfected using bleach diluted 50:50 with warm water. Cages should be rinsed and aired before ferrets are allowed to return. Bedding should also be changed, preferably daily, until lesions have resolved. Washing the bedding in a machine using hot water and detergent is effective for sanitising the bedding. If using substrate in the cage such as shredded paper, paper pellets should be discontinued during treatment. Litter, if used in a litter tray, should be changed daily as well.

ECTOPARASITES

Otodectes cynotis
Definition/overview
Very common to find ear mites (**Fig. 21.11**) (see Chapter 15).

Aetiology/pathophysiology
Mites present in the outer ear canal and feed off lymph, skin debris and blood. In severe cases they may be found in the inner ear, which may present with head tilt and/or convulsions. Ear wax is normally dark brown so in itself is not diagnostic for mites. Mites transmit easily via direct contact between ferrets, particularly if housed in a social group. The mite's life cycle is 3 weeks so treatment must be geared to multiple treatments. Ear mites may cause irritation and inflammation within the ear canal. Generally it is non-pruritic. Very few ferrets paw at their ears or shake their heads as do cats with mites. Mites may also be found on the feet and tail tip.

Clinical presentation
Ear wax contains mites, eggs. Rarely pawing or scratching at the ears, although there may be evidence of scratching of the ears by loss of hair on caudal pinna. If otitis interna present, there may be head tilt, head shaking and, in severe cases, convulsions. Otitis interna due to mites is uncommon.

Differential diagnosis
Excessive ear wax. Rarely otitis interna due to bacterial infection.

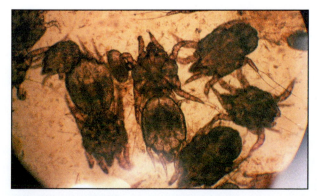

Fig. 21.11 *Otodectes cynotis.*

Diagnostic testing
Swab ear canal, microscopic examination. Otoscopic visualisation of moving mites. Heavy infestations, may be able to see mites directly.

Diagnosis
Present mites, eggs on examination.

Management/treatment
All ferrets in the group must be treated. Ivermectin has been used at 0.4 mg/kg topically. Selamectin has also been used at 10–15 mg/kg topically q30d (fleas, earmites). There are several products available for cats that are otic formulations. Ears should be swabbed out frequently. Bedding should be changed frequently while undergoing treatment.

Sarcoptes scabiei
Definition/overview
Mange mite. Dogs usually act as the source of contagion of ferrets.

Aetiology/pathophysiology
Mites burrow in tunnels in the skin, particularly in areas that are poorly furred such as in endocrine alopecia. It is a zoonotic disease.

Clinical presentation
Intense pruritis with generalised alopecia or localised lesions of the toes and feet. Lesions are prominent on sparsely haired sites, such as the caudal ventrum/inguinal area. There may be secondary dermatitis if the skin has become lacerated due to the scratching of the skin.

Differential diagnosis
Bacterial dermatitis, atopy, fleas and flea hypersensitivity.

Diagnostic testing
Microscopic examination of skin scrapings, that must be fairly deep. It is not uncommon to miss them even with multiple scrapings. It is a round mite, only the first pair of legs will protrude beyond the body shape. The legs are short and end in long, unsegmented stalks with suckers.

Diagnosis
Presence of mites.

Management/treatment
Ivermectin at 0.4 mg/kg given subcutaneously and repeated every 7–14 days for three doses. All affected and in-contact ferrets should be treated. The environment including bedding and litter trays should be cleaned several times a week until cleared. Diphenhydramine and an NSAID can help with the pruritis.

Ixodes ricinus
Definition/overview
Tick infestation.

Aetiology/pathophysiology
The ferret may pick up ticks when hunting. This is unlikely to occur in pet ferrets housed indoors. *I. ricinus* may cause anaemia. Ticks can act as vectors for many diseases in many animals, but this has not been documented in pet ferrets.

Clinical presentation
Anaemia if multiple ticks found. There may be erythema and inflammation surrounding the tick.

Differential diagnosis
Many causes of anaemia including idiopathic aplastic anaemia, prolonged hyperoestrogenaemia.

Diagnostic testing
Locating the ticks themselves. May be easier to find if the ferret is wetted.

Diagnosis
Presence of the tick.

Management/treatment
Can be removed manually. Treatment with 0.4 mg/kg ivermectin is also effective for killing the tick. Anaemia will resolve on its own although supplementation with B vitamin complex may be done.

Fleas
Definition/overview
Ctenocephalides felis (cat flea) and *C. canis* (dog flea) can infest ferrets.

Aetiology/pathophysiology
Infestation with the fleas usually signals that other pets in the household have fleas. Fleas also will be present in the environment. Flea bites cause intense pruritis, particularly in those individuals where hypersensitivity to flea saliva exists. Flea bite dermatitis and hypersensitivity has been seen in ferrets.

Clinical presentation
Usually pruritis is seen generally around the neck. There may be self-inflicted trauma and lacerations to the skin. There may be traumatic hair loss and excoriation. Alopecia may be seen on the neck and thorax.

Differential diagnosis
Scabies. Bacterial dermatitis. Endocrine imbalance.

Diagnostic testing
Direct visualisation, often easiest to see on ventrum and inguinal area where the hair normally is sparse. A positive wet-paper test to identify the presence of flea faeces. A fine-toothed flea comb may also be used to comb out fleas and have the faeces drop onto a table. The black 'dirt' will turn red if sprinkled with water.

Diagnosis
Confirmation of fleas.

Management/treatment
All mammalian pets in the household must be treated as well as the environment. Topical products such as selamectin at 10–15 mg/kg or imidocloprid 0.1–0.4 mL topically along dorsum q30d. Other topical products containing pyrethrins that are safe for cats can be used. Flea collars should not be used.

Cuterebra (cuterebriasis)
Definition/overview
Usually seen in ferrets exposed to outdoors or in households that have a bot fly population.

Aetiology/pathophysiology
The bot fly lays its eggs on the ferret – the larvae are buried within the skin with a small hole for respiration. The larvae may cause localised irritation and inflammation. The skin will also be raised as the larvae grow.

Clinical presentation

The hole and swollen appearance of the skin is diagnostic. The ferret may exhibit some pruritis in the area. If multiple bots present the ferret may present with general malaise and irritation surrounding the larval respiratory hole.

Differential diagnosis

None.

Diagnostic testing

None.

Diagnosis

Presence of the hole along with the visualization of the larvae (**Fig. 21.12**).

Management/treatment

Pretreat the ferret with diphenhydramine at 1 mg/kg IM prior to enlargement of the hole. The author usually pretreats with an NSAID such as metacam at 0.2 mg/kg subcutaneously as well to minimise the discomfort involved with hole enlargement. A local anaesthetic may be used if the hole must be surgically enlarged in order to extract the larvae manually with forceps. After removal, the hole may be flushed with a dilute chlorhexidine solution, expressed then closed with tissue glue. Alternatively the hole may be left open and topical antibiotic cream applied to it for several days until healed. If there have been multiple cuterebras removed and/or there seems to be exudate and extensive inflammation, systemic antibiotics for 7–10 days should be administered. The owner should be counselled in prevention of the problem recurring. Preferably the ferret should be housed indoors where there should not be bot flies.

ERYTHEMA MULTIFORME (EM)

Definition/overview

This is an uncommon skin disease consistent with host-specific hypersensitivity reaction induced by various antigens. The reaction alters keratinocytes which makes them targets of an aberrant immune response.

Aetiology/pathophysiology

It appears to be a T cell-mediated response directed at keratinocytes that may express antigens in a novel

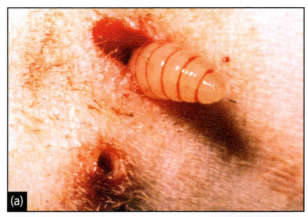
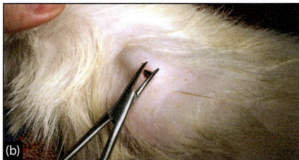
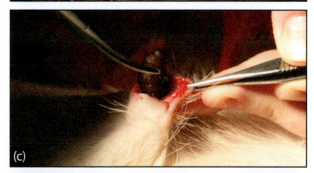
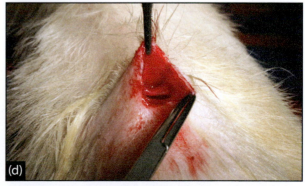

Fig. 21.12 (a) White cuterebra; (b) more typical dark cuterebra larvae and telltale hole; (c) incision to enlarge hole and grasp the larvae; (d) cavity left after removal, usually closed with sutures. (b–d, Courtesy of Vondelle McLaughlin.)

way due to drug administration, infection or neoplasia. This results in apoptosis of keratinocytes. Adverse reactions to drugs have been reported in other species. The drugs that have triggered this response in dogs include ampicillin, cephalexin, trimethoprim-sulfonamide, griseofulvin, acepromazine, enrofloxacin and lincomycin.

Clinical presentation
Lesions usually develop after 7–18 days of exposure to the causative agent; however, lesions can develop within 24 hours if the ferret has been previously exposed to the antigen. Lesions include sudden onset of scabbing and erythema of the ventral inguinal area. There have been no dermal signs typical of ferret hyperadrenocorticism. Pruritis is not present. There may be papules with varying degrees of scale and scabbing. The lesions may worsen with time and spread predominantly on the ventrum and into the axillary areas. Foot pads may thicken with hyperkeratosis and dermal inflammation between the pads. The pinnae may become inflamed and show evidence of hyperkeratosis. Lesions may also occur on the face (**Fig. 21.13**).

Differential diagnosis
Hyperadrenocorticism, contact dermatitis, generalised autoimmune dermatitis, superficial pyoderma, bacterial folliculitis, epitheliotropic lymphoma, early-stage bullous immune-mediated skin diseases such as pemphigus vulgaris, bullous pemphigoid and systemic lupus erythematosus.

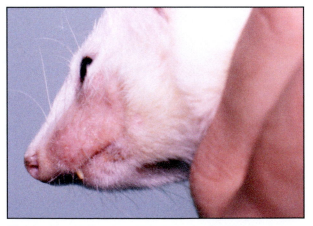

Fig. 21.13 Erythema multiforme on the face.

Diagnostic testing
Dermal tape preparation cytology will show cornified epithelial cells and occasional cocci bacteria. It may contain epidermal collarettes see with superficial pyoderma. Skin biopsy histopathology is consistent with severe manifestation of EM.

Management/treatment
Immunosuppressive drugs starting with prednisolone at 1.25 mg/kg q12h, azathioprine at 1 mg per ferret q24h, ciclosporin at 2.5 mg q12h. Additional therapy may include an antibiotic different from any suspected of initiating the problem as well as famotidine at 2.5 mg per ferret q24h to help protect the stomach from ulcers potentially caused by the continued immunosuppression.

HYPERSENSITIVITY (SEE ATOPY ABOVE)

Definition/overview
Considered atopy and may be due to food or environmental allergens.

Aetiology/pathophysiology
Reaction with inflammation to allergens. Foods have been implicated, but may be difficult to prove that is the cause. The skin may be erythematous with generalised inflammation. Usually it is bilateral, and may have areas of alopecia.

Clinical presentation
Generalised inflammation and erythema (**Fig. 21.14**). There is often pruritis and alopecia. The ferret may inflict more damage to the skin with scratching.

Differential diagnosis
Bacterial dermatitis, scabies.

Diagnostic testing
Skin scrapings for mites, although this may be negative. Recommended for confirmation of a hypersensitivity state is a full-thickness biopsy of the affected area.

Management/treatment
Food elimination trials are difficult because the ferret is often stubborn about food changes. Novel protein diets have proven problematic (urolithiasis connected,

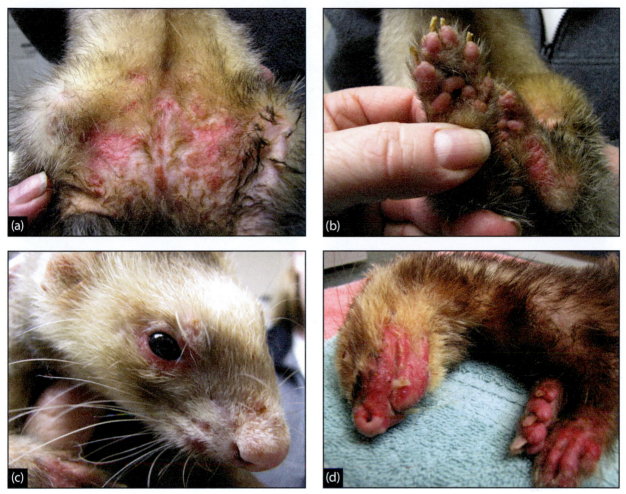

Fig. 21.14 (a) Hypersensitivity lesions on ventrum; (b) lesions of foot pads; (c) erythema of eyelids and conjunctivitis; (d) severe lesions on face and paws.

see Chapter 22). The environment needs to be examined as a possible source of allergens. NSAIDs such as metacam at 0.2 mg/kg orally once daily along with diphenhydramine at 1 mg/kg orally q12h may help temporarily with signs. Prednisone at 0.25–0.5 mg/kg orally q12h may also help in severe cases. If secondary bacterial dermatitis due to scratching, may require use of a systemic oral antibiotic. True hypersensitivity may be difficult to control if the inciting allergen(s) are present. Treatment should be geared at keeping the ferret comfortable.

NEOPLASIA

Note: many ferrets may have more than one type of cutaneous neoplasm at any given time. The more common types are listed below. In addition to these, the following have been reported in ferrets: squamous cell carcinoma, spindle cell sarcoma, mammary gland adenoma, fibroma, fibrosarcoma, xanthoma, leiomyoma and lipoma (**Fig. 21.15**). All can be diagnosed through biopsy and histopathology. Also noteworthy: in addition to cutaneous neoplasms, ferrets may have concurrent non-cutaneous neoplasia. Vaccine-induced fibrosarcomas have been reported.

Apocrine scent tumours
Definition/overview
Can be adenocarcinoma or adenoma. Usually localised in areas of concentration of scent glands such as the anal glands, head, neck, prepuce, vulva, perineum. If the prepuce is involved that is usually

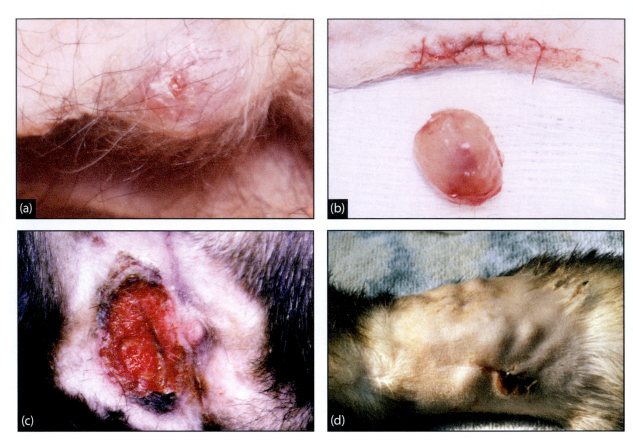

Fig. 21.15 (a, b) Dermal fibroma; (c) xanthoma; (d) multiple lipomas.

secondary to adrenal disease (see Chapter 14). This tumour may also arise from remnant anal sacculectomy that left some of the gland (**Fig. 21.16**).

Aetiology/pathophysiology
Tumours may originate in apocrine glandular tissue.

Clinical presentation
Masses that are firm and can be variable in size. Usually are freely movable.

Differential diagnosis
Any tumours of the skin.

Diagnostic testing
Fine needle aspiration cytology, tissue biopsy and histopathology.

Management/treatment
Surgical excision of the tumour. It should be sent for histopathology. If it is removed from the prepuce explore adrenal disease and usually start therapy for that (see Chapter 14). If involving anal sac area, full excision of the tissue should be done.

Basal cell tumour
Definition/overview
Fairly common mass arising from basal cells.

Aetiology/pathophysiology
Mass arising from basal cells in the skin. Usually benign and slow growing.

Clinical presentation
Discrete, solitary tumours anywhere on the body (**Fig. 21.17**). Often pedunculated or ulcerated. Non-pruritic.

Differential diagnosis
Any tumours of the skin.

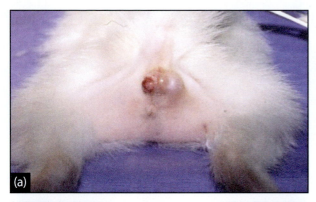

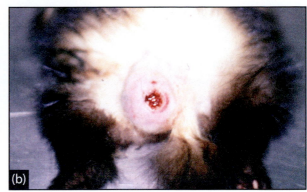

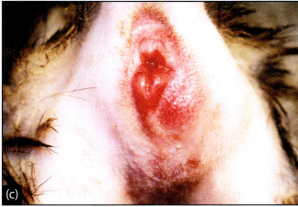

Fig. 21.16 (a, b) Apocrine scent tumours arising from anal sacs; (c) swelling on the anal sac consistent with either infection or neoplasia.

Management/treatment
Surgical excision of the mass.

Cutaneous haemangioma
Definition/overview
Mass composed of blood-filled cavernous spaces lined by well-differentiated endothelial cells that readily haemorrhage when traumatised. No sex predilection. Average age of 4.7 years in one retrospective study. Considered benign.

Aetiology/pathophysiology
Haemangiomas rarely develop into haemangiosarcomas, which appear similar to haemangiomas and, as typical for malignancies, are locally aggressive and may recur after apparently complete surgical removal.

Clinical presentation
Small, black masses or just a round red area of skin. Anywhere on body, but slight predilection for the head, face, and feet.

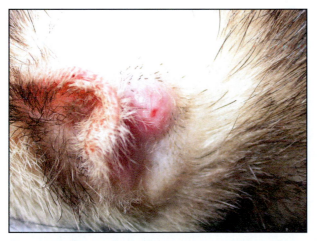

Fig. 21.17 Basal cell tumour.

Diagnostic testing
Fine needle aspiration cytology, tissue biopsy and histopathology.

Diagnosis
Confirmation of basal cells in the cytology/histopathology.

Differential diagnosis
Any tumour of the skin.

Diagnostic testing
Fine needle aspirate, biopsy, histopathology.

Diagnosis
Listed above under Definition/overview.

Management/treatment
Surgical excision of the mass. If haemangiosarcoma, risk of recurrence.

Cutaneous (epitheliotrophic) lymphoma (see Chapter 16)

Definition/overview
Lymphoma of the skin. Tumours may be associated with other lymphomas in the body. It also may just be located in skin. Arises usually from a lymph node or lymphatic tissue. It may be a solitary mass or there may be multiple masses.

Aetiology/pathophysiology
Arising from lymphatic tissue, most commonly associated with a node or lymphatic tissue. Epitheliotrophic lymphomas are usually T cell. In one retrospective study, 75% were in males with an average age of 4.6 years. Females affected later in life with an average of 7 years.

Clinical presentation
Nodules, sometimes ulcerated. There may be swelling, pruritis, alopecia, erythema, scaling. Affecting commonly feet and extremities. Has also been seen in periocular tissue (**Fig. 21.18**).

Differential diagnosis
Any tumours of the skin.

Diagnostic testing
Fine needle aspirate, biopsy and histopathology.

Management/treatment
Surgical excision of the mass(es) and send for histopathology. Prognosis is guarded as more may occur. Ferrets may live for a few months after diagnosis. Treatment with corticosteroids is rarely successful.

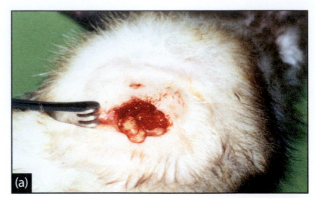

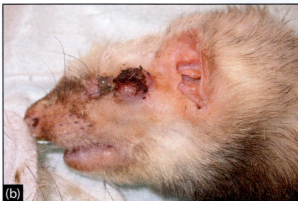

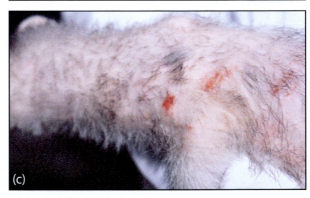

Fig. 21.18 **(a, b) Cutaneous lymphosarcoma; (c) lymphoblastic lymphoma.**

Care should be supportive to keep the ferret comfortable. Isotretinoin has been beneficial in some cases. Watch for signs of systemic lymphoma (see Chapter 16). If preputial mass, use protocol for adrenal disease control (see Chapter 14).

Leiomyosarcomas

Definition/overview
Tumour arising from arrector pili smooth muscle of the hair follicle.

Aetiology/pathophysiology

Tumours are twice as common in males as in females, can occur at any age. Considered malignant and have a high mitotic index.

Clinical presentation

Appear as raised, pink skin nodules, discrete or locally invasive. Occasionally ulcerated. Found anywhere on the body but predilection for the head, neck and limbs.

Differential diagnosis

Any tumour of the skin.

Diagnostic testing

Fine needle aspiration, biopsy, histopathology.

Diagnosis

Confirmation of leiomyosarcoma cells.

Management/treatment

Complete surgical excision. Prognosis guarded as there may be recurrence and possible metastasis.

Mammary gland tumours

Definition/overview

Tumours may be malignant adenocarcinomas, benign adenomas or fibroadenomas.

Aetiology/pathophysiology

Several different tumour types have been found as listed above. In one study, 70% of tumours in males were benign adenomas, with 30% being malignant adenocarcinomas. Only benign tumours were found in females. Adenomas were most commonly seen in males averaging 6–7 years old. Females were younger; 2–6 years of age.

Clinical presentation

Small nodule in mammary tissue. May grow large and become ulcerated (**Fig. 21.19**).

Differential diagnosis

Any tumour of the skin.

Diagnostic testing

Fine needle aspirate, biopsy, histopathology.

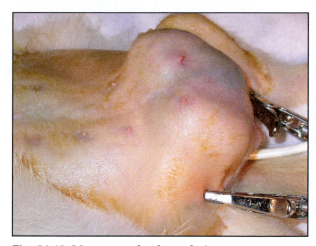

Fig. 21.19 **Mammary gland neoplasia.**

Diagnosis

Confirmation of neoplastic mammary tissue.

Management/treatment

Surgical excision. Adenocarcinomas have the potential for recurrence, particularly if surgical margins were insufficient.

Mast cell tumours

Definition/overview

Reported as 16% of all cutaneous neoplasms in one study, 33% in another. Usually benign, localised. Unlike other species where this is a systemic disease, in ferrets it is localised in the skin.

Aetiology/pathophysiology

Tumour arises from mast cells in the skin.

Clinical presentation

Small, round, slightly raised dermal mass with occasional ulcerated surface with crusts. Pruritic. Ferret may be scratching at it and causing a secondary bacterial dermatitis. Most ferrets however do not seem to notice the mass unless it is severely pruritic. Most commonly found in the shoulder, head and neck areas, but also can be found on the trunk (**Fig. 21.20**).

Differential diagnosis

Any skin tumour.

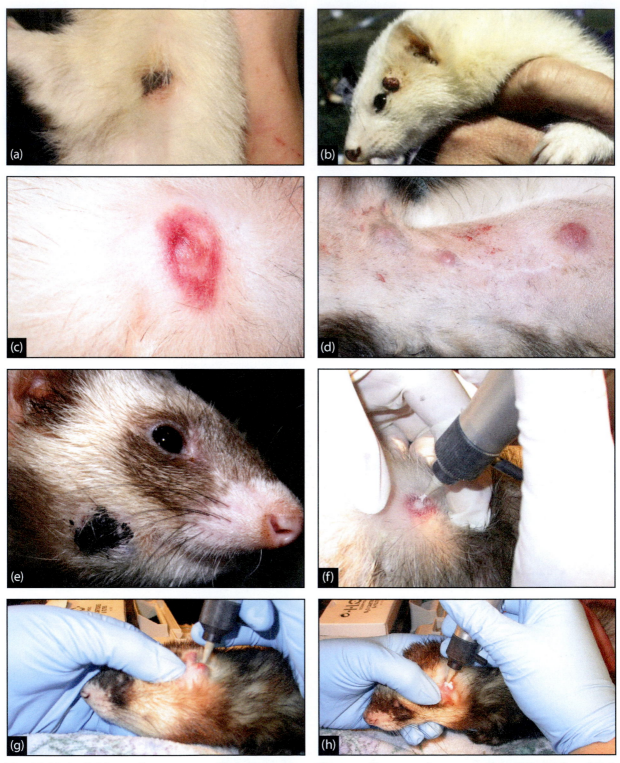

Fig. 21.20 (a–d) Mast cell tumour manifestations; (e) small mast cell tumour (courtesy of Vondelle McLaughlin); (f) cryotherapy may be used on small mast cell tumours. (g, h) cryotherapy of mast cell tumour.   *(Continued)*

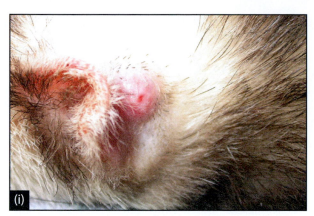

Fig. 21.20 (continued) (i) Appearance of the tumour in (g) 5 minutes post-freezing. Frozen mast cell tumours usually slough off in 5–7 days.

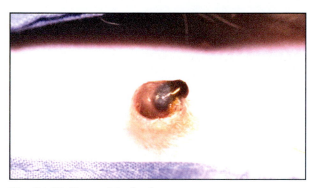

Fig. 21.21 Preputial gland mass.

Diagnostic testing
Fine needle aspirate and cytology. Biopsy and histopathology.

Diagnosis
Presence of concentration of mast cells.

Management/treatment
Surgical excision is preferred. Small tumours can be frozen off with liquid nitrogen (cryotherapy or surgery). Following freezing the tumours usually slough off in 5–7 days. For pruritis diphenhydramine at 1 mg/kg PO q12h along with an NSAID such as metacam at 0.2 mg/kg PO q24h. If owner elects not to have surgery, the above medications may help to control the itching; a topical corticosteroid or diphenhydramine cream may be used topically. Rarely there is bacterial dermatitis from laceration of the surface due to scratching, in which case a topical triple antibiotic cream can be used.

Preputial gland tumours
Definition/overview
Malignant tumours arising from the apocrine glands. Include carcinomas, adenocarcinomas, cyst-adenocarcinomas. These are present as part of the adrenal disease complex, and adrenal disease must be addressed (see Chapter 14).

Aetiology/pathophysiology
Sex steroid hormone elevations as seen with adrenal disease stimulate the apocrine glands. The tumour may be invasive into the distal urethra. Urination may be difficult and painful. Local growth is aggressive. The tumour may invade the body wall and has a moderate potential for metastasis, especially to local tissues and lymph nodes.

Clinical presentation
Often starts as a very small skin or subcutaneous nodule near the preputial orifice, which develops rapidly into a large, firm nodule. Tumour may be freely movable (early) becoming adherent to the body wall as it progresses and invades surrounding tissue (**Fig. 21.21**).

Differential diagnosis
Distinctive, no real differentials.

Diagnostic testing
Fine needle aspirate, biopsy, histopathology. Diagnostic testing for adrenal disease (see Chapter 14).

Diagnosis
Histological confirmation of apocrine appearance of cells with prominent apical protrusions.

Management/treatment
Early, wide, and deep surgical excision is necessary. Concurrent treatment for adrenal disease management must be done as well (see Chapter 14). In many cases, penile amputation and urethrostomy must be performed to obtain clean margins and prevent recurrence. Despite aggressive therapy reported including radiation, many reoccur.

Sebaceous epithelioma

Definition/overview
Reported as 58% of cutaneous neoplasms in one study of 57 neoplasms. Reported as 30% in another study. Usually benign, localised. Is also considered to be a basal cell tumour with sebaceous and squamous differentiation.

Aetiology/pathophysiology
Average age at diagnosis was 5.2 years and 70% were in females in the above study of 57 ferrets. Tumour arises from pluripotential basaloid epithelial cells of sebaceous glands.

Clinical presentation
Pedunculated or plaque-like mass, most likely to be on the face, ear, tail, limb, flank, but seem to be more common on the head and neck (**Fig. 21.22**). Surface can become ulcerated with necrotic centre. Non-pruritic.

Differential diagnosis
Any tumour of the skin, particularly pure basal cell tumours.

Diagnostic testing
Fine needle aspirate, biopsy and histopathology.

Diagnosis
Results of cytology, histopathology.

Management/treatment
Surgical excision is curative.

PYODERMA (BACTERIAL DERMATITIS)

Definition/overview
Infection and inflammation of the skin.

Aetiology/pathophysiology
Usually secondary to trauma, bite wounds, rough playing, ectoparasites. Most commonly caused by *Staphylococcus* sp. or *Streptococcus* sp. Can be superficial or deep. May be extensive with abscesses and cellulitis. Occasionally is pruritic. Ferret may cause further damage with scratching or licking.

Clinical presentation
Punctate or diffuse inflammation, laceration, pustules, or small abscessed pockets of skin. May be anywhere on body, but if from fighting or rough play, the shoulder and neck areas are most common (**Fig. 21.23**).

Differential diagnosis
Abscesses, neoplasia, hypersensitivity (due to pruritis, secondary dermatitis from trauma).

Diagnostic testing
Culture and sensitivity, cytology, biopsy and histopathology.

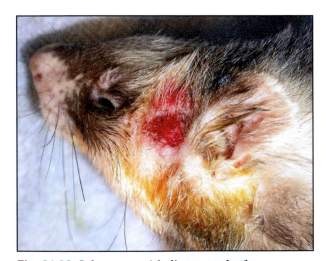

Fig. 21.22 **Sebaceous epithelioma on the face.**

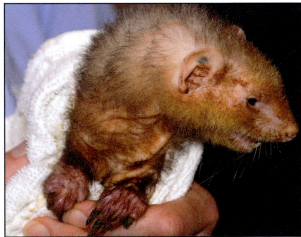

Fig. 21.23 **Pyoderma. (Courtesy of Vondelle McLaughlin.)**

Management/treatment

Determine the cause of the pyoderma. If fighting, prevent social contact with individual. Otherwise, treat for secondary bacterial infection with appropriate antimicrobials. NSAIDs will help with inflammation and discomfort. Topical treatment with antimicrobial cream may help if application can be made without the ferret licking it off too quickly.

VIRAL: CANINE DISTEMPER

Definition/overview

Rash and/or hyperkeratosis occurring with infection of canine distemper (see Chapter 20).

Aetiology/pathophysiology

Canine distemper is a paramyxovirus and is acutely susceptible. Mortality can reach as high as 100%, but treatment and vaccination in the face of an outbreak can limit mortality. Transmission is direct contact, aerosols and fomites.

Clinical presentation

Seven to 10 days following infection, ferrets may exhibit anorexia, fever, and a mucopurulent ocular–nasal discharge. There is a characteristic rash under the chin and in the inguinal area at 10–15 days. Foot pads and nasal pads often swell and exhibit hyperkeratosis (**Fig. 21.24**). There will be brown, crusted lesions on the chin, nose and perianal area.

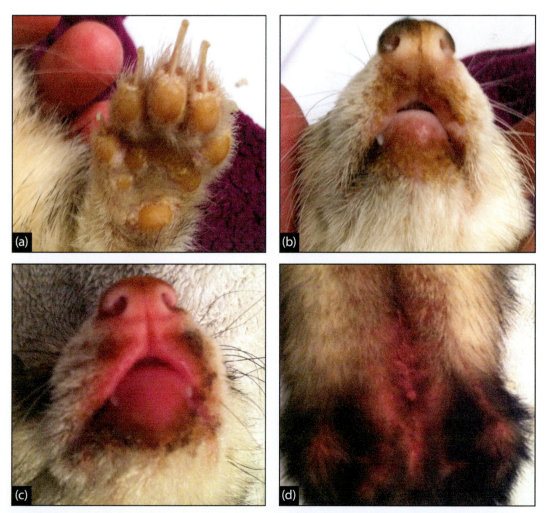

Fig. 21.24 **(a) Hyperkeratosis of footpads seen with canine distemper; (b, c) facial lesions of canine distemper; (d) erythema of ventrum seen with canine distemper. (Courtesy of Vondelle McLaughlin.)**

Terminally ferrets develop nervous signs, convulsions and death.

Differential diagnosis
Facial rash may be similar to other forms of dermatitis, atopy, autoimmune dermatitis.

Diagnostic testing
Confirmation of distemper through PCR and/or serology. Biopsy and histopathology of affected areas.

Diagnosis
History, clinical signs, confirmation of testing as listed above.

Management/treatment
Vaccinate (boost) any exposed ferrets (see Chapter 20). Treatment may be tried with interferon (following cat dosage regimens), vitamin A and vitamin C, plus supportive care (antimicrobials for rash/dermatitis, NSAIDs for comfort). In one outbreak in a shelter, the author reports mortality rate was approximately 65% with treatment regimen above.

CHAPTER 22

DISORDERS OF THE UROGENITAL SYSTEM

Cathy A. Johnson-Delaney

REPRODUCTIVE TRACT GENERAL NOTES (SEE CHAPTERS 3, 6)

Primary reproductive tract disease is uncommon in the USA where ferrets are routinely desexed at 5–6 weeks of age. Outside the USA, most ferrets are gonadectomised at 5–6 months of age if at all, therefore disease of reproductive organs and prolonged oestrus seasons are much more common.

Puberty occurs at 4–12 months of age depending on month born. Generally jills come into season the spring after they are born. Onset is earlier where ferrets are exposed to long days of more than 12 hours of light. Gonadal activity is seasonal and the breeding seasons occur from September to December in the southern hemisphere and March to August in the northern hemisphere, with peak breeding activity in April. Ferrets are long-day breeders and more than 12 hours of light promotes reproductive activity.

Male reproductive season: plasma testosterone levels begin increasing in December in the northern hemisphere and reach a peak plateau maintained from the end of February until late July. Increases in testicular size begin in January and peak in April (**Fig. 22.1**). Stages and cycle duration of spermatogenesis are similar to those of other carnivores.

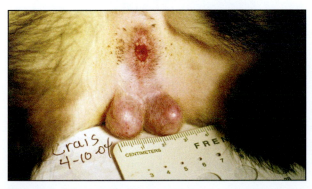

Fig. 22.1 Intact male in season.

AGALACTIA

Definition/overview
The failure of the jill to lactate enough milk for a normal litter (eight kits average).

Aetiology/pathophysiology
The jill may be stressed because of environmental factors such as overcrowding, noise, visits from strangers, repeated handling of kits and disturbance of the 'nest', overheating (temperature exceeding 21°C), systemic disease, chronic mastitis or being on a poor diet. It is more common in litters of fewer than five kits. Jills do not nurse the kits until all are born so dystocia or prolonged delivery may delay nursing and predispose the jill to lactation failure.

Clinical presentation
The kits may be thin, vocalising and moving around restlessly. The mammary glands may not be enlarged. When testing for milk, no milk can be palpated from the nipples. There may also be hardening of the glands as is seen at the end of the normal lactation period.

Differential diagnosis
Mastitis.

Diagnostic testing
Palpating gently to try to express milk from the nipple.

Diagnosis
No milk on palpation of nipple and gland.

Management/treatment
The kits will need to be hand fed using kitten milk replacer (see Chapter 26). The initial stressor that

probably led to the agalactia should be addressed. The jill should be fed an optimal diet and treated for any other disease present.

CONGENITAL ABNORMALITIES

Definition/overview

Segmental atresia of the uterus that is associated with hydrometra has been reported. Congenital persistant cloaca has been described. This is confluence of rectum, vagina and urethra into a single, common chamber. There may be concurrent caudal spinal agenesis (see Chapter 17). Dysplasia of the kidneys has also been seen with this abnormality. Cryptorchidism occurs not infrequently in males.

Aetiology/pathophysiology

There are theories that there may have been teratogen exposure and/or a genetic mutation. Inheritable, toxic, nutritional and infectious causes have been triggers for several anorectal, urogenital and skeletal anomalies in other animals. Persistent cloaca forms early in embryogenesis where a common chamber (cloaca) is normally present and both the urogenital sinus (ventrally) and the rectum (dorsally) develop from its partitions with the extension of the urorectal septum. The external genitalia develop from the primitive cloacal region. A septum defines the caudal intestinal tract dorsally, and the urogenital sinus ventrally. Any defect in mesodermal proliferation prohibiting the caudal migration of the urorectal septum inhibits the cleavage of the cloaca, resulting in the formation of the persistent cloaca. Cryptorchidism occurs when one testicle does not descend. The retained testicle becomes poorly developed although it may be a site of neoplasia as the ferret ages (**Fig. 22.2**).

Clinical presentation

There may be no external signs of the segmental atresia of the uterus with hydrometra, although the jill may have a swollen vulva and appear to be in oestrus (**Figs 22.3, 22.4**). Malformation of the urogenital region is seen with persistent cloaca. There may be wetted and faeces-soiled fur in the urogenital area and ventral tail. There may also be exudate if secondary infection is present.

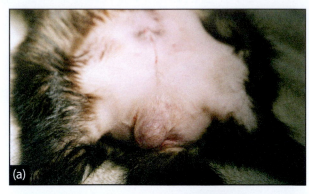

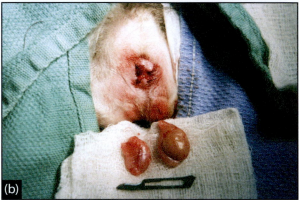

(a)

(b)

Fig. 22.2 **(a, b) Cryptorchidism.**

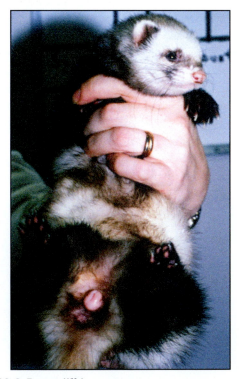

Fig. 22.3 **Intact jill in oestrus.**

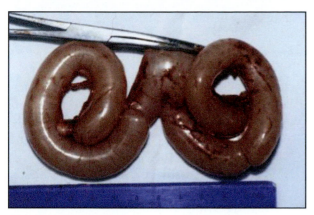

Fig. 22.4 Hydrometra.

Differential diagnosis
Segmental atresia with hydrometra: pregnancy, pyometra. There is none for the persistent cloaca.

Diagnostic testing
Ultrasound can be used to diagnose fluid swelling of the uterus. For persistent cloaca, radiographs with an excretory urogram may show kidney anomalies as well as the cloaca filling abnormalities. If there are caudal vertebral abnormalities these will show in radiographs. If secondary infection with exudate from the orifice is present, a culture may be taken.

Diagnosis
Abnormalities of the uterus can be determined with exploratory laparotomy and hysterectomy. Persistent cloaca on visual and radiographic evidence.

Management/treatment
Ovariohysterectomy of the abnormal uterus is curative (see Chapter 25). For persistent cloaca the prognosis is grave. It would be difficult to do reconstructive surgery owing to the anatomy lying largely in the pelvic canal.

DYSTOCIA

Definition/overview
Problems in parturition, an inability to give birth.

Aetiology/pathophysiology
This is not a common problem. Most jills can deliver the kits with no problems, unless there is a very large litter. Problems that may complicate parturition include oversized fetus with congenital defects such as spina bifida. A very small jill may have problems with normal-sized fetus delivery.

Clinical presentation
Generally the jill will be straining but may become exhausted and unable to continue labour. There may be large fetuses or a large litter (litter size can be 2–17, mean eight kits).

Differential diagnosis
None.

Diagnostic testing
A radiograph can identify the number of fetuses and potential size differences that are causing the dystocia. Ultrasound can be useful to identify heartbeats and if there is fetal death.

Diagnosis
The inability for the jill to deliver the kits.

Management/treatment
A Caesarian (C-) section should be performed. It is a straightforward surgery as is done in other species. A course of antibiotics along with NSAIDs for pain postsurgery should be given. An antimicrobial such as amoxicillin should not be a problem for nursing kits. This jill probably should have an ovariohysterectomy at the time of the C-section.

MAMMARY GLAND HYPERPLASIA

Definition/overview
Hyperplastic changes to the mammary tissue.

Aetiology/pathophysiology
Changes to the mammary glands due to elevated sex steroids concurrent with adrenal disease (see Chapter 14).

Clinical presentation
Unilateral or bilateral lobulated mammary masses. There may be concurrent alopecia and other changes associated with adrenal disease (see Chapters 14, 21).

Differential diagnosis

Mastitis, mammary adenoma or adenocarcinoma, skin-related neoplasia.

Diagnostic testing

Fine needle aspirate or biopsy, histopathology. Adrenal disease testing: serum hormone levels, ultrasonography, radiology.

Diagnosis

Histopathology: there will be multilobular hyperplastic nodules. The nodules are composed of ducts with hyperplastic epithelial lining cells and some stromal connective tissue. Many ducts will contain proteinaceous material.

Management/treatment

Surgical excision of the masses. Treatment for adrenal disease (see Chapter 14).

MASTITIS

Definition/overview

Inflammation and/or infection of the mammary glands in the intact, nursing jill.

Aetiology/pathophysiology

Generally there is laceration or damage by the nursing kits to the mammary glands. This in turn causes inflammation and/or infection of individual glands, although the disease can progress following the channels between the glands. There is a published report of mastitis caused by haemolytic *Escherichia coli* in which the glands were gangrenous.

Clinical presentation

The glands appear swollen, firm, bruised or discoloured or erythematous, and occasionally ulcerated. There is exudate, which may be expressed out of the nipple. The glands have raised temperature and are painful. The jill may be septicaemic and become moribund.

Differential diagnosis

Neoplasia.

Diagnostic testing

Expression of exudates for culture and sensitivity, fine needle aspirate for cytology.

Diagnosis

Positive on cytology for infection and inflammation without neoplastic cells.

Management/treatment

NSAIDs for the pain and inflammation, antimicrobials depending on culture results but generally a broad-spectrum antimicrobial should be used. Warm compresses applied to the glands may give comfort, and also help with expression of the exudates through the nipple. Prognosis is guarded due to the likelihood of septicaemia. In extreme cases surgical excision may be necessary. The kits should be removed from the jill and hand fed (see Chapter 5).

METRITIS

Definition/overview

Inflammation of the endometrium of the uterus.

Aetiology/pathophysiology

This develops in the immediate postpartum period. It can also develop after abortions or breeding. It may be associated with retained placentas or foetuses.

Clinical presentation

The uterus is distended. There may be reddish-coloured vaginal discharge (**Fig. 22.5**).

Differential diagnosis

Pyometra, neoplasia.

Diagnostic testing

Radiographs, ultrasonography. Histopathology is done of tissue postovariohysterectomy.

Management/treatment

Ovariohysterectomy is curative. Medical management can be tried using an analgesic and systemic antimicrobials. Prostaglandin F2-alpha (Lutalyse, 0.5 mg IM) to evacuate the uterus, and systemic

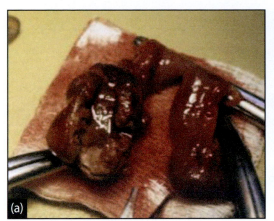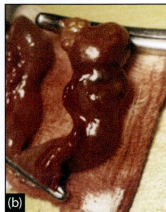

Fig. 22.5 (a, b) Metritis.

antimicrobials. Complications may be ascending cystitis and secondary urolithiasis due to the discharges in the vaginal vault.

NEOPLASIA

Ovarian
Definition/overview
Ovarian neoplasia and preneoplastic changes occur in ovaries.

Aetiology/pathophysiology
In jills, smooth muscle hyperplasia was found in a large number of ovaries in a published report. Leiomyomas were found in a significant number of ovaries, sometimes unilaterally or bilaterally. They may be solitary or multiple, reaching a diameter of 1.8 cm. Most are smaller. It is visible macroscopically as an opaque white solid mass against the pinkish-grey ovarian tissue. They are well defined and show ovarian tissue stretched over their surface. Occasionally the myoma is embedded in the ovary. The intraovarian myomatous tissue may be continuous with the hyperplastic smooth muscle tissue. Hydrometra (aseptic fluid within the uterus) and a persistent corpora lutea are seen.

Clinical presentation
There may be no outward signs that these changes have occurred. There may be signs of endocrine alopecia.

Differential diagnosis
Neoplasia.

Diagnostic testing
Ultrasonography of the ovaries may show nodules. Histopathology of the ovary, obtained at ovariohysterectomy.

Diagnosis
Confirmation of hyperplastic or neoplastic changes in the ovary.

Management/treatment
Ovariohysterectomy is curative.

Testicular
Definition/overview
Neoplastic change in testicles. Seen more commonly if cryptorchid.

Aetiology/pathophysiology
Seen in middle-aged to older intact hobs. Reported neoplasms include Leydig or interstitial cell tumours, seminoma, Sertoli cell tumour and carcinomas of the rete testis. Metastasis to the liver has been reported in one ferret with a Sertoli cell tumour.

Clinical presentation
Unilateral or bilateral enlargement of the testicle(s). Swelling may be firm, fluctuant or soft. There may be increases in serum sex steroids (**Fig. 22.6**).

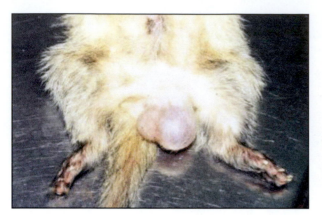

Fig. 22.6 Enlarged neoplastic testicle.

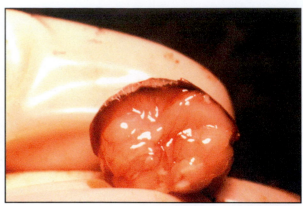

Fig. 22.7 Testicular neoplasia.

There may be increased sexual behaviour, aggression, increased dermal sebaceous gland activity that creates a greasy coat and increased musky odour. There may also be total body alopecia and severe pruritis described in a ferret with Sertoli cell tumour, presumably due to hyperoestrogenism.

Differential diagnosis
Orchitis although this has not been reported in ferrets.

Diagnostic testing
Fine needle aspiration, cytology. Biopsy, histopathology.

Diagnosis
Neoplastic cells (**Fig. 22.7**).

Management/treatment
Castration is usually curative unless there has been systemic metastasis. Histopathology of the testis to determine type of neoplasia. Thoracic radiographs are indicated if there is thought to be a risk of metastasis.

Uterine
Definition/overview
Neoplastic and preneoplastic changes in the uterus.

Aetiology/pathophysiology
Uterine tumours may be adenomas, adenocarcinomas, leiomyomas. Additionally there may be hyperplastic changes.

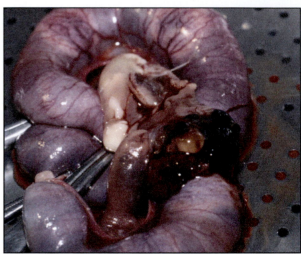

Fig. 22.8 Neoplastic uterus.

Clinical presentation
There may be no outward signs in the jill. Occasionally there may be some bleeding or exudates that may also be found with pyometra (**Fig. 22.8**).

Differential diagnosis
Pyometra.

Diagnostic testing
Ultrasonography of the uterus. Cytology of any secretions. The fluid may also be cultured as there may be secondary bacterial infection in the diseased uterus. On taking the tissue, histopathology. If neoplasia is suspected, a chest film may be indicated to rule out metastasis prior to the decision to do ovariohysterectomy.

Diagnosis

Presence of changes. Full diagnosis is usually made after ovariohysterectomy.

Management/treatment

Ovariohysterectomy is curative. These neoplasias rarely metastasise although screening with thoracic films periodically may be indicative.

OESTRUS UNBRED APLASTIC ANAEMIA

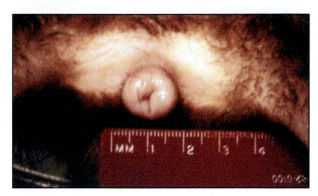

Fig. 22.9 **Oestrus vulva.**

Definition/overview

If a jill comes into oestrus and is not bred, it can lead to a fatal aplastic anaemia due to the prolonged high oestrogen levels. Ferrets are seasonally monoestrus. The normal breeding season is from March to August in the northern hemisphere. The ferret is a copulatory ovulator. The ferret will remain in oestrus up to 120 days or more if not bred.

Aetiology/pathophysiology

High oestrogen levels suppress bone marrow production of red blood cells resulting in what could become a fatal anaemia. This may take several months to develop. In addition, there may be thrombocytopaenia, granulocytopaenia and hypocellularity of the bone marrow. The anaemia is characterised by normocytic and normochromic erythrocytes and lack of a regenerative response. Nucleated red blood cells may be detected in peripheral blood. The increase in nucleated red blood cells is disproportionate to the reticulocyte response attributed to the release from sites of extramedullary haematopoiesis, usually from the spleen. The leucopaenia may be characterised as severe neutropaenia and eosinopaenia. The absolute lymphocytes count is usually in the normal range. There may be lowered plasma protein levels.

Clinical presentation

The vulva is swollen and has been for the duration of oestrus (**Fig. 22.9**). The mucous membranes will be pale. There may be bilateral symmetrical alopecia of the trunk but extending to the extremities as time progresses. They may be anorexic, depressed and lethargic. There may be a soft, left-sided protomesosystolic heart murmur compatible with anaemia. Haemorrhages may be found as ecchymoses in the skin, petechiae on the conjunctiva. There may be melena, but that may be secondary to GI ulceration brought on by stress and the possible thrombocytopaenia.

Differential diagnosis

In the intact jill, there really is no a differential. The clinical presentation is similar to adrenal disease in the sprite, although with adrenal disease there is not usually the anaemia.

Diagnostic testing

A complete blood count will measure the anaemia. There is a hormone panel that can be run to look at the levels of oestrogen, but this is usually unnecessary based on history and clinical signs. A bone marrow biopsy may be performed to look at the potential for red cell production. Generally the bone marrow appears to have the necessary precursor cells, but may also appear aplastic.

Diagnosis

Results of the CBC to confirm anaemia. Confirmation of aplasticity of bone marrow. Physical presentation along with history of not breeding (oestrus not terminated with breeding).

Management/treatment

Ovariohysterectomy of the jill will prevent further development of the anaemia. The ferret may need a blood transfusion prior to surgery to boost the red blood cell count. Additionally the use of epoeitin may be administered to boost red cell production. The author has performed this surgery on ferrets with a haematocrit of under 20 without problems. Generally the haematocrit begins to rise soon after ovariohysterectomy is performed.

PENILE LESIONS

Definition/overview
Trauma to the penis from bedding, scraping of penis on flooring, or fracture to the os penis tip.

Aetiology/pathophysiology
Seen in ferrets kept on hay bedding as the grass awns may catch in the prepuce. Ferrets that move along the ground pressing their groin down to mark their territory may scrape the prepuce. The os penis tip may be fractured from trauma including falling.

Clinical presentation
Swelling and laceration of prepuce. Foreign material (grass awns) may be present in the prepuce. If fracture of os penis, there may be bruising of the preputial area (**Fig. 22.10**). Frequently, fractured os penis is an incidental finding on radiographs (**Fig. 22.11**).

Differential diagnosis
Preputial neoplasia.

Diagnostic testing
Visualisation, radiographs. Fine needle aspiration and cytology may determine if there is infection.

Diagnosis
Presence of foreign material in prepuce. Radiographic confirmation of fractured os penis.

Management/treatment
Removal of foreign material. Topical antibacterial cream. Systemic NSAIDs and antimicrobials if abscessation. No treatment for fractured os penis. Watch to make sure the ferret urinates freely.

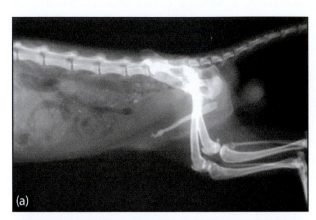

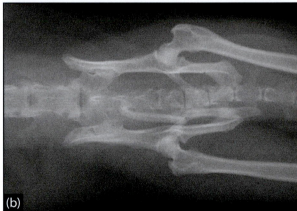

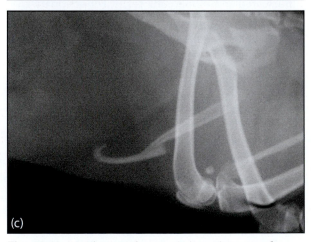

Fig. 22.11 (a) Abnormal os penis in an intact male; (b) VD radiograph mid-shaft fracture of the os penis; (c) lateral view same animal as (b).

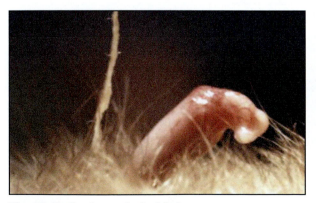

Fig. 22.10 Penis caught in fabric.

POSTPARTURIENT HYPOCALCAEMIA

Definition/overview
Postparturient hypocalcaemia is also called 'milk fever', or decreased blood calcium following parturition.

Aetiology/pathophysiology
Has been reported in primiparous jills 3–4 weeks postpartum.

Clinical presentation
Posterior paresis, sensitivity to stimuli and seizures.

Differential diagnosis
Systemic bacteraemia.

Diagnostic testing
Hypocalcaemic on blood chemistry.

Diagnosis
Hypocalcaemia along with presentation of nursing kits.

Management/treatment
Administration of oral and systemic calcium leads to rapid reversal of symptoms.

PREGNANCY TOXAEMIA

Definition/overview
Observed in late gestation. Syndrome of abnormal energy metabolism.

Aetiology/pathophysiology
Particularly seen in young, primiparous jills. There is a negative energy balance that leads to abnormal energy metabolism. This leads to hyperlipidaemia, hypoglycaemia, ketosis and hepatic lipidosis in the last 10 days of gestation. The energy deficiency is caused by either inadequate dietary intake or excess demand for nutrients due to a large litter (15 or even 20 kits). Stress ulceration of the GI tract may be a complication.

Clinical presentation
Acute onset of severe lethargy, anorexia, dehydration, weight loss and excessive shedding in late gestation. There may be diarrhoea and melena. It can also be a cause of sudden death of the jill.

Differential diagnosis
Systemic bacteraemia, pyometra, hepatic lipidosis due to anorexia, gastric ulceration.

Diagnostic testing
Haematology and serum chemistry. Radiographs to check fetuses. Ultrasonography may also be useful to determine integrity of the uterus and fetal life signs. Urinalysis.

Diagnosis
Ketonuria. There may be azotaemia, hypoproteinaemia, elevated liver enzyme activity. Hypocalcaemia, hyperbilirubinaemia, hypoglycaemia and anaemia may be found.

Management/treatment
Caesarean section. Aggressive supportive care including fluid therapy with electrolyte balancing. Nutritional support. An oesophagostomy tube may be needed for frequent force feedings if the jill won't take hand feeding or syringe feeding of dook soup (see Appendix 6). Gastroprotectants due to likelihood of GI ulceration. Broad-spectrum antimicrobials. If the jill survives she will probably be agalactic so surviving kits need to be hand nursed or cross fostered. Prognosis is guarded. Prevention should be stressed to breeders. This includes proper nutrition and minimisation of stressors for the jills during gestation. They need to provide fresh, easily accessible water as jills may stop eating if inadequate water is provided. Close monitoring of diet and water intake should be done during gestation.

PREPUTIAL LESIONS (SEE ALSO BELOW, PREPUTIAL TUMOURS)

Definition/overview
Swellings or masses involving the prepuce and preputial glands.

Aetiology/pathophysiology
Preputial glands and tissue may be stimulated hormonally as part of adrenal disease (see Chapter 14).

The abnormal tissue may become infected. If neo-plastic, it is often locally invasive and may extend into the abdominal wall.

Clinical presentation
Swelling of the tissues of the prepuce. It may be firm and attached to the body wall (**Fig. 22.12**).

PROSTATIC LESIONS: SEE URINARY SECTION

PSEUDOPREGNANCY

Definition/overview
False pregnancy.

Aetiology/pathophysiology
This is caused by failure of implantation that is associated with reduced light intensity 30 days before the start of breeding or failure to conceive. This can happen with mating to a vasectomised hob or an infertile male (usually young, less than 6 months old) to terminate oestrus. It has also been seen with termination of oestrus by administration of hCG.

Clinical presentation
Physical and behavioural changes normally seen with pregnancy such as weight gain, mammary gland enlargement and nesting behaviour. An important difference is that pseudopregnant jills develop a full, thick hair coat approximately 1.5 weeks before par-turition whereas pregnant jills lose coat and develop hairless rings around their teats. After whelping pseudopregnant jills return to oestrus if it is early in the breeding season. They become quiescent if it is late in the breeding season.

Differential diagnosis
Pregnancy.

Diagnostic testing
Radiographs, ultrasonography.

Diagnosis
No fetuses.

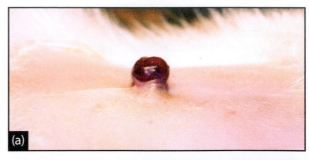

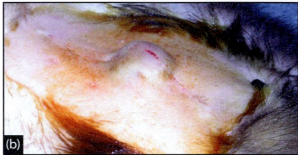

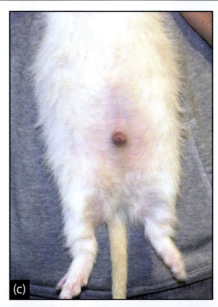

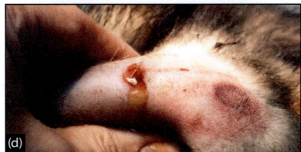

Fig. 22.12 (a–c) Preputial tissue enlargement; (d) infection involving the preputial tissue.

Management/treatment

Ensure jills are exposed to maximum light intensity during the spring. Artificially extend light hours in late summer. Use mature, sperm-tested hobs for mating. Older males will have higher sperm counts. It may not be preventable if mating with a v-hob is done to terminate oestrus as a breeding colony procedure.

PYOMETRA AND MUCOMETRA

Definition/overview

In the jill, pyometra may occur as a problem of breeding and not becoming pregnant. Stump pyometra seen in ovariectomised sprites is more common and is one of the common manifestations of adrenal disease (**Fig. 22.13**).

Aetiology/pathophysiology

Infection of the stump or uterus is an ascending bacterial disease. Various bacteria have been documented: *E. coli*, *Staphylococcus*, *Streptococcus* and *Corynebacterium* species. It has been proposed that pyometra in the breeding ferret may be under the influence of oestrogens and not progestins. Pyometra may be open or closed.

Clinical presentation

There may be purulent exudate discharging from the vulva. General signs of lethargy, depression, sometimes pyrexia. An enlarged uterus may be palpable or viewed on ultrasound, radiographs (**Fig. 22.14**). There may be some degree of endocrine alopecia.

Differential diagnosis

Vaginal infection, adrenal disease (sprites).

Diagnostic testing

Radiographs, ultrasonography. Vaginal swab with cytology, microbiology. Visual examination of vaginal vault and cervix may be done endoscopically to determine where secretion is coming from.

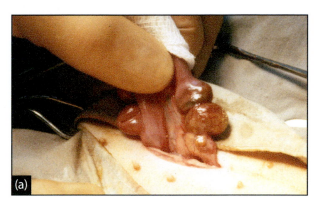

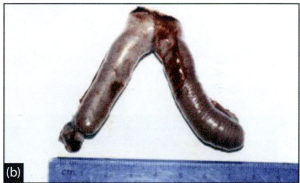

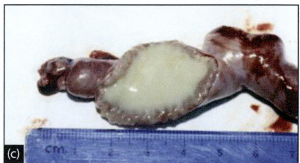

Fig. 22.14 (a) Exteriorising the uterus during ovariohysterectomy; (b) uterus, pyometra; (c) opened uterus showing exudate.

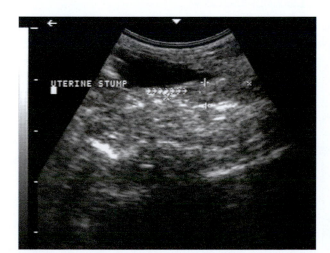

Fig. 22.13 Ultrasonography of uterine stump pyometra.

Diagnosis

Positive exudates for bacterial infection.

Management/treatment

Antimicrobial administration. Surgical excision of the uterus (ovariohysterectomy). Surgical excision of the stump, although that may resolve with treatment of adrenal disease (see Chapter 14).

VAGINITIS

Definition/overview

Inflammation of the vagina. There may also be bacterial infection present.

Aetiology/pathophysiology

It is associated with chronic and/or severe vulvar swelling such as hyperoestrogenism (adrenal disease, persistent oestrus, ovarian remnant disease). Vulvar swelling may also develop with cystitis, crystalluria or aggressive hob mating behaviour. Poor husbandry and inadequate sanitation may exacerbate vaginitis in jills housed on hay, straw, shavings. Bacteria implicated include *E. coli*, *Staphylococcus*, *Streptococcus*, *Proteus* or *Klebsiella* spp.

Clinical presentation

Vulva is swollen with purulent exudates present. There is discomfort as well (**Fig. 22.15**).

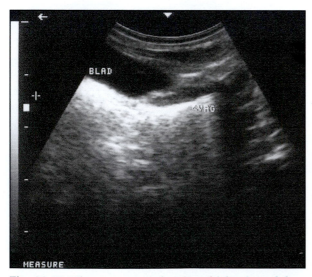

Fig. 22.15 Ultrasonogram showing thickening of the vaginal wall consistent with vaginitis.

Differential diagnosis

Oestrus, stump pyometra disease, pyometra, adrenal disease.

Diagnostic testing

Culture and sensitivity of the discharge. Endoscopic examination of the vaginal vault. Ultrasound and radiographs to rule out adrenal disease (see Chapter 14).

Diagnosis

Inflammation/infection of the vaginal vault.

Management/treatment

Antimicrobials systemically. The vault may also be treated topically with a triple antibiotic ointment applied within the vault. NSAIDs systemically for the pain and inflammation. If there is other underlying disease such as adrenal disease it should be addressed (see Chapter 14).

URINARY TRACT

Radiographic kidney measurements have been evaluated as a tool to assess kidneys (see Appendix 9). Scout radiographs, excretory urograms, ultrasonography and urinalysis are the most common techniques for assessing the urinary tract.

Aleutian disease

Definition/overview

A parvovirus (see Chapter 16). Systemic disease may be associated with disease in urinary tract.

Aetiology/pathophysiology

Many are asymptomatic carriers. Can cause deposits in the kidney as membranous glomerulonephritis and tubular interstitial nephritis and possibly renal failure. There may also be liver failure, intestinal disease including melena and central nervous system disease.

Clinical presentation

Chronic wasting and ataxia, attributed to immune complex deposition. Renal failure.

Differential diagnosis

Neoplasia, nephrosis/nephritis.

Diagnostic testing

Serology, PCR for Aleutian disease. General haematology and serum chemistry, radiographs, ultrasound looking for causes of the weight loss, ataxia, renal failure.

Diagnosis

Serologically, PCR positive for Aleutian disease (see Chapter 16). Presence of renal failure.

Management/treatment

Supportive care including fluid therapy. Prognosis is poor.

Cystitis and urolithiasis

Definition/overview

Inflammation and/or infection of the bladder with or without urolithiasis. Stones recovered from ferrets have been struvite (magnesium ammonium phosphate) or cysteine (**Fig. 22.16**).

Aetiology/pathophysiology

The urine of ferrets is acidic (pH normally of 5). With infection the bacteria may cause the urine to become alkaline, which in turn may contribute to more bacterial growth. Often cystitis occurs due to presence of urolithiasis or due to incomplete voiding such as seen in males with enlarged prostates. Uroliths are usually struvite, except for ferrets on a no-grain, novel protein or diet with legumes such as peas. Ferrets on these no-grain diets seem to have cysteine stones.

Clinical presentation

The ferret may be straining to urinate. The urine may be blood tinged. In severe cases the ferret may be lethargic and have an enlarged bladder due to incomplete voiding (**Figs 22.17, 22.18**). Male ferrets may become blocked similar to the problems seen in cats. There may be mucus plugs or urolithiasis in males that plug the urethra. There is usually pain even on gentle palpation of the bladder.

Differential diagnosis

Presence of urolithiasis in ureter, bladder, urethra. Clinical signs due to prostate enlargement and adrenal disease.

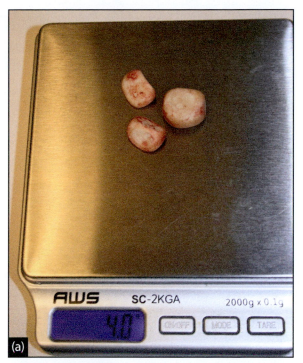

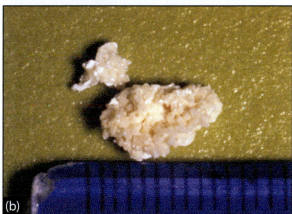

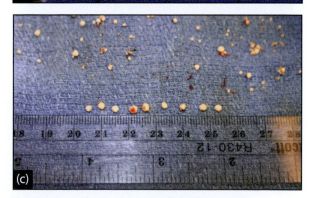

Fig. 22.16 (a, b) Cysteine uroliths; (c) struvite uroliths. (Courtesy of Vondelle McLaughlin.)

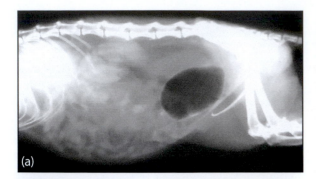

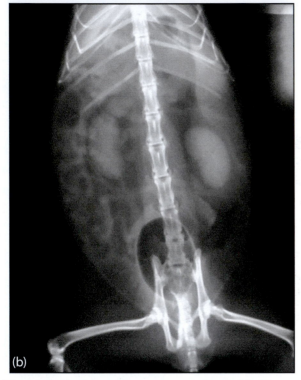

Fig. 22.17 (a, b) Double contrast study of a bladder with thickened walls indicative of cystitis.

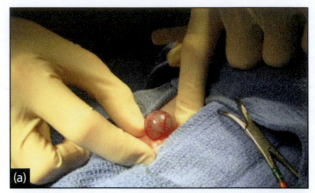

Fig. 22.18 (a) Cystitis bladder exteriorised for stone removal; (b) cystotomy.

Diagnostic testing

Urinalysis best obtained with cystocentesis. Ultrasonography can look at the bladder wall and prostate and usually visualises uroliths. Radiographs to find uroliths (**Fig. 22.19**). Content of the uroliths can be determined by laboratory testing.

Management/treatment

Surgery is necessary to relieve plugs or stones. Catheterisation may be necessary in the males if urethra is blocked. Technique for unblocking the

ferret may include retrograde flushing of stones back into the bladder where they can be surgically removed. The technique is essentially the same as in cats (**Fig. 22.20**). Antimicrobials, NSAIDs for symptoms and postoperatively.

If prostate enlargement is present, it is due to adrenal disease. Treat the adrenal disease (see Chapter 14). Change ferret diet to a traditional diet, not the current commercial no-grain diet (see Chapter 5). Treatment of struvite lithiasis has been reported by supplementing phosphoric acid (H_3PO_4) into the feed.

Glomerulosclerosis and renal hypertension

Definition/overview

Sclerosis of the glomeruli. Renal hypertension is a sequela as it is in other species.

Aetiology/pathophysiology

Condition is probably age related but may be accompanying nephrosis or nephritis. Because of the changes, there is some vascular compromise but there are

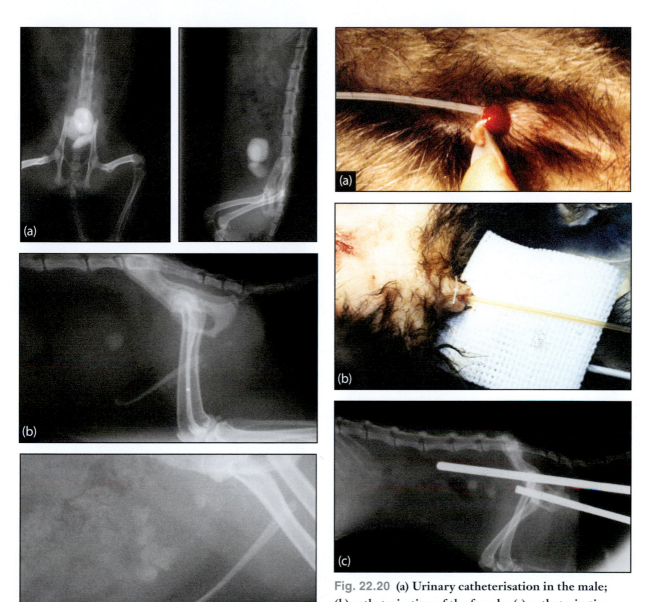

Fig. 22.19 (a, b) Lateral radiographs of cysteine urolithiasis (courtesy of Vondelle McLaughlin); (c) lateral radiograph of struvite urolithiasis.

Fig. 22.20 (a) Urinary catheterisation in the male; (b) catheterisation of the female; (c) catheterisation showing placement and uroliths.

changes in the renin–angiotensingenerating enzymes as cells are located in the juxtaglomerular region.

Clinical presentation
There may be renal disease or failure. Blood pressure may be elevated above 150 mmHg systolic.

Glomerulosclerosis may have no outward signs. Unless blood pressure is taken it may not be considered antemortem.

Differential diagnosis
Cardiac disease and hypertension. Renal disease or failure from other causes.

Diagnostic testing
Blood chemistry, peripheral blood pressure. Ultrasound of kidneys. Radiographs.

Diagnosis

Elevations in BUN, creatinine, elevated blood pressure. Or it may be unable to be detected clinically.

Management/treatment

When kidney disease is present, there is a likelihood of renal hypertension and use of an ACE inhibitor should be started. If this is not sufficient to bring down peripheral blood pressure when hypertension has been found, amlidopine or spironolactone may be added to the regimen for concurrent heart disease. Cardiac disease and renal disease are frequently linked with age-related changes.

Hydronephrosis

Definition/overview

Compression of the renal parenchyma via urine build-up within the renal capsule.

Aetiology/pathophysiology

This seems to be a congenital disease as it may be found in young ferrets. It can be unilateral or bilateral. Renal function is compromised. With renal cysts, renal function is not generally compromised. The capsule fills with urine, compressing the renal parenchyma and leading to renal failure.

Clinical presentation

Grossly enlarged abdomen (**Fig. 22.21**). Upon palpation the kidney is greatly enlarged.

Differential diagnosis

Neoplasia, renal cyst.

Diagnostic testing

Radiographs, ultrasonography, ultrasound-guided centesis with urinalysis. Haematology and blood chemistry. Excretory urogram (**Fig. 22.22**).

Diagnosis

Results of the pyelogram for renal function, ultrasonography to look at the kidney.

Management/treatment

If unilateral and the contralateral kidney appears normal on ultrasound and pyelogram, surgery may be done to remove the hydronephrotic kidney if it is causing discomfort to the ferret (**Fig. 22.23**). It can be drained via ultrasound-guided centesis but it will fill again. If bilateral, prognosis is poor. Palliative therapy for comfort of the ferret is all that can be done. The ferret will go into renal failure as the tissue is compressed. The author has used omega 3–6, enalapril and a Chinese herbal, rehmannia-6, for kidney function support.

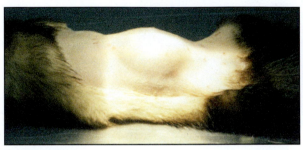

Fig. 22.21 Enlarged abdomen due to hydronephrosis.

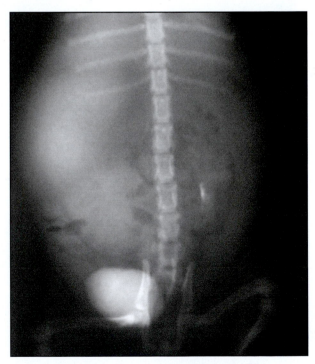

Fig. 22.22 Excretory urogram in a 9-week-old ferret showing normal filling of the left kidney and diffuse dye uptake with an enlarged kidney due to a complication from the ovariohysterectomy. The ureter had been ligated.

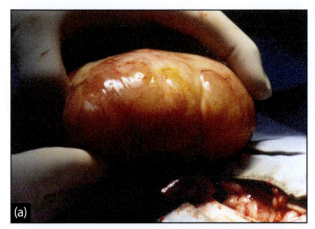

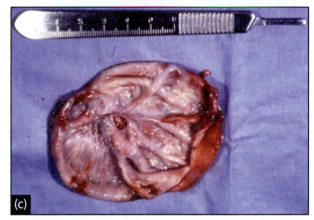

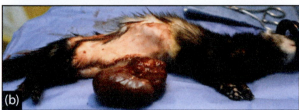

Fig. 22.23 (a) Nephrectomy; (b) comparison of the hydronephrotic kidney to the body postnephrectomy; (c) opened hydronephrotic kidney.

Preputial tumour

Definition/overview
Neoplasia present in the preputial tissue. Relatively long os penis, J-hook shaped. Urethral opening may be difficult to visualise.

Aetiology/pathophysiology
Tumour generally due to developing adrenal disease. The mass may be invasive to tissues around the prepuce. Occasionally this mass makes it difficult for the

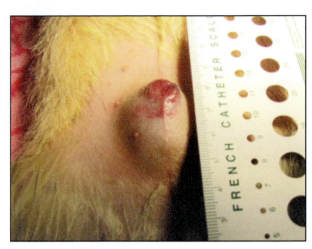

Fig. 22.24 Preputial mass.

ferret to void, resulting in a cystitis. The urine may cause the surface of the tumour to become ulcerated and painful.

Clinical presentation
There is a mass associated with the prepuce. It may be freely movable initially but seems to be quick to invade deeper tissue and the body wall. On palpation it may be painful. The surface may be ulcerated and secondarily infected (**Fig. 22.24**).

Differential diagnosis
Neoplasia.

Diagnostic testing
Fine needle aspirate, biopsy, histopathology. Ultrasonography is useful to see if the tumour has invaded the body wall. The adrenals can also be looked at as well as the prostate. Radiographs may be useful.

Diagnosis
Presence of the mass at the prepuce.

Management/treatment
Surgical excision as soon as possible is warranted, particularly to get deep tissue if invasive to the body wall. Treatment for adrenal disease should be started (see Chapter 14). If cystitis is present, antimicrobials should be given. NSAIDs will help with inflammation and analgesia postsurgically. The urethra may need to be catheterised if urine flow is obstructed.

Prostate enlargement, prostatitis, prostate abscess, prostatic cysts

Definition/overview

Prostate enlargement is part of the adrenal disease complex (see Chapter 14).

Aetiology/pathophysiology

The prostate may be cystic or hypertrophic or a combination. The cysts are frequently secondarily infected. The urethra may be compressed making it difficult to void. In severe cases the urethra is blocked completely. It may be blocked internally with prostate cells and secretions or it may be compressed by the prostate tissue. Secondary cystitis and atonic bladder may be present. It can be life threatening if urine flow is not restored.

Clinical presentation

Stranguria, dysuria are the first signs. As it progresses the bladder may be distended and the ferret may be unable to urinate. There may be pain associated with the straining and on palpation of the pelvic area.

Differential diagnosis

Urolithiasis, cystitis.

Diagnostic testing

Ultrasonography to look at the prostate, bladder, urethra (**Fig. 22.25**). Radiographs to look at urinary tract. Prostate cysts can be aspirated (ultrasound guided), cytology, culture, histology.

Diagnosis

Presence of enlarged prostate.

Management/treatment

Large cysts can be drained (ultrasound guided). To restore urine flow it may be necessary to treat with a relaxant such as a benzodiazepine plus opioid analgesic and anti-inflammatory corticosteroid along with antimicrobials. It may also be necessary to catheterise the urethra. Opening to urethra may be difficult to locate; can catheterise with #3–5 (the author uses #5 with a guitar string stylet) and lidocaine flush while doing it. Surgery to open the cysts may also be necessary. Large cysts have successfully been marsupialised. Treatment for adrenal disease must be instigated (see Chapter 14). Direct medications such as finasteride and bicalutamide will help shrink hypertrophy due to direct action on androgenic receptors on the prostate tissue. Prognosis is guarded. Restoration of urinary tract function is key.

Neoplasia

Definition/overview

Neoplasia within the urinary tract. Most commonly it is renal or bladder (**Fig. 22.26**).

Aetiology/pathophysiology

Renal lymphoma/lymphosarcoma is the most common neoplasia in the urinary system. Bladder carcinoma has been diagnosed.

Clinical presentation

The ferret may be presented with general malaise, anorexia and loss of weight and condition. The kidneys may be sensitive on palpation. The kidneys may palpate enlarged or irregularly shaped. If the bladder has a tumour, it may be distended and painful.

Differential diagnosis

Nephritis/nephrosis, infection/inflammation urinary tract included cystitis and urolithiasis.

Diagnostic testing

Radiographs, ultrasonography. Fine needle aspirate with histopathology of the kidney. Urinalysis, haematology, chemistry.

Diagnosis

Presence of neoplastic cells in the biopsy, occasionally neoplastic cells will present in the urine.

Management/treatment

If unilateral, nephrectomy of neoplastic kidney; however, the kidney may be the secondary site of a metastatic neoplastic process such as lymphoma. Prognosis is poor. If lymphoma, protocols have been established for ferrets based on the feline regimen. These do not work very well. Prednisone alone may work as well and not reduce the quality of life for the ferret. Bladder neoplasia could possibly be treated

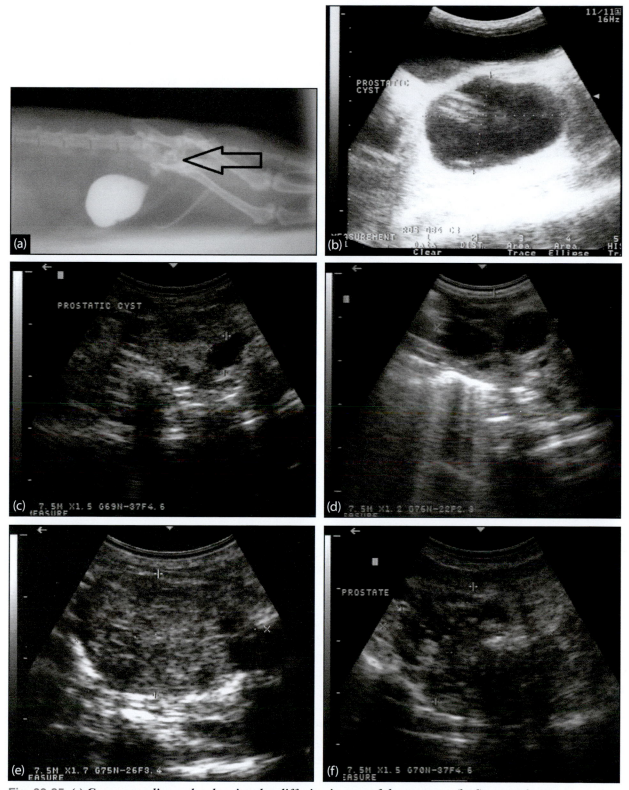

Fig. 22.25 (a) Contrast radiography showing dye diffusion in area of the prostate; (b–d) prostatic cysts; (e, f) enlarged prostate.

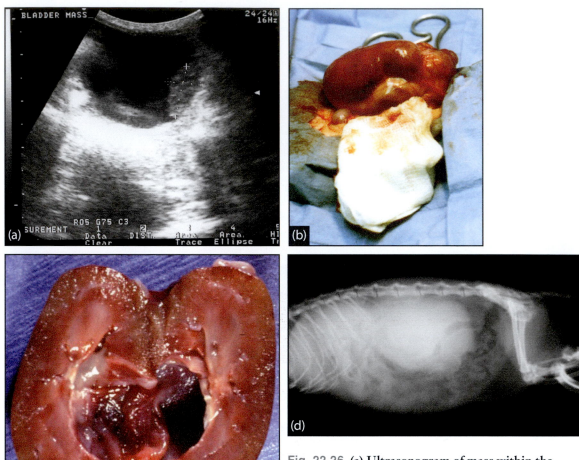

Fig. 22.26 (a) Ultrasonogram of mass within the urinary bladder; (b) exteriorisation of neoplastic kidney during nephrectomy; (c) renal leiomyosarcoma; (d) lateral radiograph of a renal mass.

with a cystotomy and removal of the diseased tissue, but rarely has this been performed.

Nephrocalcinosis

Definition/overview
Presence of calcium deposition in the kidney (**Fig. 22.27**).

Aetiology/pathophysiology
Areas of hyperechogenicity in the renal medulla were found in 40–58% of European pet ferrets. It was not found in laboratory ferrets. There were calcium deposits in the renal tubules consistent with renal calcification. There were crystalline structures within renal parenchyma that could not be found sonographically and were believed to be urates. Probably due to dietary imbalance of calcium and phosphorus.

Clinical presentation
None reported.

Differential diagnosis
None.

Diagnostic testing
Radiographs, ultrasonography. Biopsy with histopathology.

Diagnosis
Presence of calcium deposition in the kidney.

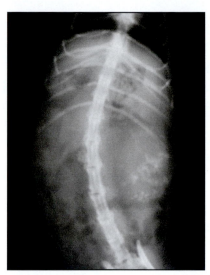

Fig. 22.27 Calcium deposits in the left kidney consistent with nephrocalcinosis.

Management/treatment
Switch ferret to a good commercial diet that has been validated by feeding trials not to have caused this condition.

Nephrosis, nephritis
Definition/overview
Changes within the kidney. Nephrosis generally is a degenerative disease seen in geriatric ferrets and may be found incidentally at necropsy. Ferrets can have an inflammatory, immune-mediated/infected nephritis but this may only be picked up on necropsy as no outward signs may be seen.

Aetiology/pathophysiology
Ascending infection or secondary infection from a systemic infection may affect the kidney. Nephrosis may just be changes in the kidney due to aging. It may lead to end-stage kidney disease with elevated BUN and creatinine, electrolyte imbalance. Immune mediated/complex disease may eventually result in renal failure.

Clinical presentation
Nephritis may present as a non-specific illness – anorexia, lethargy and tender kidneys on palpation. Occasionally there may be fever and leucocytosis. The urinalysis may show blood, leucocytes and possibly bacteria (cystocentesis). Nephrosis is silent until there is end-stage kidney failure.

Differential diagnosis
For nephritis, any infection of the urinary tract. Renal failure due to age, neoplasia for the nephrosis.

Diagnostic testing
Radiographs, ultrasonography, urinalysis, haematology and chemistry. Fine needle aspirate or biopsy with histopathology. Urine culture and sensitivity obtained via cystocentesis. The cytology of the urine should be done.

Diagnosis
Presence of inflammation/infection of the kidney (nephritis). Nephrosis diagnosis is via histopathology.

Management/treatment
Nephritis can be managed with antimicrobials, fluid therapy and supportive care. Nephrosis and renal disease may be helped with omega 3–6 fatty acids. There is some indication that rehmannia-6 may help with kidney disease. The author uses a combination of omega 3–6 fatty acids, enalapril (it may be assumed that ferrets develop renal hypertension similar to other species with renal disease), and rehmannia-6. Fluid therapy may be necessary for dieresis and electrolyte rebalancing.

Pyelonephritis
Definition/overview
Infection of the kidney(s).

Aetiology/pathophysiology
Usually due to an ascending infection of the urinary tract. May also be found if systemic septicaemia.

Clinical presentation
Pain in region of kidney(s). Other signs similar to lower urinary tract infection including frequent urinary, haematuria, pyelouria.

Differential diagnosis
Lower urinary tract disease including urolithiasis, cystitis. Neoplasia of the kidneys. Large cysts within the kidneys.

Diagnostic testing
Urinalysis – may see renal cells. Excretory urogram. Ultrasound. Fine needle aspirate of the kidney (ultrasound guided).

Diagnosis

Presence of bacteria and inflammatory reaction on biopsy. Renal cells in urine suggestive of pylonephritis.

Management/treatment

Antibiotics. For pain an analgesic such as buprenorphine or tramadol needed for the first few days of antibiotic therapy. Repeated urinalysis to verify clearance of bacteria, RBCs and WBCs and renal cells. Repeated excretory urogram and ultrasound to verify kidney tissue and function returning to healthy state.

Renal cysts

Definition/overview

Cysts may develop in the kidney parenchyma.

Aetiology/pathophysiology

Some are present at birth, indicating congenital formation. The cysts may be an incidental finding on ultrasound; some may become extremely large but generally expand rather than compress kidney tissue (**Fig. 22.28**). Rarely is any kidney disease indicated by BUN and creatinine (normal values). They may be classified as either perinephric pseudocysts or polycystic kidneys.

Clinical presentation

If large, the kidney(s) may palpate enlarged or misshapen. Small cysts are asymptomatic and rarely malform the kidney.

Differential diagnosis

Hydronephrosis, neoplasia.

Diagnostic testing

Radiography, ultrasonography, ultrasound-guided fluid drainage and urinalysis with cytology.

Diagnosis

Presence of the cysts on radiography or better visualised on ultrasound. Fluid aspirated from perinephric cysts may be distinguished from urine by measuring creatinine concentrations. Polycystic kidneys may have fluid more consistent with urine.

Management/treatment

Large cysts may be drained for comfort for the ferret. They may fill again. In severe cases surgery is warranted to resect the renal capsule to prevent further filling. The cyst walls can be removed using bipolar radiosurgery. The cyst cavity can be packed with perirenal fat and closed. Small cysts found incidentally on ultrasound should be measured and rechecked every few months via ultrasound to watch for expansion and compression of the renal parenchyma. If these enlarge it may be necessary to drain them as well.

Renal failure

Definition/overview

Failure of function of kidneys.

Aetiology/pathophysiology

See other diseases in this section as possible causes. Aging plays a large role. Theoretically different pharmaceuticals, like heavy use of NSAIDs, have been linked with kidney failure in other species but not documented as a cause in ferrets.

Clinical presentation

Ferret may be losing weight and condition. Frequent bouts of nausea manifested by gagging and pawing at the mouth, foamy vomiting. There may be hindquarter weakness, dehydration, and either large amounts of urine or lack of urine. There may be oral ulcers and halitosis. Mucous membranes may be pale and dry. Signs may be non-specific without laboratory testing.

Differential diagnosis

Insulinoma, lymphoma, gastric ulcers, dental disease. Any causes of stress, dehydration, generalised weakness and 'poor doing' (neoplasia, cardiac disease).

Diagnostic testing

Complete blood work including haematology, serum chemistry. Urinalysis including specific gravity and cytology. A water deprivation test could be performed if the urine is isouric (this is rarely done as the ferret is usually dehydrated). Kidney biopsy/fine needle aspirate (ultrasound guided), ultrasonography of the kidneys. Radiographs.

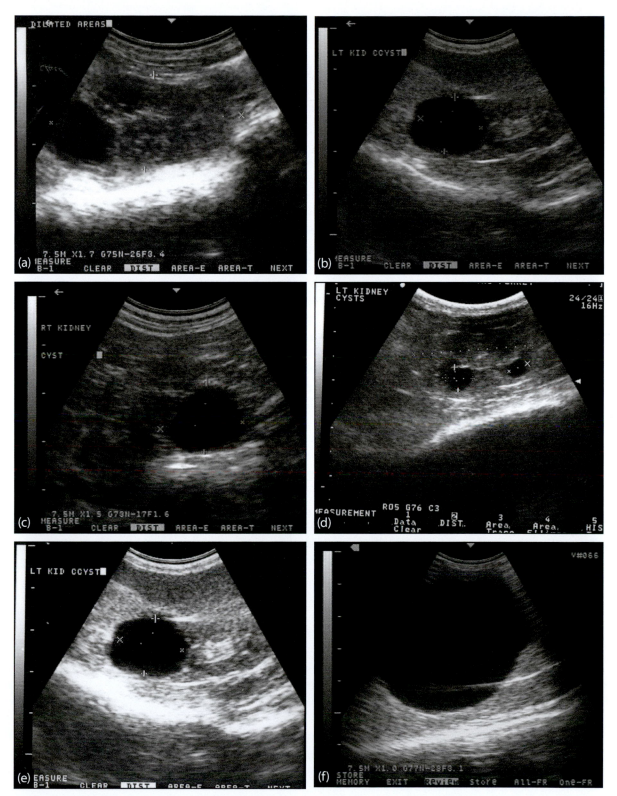

Fig. 22.28 (a–e) Ultrasonography of incidental finding of renal cysts; (f) severe renal cyst that was drained repeatedly with ultrasound-guided drainage.

Diagnosis

Elevated BUN, creatinine and imbalance in calcium/phosphorus (usually high phosphorus). Urinalysis specific gravity may be isouric and may indicate lack of dilution or concentration ability. Ultrasound and radiographs may show kidney size/shape irregularities. Ultrasound may also show changes in the kidney tissue. Biopsy/fine needle aspirate may be definitive.

Management/treatment

Prognosis is poor. Fluid therapy to correct dehydration and electrolyte imbalances may temporarily alleviate some clinical signs. Theoretically the ferret needs to be placed on dialysis, which can be done peritoneally. Daily fluid calculation (50–100 mL/kg/day) can be administered into the abdomen, waiting 30–60 minutes then aspirating as much fluid as possible out of the abdomen. The ferret should be on antibiotics while undergoing peritoneal dialysis. Analgesics may be used as the injections may be painful. Dialysis is done at least every other day. In severe cases it may be done daily. Carafate may be used to help soothe oral ulceration and help with nausea. Famotidine is generally used to aid in prevention of nausea and gastric ulcers.

Urethral obstruction (see also Cystitis/urolithiasis and Prostate disease)

Definition/overview

Blockage of the urethra. This is usually critical in males due to the long urethra. Blockage frequently occurs where the urethra bends around the pelvis.

Aetiology/pathophysiology

Stone formation may be struvite or cysteine. Stones are formed in the bladder. Small stones pass into the urethra. Mucoid plugs/prostate cells can also block the urethra and are consistent with prostate changes due to adrenal disease. In intact males this mucoid plug blockage has been seen by the author.

Clinical presentation

Stranguria and pain. The ferret may also be nauseated and anorexic. May show ataxia or reluctance to move.

Differential diagnosis

Blockage by neoplasia of tissue surrounding the urethra, including prostate hyperplasia, cysts.

Diagnostic testing

Radiographs – scout and excretory urogram. Ultrasonography of prostate and bladder. Catheterisation of the urethra may not be able to get through the prostate if it is enlarged (**Fig. 22.29**).

Diagnosis

Visualisation of obstruction.

Management/treatment

Urinary catheter passage with retrograde flushing of the urethra, cystotomy to remove stones. If prostate disease, likely adrenal disease and treatment should be initiated (see Chapter 14). Usually antibiotics and analgesics are prescribed for symptoms of secondary infection and discomfort associated with flushing and/or surgery. In cases where the blockage is distal to the pelvic brim and cannot be resolved, a perineal urethrostomy may be performed, as is done in cats.

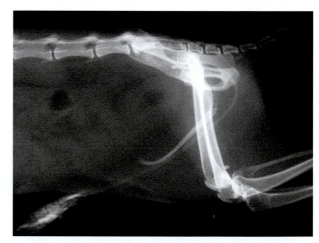

Fig. 22.29 Catheter has been passed to the level of the prostate but could not be passed further. Contrast agent pooled on the abdominal fur.

MISCELLANEOUS CONDITIONS

INTRODUCTION

There are a number of conditions in ferrets that need to be documented in this book, but which do not fit easily within the book framework. For instance, the fact that some ferrets snore! Ferrets also get hiccups, which can be alleviated by getting them to drink, lick a dab of nutrient gel or eat, or get a mid-body section massage (area of the diaphragm).

The following are multi-system diseases or emerging diseases with which practitioners should be acquainted.

CRYPTOCOCCOSIS

Definition/overview

Cryptococcosis is a sporadic but not uncommon fungal infection in humans and animals. The most common nomenclature for it is *Cryptococcus neoformans*, although with DNA sequencing more specific variations are being found. There are reports in the literature of *Cryptococcus* infection in ferrets. Environmental sources include soil and trees from a geographical area (such as western British Columbia, Canada) and one case from central Massachusetts where reporting of this fungi is rare. The Canadian ferrets were occasionally walked outdoors, whereas the Massachusetts case was completely housed indoors. It has been reported worldwide, and often in association with eucalyptus forests – Australia has many reports in animals and people.

Clinical presentation

The author had a ferret case of cryptococcosis presenting as a lump in the skin (**Fig. 23.1**). When the mass was removed and presented for histopathology, it was diagnosed as cryptococcosis. The lump was completely excised. No other masses were detected and the lungs on radiograph were clear. No further treatment was done. It was unknown how the ferret contracted the disease.

In the literature reports, one ferret had respiratory tract signs including nasal discharge and rhinitis, and the other had signs of acute abdominal discomfort and a palpable abdominal mass. One ferret showed retching with increased respiratory effort and tachypnoea (pneumonia) as well as weight loss. It had splenomegaly.

Diagnostic testing

Haematology and biochemistry, radiographs, cytology and histopathology, ultrasonography, culture and antigen serology.

Diagnosis

The one ferret that had retching and respiratory signs had lymphopenia, lactic acidosis, hypoglycaemia, hypocalcaemia, hypoalbuminaemia and hyperglobulinaemia. Radiographic findings showed a pulmonary bronchointerstitial pattern. Abdominal ultrasonography revealed a suspected pancreatic

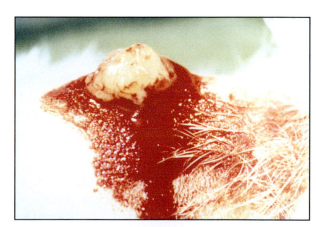

Fig. 23.1 **Cryptococcosis of the skin.**

mass and mesenteric lymphadenopathy. This ferret at necropsy had *Cryptococcus* in lungs, brain, spleen and multiple lymph nodes. Lymph node cytology and histopathology from all the ferrets yielded *Cryptococcus*-like organisms. In the retching ferret case, formalin-fixed lung tissue was submitted for DNA extraction, and the organism identified as *Cryptococcus neoformans* var. *grubii*. The other two ferrets in the literature had serum samples that were positive with one ferret having a titre of 1:20,000, which was the maximum dilution performed.

Management/treatment

If dermal lesions only, it may be possible for total excision, but one should consider systemic antifungal treatment as well. Itraconazole at 10 mg/kg PO q12h and amphotericin B at 0.25 mg/kg diluted in 5% dextrose IV q24h. Amphotericin B has also been given SC, which slows its absorption but may be less nephrotoxic. Prognosis is poor for the respiratory signs or for disseminated cryptococcosis. Direct transmission between animals and humans has not been documented; however, infected animals in the household can shed the organism into the environment, potentiating its spread. Owners of affected pets should be advised that the pets can act as sentinel animals for the detection of *Cryptococcus* spp. that are pathogenic to humans in their immediate environment.

GYROVIRUS

Definition/overview

Gyrovirus (GyV) is in the family Circoviridae. Gyrovirus has an average size of 19–27 nanometers. It is non-enveloped and has an icosahedral capsid with T = 1 symmetry. The unique, single-protein, trumpet-shaped capsomeres of GyV are arranged into 12 pentomers yielding a capsid 50 units in size. The genome is circular, non-segmented, and 2290–2320 nucleotides long. A known GyV in chickens causes anaemia (chicken anaemia virus, CAV). Birds are natural hosts. It has been described worldwide in areas where chickens are produced. CAV causes severe anaemia, haemorrhaging and depletion of lymphoid tissue through the destruction of bone marrow erythroblastoid cells. The disease affects many young chicks not protected by maternal antibodies. Age resistance to disease begins at about 1 week, but can be overcome by coinfection with immunosuppressive diseases such as bursal disease virus, Marek's disease and others. Recently a second chicken GyV has been found. Human GyV has recently been discovered. Two species have been described: human GyV1 and human GyV3. Human GyV1 appears to be the same virus as avian GyV2. A fourth virus, GyV4, has been isolated from human stool and chicken meat.

The GyV was found in the faeces of a pet ferret in Hungary that had enlargement of lymph nodes and organs. There was no demonstrated association between GyV shedding from ferrets and observed background disease. The virus was sequenced and found to be a novel GyV3 strain. Because of the evidence for genetic diversity among gyroviruses and the fact that ferrets shed the virus in faeces, there is a possibility that the ferret GyV3 might be transmissible to heterologous hosts, e.g. humans.

At present, there is no commercial test for this virus so prevalence is unknown. At this time it is unknown if the virus actually causes disease in the ferret.

HEPATITIS E

Definition/overview

Hepatitis E virus (HEV) is a newly identified human virus. It is a single stranded, RNA virus in the family Hepeviridae, genus *Hepevirus*. It causes acute hepatitis in humans. Mortality rates are less than or equal to 20% in pregnant women. Transmission is faecal–oral. It is recognised as a zoonosis because transmission of the virus from deer, swine and wild boars to humans has been documented. HEV or HEV-like viruses have also been found in monkeys, rabbits, trout, mongooses and bats. The genus *Hepevirus* includes 3 additional species: avian HEV, bat HEV, and rat/ferret HEV. It is not known if these three can be transmitted to humans.

HEV was identified in the stool of laboratory ferrets in Japan as part of screening prior to influenza research. The ferrets came from a USA source. It has also been identified in the stool of laboratory ferrets in the Netherlands, from multiple sources. Some pet ferrets in the Netherlands have tested positive with no overt signs of disease.

The Japan virus shared only 82.4–82.5% nucleotide sequence with strains found in the Netherlands. The conclusion is that the ferret HEV genome is genetically diverse. Genetic work being done on the virus so far links it more closely to the rat virus than that of genotypes established as zoonotic. There are no reports at this time of zoonotic disease resulting from exposure to infected ferrets. A recent report has found that ferret HEV infection is responsible for liver damage. There are three patterns: subclinical infection, acute hepatitis and persistent infection. Alanine aminotransferase (ALT) levels were elevated in over 65% of the ferrets. The authors concluded that ferret HEV infection did induce acute hepatitis and set up persistent infection. The ferret may be suitable as an animal model for immunological and pathological studies of hepatitis E. It is also not known how widespread the virus is.

Diagnostic testing

A commercial laboratory (Research Associates Laboratory, Dallas, TX) designed a capsid protein with a taq-man probe. This is used to perform quantitative real time-PCR with tests compared to a known negative control. The need so far is to find a positive control to make sure the test is valid. The author sampled 100 adult ferrets from two facilities along with two shipments of 8-week-old ferrets (211) and all have been negative on this test.

The future: there is still a need to find a positive control ferret to validate the test. It is unknown if this is in the pet ferrets sold in the USA. Continued vigilance is needed to find out the clinical implications and pathology concerning infection with this virus.

HISTOPLASMOSIS

Definition/overview

This disease has recently been described. It is a fungal disease that tends to grow in avian nitrogen-rich faeces. Ferrets and humans can be exposed via the environment. In the report, the ferrets lived with a bird.

Clinical presentation

The ferret had a 6-month history of green, mucoid diarrhoea that was unresponsive to amoxicillin with clavulinic acid, metronidazole, and omeprazole and presented for profound depression, dyspnoea, fever and seizures. There was a profound thrombocytopaenia ($10,000 \times 10^9/L$), reactive lymphocytes, echinocytes and schistocytes. The ferret had hypocalcaemia (7.9 mg/mL [2.1 mmol/L]), hypoalbuminaemia (3.8 g/dL [38 g/L]), and bilirubinuria. Radiographs showed a mild diffuse bronchial pattern. There was splenomegaly and hepatomegaly. At necropsy, there was profound hepatomegaly, lungs estimated to be 60% filled with fluid and granulomatous cells. The spleen was enlarged and pale.

Diagnostic testing

An exploratory laparotomy was done and liver biopsies obtained from the liver that appeared tan and leathery looking. The rest of the abdomen was unremarkable. Further testing included serum AGID antibodies, urine EIA and PCR of the environment.

Diagnosis

On histopathology of the liver, there was histiocytic, lymphocytic inflammation. *Histoplasma capsulatum* was seen using PAS and GMS staining. At necropsy the organisms were found in the liver, lung, spleen, brain and multiple lymph nodes and bone marrow. The urine was EIA positive, although serum AGID for antibodies was negative. All ferrets in the household had positive urine. The cage-mate ferrets were asymptomatic.

Management/treatment

Itraconazole at 5–10 mg/kg PO q12h, amphotericin B nebulisation has been tried. The symptomatic case was euthanased due to worsening dyspnoea despite supportive care. The three asymptomatic ferrets responded well to long-term itraconazole treatment at 5 mg/kg PO q12h for 2–3 months. There was resolution of soft stools and decreasing EIA titres. Prevent build-up of avian droppings in the household. Histoplasmosis can be contracted by the humans in the household.

MYCOBACTERIOSIS

Definition/overview

In the literature, mycobacteriosis has been diagnosed in Japan, Australia and New Zealand, although the author has seen cases in practice in the USA. Mycobacteriosis was not typed out in the Japan case, but reported as *Mycobacterium genavense* in two aged ferrets with conjunctival lesions in Australia. Feral ferrets in New Zealand are seen as hosts as well as sentinels for *Mycobacterum bovis* infection. *M. avium* complex and *M. triplex* have also been isolated. Because of the zoonotic risks with *Mycobacterium* spp., cases in pets become problematic as to whether or not to treat.

Aetiology/pathophysiology

Transmission is probably both through inhalation and/or ingestion of the organisms from the environment or exposure to other infected animals. There is the risk of ferret–ferret transmission. In New Zealand they have also established ferret–other wildlife and livestock transmission. Ferrets in New Zealand play a complex role in the tuberculosis (TB) cycle: they are capable of contracting, amplifying and transmitting *M. bovis* infection. The brush-tail possum (*Trichosurus vulpecula*) is the main host of the disease and ferrets are thought to contract the disease from feeding on tuberculous carcasses.

Clinical presentation

In the Japan case, the ferret had a 2-month history of anorexia, vomiting and occasional diarrhoea and weight loss. On palpation there was a mass in the cranial abdomen. Radiographic findings were of gas retention in the stomach and intestines. A barium study of the GI tract demonstrated a slightly delayed gastric emptying time. Abdominal ultrasonography revealed thickening of the gastric wall and abdominal lymphadomegaly. This ferret also had an enlargement of the lymph node of the glans nictitans, but that link to mycobacteriosis was not explored. Of the reported ferrets with conjunctivitis, one had generalised peripheral lymph node enlargement and proliferative lesions of the conjunctiva of the nictitating membrane. The other had conjunctival swelling, serous ocular discharge and swelling of the subcutaneous tissues of the nasal bridge. In New Zealand, the infected ferrets typically have gross tuberculous lesions most commonly in the lymph nodes draining the alimentary tract. It is rarely found in the lungs. This is consistent with infection through ingestion of infected material.

Differential diagnosis

Any bacterial or viral aetiology for gastroenteritis, weight loss, lymphadenopathy, conjunctivitis, particularly if the lymph node of the glans nictitans is involved.

Diagnostic testing

Cytology, biopsy, histopathology, identification of the organisms in tissue or faeces via PCR, culture. Radiographs, ultrasonography as well as CBC and serum biochemistry also performed in clinical cases.

Diagnosis

In the Japan case, an exploratory laparotomy with subsequent cytology and histopathology was performed. Characteristic macrophages containing rod-shaped to filamentous non-staining bacterial organisms were found. On histopathology, there was severe multifocal to diffuse infiltration of inflammatory cells, consisting mainly of macrophages and epithelioid cells with a small number of lymphocytes and neutrophils, throughout the lamina propria into the muscular layer. The macrophages and epithelioid cells contained intracytoplasmic, filamentous, pale to slightly basophilic bacteria that were intensely positive with Ziehl–Neelsen stain. Similar granulomatous lesions were found in the lymph node and liver. In the conjunctival cases, cytology, histopathology and sequence analysis of the 16S rRNA gene amplified using PCR was performed. The New Zealand ferrets were diagnosed at necropsy showing macroscopic alimentary tract TB lesions characterised by enlargement and erythema of the nodes, along with gross lymphadenopathy and extensive liquefactive necrosis.

Management/treatment

Because of the zoonotic risk, treatment options need to be discussed with the owner. In the literature cases, no transmission was noted from ferret to human. In the Japan case, the ferret was treated with a regimen of rifampicin (10 mg/kg PO q12h), azithromycin (10 mg/kg PO q12h), enrofloxacin (5 mg/kg PO q24h) and prednisolone (0.25–1.0 mg/kg PO q24h), along with other supportive medications for hepatic and intestinal disorders. These were not specified in the report. This ferret did not significantly improve with treatment and developed progressive anaemia and leucopaenia in addition to icterus, severe splenomegaly and ascites. The ferret improved slightly following a blood transfusion on day 194, haematopoietic stimulants, such as erythropoietin and supportive therapies, such as force feeding and subcutaneous fluids. The ferret died 220 days after the initial presentation. No necropsy was performed. One of the conjunctival cases was treated with rifampicin, clofazimine and clarithromycin and was considered cured. The second ferret was treated successfully with rifampicin alone. Both of these ferrets died later of different disease conditions. New Zealand is trying to manage the mycobacteriosis by culling of ferrets and brush-tail possums.

PSEUDOMONAS LUTEOLA

Definition/overview (see also Chapter 20)

Pseudomonas luteola is a motile, aerobic, gram-negative rod with yellow-orange pigmentation when grown on blood agar. It is frequently found in water, soil and other damp environments. It has a polysaccharide capsule and multitrichous polar flagella.

Aetiology/pathophysiology

In humans, it may cause septicaemia, peritonitis and endocarditis when there is an underlying disease present. The organism may also act as a nosocomial agent and infect critically ill patients that have had surgery or have indwelling devices inserted. It has been associated with immunosuppressive therapy, chronic renal failure and malignancy. In ferrets, it has been linked with pyogranulomatous pleuropneumonia, mediastinitis and panniculitis. Panniculitis is inflammation of the subcutaneous adipose tissue characterised by the development of single or multiple cutaneous nodules.

Clinical presentation

In three ferrets with pleuropneumonia and mediastinitis there was depression, dehydration, anorexia, hyperthermia and acute onset dyspnoea. One ferret's main symptom was coughing. Complete blood counts and serum biochemical examinations revealed anaemia, severe neutrophilic leucocytosis with toxic neutrophils, hyperglycaemia and hypoalbuminaemia. One ferret also had hyperglobulinaemia. Another report was of three ferrets that presented with pyogranulomatous subcutaneous inflammation affecting the inguinal, preputial and femoral regions.

Differential diagnosis

Any bacterial pneumonia, influenza, canine distemper, ferret systemic coronavirus. *Pneumocystis* spp. were tested for in two of the cases and were negative. Ferrets have been used as animal models for *Pneumocystis carinii* infection in the laboratory although spontaneous cases have not been published to the author's knowledge.

Diagnostic testing

CBC and serum chemistry. Radiographs of the thorax, which included a unilateral pleural effusion and mediastinal mass displacing the trachea dorsally. Ultrasonography in one ferret revealed a large quantity of hypoechoic effusion within the thorax and a heterogeneous ill-defined soft-tissue mass in the left mediastinum. Thoracentesis yielded purulent fluid. Histopathology of panniculitis tissue revealed the organism staining positively by PAS reaction. Necropsy was performed on several of the ferrets above, with H&E, Ziehl–Neelsen (ZN) and PAS stains done on processed tissue. The mediastinal mass observed radiographically correlated with a severe mediastinal lymphadenopathy with abundant purulent exudate on the cut surface. One ferret had a large white mass in the mediastinum that encircled the trachea, oesophagus and regional lymph nodes. Microscopic examination of the mediastinal lymph nodes revealed a severe, multi-focal to diffuse, necrotising and neutrophilic to pyogranulomatous inflammation with variable infiltration of macrophages and lymphoplasmacytic cells. There were abundant colonies of rod-shaped eosinophilic and gram-negative microorganisms with a clear and wide halo (capsule). In the lungs, small white nodules were observed grossly consisting of multifocal peribronchiolar aggregates of foamy macrophages.

Transmission electron microscopy (TEM) was performed on pleural exudate and formalin-fixed lung and lymph nodes. Culture of the exudate obtained on thoracentesis. Cytology was also performed on the exudate that showed an abundance of clusters of rod-shaped to serpentine microorganisms.

Diagnosis

Confirmation of the organism by the various tests listed above.

Management/treatment

Ferrets were treated with oxygen supplementation, crystalloid fluids, antibiotics (enrofloxacin, clindamycin and metronidazole), itraconazole, buprenorphine, ranitidine and sucralfate. The animals died within 2–5 days of presentation. One ferret was euthanased upon presentation. Treatment in all of the cases was not effective. It is likely the ferrets were infected via the respiratory route from environmental bacteria, but the origin of the infection or the incubation time are unknown.

CHAPTER 24

ANALGESIA AND ANAESTHESIA

Cathy A. Johnson-Delaney

INTRODUCTION

Ferrets are very sensitive to stress and pain, although outward manifestations may be subtle if the practitioner is unfamiliar with ferret behaviour, posture and facial expressions. Signs of pain are listed in *Box 24.1* (**Fig. 24.1**). The reader is directed to: *Ferrets: anaesthesia and analgesia*, in Emma Keeble, Anna Meredith (eds), *BSAVA Manual of Rodents and Ferrets*, 2009, for more information.

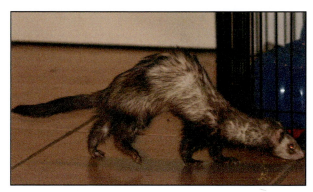

Fig. 24.1 **Ferret in pain. (Courtesy of Vondelle McLaughlin.)**

Box 24.1 **Signs of pain**

- Abnormal emotional behaviours including biting in a previously very gentle ferret, or wanting cuddling and burrowing into owner's clothing while being held.
- Anorexia or refusal to eat unless hand fed.
- Bruxism.
- Changes in gait.
- Chronic dehydration.
- Collapse.
- Cringing when touched.
- Facial expression: a dull look in the eyes, glassy eyes, seeming 'far away' although conscious.
- Hypersalivation.
- Lack of playing and/or ignoring favourite toys/treats.
- Pawing at mouth.
- Refusal/reluctance to move.
- Reluctance to wake.
- Tarry stools.
- Tension in forehead skin.
- Trembling.
- Vocalisations when touched or moved and/or during urination/bowel movement.
- Withdrawal from other ferrets or humans.

ANALGESIA

Choosing an analgesic involves consideration of the type of pain being treated, route of administration, formulation, duration of action (frequency of administration), owner compliance, side-effects and contraindications from other medications or medical conditions. Acute pain such as that from trauma or postsurgery can be treated with local anaesthetics, opiates for 1–3 days, coupled with an NSAID for up to 7 days depending on severity of injury or surgical incision. Chronic pain as seen with neoplasia may need long-term pain control that the owner may need to administer based on clinical signs. The clinician needs to educate the owner on signs in their ferret and what the different medications will do, as well as work out dosage and frequency schedules. Most owners are in tune with their ferrets and can become astute in the subtle signs of pain. Because of the ferret having a propensity to develop GI ulcers and acid reflux disease, GI protectant and antihistamine/antacid therapy should accompany administration of NSAIDs. The author encourages treatment of all ill, stressed, or postsurgical ferrets with one of the GI antihistamines for the duration of the medical problem.

Commonly used analgesics are listed in *Table 24.1*.

Recently, the use of Class IIIb and IV lasers for the treatment of pain has come to the forefront, not only for analgesia and anti-inflammatory

Table 24.1 Commonly used analgesics

DRUG	DOSAGE, ROUTE, FREQUENCY	COMMENTS
Aspirin	10–20 mg/kg PO q24h	Analgesic, anti-inflammatory, antipyretic. Give with food, use with H2 blocker
Bupivacine	1–1.5 mg/kg local delivery, SC area of incision, once	Local anaesthetic, effects may last several hours. Caution when using it for oral surgery
	1.1 mg/kg epidural, once	Can be combined with morphine for more complete analgesia. May alter hindlimb motor function for up to 12 hours
Buprenorphine	0.01–0.05 mg/kg IM, IV, SC q8–12h	Minimal sedative effect. Can be used concurrently with an NSAID
Butorphanol	0.05–0.5 mg/kg IM, SC q8–12h; 0.1–0.5 mg/kg IM, IV, SC q4–6h	Some sedative effect. Often part of preanaesthetic regimen when sedation needed. Can be used with benzodiazepines, NSAIDs
Carprofen	1–5 mg/kg PO q12–24h	NSAID; use with H2 blocker
Fentanyl citrate	1.25–5 µg/kg/h IV via CRI	Postoperative analgesia
	10–30 µg/kg/h IV via CRI	Perioperative analgesia after loading dose of 5–10 µg/kg IV
Flunixin	0.3 mg/kg SC, PO q24h	NSAID, not recommended due to potential for renal damage. Use for less than 3 days. Use with H2 blocker
Gabapentin	3–5 mg/kg PO q8–24h	Neurotropic pain. May cause sedation at higher doses
Hydromorphone	0.1–0.2 mg/kg IM, IV, SC q6–8h	Opioid
Ibuprofen	1 mg/kg PO q12–24h	NSAID. Has caused toxicosis at higher doses (see Chapter 29). Use with H2 blocker
Ketamine	0.1–0.4 mg/kg/h IV via CRI	Postoperative analgesia
	0.3–1.2 mg/kg/h IV via CRI	Perioperative analgesia after 2–5 mg/kg IV loading dose
Ketoprofen	0.5–3 mg/kg IM, PO, SC q24h	NSAID. Caution with gastritis or enteritis or for longer than 5 days. Use with H2 blocker
Lidocaine	1–2 mg/kg total, volume delivered in local area infiltrate or ring block, once	Local anaesthetic. Use either 1% or 2%, duration of action approximately 15–30 minutes. May be combined with bupivacaine (particularly for dental blocks)
	4.4 mg/kg epidural, once	Epidural block, can be combined with morphine for more immediate and complete analgesia
Meloxicam	0.2 mg/kg IM, PO, SC q24h	NSAID, use with H2 blocker
Meperidine	5–10 mg/kg IM, IV, SC q2–4h	Analgesic, short duration. May cause drowsiness in some
Morphine	0.1 mg/kg epidural, once	Effects may last 12–24h. Epidural for surgical anaesthesia/analgesia. Can be combined with either lidocaine or bupivacaine for immediate and more complete analgesia
	0.5–5 mg/kg IM, SC q2–6h	Analgesic. Short duration of action. Usually used just once preoperative dose
Nalbuphine	0.5–1.5 mg/kg IM, IV q2–3h	Analgesic. Short duration of action
Oxymorphone	0.05–0.2 mg/kg IM, IV, SC q8–12h	Analgesic
Pentazocine	5–10 mg/kg IM q4h	Analgesic
Tramadol	1–5 mg/kg PO q12–24	Analgesic for mild to severe pain (higher dose). Synergistic with NSAIDs. Can be used long-term for pain associated with neoplasia

Key: CRI, constant rate infusion; H2, histamine type 2; IM, intramuscular; IV, intravenous; NSAID, non-steroidal anti-inflammatory drug; PO, per os; SC, subcutaneous.

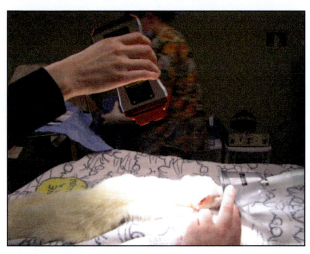

Fig. 24.2 **Laser application to sutured incision line.**

properties, but as an aid to healing incisions and wounds (**Fig. 24.2**). It should not be used on neoplasia because of the stimulation of cell growth. Use in or around endocrine tissue is also contraindicated due to potential angiogenesis. Because of the vasodilatory effect of near-infrared light, laser use is not recommended for any condition with concurrent haemorrhage or anticoagulation therapy. Lasers are not recommended in ferrets receiving steroid treatments. Many of the lasers on the market are now coming with small animal and even exotics settings for the different wavelengths and duration of treatment. Class IIIb lasers are low-power, typically producing less than 500 mW of energy. These have been used for osteoarthritis or myositis. Class IV lasers are high-power, producing greater than 500 mW of energy and visible infrared light with a wavelength of 635–1,064 nm. These can be used for tissue repair as they can penetrate 5 cm into tissue. Although mostly anecdotal for therapy response, work has been done in rats and has shown to be effective for pain including musculoskeletal, chronic atopy, inflammation and healing acceleration.

SEDATION AND ANAESTHESIA

Many of the agents for sedation and anaesthesia used in small animal practice can be used in ferrets. In all cases, agents that have the least cardiovascular depression are preferable as many ferrets have

subclinical cardiomyopathy. A balanced approach to sedation and anaesthesia is preferable for dental procedures and general surgeries. This includes pre-emptive pain control: systemic analgesic, local anesthetics, and for abdominal or hindquarters surgery, epidural anaesthetic and analgesia. A sedated or anaesthetised ferret should be supported with a heating system to maintain body temperature (**Fig. 24.3**).

Monitoring of the ferret includes blood pressure (on forelimb/wrist or tail), ECG, respirations (rate and depth, character), temperature, reflexes to judge anaesthesia depth (corneal, blink, swallowing, rectal tone, toe pinch) and degree of muscle relaxation (**Fig. 24.4**). Continuous audio Doppler can be done by placing the transducers over the femoral pulse (**Fig. 24.5**). Capnography can be used when the ferret is intubated. Capnography is preferable to pulse oximetry as an indicator of perfusion and

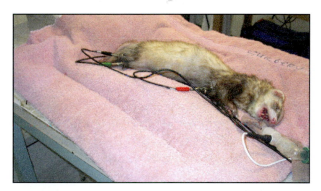

Fig. 24.3 **Anaesthetised ferret on a specially made forced heated air convection system towel. ECG leads are connected.**

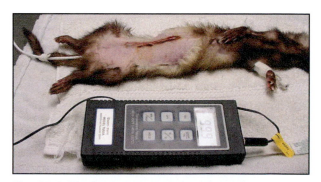

Fig. 24.4 **Monitoring temperature through surgery and recovery using an electronic rectal temperature probe.**

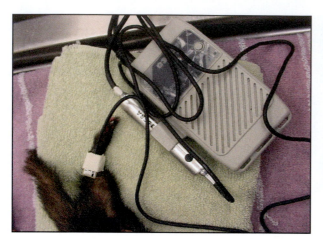

Fig. 24.5 Continuous audio Doppler for pulse can be achieved with the transducer fixed to the hindlimb using the femoral pulse.

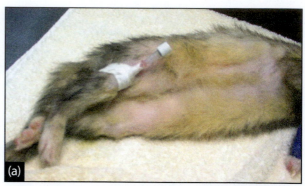

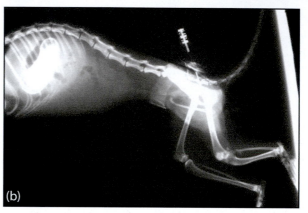

Fig. 24.6 (a) Intraosseous catheter in the tibia for administration of fluids; (b) placement of intraosseous catheter in the femur.

gas exchange. Pulse oximetry can be used although those designed for cats and dogs are frequently too large to attach to the ferret's tongue, cheek or ear. Ideally IV fluid therapy should be provided whenever there is to be general anaesthesia. Except for short minor procedures, an IV catheter should be placed. A 24 gauge is the most commonly placed catheter in the cephalic vein. If the surgery is to be extensive with potentially a lot of blood loss, a jugular catheter (22G) is an alternative. Another possibility is that of an intraosseous catheter (also 22G) (**Fig. 24.6**). To place the jugular catheter, a cut-down to expose the jugular vein may be necessary as the neck can be muscular with thick subcutaneous fat and tough skin.

Warm isotonic fluids should be provided. If the blood pressure drops during the procedure, with a catheter in place colloids can be administered. A blood transfusion may be necessary if there is significant blood loss and the ferret cannot maintain a haematocrit greater than 25%. Subcutaneous administration may be used when IV catheter placement is not possible and may be sufficient for minor surgeries lasting less than 30 minutes or for those with minimal expected blood loss.

Ferrets have a strong vagal reflex and may also demonstrate arrhythmias and apnoea in response to gas anaesthesia. In addition, because of strong oesophageal reflux during stress and gastric irritation and subsequent histamine release, and in many ferrets pre-existing gastrointestinal ulceration, the author has found that premedication with both famotidine and diphenhydramine along with atropine minimises intraoperative and postoperative complications due to these physiological responses. Ferrets should be fasted for 2–4 hours prior to surgery except those with islet cell neoplasia, for which the fast must be monitored and should be under 2 hours.

Induction

After sedation, ferrets can be masked until sufficiently anaesthetised to allow endotracheal intubation (**Fig. 24.7**). Alternatively, an injectable agent such as etomidate or ketamine can be used IV titrated to effect. An aggressive ferret may need to be restrained using thick leather gloves (e.g. leather primate handling gloves or thick gardening gloves) to even administer the sedatives. If an induction chamber is used, it is still preferable to administer

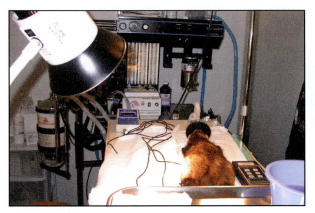

Fig. 24.7 Ferret being induced with inhalant anaesthetic. Note placement on a heating towel and ECG monitoring set up.

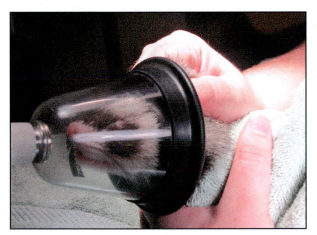

Fig. 24.8 Mask induction with the ferret scruffed and in a rolled towel.

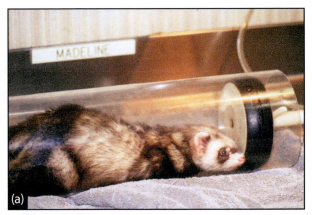

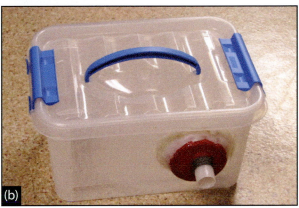

Fig. 24.9 (a, b) Custom-made induction chambers.

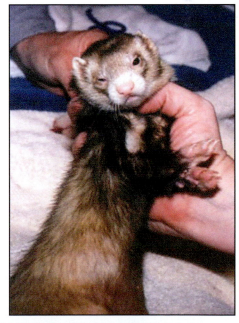

Fig. 24.10 Sedated ferret ready for inhalant anaesthetic.

midazolam to decrease the anxiety and keep blood pressure and heart rate at physiologically normal levels.

Anaesthetic induction by mask alone should be avoided as the increased anxiety, panic and subsequent increases in heart rate, blood pressure and other stress-related physiological changes can make it difficult to maintain homeostasis during surgery and postoperatively (**Fig. 24.8**). Ferrets can also be anaesthetised using a chamber, but at least a benzodiazepine should be on board to prevent anxiety-related stress (**Fig. 24.9**). Pre-emptive analgesia before any surgery is necessary and may also serve as the preoperative sedative that allows for smoother induction (**Fig. 24.10**). For example butorphanol at

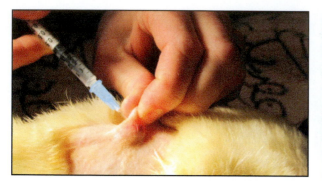

Fig. 24.11 **Local incision line block using lidocaine.**

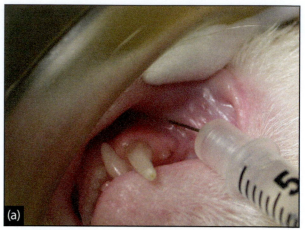

(a)

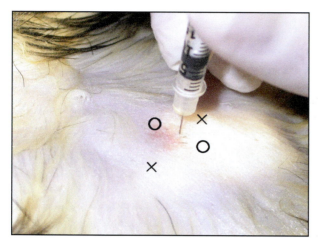

Fig. 24.12 **Epidural injection going inbetween the wings of the ileum (crosses), pelvis, on midline between the last lumbar vertebral bodies (circles).**

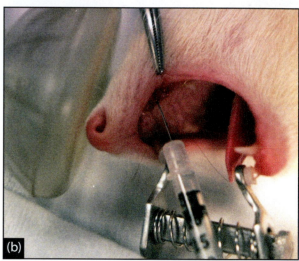

(b)

Fig. 24.13 **(a) Orbital blocking at the site of the infraorbital foramina; (b) infiltration of gingiva in the location of the extraction.**

0.2–0.4 mg/kg subcutaneously 20–30 minutes prior to gas induction provides this function. Use of a benzodiazepine decreases anxiety and increases muscle relaxation, both of which contribute to a smooth induction. Midazolam at 0.25–0.3 mg/kg IM or IV can be given 15–20 minutes prior to induction with an inhalant anaesthetic. It is often necessary to use a small amount of lidocaine (0.1 mL of 1% or 2%) to paralyse the larynx to accomplish intubation, as with cats. With sufficient premedication, this can usually be accomplished with a flow rate of 1–2 L/min and a 4–5% isoflurane or sevoflurane concentration. The animal relaxes in 2–5 minutes. Epidural administration or local incision line analgesia/anaesthetic is done once the ferret is anaesthetised but prior to abdominal surgery preparation (**Figs 24.11, 24.12**). Dental blocks using lidocaine

or lidocaine/bupivacaine can be done at this time (**Fig. 24.13**). The maintenance level of isoflurane or sevoflurane with a non-rebreathing system at 0.6–1.0 L/min is 1.75–2.5%.

All ferrets should be intubated except for in the most minor procedures. Use of 1.5- to 4.5-French endotracheal tubes is sufficient for most ferrets (**Fig. 24.14**). The endotracheal tube can be secured by tying it with gauze bandage material cinched around the tube as it exits the mouth and a length looped around each forelimb above the elbow (**Fig. 24.15**). If a cephalic catheter is in place, the gauze loop on that leg should be placed distal to the catheter. This method of securing the endotracheal

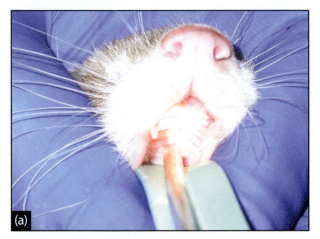

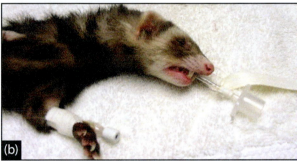

Fig. 24.14 (a) Using a laryngoscope (example Miller blade size 1, pictured) to visualise the epiglottis and intubate; (b) intubated ferret with cephalic catheter.

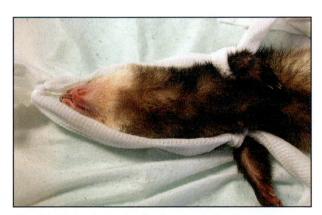

Fig. 24.15 Endotracheal tube secured using gauze bandage material looped around each forelimb.

tube works well with the ferret in dorsal recumbency, as ferrets have such a short muzzle and elongated skull and neck that methods used to secure the tube in dogs or cats do not work well in the ferret. If apnoea occurs, doxapram (2–5 mg/kg IV, IM) may

be administered as needed to stabilise respirations. The author uses the guidelines of 185–225 bpm and systolic blood pressure above 90 mmHg with a preanaesthetic respiration rate (varies per ferret) for maintenance through any surgery.

In the author's opinion, xylazine or acepromazine should not be used for ferret anaesthesia or sedation due the vasodilatory effects and depression of cardiac functions (xylazine). Blood pressure can be severely depressed with xylazine even in a normal healthy ferret. In a ferret with heart disease it can lead to fatalities. Using a balanced anaesthesia approach that includes antianxiety/relaxants, analgesics and anaesthetics can reduce the depression in cardiac parameters seen with just using anaesthetic agents either injectable or inhalant. Ketamine should be used in combination with either diazepam or midazolam. Ketamine alone does not provide adequate relaxation in the ferret – it seems to trigger paroxysmal sneezing, hyperreflexiveness and salivation. Ketamine may not provide adequate analgesia by itself for surgical procedures. If medetomidine is used, careful attention to blood pressure, supplemental oxygen and reversal as soon as possible are needed. The author currently does not use this drug in ferrets.

Agents used for ferret anaesthesia are listed in Table 24.2.

Ventilation

A standard non-rebreathing system with a flow rate of 0.6–1.0 L/min is used once intubated. If apnoea occurs, doxapram at 2–5 mg/kg IM or IV should be administered as needed to stabilise respiration. If a mechanical ventilator is used, it should be adjusted according to the estimated lung volume with the frequency of respirations set between 40 and 70 breaths per minute. Ventilators allow for better aeration and regular chest excursions. Because of this, the percentage of inhalant anaesthetic used is less than in the patient that is allowed to respire spontaneously. An ECG with respiratory monitor capabilities including capnography and pulse oximetry is extremely useful for complete monitoring. Care should be taken to minimise throat and neck manipulation as these can trigger the vagal response and the heart rate may markedly decrease

Table 24.2 Anaesthetics and drugs routinely used as part of balanced anaesthesia

DRUG	DOSAGE, ROUTE, FREQUENCY	COMMENTS
Acepromazine	0.1–0.25 mg/kg IM, SC, once	Preanaesthetic, light sedation. May cause vasodilation
	0.2–0.5 mg/kg IM, SC, once	Tranquillisation
Alphaxalone	5–15 mg/kg IM	Sedative, preanaesthetic. Has been used following an opioid and benzodiazepine
Alphadolone and alphaxalone	12–15 mg/kg IM initially, followed by multiple 6–8 mg/kg IV as needed to maintain	Anaesthetic
Atipamezole	0.4 mg/kg IM; 1 mg/kg IP, IV, SC	Reversal agent for dexmedetomidine and medetomidine. Give the same volume IP, IV, SC as dexmedetomidine or medetomidine. This equals 10 × dexmedetomine or 5 × medetomine dose in mg
Atropine	0.04–0.05 mg/kg IM, IV, SC, once	Preanaesthetic; prevent bradycardia, hypersalivation. At this dose, does not affect gut motility
Bupivacaine	1 mg/kg epidural	Epidural anaesthesia/analgesia. May be combined with morphine
	1–1.5 mg/kg SC infiltrate	Local anaesthesia for several hours
Dexmedetomidine	0.04–0.1 mg/kg IM	α2 agonist similar to medetomidine; not commonly used because of side-effects of bradycardia. Advantage is reversal if ferret has cardiac parameter effects
Diazepam	0.5–2 mg/kg IM, IV, once, effects may last 4–6 hours. Can be combined with opioids, ketamine	Benzodiazepine sedative/hypnotic, anxiolytic, muscle relaxant, anticonvulsant. Excessive sedation may occur if used with cimetidine, barbiturates, narcotics, anaesthetics. Reversal with flumazenil at 0.01–0.2 mg/kg IM
Diphenhydramine	1.25 mg/kg PO, SC, once	Antihistamine to counter histamine release during surgery. May have slight sedative effect
Etomidate	1 mg/kg IV (although may use less, to effect)	Induction, usually sufficient for intubation. No depression of cardiopulmonary parameters. Excellent for ill, critical ferrets
Famotidine	2.5 mg/ferret PO or SC	H2 blocker to prevent likelihood of GI histamine release and ulceration due to stress of surgery/manipulation of GI tract
Fentanyl/fluanisone	0.3 ml/kg IM, once	Anaesthetic
Fentanyl/droperidol	0.15 mL/kg IM, once	Deep sedation, some analgesia. Can be used for some minor procedures
Flumazenil	0.01–0.2 mg/kg IM	Reversal for benzodiazepines (diazepam, midazolam)
Glycopyrrolate	0.01 mg/kg IM, once	Part of preanaesthetic regimen to prevent bradycardia, reduces salivation
Isoflurane	Induce at higher concentrations, maintenance usually 1–3%	Inhalant anaesthetic, may produce hypotension
Ketamine	10–20 mg/kg IM, once	Mild sedation, no muscle relaxation, alone causes sneezing reflex; rarely used alone
	0.5 mg/kg IV presurgery; 10 µg/kg/min IV via CRI during surgery, 2 µg/kg/min IV via CRI for 24 h postoperatively	At these low doses may provide some analgesia if ferret has an indwelling or intraosseous catheter, on a fluid pump. Additional analgesics and/or an NSAID may be necessary

Key: CRI, constant rate infusion; GI, gastrointestinal; H2, histamine type 2; IM, intramuscular; IP, intraperitoneal; IV, intravenous; NSAID, non-steroidal anti-inflammatory drug; PO, per os; SC, subcutaneous.

(Conitnued)

Table 24.2 *(continued)* **Anaesthetics and drugs routinely used as part of balanced anaesthesia**

DRUG	DOSAGE, ROUTE, FREQUENCY	COMMENTS
Ketamine (K) + Dexmedetomidine (D)	(K) 5 mg/kg IM + (D) 0.03 mg/kg IM, once	Light anaesthesia, may be hypotensive, poor analgesia
Ketamine (K) + Diazepam (D)	(K) 10–20 mg/kg + (D) 1–2 mg/kg IM, once	Light anaesthesia, poor analgesia
	(K) 25–35 mg/kg + (D) 2–3 mg/kg IM, once	Moderate anaesthesia, poor analgesia
Ketamine (K) + Dexmedetomidine (D) + Butorphanol (B)	(K) 5 mg/kg IM + (D) 0.04 mg/kg IM + (B) 0.1 mg/kg IM, once	Induction, has analgesic properties
Ketamine (K) + Midazolam (M)	(K) 5–10 mg/kg + (M) 0.25 mg/kg IM. Give (M) 10 minutes prior to (K); once	Heavy sedation/induction. Follow with inhalant anaesthetic
Lidocaine	1–2 mg/kg total dose SC, once	Can be used for local splash blocks, dental, peripheral nerve blocks
	4.4 mg/kg epidural	Can be combined with morphine
Medetomidine	0.08–0.1 mg/kg IM, SC, once	Light sedation, rarely used alone. May cause hypotension, bradycardia. Have oxygen ready, atipamezole to reverse
Medetomidine (M) + Butorphanol (B)	(M) 0.08 mg/kg + (B) 0.1 mg/kg IM once	Anaesthesia, hypotensive, respiration depression. Have oxygen ready, atipamezole to reverse medetomidine
Midazolam	0.25–0.3 mg/kg IM, IV, once	Effects may last 2–4 hours. Benzodiazepine, sedative–hypnotic, anxiolytic, muscle relaxant, amnesiac, anticonvulsant. Hypotensive if used with meperidine. Reversal with flumazenil at 0.01–0.2 mg/kg IM
Morphine	0.1 mg/kg epidural, once	Epidural anaesthetic/analgesic. Combine with either lidocaine at 4.4 mg/kg or bupivacaine at 1.1 mg/kg for faster and more complete action
Naloxone	0.02–0.04 mg/kg IM, IV, SC, once	Reversal of opioids
Propofol	5 mg/kg IV to effect	Induction, titrate to effect
Sevoflurane	Induce at higher concentrations, maintenance at lower %. Depending on sedation premedications, induction may be obtained at 2.5–4.0%. If no premedications are used, induction is usually done at the maximum concentration (5%)	Inhalant anaesthetic. Additional analgesics need to be added
Thiopental 2%	8–12 mg/kg IV to effect, once	Induction
Tiletamine/zolazepam	12–22 mg/kg IM, once	Lower doses give sedation, higher doses light anaesthesia. Recovery is prolonged with higher doses. Rarely used in ferrets
Xylazine	0.5–1.0 mg/kg IM, SC, once	Usually in combination with ketamine at 10–20 mg/kg IM; sedation. Severe hypotension, bradycardia, arrhythmias. Not recommended for use in ferrets. Reverse xylazine with yohimbine
Yohimbine	0.2 mg/kg IV or 0.5 mg/kg IM once	Xylazine reversal

Key: CRI, constant rate infusion; GI, gastrointestinal; H2, histamine type 2; IM, intramuscular; IP, intraperitoneal; IV, intravenous; NSAID, non-steroidal anti-inflammatory drug; PO, per os; SC, subcutaneous.

or become irregular. If this occurs, the ferret needs to be stabilised back to a regular heart rate, ECG and respiration rate prior to the initial incision.

POSTOPERATIVE CONSIDERATIONS

The inhalant anaesthetic should be discontinued upon conclusion of the surgery as determined by the surgeon. The ferret can be maintained on oxygen until it is breathing spontaneously (ventilator turned off). The blood pressure, heart and respiratory rate should approximate to the preanaesthetic levels (**Fig. 24.16**). The ferret will begin moving or gagging, signalling readiness for extubation and disconnection from ECG and other probes. The temperature as well as reflexes should continue to be monitored until the ferret begins to move around. Generally ferrets will then curl up into their usual sleep position and sleep postoperatively. Heat and plenty of cloths or towels for burrowing into should be provided although that may make it more difficult for close observation.

POSTANAESTHETIC COMPLICATIONS

It has been noted that ferrets have awakened then had a massive drop in blood pressure, and have succumbed several hours after surgery. This has been seen particularly following surgeries that have manipulated the upper GI tract or when there has been significant blood loss such as in a splenectomy. The hypothesis for this is histamine release and the triggering of the vagal reflex. Death after apparent recovery may also be a consequence of low blood pressure and depressed cardiovascular function (although immediately postoperatively these may have returned to normal) coupled with mild to moderate hypothermia during the surgery.

Blood pressure drops can be minimised using drugs with minimal cardiovascular depressive effects such as midazolam and etomidate as induction medications, then lowered amounts of inhalant anaesthetic agents. Intravenous fluid therapy can be used intraoperatively to increase intravascular volumes. Fluids should always be warmed to body temperature before infusion.

The author has successfully reversed this effect when it was noted during induction or surgery by administering additional diphenhydramine, atropine and in rare cases adrenaline (epinephrine) intravenously to effect. If this massive drop in blood pressure and bradycardia occurs during induction, the ferret is recovered and the surgery aborted. If it happens during the surgery, the procedure is halted as the ferret is stabilised, then finished as quickly as possible. The recovery period must be closely monitored for 12–24 hours, with continued intravenous access available.

POSTOPERATIVE ANALGESIA

Postoperative analgesia should be administered at time points to coincide with the expected end of analgesia provided by the preoperative butorphanol or buprenorphine. NSAIDs such as meloxicam can be given at the conclusion of the surgery when the blood pressure and body temperature have returned to preanaesthetic levels. The author routinely combines the use of an opioid and an NSAID, along with famotidine for most surgeries requiring inhalant anaesthetic. Lasering of the incision line has become standard to increase circulation and healing and to minimise inflammation. Ideally the incision line should be lasered daily for a few days postoperatively.

Several examples of multimodal balanced anaesthetic/analgesic protocols are listed in *Table 24.3.*

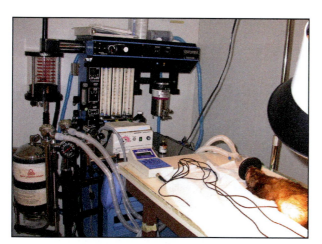

Fig. 24.16 **Recovery on oxygen via mask as long as the ferret will allow it, continued ECG monitoring until the ferret is moving around. Ferret is on a heated water blanket.**

Table 24.3 Balanced anaesthesia/analgesia regimens for selected procedures

PROCEDURE	PREOPERATIVE	INDUCTION/MAINTENANCE	POSTOPERATIVE
Cutaneous mass removal, wound repair	Famotidine 2.5 mg/kg PO or SC; diphenhydramine 1.25 mg/kg PO or SC; atropine 0.05 mg/kg SC; butorphanol 0.2 mg/kg SC; midazolam 0.25 mg/kg IM. Wait 20–25 minutes	Inhalant anaesthetic via mask or chamber. Induce at highest %, then decrease to achieve a light surgical plane. Intubation optional, may maintain for short time with mask. Eye lubricant administered. Clip, initial surgical scrub of mass, surrounding area. Locally infiltrate surgical area with lidocaine 1.5 mg/kg or bupivacaine at 1.25 mg/kg. Subcutaneous fluids should be given while being masked and prepped. When suturing is finished, give meloxicam at 0.2 mg/kg SC. If mass (neoplasia) totally removed, or for wound care, use laser on incision line to stimulate healing, decrease inflammation. Monitor during procedure with ECG, blood pressure, respirations, body temperature, pulse oximeter	Buprenorphine at 0.01–0.05 mg/kg SC at 4–6 hours post butorphanol administration. Depending on severity of mass removal or tissue excision, may continue with buprenorphine q12h × 1–2 days; meloxicam at 0.2 mg/kg PO q24h × 3–5 days. Famotidine 2.5 mg/ferret while on meloxicam. Additional incision line lasering may be done at 24 h intervals
Dental cleaning, extractions, periodontal work	Famotidine 2.5 mg/kg PO or SC; diphenhydramine 1.25 mg/kg PO or SC; atropine 0.05 mg/kg SC; butorphanol 0.2 mg/kg SC; midazolam 0.25 mg/kg IM. Wait 20–25 minutes	Mask or chamber induction with inhalant anaesthetic, transfer to mask once quieted. Induce with high %, reduce to effect. Intubate. IV catheter placement for fluid therapy. Alternatively for just cleaning, subcutaneous fluids may be given at 50 mL/kg. Eye lubricant placed. Time to take dental/skull radiographs. Lidocaine 0.1 mL to glottal area, intubate. The gingiva should be swabbed with dilute chlorhexidine oral rinse. If a tooth requires extraction, local block with lidocaine 2% at 1.5 mg/kg. Bupivacaine can be added at 1 mg/kg (foramina, root, pulp cavity, local subgingival). May get lidocaine seepage into the nasal cavity if volume is too much or there is osteolysis due to abscessation. Monitor with ECG, blood pressure, respiration, body temperature, pulse oximeter, capnography. At conclusion of procedure, discontinue inhalant. Laser the suture lines or extraction area. When the ferret begins to awaken, heart rate and blood pressure return to preoperative levels, administer meloxicam at 0.2 mg/kg SC	Buprenorphine 0.01 mg/kg SC 6 h after the butorphanol and continued q12h × 2–3 days depending on the severity and number of extractions. Meloxicam at 0.2 mg/kg PO q24h × 5–7 days. Famotidine 2.5 mg/ferret PO q24h while on meloxicam. Usually an oral antibiotic for 10–14 days is prescribed. Owner needs to swab gingiva with a dilute chlorhexidine oral rinse or a commercial children's mouth rinse without alcohol once daily for 5–7 days after surgery or as long as sutures are in place. The oral swabbing should remove any food that has adhered to the extraction sites
Laparotomy (ferret should have an IV or IO catheter in place)	Famotidine 2.5 mg/kg PO or SC; diphenhydramine 1.25 mg/kg PO or SC; atropine 0.05 mg/kg SC; buprenorphine 0.01 mg/kg SC, midazolam 0.25 mg/kg IM. Wait 20–25 minutes	Etomidate 1 mg/kg IV, lidocaine 0.1 mL of 2% squirted on glottal area, intubate. (An alternative to etomidate would be to give ketamine titrated to effect with a syringe filled with ketamine at 20 mg/kg. Another alternative would be to give alfaxalone at 6–8 mg/kg IM or at 8–12 mg/kg IV titrated to effect.) Eye lubricant placed. Begin inhalant anaesthetic at highest %, then decrease to surgical %. Clip and prep dorsal pelvic area. Epidural of morphine 0.1 mg/kg with lidocaine 4 mg/kg. Monitor with ECG, blood pressure, respirations, pulse oximetry, capnography, body temperature. Clip and surgically prep abdomen. Locally infiltrate surgical area with lidocaine 1.5 mg/kg or bupivacaine at 1.25 mg/kg. After first layer closure, splash with 0.1 mL of the lidocaine diluted to 0.5 mL with saline so that the body layers are locally anaesthetised for closing. When the incision line closed, laser the line and surrounding skin. When the ferret begins to awaken, heart rate and blood pressure return to preoperative levels, administer meloxicam at 0.2 mg/kg SC	Buprenorphine at 0.01 mg/kg SC at 6 hours post the initial administration. Dose continued at q10–12h for 2–3 days as needed. If possible, laser the incision line daily for 3–5 days. Meloxicam at 0.2 mg/kg PO q24h × 7 days. Famotidine 2.5 mg/ferret PO q24h while on meloxicam

Key: ECG; electrocardiography; IM, intramuscular; IO, intraosseous; IV, intravenous; PO, per os; SC, subcutaneous.

CHAPTER 25

COMMON SURGICAL PROCEDURES

John R. Chitty and
Cathy A. Johnson-Delaney

INTRODUCTION

Surgery is commonly indicated in ferrets, especially with their predilection for neoplastic and endocrine conditions. This chapter will endeavour to provide a practical guide to some of the more common ferret surgeries and their indications. Surgical neutering will be included, although with the advent of deslorelin implants this is performed less regularly except in the presence of pathological conditions of the reproductive organs.

SURGICAL PRINCIPLES IN THE FERRET

From a surgical perspective, ferrets are excellent candidates for internal surgery. Their long 'tubular' body makes abdominal access relatively easy; they are large enough that normal small animal surgical instruments (see below) and skills are generally sufficient; they will tolerate a reasonable degree of blood loss and are small enough that surgery is not physically demanding. Unlike herbivorous small mammals, they lack large fragile caecae, which greatly facilitates surgical access throughout the abdomen.

They are also generally good candidates for anaesthesia (see Chapter 24) and this of course means they are more likely to tolerate longer, more invasive procedures.

In general, skin preparation is similar to that performed in small animal (dog/cat) surgery, and a margin around the wound should be clipped and prepared aseptically. Hypothermia should always be considered a potential risk in this species, especially for animals that may need to be returned to outdoor enclosures relatively soon after surgery. To this end,

clipped areas should not be excessive. In addition, with respect to short-term perioperative heat loss it is recommended that surgical alcohol is not used as part of the skin preparation (although alcohol-based chlorhexidine wipe does not seem to cause excessive heat loss through evaporation).

Draping up is performed as per small animal surgery – given the size and shape of ferrets, fenestrated adhesive paper drapes appear particularly useful.

The following is a list of basic surgical equipment used by these authors for ferret abdominal surgery:

- Blade handle and No 11 blade.
- Scissors – Metzenbaum and iris (curved and straight – blunt ended).
- Mosquito forceps – fine tips; curved and straight.
- Haemostatic clips (the authors prefer the Weck Hemoclip system [Teflex Medical, Research Triangle Park, NC] due to the angle of applicators and method of closure – however, other systems are available). A range of sizes and appropriate applicators should be available.
- Olsen-Hagar needle holders.
- Forceps – Adson thumb forceps (rat-tooth); cat spay forceps.
- Allis Tissue holders.
- Retractors – the Lone Star Retractor system (CooperSurgical Inc, Trumbull CT) is light and versatile.

Postoperatively, ferrets will need a warm secluded area in which to recover. Heat should be provided throughout surgery and afterwards until they are able to thermoregulate (see Chapter 24).

Suture care

Ferrets can be difficult to manage in terms of suture care. The following may assist in reducing wound care problems:

- Sympathetic suturing patterns and materials. It is strongly advised not to tighten skin sutures excessively or use subcuticular patterns. Horizontal mattress sutures are not indicated. Where possible, sutures can be avoided with use of tissue adhesives. Where skin sutures are used, softer absorbable materials (e.g. polyglactin – the authors generally use 3/0 for subcuticular sutures) are preferred.
- Local anaesthesia. Regional and irrigation blocks will help (see Chapter 24).
- Analgesia (see Chapter 24).
- Avoidance of excessive tissue handling and bruising will reduce local pain and likely interference with the wound as well as reducing chances of localised necrosis and wound breakdown.
- Wound care – gentle daily cleaning of wounds and keeping the postoperative ferret in hygienic surroundings will assist in reducing the chances of wound infection.
- Use of a therapeutic Class IV laser on the incision line is thought to help healing and reduce inflammation. Anecdotally it seems to speed healing.
- Wound coverings, T-shirts and tubular bandages may be used to provide a mechanical covering. These can be useful where the ferret is housed with others.

Gloving up

It is now the accepted norm to 'glove up' for sterile surgery. However, examination of the literature does produce some interesting results in terms of the efficacy of this technique. A major reason for extensive gloving up in human surgery is to reduce infection from patient to surgeon (especially human immunodeficiency virus [HIV] and hepatitis viruses, that are not a concern in veterinary medicine) as much as reducing surgical site infection (SSI).

In this latter respect there are few studies. Reichman and Greenberg (2009) provides an excellent review of SSIs, and a review of some of the truths of gloving up techniques can be found via: http://www.infectioncontroltoday.com/articles/2011/04/double-gloving-myth-versus-fact.aspx.

These reviews indicate that gloving up with single layer gloves alone is insufficient in reducing SSI rates, which are mainly dependent on patient factors and use of antimicrobials. In particular, scrubbing up must be performed as thoroughly when gloving up than when not as perforation rates are so high (industry standard is for up to 1.5% microperforation rate in glove manufacture, and studies in orthopaedic and thoracic surgery show perforation rates of up to 60%, many of which are not detected by surgeons). There are concerns that gloving up may increase complacency when scrubbing up, though studies have not been performed to support this. SSIs may be reduced by double gloving, ideally with double coloured gloves as, while perforation rates are reduced, they are harder to detect. Studies show tactile sensitivity is not necessarily reduced though individual surgeons may report this.

Surgical pictures in this chapter show my operating (JRC) with bare hands rather than in gloves. This reflects the teaching I received and long-term operating in this manner means that I find a marked reduction in tactile sensitivity when using gloves. In the absence of convincing evidence as to the effect of gloving up on SSI, and comparable SSI rates to other gloved-up surgeons, I continue to operate without gloves.

However, when operating with or without gloves it is always important to perform regular clinical audit of SSI rates and to review and alter technique should a problem become apparent.

CASTRATION

Indications

Birth control. Removal of undesired male secondary sexual characteristics (e.g. scent, aggression). Testicular neoplasia, cysts (**Fig. 25.1**), etc.

Preoperative considerations

If performed, it should be done after descent of testes and after onset of sexual maturity. The earlier performed, the sooner the possible onset of adrenal disease (see Chapter 14). The long-term risk of adrenal disease associated with surgical castration should always be discussed with owners prior to surgery.

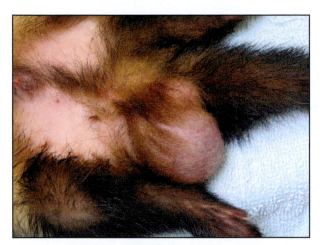

Fig. 25.1 **Testicular cyst.**

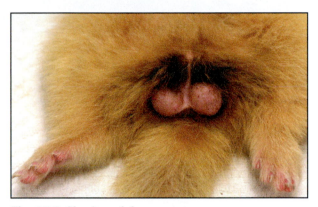

Fig. 25.2 **Shaving of the scrotum.**

Procedure

The ferret is anaesthetised and placed in dorsal recumbency. The scrotum is shaved (**Fig. 25.2**), prepared aseptically (**Fig. 25.3**) and draped. The skin is incised over the first testis and the testis withdrawn in the tunic. The tunic is then incised over the testis and the testis withdrawn from the tunic (**Fig. 25.4**). The tunic is clamped and the gubernaculum torn through. The testicular blood vessels are then clamped and ligated (polyglycolic acid 3/0) (**Figs 25.5, 25.6**). The vessels are then cut distal to ligature. The tunic is then 'stripped' and ligated as far proximal as possible. The distal tunic is removed (**Fig. 25.7**) and the proximal end released back into the inguinal canal.

The process is repeated on the other side. The two scrotal incisions (**Fig. 25.8**) are then closed with tissue glue.

Postoperative care

These authors routinely give a single dose of long-acting amoxycillin (75 mg/kg SC) and carprofen (5 mg/kg SC). The scrotal incisions should be gently bathed daily for 3–5 days. The ferret should be kept in clean conditions indoors for several days postoperatively and not worked for at least 2 weeks postcastration. Swelling (haematoma/abscess) is

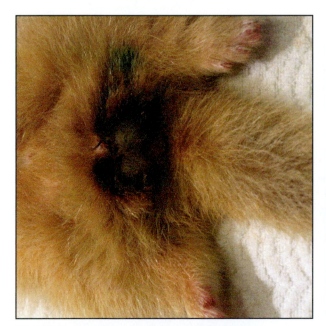

Fig. 25.3 **Aseptic preparation and draping.**

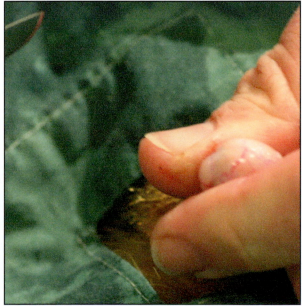

Fig. 25.4 **Incision and testis withdrawn from the tunic.**

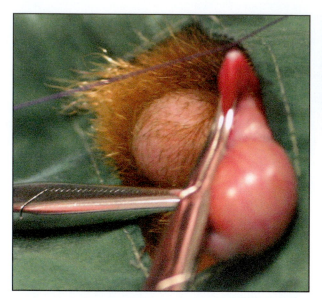

Fig. 25.5 The testicular vessels are clamped.

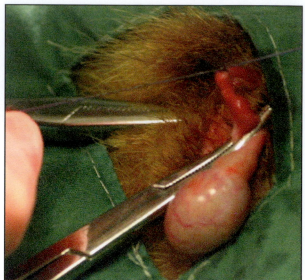

Fig. 25.6 The testicular vessels are ligated.

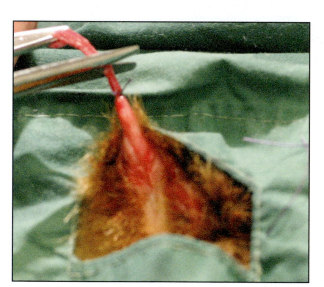

Fig. 25.7 The tunic ligated as far proximal as possible.

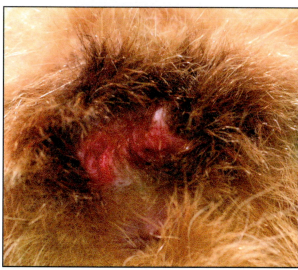

Fig. 25.8 The two scrotal incisions are closed with tissue glue.

rare but swelling should always be reported by the owner to the veterinarian.

CRYPTORCHID

Indications

Retained testes (i.e. those not descended by 1 year of age) should be removed to prevent development of neoplasia of the testes. If only one testis is retained there is an option to remove just the retained testis. It is not recommended to then use these hobs for breeding as crytorchidism has a hereditary component.

If unilaterally or bilaterally castrated it is recommended that deslorelin implants are used to prevent adrenal gland disease development.

Preoperative considerations

If possible the location of the retained testis should be determined – i.e. inguinal or abdominal. This is not always possible.

Procedure

The ferret is anaesthetised and placed in dorsal recumbency. If not already determined, the inguinal canal is palpated to see if the retained testis can be located. If located in the inguinal canal, the relevant site is clipped and prepared aseptically. The skin is incised over the testis that is then removed in the same manner as for routine castration (above). The skin is sutured using 3/0 polyglycolic acid in a simple interrupted pattern. If not located, the ventral caudal abdomen is clipped and prepared aseptically.

A 2.5–4 cm midline incision is made caudal to the umbilicus. If necessary, the penis is reflected to one side. The bladder is located and reflected ventrally. The vas deferens can then usually be identified entering the prostate region immediately distal to the bladder. The vas on the relevant side is then followed until the testis is located. When located it is removed in a similar fashion to a routine castration.

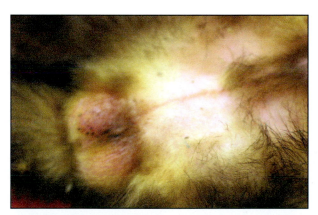

Fig. 25.9 The area just cranial to the scrotum is clipped, aseptically prepared.

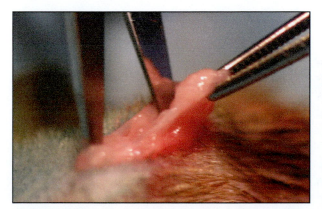

Fig. 25.10 The skin is incised and the cord is located.

Once removed, the non-retained testis can be removed if desired.

Postoperative care

This is similar to care for a routine castration. Wound care is the same as that for an exploratory coeliotomy (see below). Administration for 2–3 days of an NSAID provides analgesia and anti-inflammation control.

VASECTOMY

Indications

Breeding control, but enabling a hob to mate with jills and bring them out of season.

Preoperative considerations

Should be performed in a sexually mature animal with both testes descended. Magnifying loupes and very small/microsurgery instruments are extremely useful in performing this surgery.

Procedure

The ferret is anaesthetised and placed in dorsal recumbency. An area just cranial to the scrotum is clipped (**Fig. 25.9**) and aseptically prepared. The skin is incised (1 cm incision approx 5–10 mm cranial to the base of the scrotum – do not go too close to the testis; although it is much easier to locate the cord, it is much harder to identify and isolate the vas deferens) and the underlying fat blunt dissected (**Fig. 25.10**).

The cord is located and grasped and exteriorised (**Fig. 25.11**); care must be taken that this is

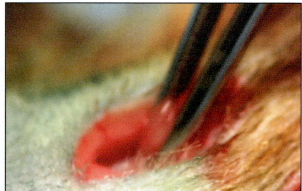

Fig. 25.11 The cord is located and exteriorised.

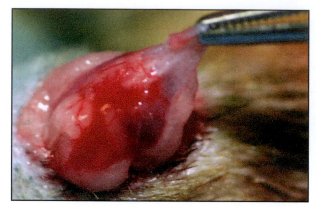

Fig. 25.12 **The vas deferens is identified and grasped.**

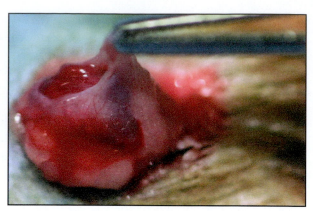

Fig. 25.13 **The tunic is incised over the vas.**

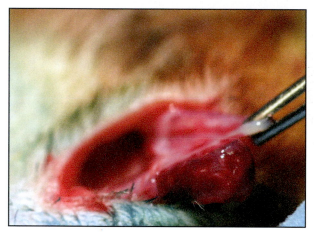

Fig. 25.14 **The vas is grasped and exteriorised.**

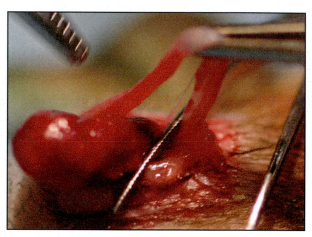

Fig. 25.15 **A section of the vas is bluntly dissected from underlying spermatic vessels.**

the spermatic cord. With gentle traction it should be possible to see the testes move within the scrotum. In addition the penis should always be identified separately – it has been reported for the penis to be identified as spermatic cord and sections of urethra removed rather than vas.

The vas deferens is identified and grasped (**Fig. 25.12**). The tunic is incised over the vas (**Fig. 25.13**) and the vas grasped (**Fig. 25.14**) and exteriorised. Care is needed to identify this as there may be a separate white fibrous cord in the ferret spermatic cord. The vas will normally have a tortuous blood vessel running over the wall. A section of vas (ideally 1–2 cm) is bluntly dissected from underlying spermatic vessels (**Fig. 25.15**). The section of vas is clamped at each end (**Fig. 25.16**).

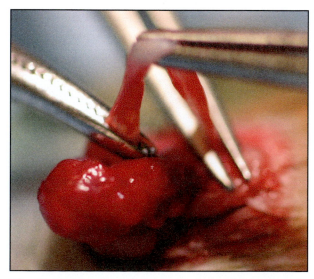

Fig. 25.16 **A section of the vas is clamped at each end.**

The section of vas is cut at each end and removed (**Fig. 25.17**). The ends of the removed section are examined – gentle pressure should slightly extrude the lining mucosa showing the structure to be tubular and therefore likely to be vas deferens. Each end is reflected and ligated (5/0 polyglycolic acid) such that the cut ends are facing away from each other (**Fig. 25.18**). The ligated ends of vas are replaced in the spermatic cord. The tunic is not ligated but the cord is replaced in the wound.

The process is repeated on the other spermatic cord. The skin wounds are sutured using 3/0 polyglycolic acid in a simple interrupted pattern (**Fig. 25.19**).

Postoperative considerations

Wound care and drugs given are as per a routine castration. Administration for 2–3 days of an NSAID provides analgesia and anti-inflammation control.

The ferret should not be put with jills for 8 weeks following vasectomy. An exception is when the owner has a jill he does not mind getting pregnant, in which case the vasectomised hob may be placed with her 2–4 weeks after vasectomy and he can then be mixed with other jills 6 weeks postvasectomy.

Removed sections of vas should be placed on labelled pieces of white card (for orientation) and placed in 10% formol saline. These can be sent for histopathology immediately (in which case the client should be advised of additional fees), or retained for 1 year in case of queries over the accuracy of the vasectomy technique.

The major complication is a return to fertility. All owners should be warned that recanalisation may occur in any species following vasectomy and may occur at any point from 2 years postvasectomy.

EXPLORATORY COELIOTOMY

Indications

Coeliotomy is frequently indicated in ferrets with a preponderance to internal neoplasia, splenic disorders, reproductive disease and gut disease that may require biopsy. The basic coeliotomy approach is the same for each, with only the position and length of incision varying with surgical indication.

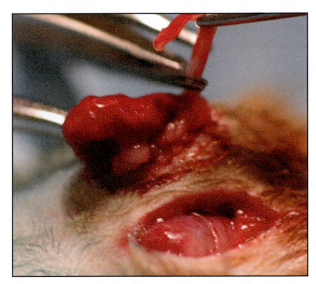

Fig. 25.17 **A section of vas is cut at each end and removed.**

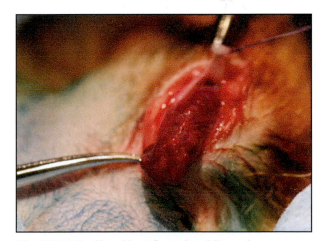

Fig. 25.18 **Each end is reflected and ligated.**

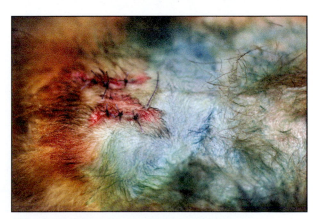

Fig. 25.19 **The skin wounds are sutured.**

Procedure

The ferret is anaesthetised and placed in dorsal recumbency. The ventral midline is clipped and aseptically prepared (**Fig. 25.20**). The area is draped (the authors' preference is for disposable adhesive paper cat or bitch spay fenestrated drapes). The skin is incised in the ventral midline (**Fig. 25.21**). The linea alba is located, tented and incised using scissors (**Fig. 25.22**).

Once opened, exposure of the abdomen may be increased by using retractors – the authors' preference is the Lone Star Retractor system (CooperSurgical Inc, Trumbull, CT). Good lighting is essential and well-directed surgical lights are of immense value.

If performing a full exploratory then the incision should be sufficiently long to give good access to the whole abdomen. In males, this will generally require lateral reflection of the penis. A four-quadrant approach to the exploratory should be adopted.

After surgery, the abdomen should be thoroughly irrigated with warmed saline ('the solution to pollution is dilution') (**Fig. 25.23**).

Closure is similar to other species. The linea alba is closed using simple interrupted sutures (3/0 polyglycolic acid or polydioxanone) (**Fig. 25.24**). A local 'splash block' may be placed before skin closure. The skin is sutured using a simple continuous intradermal polyglycolic acid 3/0 suture (**Fig. 25.25**). A buried knot (e.g. Aberdeen knot) may be used if desired. Tissue glue is then placed over the wound.

Postoperative care

Postoperative complications are unusual with adequate exercise, restriction of the patient immediately postoperatively and good wound care. The ferret should be given a broad-spectrum antibiotic for 5–7 days as well as adequate analgesia. Typically this may be the use of an opioid for 48–72 hours such as buprenorphine, along with an NSAID for 3–5 days or as long as needed for discomfort.

NEPHRECTOMY

Indications

Kidney enlargement due to hydronephrosis, renaliths that have obstructed the renal pelvis and ureters, severe renal cysts or neoplasia (see Chapter 22).

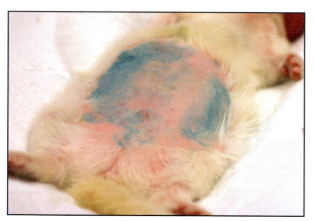

Fig. 25.20 **Ventral midline is clipped and aseptically prepared.**

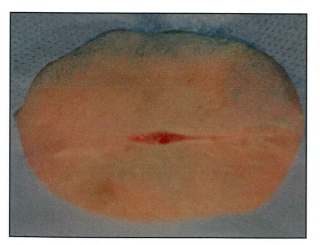

Fig. 25.21 **The skin is incised in the ventral midline.**

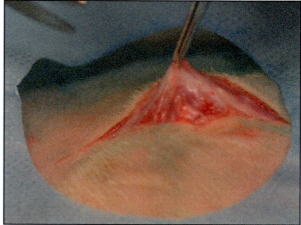

Fig. 25.22 **The linea alba is located, tented and incised.**

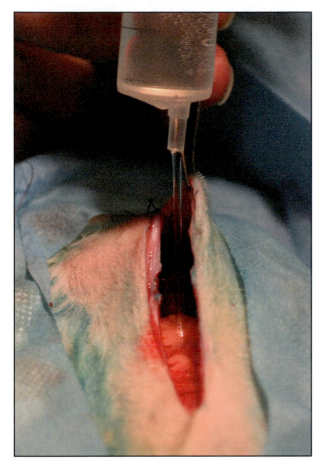

Fig. 25.23 **The abdomen should be thoroughly irrigated with warmed saline.**

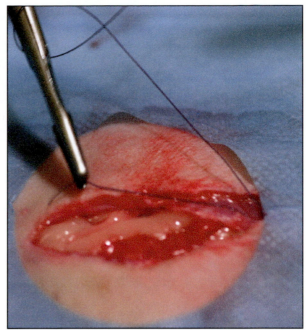

Fig. 25.24 **The linea alba is closed using simple interrupted sutures.**

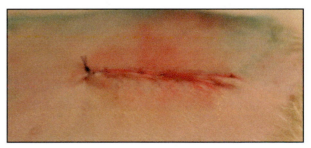

Fig. 25.25 **The skin is sutured using a simple continuous intradermal suture.**

Preoperative considerations

Prior to nephrectomy, kidney function needs to be assessed through haematology, chemistry and urinalysis. Imaging including radiographs and ultrasound should be performed to try to characterise the pathology. An excretory urogram should be run to assess function of the contralateral kidney.

The ferret should receive preanaesthetic drugs and an analgesic before inhalant anaesthetic (see Chapter 24). An IV or IO catheter should be placed to aid in managing blood pressure throughout the surgery, although the authors have rarely seen hypotension develop directly due to the kidney removal.

Procedure

The ferret is placed in dorsal recumbency and the abdomen clipped and aseptically prepared as for exploratory coeliotomy. The incision is made on the midline parallel to the kidney for removal. The peritoneum over the caudal pole of the kidney is grasped with tissue forceps and incised with scissors to mobilise the kidney. The kidney is gently elevated through the incision, allowing for the identification of the renal artery and vein and the ureter (**Figs 25.26, 25.27**).

The vessels are clamped individually using vascular clips and ligated. The ureter is clamped with vascular clips and ligated. Alternatively 4-0 suture can be used for ligatures. The abdomen is irrigated with warm saline and routinely closed (**Fig. 25.28**).

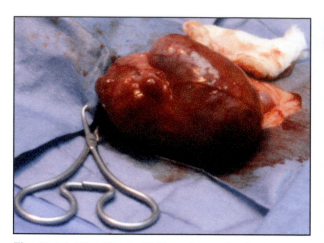

Fig. 25.26 **The diseased kidney is exteriorised for attachment visualisation.**

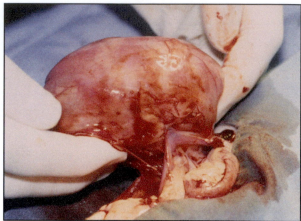

Fig. 25.27 **The vasculature and ureter are identified for ligation.**

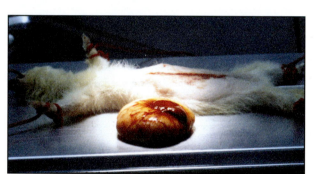

Fig. 25.28 **The abdomen is routinely closed. The ferret should be closely monitored postoperatively as there may be a drop in blood pressure.**

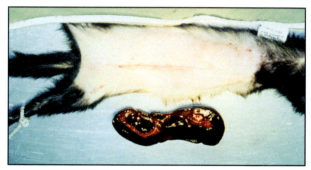

Fig. 25.29 **Postoperative comparison of size of the spleen to the ferret.**

Postoperative care

Immediately postoperatively blood pressure should be monitored as well as perfusion. Broad-spectrum antibiotic therapy for 7–10 days is instigated. Analgesia should include an opioid such as buprenorphine as well as an NSAID. Usually the opioid is continued for 1–3 days postoperatively and the NSAID for 3–5 days. Pain assessment of each patient dictates duration of pain control.

SPLENECTOMY

Indications

Splenomegaly (see Chapter 16) in the ferret is very common, and may be present as a result of any chronic disease syndromes. It may become a major centre of haematopoiesis, particularly if a neoplastic process is involved. The spleen may also become neoplastic itself (lymphoma is the primary tumour), or cystic. Occasionally a spleen will become grossly enlarged in an older ferret and, because of its size, becomes uncomfortable. This is also an indication for removal (**Fig. 25.29**). Ultrasonography of the spleen will frequently enable the clinician to ascertain a neoplastic process versus one primarily of extramedullary haematopoiesis. Cysts within enlarged spleens are usually blood filled, and may be aspirated under ultrasound guidance. These frequently reoccur, which may be an indication for splenectomy. Prior to splenectomy in any ferret, a CBC and serum chemistry should be done. A bone marrow aspirate also needs to be taken to determine if the ferret's bone marrow is capable of producing red cells following the splenectomy. Many times it is not, and the ferret will succumb to a non-regenerative anaemia several weeks after splenectomy.

Procedure

The surgery itself is similar to that in the cat or dog. Vasculature is easily visualised, and ligated. It is advisable to submit a sample for histopathology. Ligation of vessels can also be done with haemoclips. The abdomen should be lavaged with warm saline prior to closure.

Postoperative care

Postsplenectomy therapies may include blood transfusions (all ferrets are one blood type so any healthy donor ferret can be used), erythropoietin therapy, vitamin supplementation and supportive care. Postoperative analgesics should be continued for 3–5 days, and famotidine or ranitidine should be given to decrease acid secretion. The haematocrit should be monitored weekly for the first few weeks until it is assured that the bone marrow is producing red cells. Adjunctive therapy of erythropoietin and blood transfusions may be needed for 1–2 weeks postoperatively if the histopathology confirms the splenomegaly was primarily extramedullary hematopoiesis.

OVARIOHYSTERECTOMY

Indications

Birth control. Prevention and treatment of oestrogen-associated pancytopaenia (in the latter case, it is strongly advised to bring the ferret out of season using proligestone, and to stabilise blood counts with transfusion prior to surgery). Treatment of cystic endometrial hyperplasia (**Fig. 25.30**) or pyometra (**Fig. 25.31**). Treatment of ovarian/uterine neoplasia (**Fig. 25.32**).

Preoperative considerations

The surgery can be performed preferably from 12 weeks of age – however, the earlier performed, the sooner the onset of adrenal disease. Most pet ferrets in the USA have been spayed at 5–6 weeks of age.

As with castration, increased risk of adrenal disease associated with surgical neutering should be discussed with owners prior to surgery.

If looking for ovarian remnants (e.g. return to oestrus following surgery) then the procedure is carried out in a similar manner to that described below. The ovaries are located immediately caudal to the kidneys. However, the ferret should not be brought out of season prior to surgery. While this increases risk of haemorrhage, it makes finding the ovarian remnants much easier as they will be larger and contain follicles. If treated prior to surgery, they can be extremely hard to find, especially in fat animals.

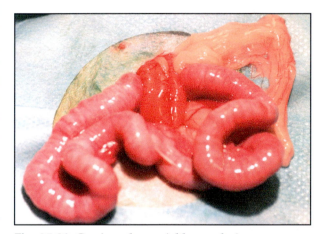

Fig. 25.30 **Cystic endometrial hyperplasia.**

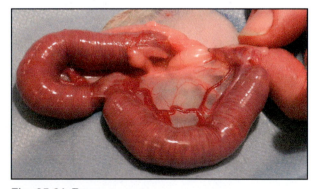

Fig. 25.31 **Pyometra.**

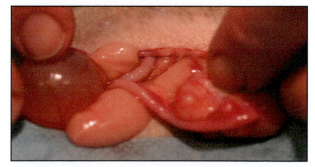

Fig. 25.32 **The left horn is exteriorised and traced cranially to the left ovary. This left ovary is neoplastic.**

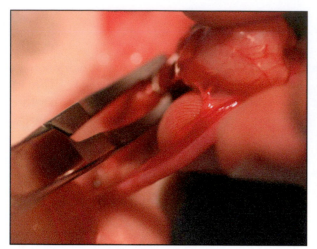

Fig. 25.33 The ovarian blood vessels are identified and ligated. Surgical clips may be used.

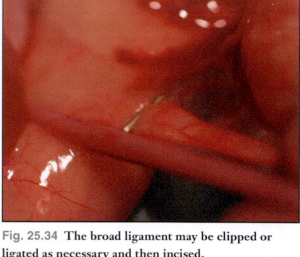

Fig. 25.34 The broad ligament may be clipped or ligated as necessary and then incised.

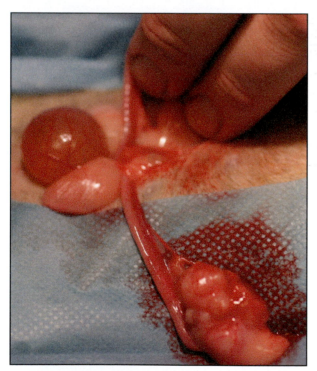

Fig. 25.35 The procedure is repeated for the right ovary.

Fig. 25.36 The right uterine horn is exteriorised and traced cranially to the right ovary.

The left horn is exteriorised and traced cranially allowing identification of the left ovary. This is gently exteriorised (**Fig. 25.32**).

The ovarian blood vessel is identified and ligated (3/0 polydioxanone) or clipped using titanium ligating clips (**Fig. 25.33**) and then incised. The broad ligament may be clipped or ligated as necessary (**Fig. 25.34**) and then incised. The procedure is repeated for the right ovary (**Figs 25.35–25.37**).

The uterus is then reflected caudally and ligated at the base using 3/0 polydioxanone (**Fig. 25.38**). Ideally this should be distal to the cervix. However, sometimes

Procedure

The ferret is anaesthetised and placed in dorsal recumbency. The ventrum is clipped and prepared aseptically. The skin is incised – 2 cm incision extending caudally from 0.5 cm caudal to the umbilicus. The linea alba is opened. The bladder is identified and reflected ventrally revealing the uterus.

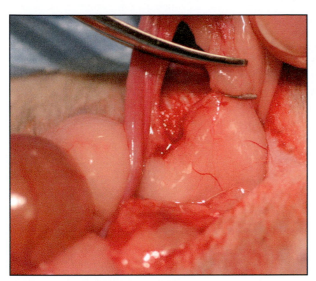

Fig. 25.37 **The ovary is identified, and the ligaments clipped and ligated.**

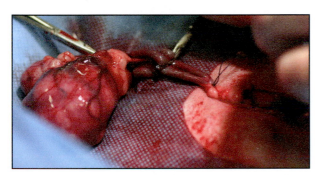

Fig. 25.38 **Uterine clamping and ligature.**

in routine spays (as in cats) the uterine body will be ligated leaving the cervix and remnant of uterus. This does not appear to cause clinical problems. In cases of cystic endometrial hyperplasia, uterine neoplasia and pyometra, all uterine tissue should be removed.

Intra-abdominal fluid is given (30 mL/kg warmed saline) (**Fig. 25.23**). The wound is closed as described above.

Postoperative care
The wound should be cleaned daily with saline until healed. The ferret should be kept indoors and restricted for 2 days postoperatively. The authors give 75 mg/kg amoxicillin long-acting and 0.2 mg/kg meloxicam SC perioperatively along with saline SC at 30 mL/kg. Ferrets are discharged with a 3-day course of meloxicam (0.2 mg/kg PO q12h).

LEFT ADRENALECTOMY

Indications
Diagnosis and treatment of left adrenal gland disease (see Chapter 14).

Preoperative considerations
Ideally the left adrenal will have been confirmed as enlarged by ultrasonography. However, in some cases this cannot be done, and adrenal size is determined on direct visual appearance at exploratory coeliotomy.

Concurrent disease should be ruled out or treated prior to surgery.

Procedure
The ferret is anaesthetised and placed in dorsal recumbency. The ventrum is clipped and prepared aseptically. The skin is incised – 3–4 cm incision extending caudally from the xiphisternum (**Fig. 25.39**). The linea alba is incised. The intestine and spleen are reflected (exteriorised if necessary, in which case they should be moistened with saline throughout). The adrenal is located at the cranial pole of the left kidney (**Fig. 25.40**).

The fat surrounding the adrenal is elevated and carefully dissected away to reveal the gland (**Fig. 25.41**). Blood vessels (typically originating from either aorta/vena cava or renal artery/vein, or both) are identified and ligated using titanium vascular clips (**Fig. 25.42**). Once vessels are ligated the tissue around the gland is incised and

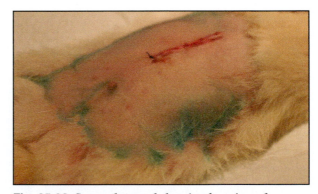

Fig. 25.39 **Sutured wound showing location of incision.**

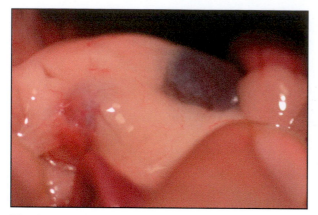

Fig. 25.40 **The left adrenal gland is located at the cranial pole of the left kidney.**

the gland removed **(Fig. 25.43)**. This leaves a cavity in the fat **(Fig. 25.44)**. The cavity is closed using a single horizontal mattress suture (3/0 polyglycolic acid) **(Fig. 25.45)**.

The right adrenal is checked (see below). In males, prostate size is checked by palpation. Warmed fluid is added to the abdomen and the wound closed as described for coeliotomy.

Postoperative care

The authors give 75 mg/kg amoxicillin long-acting, 0.02 mg/kg buprenorphine and 0.2 mg/kg meloxicam SC perioperatively along with saline SC at 30 mL/kg. Ferrets are hospitalised overnight and then discharged with a 3-day course of meloxicam

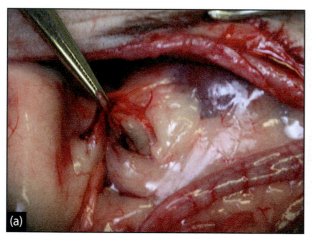

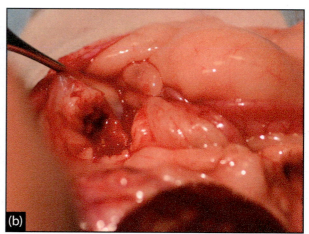

Fig. 25.41 **(a, b) The fat surrounding the adrenal gland is elevated and carefully dissected away to reveal the gland.**

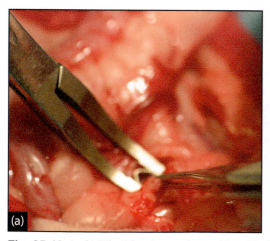

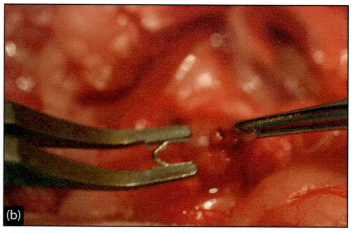

Fig. 25.42 **(a, b) The blood vessels are identified and ligated using titanium vascular clips.**

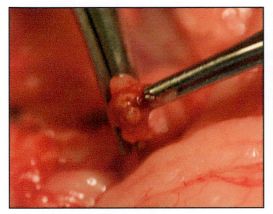

Fig. 25.43 **The tissue around the gland is incised and the gland removed.**

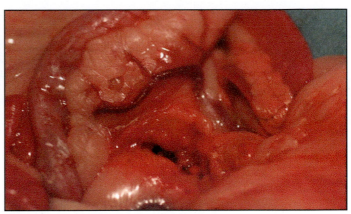

Fig. 25.44 **Cavity in the fat.**

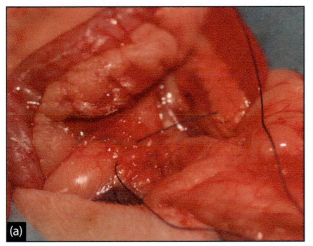

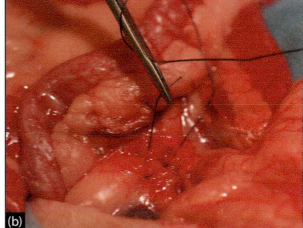

Fig. 25.45 **(a, b) The cavity is closed using a single horizontal mattress suture.**

(0.2 mg/kg PO q12h). Perioperatively a deslorelin implant is placed subcutaneously unless both adrenals are completely removed or the prostate is enlarged. If the prostate is enlarged, a course of osaterone acetate (Ypozane, Virbac, Bury St Edmunds, UK) is given at 0.25–0.5mg/kg q24h for 7 days. A deslorelin implant can then be placed if required.

Owners should be warned to expect considerable skin bruising (**Fig. 25.46**) – this reflects the frequently raised oestrogen levels and possibly thrombocytopaenia as the result of bone marrow suppression and does not seem to imply pain.

Wound care is as described earlier.

The removed gland should be submitted for histopathology.

RIGHT ADRENALECTOMY

Indications
Diagnosis and treatment of right adrenal gland disease (see Chapter 14).

Preoperative considerations
Ideally the right adrenal will have been confirmed as enlarged by ultrasonography. However, in some cases this cannot be done, and adrenal size is determined on direct visual appearance. Concurrent disease should be ruled out or treated prior to surgery.

Removal of the right adrenal carries considerable risk as a section of vena cava is almost always removed. While a collateral circulation will rapidly

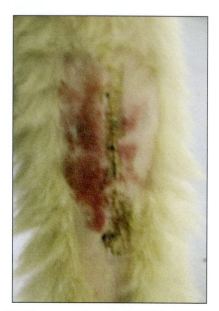

Fig. 25.46 **There may be considerable skin bruising postoperatively due to elevated oestrogen levels and possible thrombocytopaenia resulting from bone marrow suppression.**

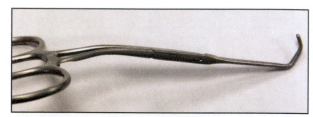

Fig. 25.47 **A Bennett (Satinsky) vascular clamp.**

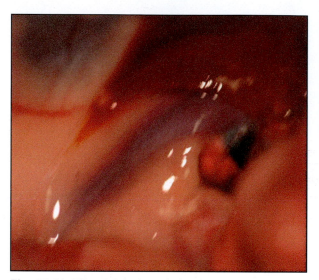

Fig. 25.48 **The right adrenal gland showing close association with liver and vena cava. In this case the adrenal was invading the vena cava.**

form via the vertebral venous sinus and azygous vein, death rates are approximately 25% postsurgery, presumably related to increases in caval pressure (Bennett *et al.*, 2008).

The technique described below is that used by the authors and is the 'traditional' technique. However, a novel technique described by Driggers (2008) exists, utilising a 5 mm ameroid constrictor ring placed round the adrenal gland. Once placed, a second surgery is performed 1–3 months later to remove the entire block of vena cava, gland and caudate process of the liver (surrounded by constrictor ring). This was reported as having high success (8 cases of 9) and no mortality.

Blood pressure should be monitored peri- and postoperatively.

Procedure

Approach as for left adrenalectomy. Reflect tissues and check left adrenal first. Perform left adrenalectomy if required. Reflect tissues to the left (or exteriorise if necessary) and identify the right adrenal gland. If the gland has not entered the vena cava then it is sometimes possible to place very small

vascular clips along the vena cava between gland and vena cava. The gland may then be dissected clear. If the gland has entered the vena cava then a section of vein needs removing along with the gland. The gland is isolated from the caudate process of the liver and surrounding fat using vascular clips. A Bennett (Satinsky) clamp (**Fig. 25.47**) is placed around the gland and occludes the vena cava cranial and caudal to the gland. Vascular clips (or 3/0 polydioxanone ligatures) are placed around the vena cava cranial and caudal to the clamp. The clamp is withdrawn, vena cava cut and section of vein and gland removed (**Fig. 25.48**). Fluid is placed in the abdomen, and the abdomen closed routinely (**Fig. 24.23**).

Postoperative care

The authors give 75 mg/kg amoxicillin long-acting, 0.02 mg/kg buprenorphine and 0.2 mg/kg meloxicam SC perioperatively along with saline SC at 30 mL/kg.

Ferrets are hospitalised for 48 hours, receiving analgesia as required and monitoring of blood pressure and then discharged with a 3-day course of meloxicam (0.2 mg/kg PO q12h). Perioperatively a deslorelin implant is placed subcutaneously unless both adrenals are completely removed or the prostate is enlarged. If the prostate is enlarged, a course of osaterone acetate (Ypozane, Virbac, Bury St Edmunds, UK) is given at 0.25–0.5 mg/kg SID for 7 days. A deslorelin implant can then be placed if required.

Owners should be warned to expect considerable skin bruising (**Fig. 25.46**) – this reflects the frequently raised oestrogen levels and does not seem to imply pain.

Wound care is as described earlier.

The removed gland should be submitted for histopathology.

INSULINOMA

Indications
Surgical treatment of insulinoma (see Chapter 14).

Preoperative considerations
Blood glucose levels should be stabilised prior to surgery (see Chapter 11). Concurrent disease should be identified and controlled.

Procedure
The ferret is anaesthetised and placed in dorsal recumbency. Skin preparation and incision as per left adrenalectomy. The pancreas is identified and the extent of diseased tissue ascertained (**Fig. 25.49**). In the case of single nodules (**Fig. 25.50**) only the nodule needs removal. In the case of diffuse thickening (in the UK many cases appear hyperplastic rather than neoplastic) or where there are multiple or large nodules (**Fig. 25.51**), a whole lobe may need removal. In either case, diseased tissue is identified and isolated using vascular clips. Alternatively radiosurgery or a harmonic scalpel can be used to dissect away from surrounding pancreas. Omentum is sutured over the pancreatic 'wound' using simple interrupted polyglactic acid 3/0 placed into the capsule of the pancreas. Fluid is placed intra-abdominally and the wound closed as for exploratory coeliotomy (**Fig. 25.23**).

Postoperative care
The authors give 75 mg/kg amoxicillin long-acting, 0.02 mg/kg buprenorphine and 0.2 mg/kg meloxicam SC perioperatively along with glucose–saline SC at 30 mL/kg. Ferrets are hospitalised for 48 hours, receiving analgesia as required and monitoring of

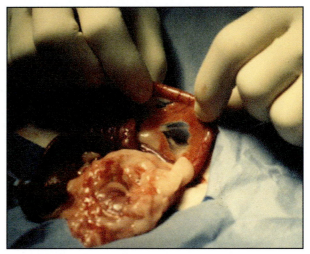

Fig. 25.49 **Exteriorising the pancreas for examination.**

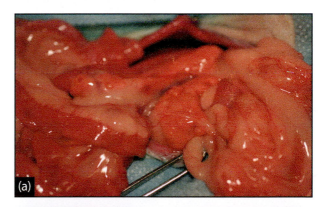

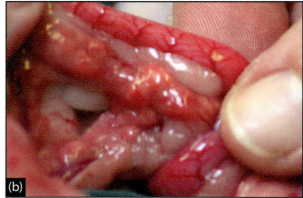

Fig. 25.50 **(a, b) Single nodules can be removed.**

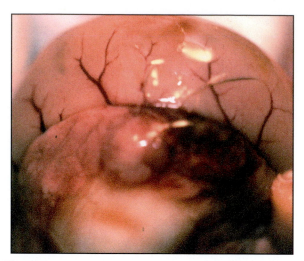

Fig. 25.51 **A whole lobe may need to be removed if there are multiple nodules.**

blood glucose. Two days postoperatively predniso-lone is started at 1 mg/kg PO BID. Insulinomas are rarely fully resected and frequently recur.

Owners are taught how to monitor blood glucose and prednisolone doses are tapered to effect.

In one case, the author has seen hyperglycaemia develop post pancreatic lobectomy. This is presumed to be due to atrophy of the islets in the unaffected lobe. Management as per an unstable diabetic using diets low in simple carbohydrates and use of porcine insulin (Caninsulin, MSD Animal Health, Milton Keynes, UK – approximately 30% amorphous zinc insulin and 70% crystalline zinc insulin in a suspension). Insulin doses are reduced as blood glucose levels fall, and the animal is hospitalised for 14 days.

CYSTOTOMY

Indications (see Chapter 22)
Cystic calculi (**Fig. 25.52**). Bladder tumours.

Preoperative considerations
All cases should be radiographed preoperatively to determine size/number/position of calculi. If radio-graphed several days previous to surgery then cases should be reradiographed immediately prior to sur-gery as uroliths are sometimes passed in this period.

Any concurrent problems (especially renal func-tion) should be evaluated and stabilised as far as possible prior to surgery.

If renal function is compromised, intravenous or intraosseous fluid support is required.

Procedure
The basic technique is identical to that utilised in other small mammals and cats. The approach is as per coeliotomy (see above) with the incision site mid-line from pubis extending 2 cm cranially. In males the site is similar but the skin incision must be slightly paramedian with the penis reflected laterally.

Many texts advise reflecting the bladder crani-ally and incising the dorsal surface of the bladder. However, this induces a flexion in the neck of the bladder and may make it impossible to access uro-liths in this region. The authors recommend incis-ing the ventral surface of the bladder (incision large enough to admit fine-tipped forceps and withdraw the largest urolith) (**Figs 25.53, 25.54**). Prior to incision, the abdomen is thoroughly packed off with moistened laparotomy sponges or large gauze sponges, and if the bladder is very distended, urine

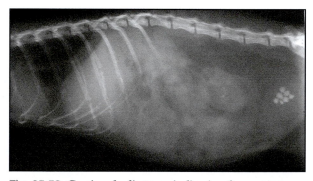

Fig. 25.52 **Cystic calculi are an indication for cystotomy.**

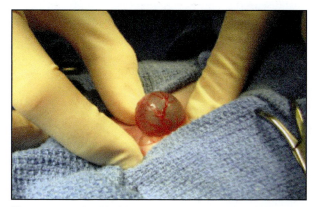

Fig. 25.53 **The bladder is exteriorised. The abdomen is well packed off with moistened sponges.**

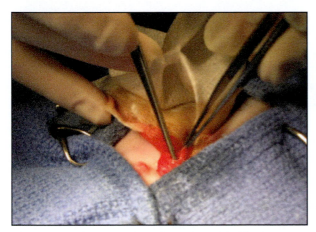

Fig. 25.54 **The ventral surface of the bladder is incised for removal of the uroliths.**

should be withdrawn using a needle (21G) and syringe prior to opening.

Once uroliths are removed, the bladder should be thoroughly irrigated with saline. The bladder wall is usually thickened so can be closed in two layers (both simple continuous using 4/0 polyglycolic acid) – mucosa and muscularis/serosa.

The abdomen is irrigated with saline and the wound closed in the normal manner.

Postoperative care

The authors give 75 mg/kg amoxicillin long-acting, 0.02 mg/kg buprenorphine and 0.2 mg/kg meloxicam SC perioperatively along with saline SC (or continuation of IV/IO fluids) at 30 mL/kg. Ferrets are hospitalised for 48 hours, receiving analgesia as required and monitoring of renal function and urine output.

Owners are advised to feed a wet diet rather than dry.

Uroliths should be submitted for analysis and the ferret subsequently may be placed on an appropriate feline urolith diet, although this has not been proven in ferrets and nutritionally may not meet the needs long term. Recently there has been an increase in cysteine uroliths connected with some grain-free diets. The ferret should be returned to a recommended commercial ferret diet (see Chapter 5).

Bladder lesions may be biopsied at cystotomy (using a pinch biopsy technique). In the case of tumours, meloxicam may be continued permanently at the above dose rate.

PROSTATIC (PARAURETHRAL) CYST REDUCTION

Indications

Paraurethral cysts are a secondary problem caused by adrenal disease and the production of sex steroids (see Chapters 14, 22). The prostate tissue surrounds the urethra and enlarges and/or becomes cystic, effectively causing dysuria and in some cases complete blockage (**Fig. 25.55**). If the prostatic tissue is enlarged enough, it may be palpated just caudal to the bladder, anterior to the pubis. Ultrasound examination can determine the extent of the prostatic tissue and cysts (**Fig. 25.56**). If the urinary tract becomes totally obstructed, the blockage must be alleviated by passing a catheter. The procedure (see Chapter 10) can use a tomcat catheter or 3-French red rubber catheter, and gently massaged perineally as is done in the dog. The catheter may not be able to pass the obstruction: gentle flushing with warmed saline and dilute lidocaine may cause material to pass into the bladder and relieve the obstruction. In some instances a cystotomy may be needed to introduce the catheter through the prostatic tissue.

Procedure

As this is part of the adrenal disease complex, adrenalectomy should be considered and concurrent medical therapy to block sex steroid production and/or steroid receptors on the prostatic tissue should be initiated.

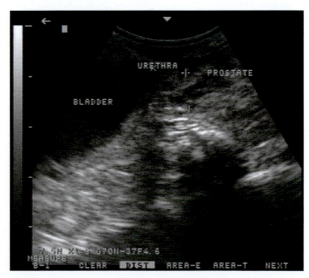

Fig. 25.55 **Ultrasonogram of the prostate, urethra and bladder.**

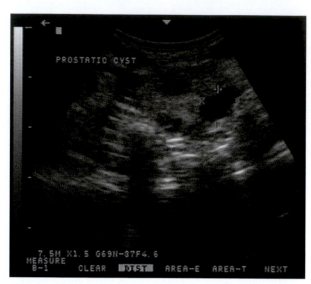

Fig. 25.56 Ultrasonogram of a cystic enlarged prostate.

Pain and inflammation control are critical as the ferret in pain will have urethral spasms and dysuria due to the reluctance to squat or compress the abdomen. Occasionally a benzodiazepine may be used to relax the ferret and, along with pain control, the ferret may be able to urinate despite the enlarged prostate and pressure on the urethra.

The prostatic cysts may be aspirated (ultrasound guided). The perineal and caudal abdomen should be clipped and aseptically prepared. The ferret should be anaesthetised, and have an analgesic previously administered.

A 22-gauge needle and 3 mL syringe can aspirate the flocculent material. Leakage from aspirated cysts does not seem to cause any problems. If cysts have not regressed using medical therapy and previous ultrasound-guided aspiration, and blockages are reoccurring, a coeliotomy is performed.

Marsupialisation of larger cysts has been described. Surgical drainage then packing the cavity with omentum has also been described for reduction of the cysts.

If the abdomen has been opened, it should be closed as for exploratory laparotomy above.

Postoperative care

The cysts will regress with decreased sex steroid levels. Usually the ferret is kept on broad-spectrum antibiotics, and anti-inflammatory drugs such as an NSAID until the dysuria is resolved. It has been proposed that in severe cases, prescrotal, perineal urethrostomy can be performed, although the authors have not needed to do this.

GASTROTOMY/ENTEROTOMY (SEE CHAPTER 13)

Indications
Biopsy of suspected lesions. Foreign body removal.

Procedure
The technique is identical to that used in other small mammals and cats. A coeliotomy approach (described above) is used with incision length determined by the region of gut to be approached and whether the procedure is exploratory/biopsy or to remove a foreign body. Prior to procedure, patients should be stabilised, and have concurrent disease evaluated/stabilised.

All cases should be radiographed and, ideally, have ultrasound before surgery. Intravenous or intraosseous fluids should be started prior to surgery and continued after. Choice of fluid should be determined by plasma electrolyte measurements.

Areas of necrosis should be resected. It should be remembered that ferrets have a very short intestine so they may only tolerate small lengths of gut being resected. Anastomosis techniques used in cats may be applied to ferrets.

Gut operative areas should be isolated using bowel clamps. Closure of gut is similar to that described for the bladder (see above) with a two-layer simple continuous technique. Inverting patterns should be avoided in the intestine due to the small lumen. After closure, patency of the wound is checked by injecting a small volume of saline into the gut proximal to the wound but within the part closed off by the clamps. Omentum should be sutured loosely over the wound prior to returning it to the abdomen.

Postoperative care
The authors give 12.5 mg/kg clavulanate-amoxicillin SC q24h (from 24 h preoperatively – alternatively given IV perioperatively, then continued by the SC route), 0.02 mg/kg buprenorphine and 0.2 mg/kg meloxicam SC perioperatively.

Ferrets are hospitalised for several days following intestinal surgery, with monitoring of faecal/urinary output and vomition. Blood glucose should also be monitored. They are given nil by mouth for 12 hours following surgery. Liquid critical care diet is then given little and often over the next 24 hours prior to the gradual reintroduction of normal diet.

LYMPH NODE BIOPSY

Indications
Lymph node enlargement, especially if non-responsive to broad-spectrum antibiosis.

Procedure
Three techniques may be indicated:

1. Fine needle aspirate:
   - The skin over the lymph node is clipped and aseptically prepared.
   - Grasping the lymph node, a 23G 5/8" needle is inserted. Using a 5 mL syringe, negative pressure is applied. The needle is withdrawn and smears prepared.
   - *Advantages:* no anaesthesia is required; unlikely to cause complications; quick and simple; easy to sample multiple nodes.
   - *Disadvantages:* absence of tissue architecture on smears may reduce diagnostic capability; easy to sample surrounding fat rather than lymph gland.
2. Trucut biopsy:
   - The ferret is anaesthetised (or sedated and local infiltrated under skin over lymph node).
   - The skin over the node is clipped and aseptically prepared.
   - A scalpel blade is used to make a stab incision over the node. Grasping the node, a Trucut biopsy needle is inserted into the node and 2–3 sections removed.
   - The skin wound is glued. Any haemorrhage is controlled by pressure.
   - *Advantages:* more likely to obtain diagnostic sample; relatively non-invasive.
   - *Disadvantages:* cost of Trucut biopsy device; may still obtain unrepresentative sample; small chance of haemorrhage.

3. Lymph node removal:
   - Ideally for popliteal, axillary or inguinal glands – submandibular glands may be too closely associated with blood vessels and nerves.
   - The ferret is anaesthetised and the skin over the gland is clipped and aseptically prepared.
   - Skin is incised over the node.
   - The node is identified and bluntly dissected from surrounding tissue. Any blood vessels are ligated using 3/0 polyglycolic acid (**Fig. 25.57**).
   - The removed node is placed in 10% formol saline.
   - Subcutaneous tissues and skin are closed with polyglycolic acid 3/0 – the former closed using a simple continuous pattern, the latter with a simple continuous subdermal suture. Tissue glue is then placed over the wound.

Postoperative care
The authors routinely give a single dose of long-acting amoxycillin (75 mg/kg SC) and carprofen (5 mg/kg SC) and advise daily cleaning of the wound.

- *Advantages:* best preservation of tissue architecture so much more likely to be diagnostic.
- *Disadvantages:* full surgical procedure with increased cost, anaesthetic risk and complication rates.

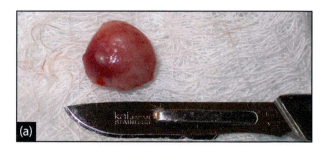

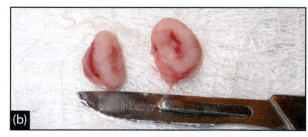

Fig. 25.57 (a) The lymph node is removed using blunt dissection; (b) cut node to submit for histopathology.

SURGICAL BIOPSY

With a species predisposition to neoplasia, biopsy of lesions is frequently indicated.

Skin mass

Skin masses are extremely common with both malignant and benign tumours being seen, along with non-neoplastic cysts, granulomas and abscesses (**Fig. 25.58**). The methods described earlier for lymph node biopsy may all be appropriate for skin masses, with similar surgical approaches and advantages/disadvantages.

In addition, the following may also be considered:

- Ulcerated lesions:
  - Surface smears may sometimes be of assistance. However, secondary infection may obscure the primary lesion (**Fig. 25.59**).
  - Complete surgical removal. This is often used as it may combine surgical cure with diagnosis. However, further surgery may well be needed for malignant masses as insufficient margins may be taken initially. This is best used for masses that are strongly suspected to be benign, or for lesions on extremities (**Fig. 25.59**), i.e. tail or toes, where any removal will necessitate amputation of the tail or toe and so it is unlikely that full surgical resection will not be achieved.

Abdominal organ or mass

Abdominal enlargements are common. Diagnosis is generally by means of palpation, radiography or ultrasonography. However, this will often simply confirm the presence of organomegaly or a mass without giving specific diagnosis. For this, biopsy is required. The simplest means of biopsy is ultrasound-guided fine needle aspirate. Anaesthesia or sedation is almost always required and the skin over the mass should be aseptically prepared.

The advantages and disadvantages of this are similar to fine needle aspirates of lymph nodes (described above).

For liver biopsy, or solid (i.e. no fluid obvious on scan) masses, ultrasound-guided Trucut biopsy may be performed. This gives a larger and therefore more

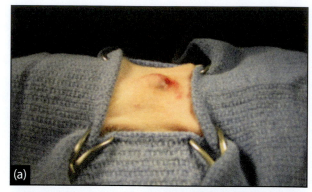
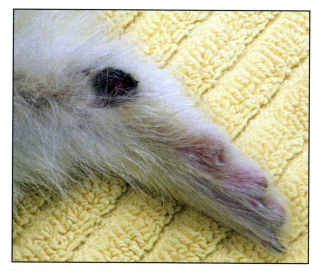

Fig. 25.58 (a) the skin mass is prepped for excision; (b) incision finished closure with tissue glue and therapeutic laser applied for improved healing.

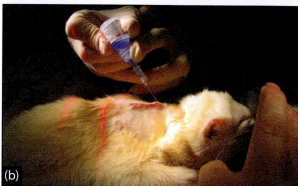

Fig. 25.59 An ulcerated lesion on the distal limb. Surface cytology simply confirmed a superficial secondary infection. The most effective means of biopsy was complete surgical removal using radiosurgery, confirming a benign cystadenoma.

likely diagnostic biopsy. However, there is a much greater risk of iatrogenic damage and/or haemorrhage. This technique should only be attempted by experienced ultrasonographers and the ferret should be preprepared for exploratory coeliotomy (see above) as emergency surgery may be required if there is a complication (haemorrhage or entry into a fluid-filled viscus).

Otherwise, exploratory coeliotomy is required. The great advantage of this is that it is easier to assess:

- Size and extent of lesion/mass.
- Determination of whether or not the mass is operable.
- Removal of the mass as part of the diagnostic process.
- Biopsy under visual control that will greatly reduce risks of iatrogenic damage.
- Ability to control haemorrhage.

Biopsy techniques that may be employed are:

- Fine needle aspirate – solid lesions (**Fig. 25.60**).
- Trucut – kidney, spleen, solid lesions.
- Pinch biopsies – liver, solid lesions.
- Wedge biopsies – liver (**Fig. 25.61**), spleen (ideally with radiosurgery), pancreas.
- Resection/removal – masses, lymph nodes, adrenal glands (**Fig. 25.62**).
- Punch biopsy – stomach, gut, spleen.

The major disadvantage is that exploratory coeliotomy is a major procedure to undertake as a diagnostic procedure unless there is a good chance of achieving surgical cure and/or other methods have failed to produce definitive diagnosis.

It is also likely that where non-removable masses are discovered, intraoperative euthanasia may need to be offered as it can be hard to justify any postoperative pain for an animal with a hopeless prognosis.

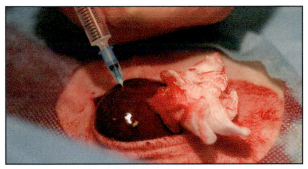

Fig. 25.60 **Fine needle aspirate of splenic mass taken at exploratory laparotomy.**

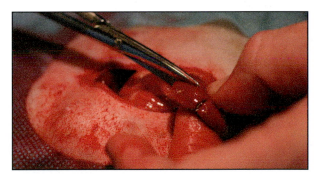

Fig. 25.61 **Wedge biopsy of liver using haemoclips to isolate a wedge of tissue that is then resected.**

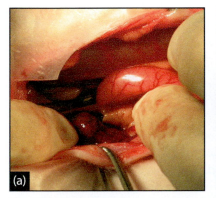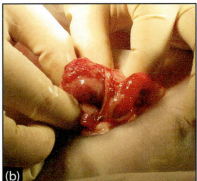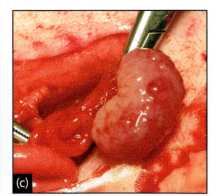

Fig. 25.62 **(a) A small mass is found; (b) the mass can be exteriorised prior to excision; (c) the mass is exteriorised and separated from vasculature for excision.**

To this end, recent advantages in laparoscopic techniques mean that many exploratory procedures and some organ biopsies may be carried out using a 2-port system and 3 mm equipment with electrocautery or radiosurgical devices.

LUMPECTOMY

Most considerations when removing masses are considered earlier in the section on biopsy techniques. In general, the techniques used to remove masses are the same as used in other species (**Fig. 25.63**). One difference that may exist is the large number of distal limb masses in ferrets compared to other companion animal species. Restricted tissue in these sites may impair the

ability to achieve either adequate surgical margins or to close wounds. Therefore, radiosurgery or other forms of cautery may be used where lesions are known to be benign, or amputation of tail or toe may be the only means to adequately remove a mass (**Fig. 25.64**).

Preputial masses

Preputial masses appear relatively common in ferrets (**Fig. 25.65**). Histologically these are most commonly adenomata or adenocarcinomas (Antinoff & Williams, 2012). However, carcinoma and cystadenomacarcinoma are also reported (Reavill *et al.*, 2010). Tumours are associated with the apocrine glands of this region and activity of these glands may be expected to reflect hormonal activity in these animals (Protain *et al.*, 2009).

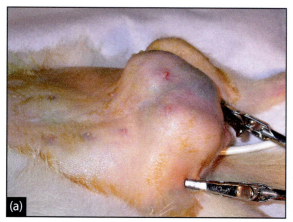
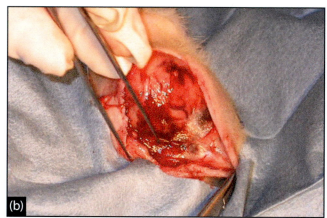

Fig. 25.63 (a) Mammary masses consistent with mammary adenomas; (b) incision is made over the mass, which is bluntly dissected out.

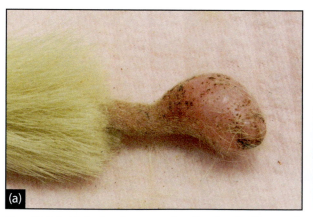
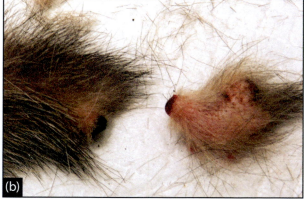

Fig. 25.64 (a) A chordoma on the distal tail; (b) complete surgical removal of the chordoma – it was removed with a simple tail tip amputation and cautery of the tail end. The authors prefer not to suture tail amputation sites when only the distal tip is removed. Ferrets often find the sutures irritating and these sites frequently break down. Proximal tail amputations should be sutured as per a cat tail amputation.

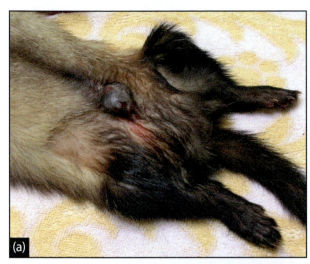

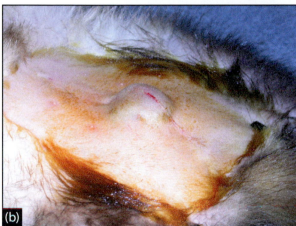

Fig. 25.65 (a, b) Preputial masses.

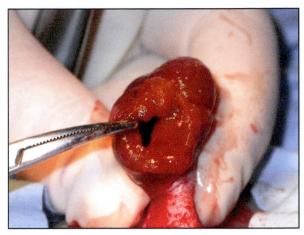

Fig. 25.66 **A preputial mass being excised. This one was cavitated.**

Being frequently seen in neutered animals it is certainly possible that they may be associated with adrenal gland disease, which is the authors' clinical experience. That said, it should be remembered that adrenal gland disease is extremely common in these animals and so may be coincidental. One such tumour treated by the authors did respond to deslorelin implants. However, others have not.

Malignant tumours tend to be extremely invasive and respond poorly to therapy, whether radiation (Miller *et al.*, 1985) or surgery.

Surgically the problem is achieving sufficiently wide surgical margins – at least 1 cm (van Zeeland *et al.*, 2014) to prevent recurrence (**Fig. 25.66**). Simple excision is rarely sufficient except for benign masses (where subsequent penile exposure may result in damage or infection of the mucosa). Fisher (2002)

and van Zeeland *et al.* (2014) describe penile amputation and urethrostomy as a means of treating these tumours. While this technique does achieve the required margins, it has to be questioned in terms of potential complications and careful owner preparation would be required before carrying out such surgery.

ORTHOPAEDIC SURGERY

In the authors' practices, orthopaedic cases are unusual, with the majority of cases occurring due to falling injuries. The most common presentations include:

- Dislocation of the hip.
- Dislocation of the elbow.
- Long bone fractures.
- Stifle ligament damage.

Spinal injuries and intervertebral disc disease are more frequent than any of these, but are usually not surgical cases – a consequence of size and anatomy. These are usually managed medically (see Chapters 17, 18).

Dislocation of the hip

This typically occurs as a result of falling with one hindlimb held/trapped. The hip joint is easily replaced but is also easily redislocated. An Ehmer sling can be attempted, but is unlikely to be retained due to the twin problems of restricting ferret activity, and restricting their chewing at bandages.

Therefore, manual relocation should be attempted and the ferret should be placed in a restricted one-level space with no wire or other materials for them to climb. If harness- or lead-trained then they should receive short walks several times a day (after the first 3 days' complete restriction) as this may reduce some tendency to self-exercise and become frustrated. NSAIDs should be given.

Typically a false joint will form in 2–4 weeks and ferrets cope well with this.

Should the joint be too unstable, then there are two main options:

- Femoral head and neck excision arthroplasty. This can be carried out in a manner similar to that in other pet species and is relatively simple due to the lack of muscle bulk around the hip joint in ferrets. Postoperative care is as described above.
- Amputation of the limb (see below).

Dislocation of the elbow

This typically occurs as a result of falling with one forelimb held/trapped. As with the hip, this is easily replaced manually, but is much less stable and so rarely will be retained.

Various techniques are described for longer-term stabilisation, including transarticular pinning and transarticular external fixation. External coaptation is unlikely to be successful due to the shape of the limb.

As with the hindlimb, where surgery is not feasible or successful, amputation is an option.

Long bone fractures

Typically these are a consequence of falling and most frequently involve the femur, radius/ulna or tibia. As in all fractures, the individual injury should be assessed and a repair method used appropriate to that injury in that animal. In general, though, ferrets appear good orthopaedic surgery candidates and usually have good bone density for holding implants. Typically most fractures can be repaired using a Type 1 external fixator usually tied into an intramedullary pin. Techniques for pin placement are similar to those used in other small mammals and cats.

After surgery, the ferret should be restricted (as described above) and given analgesia (opiate and NSAID for 2 days, then NSAID until implants removed). Most fractures will repair in 3–4 weeks and radiographs should be taken weekly though the repair process.

External fixators do require considerable protection from the ferret and should be well padded and bandaged while still allowing exposure of the pin entry sites to facilitate cleaning.

If the fracture is not amenable to surgery, or the repair technique is unsuccessful then amputation should be considered.

Stifle ligament damage

The authors have seen a single case of stifle ligament disruption involving rupture of cranial cruciate and lateral collateral ligaments. This occurred as a result of hindlimb entrapment in a swinging rope and suspension via the single limb.

In an animal of this size, restriction (see earlier) and anti-inflammatory drugs would be expected to be successful. However, where the joint is too unstable, surgery is required to stabilise. A single lateral suture using 0 polydioxanone was placed (**Fig. 25.67**) in a manner as described for similar injuries in cats. The ferret was restricted without climbing for 2 weeks with successful results and return to full limb function.

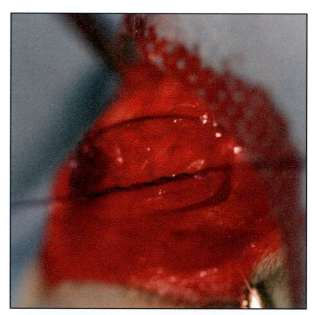

Fig. 25.67 **A single lateral suture is placed in the stifle joint to stabilise it.**

AMPUTATION

Indications

Ferrets cope extremely well following amputation of a limb. However, this technique should be regarded as a salvage technique and reserved for these cases:

- Orthopaedic injuries that are either not amenable to surgery (excessively complicated or open/contaminated fractures; or where there is considerable joint disruption) or where surgery has failed or not been tolerated by the ferret or where repair is beyond the owner's means (financial or nursing time).
- Neoplasia of the distal limb, to allow removal with adequate surgical margins.
- Where there is no concurrent spinal disease, or disease/injury to contralateral limbs. Whole body/limb radiographs must always be taken as a part of the presurgical evaluation.

Procedure

This is essentially the same as in other species. Hindlimb amputation is described – forelimb amputation is similar but with the limb removed at distal humeral level.

The ferret is anaesthetised and placed in lateral recumbency, affected limb uppermost. The affected limb is clipped and aseptically prepared from mid-tibia to hip. A circumferential skin incision is made just distal to the stifle. The skin is reflected proximally.

The muscles are incised immediately proximal to the stifle joint. Large blood vessels are normally located in the caudal muscle mass – ideally these should be located and ligated prior to incision. The muscle ends are reflected proximally to expose the femur.

The distal femur is cut using small bone cutters. Any 'splintering' of the bone should be tidied and bone fragments removed from the wound. The two muscle ends are then sutured over the bone end using 2/0 polyglycolic acid in a horizontal mattress pattern. The skin is then sutured using 3/0 polyglycolic acid in a simple continuous intradermal pattern. Tissue glue is then placed over the wound.

Postoperative care

The authors give clavulanate/amoxicillin at 12.5 mg/kg q12h for 5 days. Analgesia (single subcutaneous dose of 5 mg/kg carprofen) is given perioperatively. The ferret is restricted for 5 days and then exercise is gradually increased. Climbing is prevented for 10–14 days to allow the animal to 'learn' without falling. The wound should be bathed daily with saline until healed.

Complications are unusual but may involve wound breakdown or infection. In these cases, medical management usually suffices or reamputation at a higher level.

ANAL SACCULECTOMY

Indications

In the UK, this is considered an unethical surgery unless there is a medical reason for it such as an infected impaction or tumour. In the USA, most ferrets in the pet trade have had this done at 5–6 weeks of age. There may be incomplete removal or partial regrowth of the gland, which in most cases needs to have surgery to remove the offending tissue (**Figs 25.68, 25.69**). These conditions may be painful and become secondarily infected. If the ferret comes from a hobby breeder, this surgery may be done on request by the owner at the time of neuter or spay. Removal of the glands eliminates the odour of anal sac secretions, but ferrets still will have some odour from sebaceous and aprocrine tubular glands located in the perianal area.

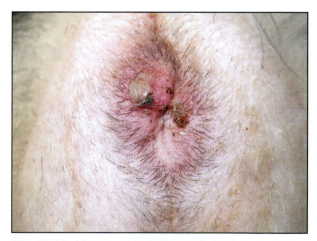

Fig. 25.68 Abscess of remnant anal gland.

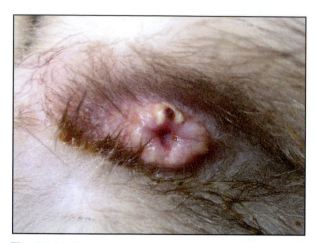

Fig. 25.69 **Previous incomplete excision of the gland.**

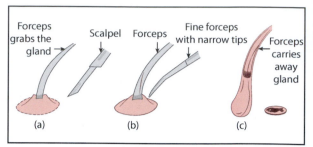

Fig. 25.71 **Procedure for removing an anal gland. (a) The duct is clamped, and a small elliptical incision is performed around the tip of the forceps; (b) a forceps is used to gently dissect tissue around the gland. Muscle and glandular tissue surrounding the sac is scraped away with forceps or a scalpel blade; (c) gentle traction is performed along with blunt dissection to free the gland.**

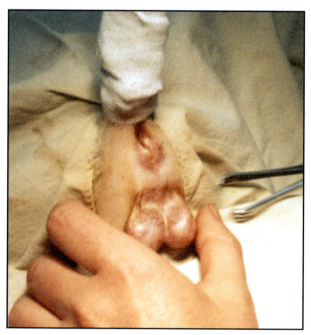

Fig. 25.70 **Positioning for anal sacculectomy or correction. This same positioning is used for castration and vasectomy.**

Preoperative considerations

The ferret should receive preanaesthetic drugs and an analgesic before inhalant anaesthetic (see Chapter 24). The ferret is intubated and maintained for general surgery. The ferret should be placed on a heated pad. The ferret may be positioned at the end of a table in either dorsal recumbency with the tail dropped down and the hind legs drawn cranially, or in ventral recumbency with the tail drawn forward. The authors prefer ventral recumbency as this keeps the glands in normal anatomical position (**Fig. 25.70**). The perineal area including the scrotum should be clipped and aseptically prepared and draped. If neutering is being done at the same time, it should be done first before the anal sacs.

Procedure

The opening of the ducts and adjacent 2 mm of skin and mucous membrane on the anus should be located and clamped closed with mosquito forceps or delicate allis forceps. This will decrease the leakage of glandular secretion during the procedure. A superficial circumferential incision is made around the tips of the forceps using a No. 15 Bard-Parker scalpel blade (**Fig. 25.71**). The skin and mucosa are reflected from the duct by using a gentle scraping action with the blade.

Using a mosquito forceps directed cranio-laterally from the incision, follow along the curve of the gland. The sphincter muscle and glandular tissue surrounding the gland can be gently removed with scraping using the scalpel blade or the tip of the forceps.

The wall of the gland appears yellowish and is thin. Glandular secretions are yellow.

With gentle traction on the clamped duct, the gland can be dissected out and removed (**Fig. 25.72**).

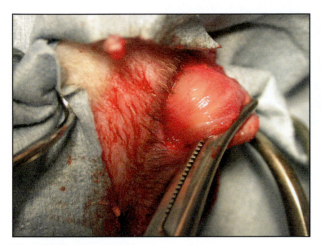

Fig. 25.72 **The gland is removed.**

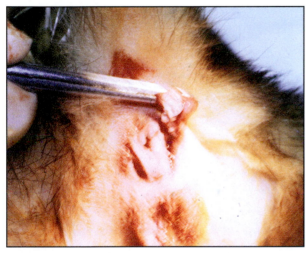

Fig. 25.73 **If the gland ruptures, surgical extirpation to remove the gland walls is done.**

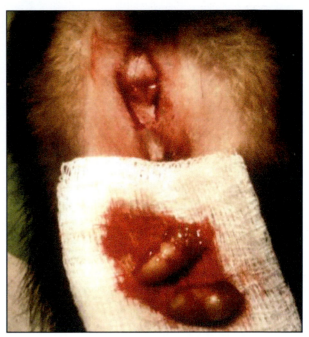

Fig. 25.74 **An alternative removal route involves the skin over each gland to be incised, and blunt dissection used to free the gland. The duct is clamped to prevent leakage.**

If the gland is ruptured, surgical extirpation can still be done, although locating and removing all of the gland's walls may be difficult (**Fig. 25.73**). The odour from an incised or ruptured sac is irritating and foul. The removed glands should be placed in a ziplock-sealing plastic bag for disposal so that the hospital is not overwhelmed with the odour.

Intraoperative haemorrhage is minimal, but can be staunched using sterile cotton buds.

Some surgeons do not close the holes, but the authors prefer to place 1–3 sutures or use tissue glue to close the tissue on each side.

A second technique for anal sacculectomy further decreases potential damage to the muscles of the rectum and sphincter. A ferret is prepared as above, but the incision is made over the body of the gland in the skin, approximately 1 cm from the opening of the duct (**Fig. 25.74**). It is helpful to apply a clamp to the duct to keep the secretion from leaking and keep the gland full. Blunt dissection with haemostats is then done around the body of the gland caudal to the attachment of the duct to the sphincter mucosa. The attachment can be ligated and cut from 'inside' the skin/mucosa. The skin is closed with either tissue glue or 1–3 sutures.

Postoperative care

Postoperative care includes use of an NSAID for 3–5 days postsurgery. Usually there are no serious postoperative sequelae, but complications such as persistent minor haemorrhage and bruising can develop. There are potential complications of prolapsed rectum and faecal incontinence if trauma to the anal sphincter muscles is excessive.

RECTAL PROLAPSE

Indications

This is most often the sequela to the anal sacculectomy done in kits where too much tissue was removed from the sphincter or the sphincter was damaged (**Fig. 25.75**). Rarely does it happen as a sequela to diarrhoea or neoplasia. In an adult ferret with a prolapse occurring due to tenesmus or diarrhoea, the classic purse-string suture along with appropriate antibiotics and NSAIDs is usually enough for correction as with other mammals. The kits, however, need to have a more extensive surgery to cinch up the anus (**Fig. 25.76**). The authors term this 'recto–anal reconstruction' rather than just prolapse reduction.

Presurgical considerations

A faecal analysis should be done to eliminate the possibility of coccidia or cryptosporidia as aetiology of the prolapse. The ferret should be placed on appropriate anticoccidial treatment if present. Otherwise, a broad-spectrum antibiotic such as oral amoxicillin should be started.

Procedure

The perirectal area is clipped and the skin aseptically prepped. The prolapsed tissue is also cleansed, usually with a chlorhexidine or iodine surgical scrub. The tail is reflected dorsocranially (**Fig. 25.77**). Two or four 'wedge' skin removals are made to reduce the anus size (**Fig. 25.78**).

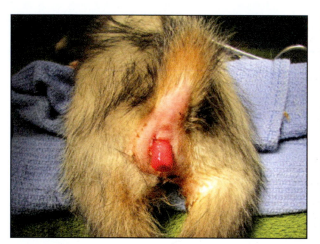

Fig. 25.75 **Prolapsed rectum in an 8-week-old kit.**

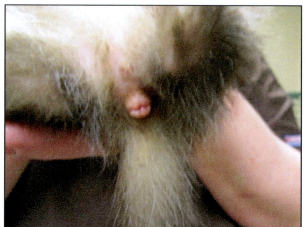

Fig. 25.76 **Prolapsed rectum less severe in an 8-week-old kit.**

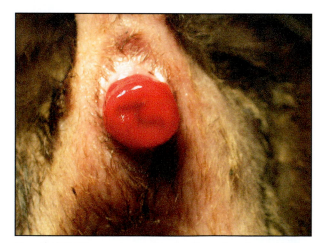

Fig. 25.77 **The perianal skin is clipped and prepped with an antiseptic solution.**

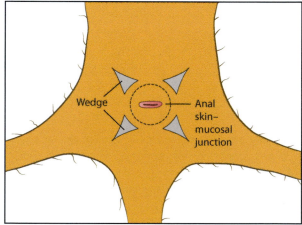

Fig. 25.78 **Diagram illustrating the possible four wedges of tissue to take to tighten the anal opening.**

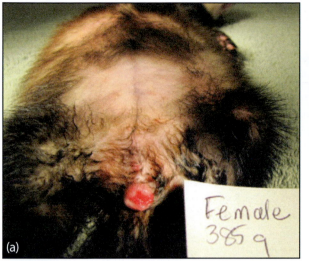
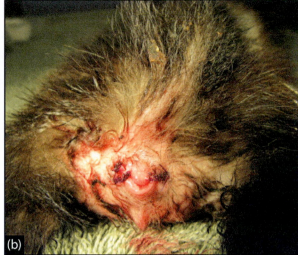

Fig. 25.79 (a) Prolapsed rectum and (b) repair.

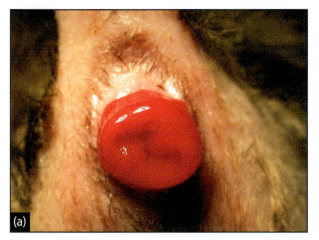
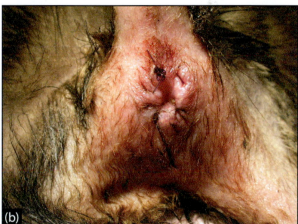

Fig. 25.80 (a) Prolapsed rectum and (b) repair.

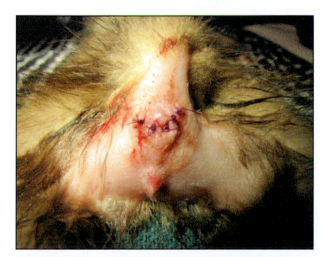

Fig. 25.81 A sutured repair using two wedges.

Examples of the prolapse and repair are shown in **Figs 25.79**, **25.80**.

The sutures are 4-0 suture – either absorbable or non-absorbable can be used, although the authors use absorbable (**Fig. 25.81**). Suture removal is at 10–14 days, although many of the sutures may have fallen out before then.

Postoperative care

Postoperative care generally includes continuing with a broad-spectrum antibiotic for 10 days and an NSAID for 3 days concurrently with a stomach protectant such as famotidine. The authors have rarely seen any complications with this surgery. The rectum/anus returns to full function and cosmetically looks normal.

CHAPTER 26

PAEDIATRICS

Cathy A. Johnson-Delaney

NORMAL KITS: GROWTH AND BIOLOGY (SEE CHAPTER 6)

- Gestation: 41 days (39–42 days). There is kit mortality at day 43 if not delivered. Gestation is often shorter in primiparous jills.
- Parturition: whelping.
- Parturition duration: 2–3 hours.
- Litter size: average 8–9 kits (range 7–15).
- Altricial.
- Newborn kit is covered in fine white hair (**Figs 26.1–26.3**).

- At 3 days of age kits begin to change hair coats. Albinos retain white hair coats; ferrets of other colours acquire grey coats (**Fig. 26.4**).
- They have a subcutaneous fat pad on the dorsal surface of the neck.
- Little ability to maintain normal body temperature for first 3 weeks of life.
- Normal litter lies close to the jill, nursing and sleeping except when the jill leaves the nest.

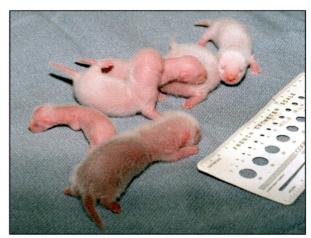

Fig. 26.3 **Litter, with one considerably smaller.**

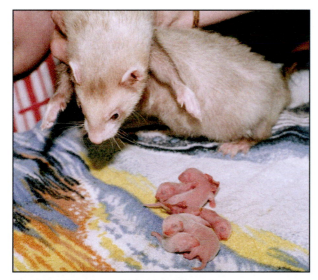

Fig. 26.1 **Newborn kits with jill.**

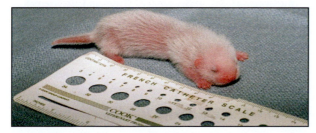

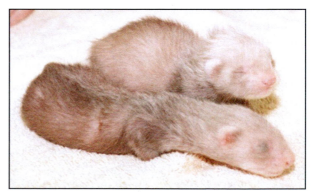

Fig. 26.2 **Individual newborn kit.**

Fig. 26.4 **Seven-day-old kits; the coats are changing colour.**

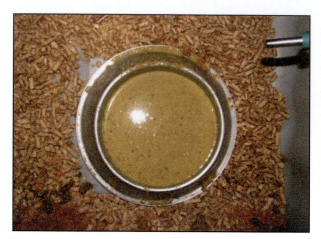

Fig. 26.5 Gruel made with regular ferret food soaked can be offered to kits starting at 2–3 weeks of age.

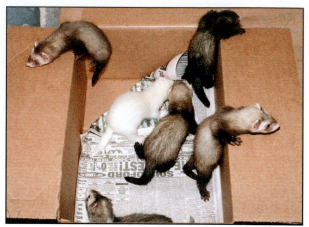

Fig. 26.6 Eight-week-old weaned ferrets.

- At 3 weeks of age begin exploring.
- Eyes open at day 30–35 although eyes may open as early as day 25.
- Hear sound at about 32 days of age.
- Deciduous teeth erupt at 14 days; emerge completely through gingiva at 18 days.
- Permanent canine teeth appear at 47–52 days, before shedding of deciduous canines at 56–70 days.
- May begin taking solid food at 2–3 weeks of age (**Fig. 26.5**).
- Jill stimulates the kit for urination/defaecation until they are eating solid food exclusively (weaned).
- Weaned at 6–8 weeks (**Fig. 26.6**).
- Weigh 8–10 g at birth (range 6–12 g).
- Bodyweight 30 g at 1 week.
- Bodyweight 60–80 g at 2 weeks.

REARING

For abandoned, orphaned or ill kits, provide supplemental heat. Keep a temperature gradient in the nest box of 30–40°C. Hypothermic kits do not nurse, so administer a few drops of 50% dextrose solution by mouth or rub a small drop of corn syrup on the gingiva. Then give warmed subcutaneous fluids (50–100 mL/kg). Feed the kit only once it is normothermic (38.5–39°C).

Neonatal ferrets are difficult to hand rear due to their needing to be fed very frequently (every 2 hours

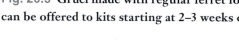

Table 26.1 **Composition of ferret milk**

POSTPARTUM (DAYS)	MEAN % FAT	MEAN % PROTEIN	MEAN % LACTOSE
5	7.8–8.5	7.2–8.8	2.7–4.2
11	9.3–10.5	6.3–7.9	2.8–4.4
19	8.9–10.8	6.0–8.3	3.8–4.2
25	8.8–9.5	5.0–7.9	3.3–4.2
33	9.2–10.3	8.6–9.8	3.0–4.1
39	9.0–13.0	8.4–10.6	1.5–3.2

including at night). Ferret milk should be fed for the first 7–10 days. Days 10–21, kits may be offered puppy or kitten milk replacer 4–6 times daily. Some authors recommend enriching milk replacer with cream until the fat content is 20%.

The composition of ferret milk varies over the course of lactation (*Table 26.1*).

Because hand-rearing is so challenging, consider supplemental hand-feedings when the jill's milk production is reduced because of illness. The stimulus of nursing may promote lactation as the jill improves. Another important alternative is cross-fostering. It is best to breed jills in pairs so one may serve as a foster mother if problems arise. Most jills accept kits of any size or age at any stage of lactation. Merely remove kits from both litters for a short time, mix the two litters together and then replace all kits with the foster mother.

Nursing techniques and amounts to feed

Kits need to be taught how to feed from a nipple or syringe. Wrap the kit's body in a towel, with its head protruding. The kit should not be on its back. Hold it at an angle it would naturally assume if suckling. It is best with gentle handling and softly talking to it. With a drop of milk on the tip of the cannula/nipple place it gently into the kit's mouth, slightly off centre. This may take time at the first feeding. If the nipple is forced the kit will struggle. If the bottle and nipple are not working, use a 1–3 cc syringe with a feeding tip. Dribble the liquid in very gradually and be careful not to choke the kit. The milk should be warmed to approximately 37–38°C.

Feed every 2 hours including nights with neonates, and gradually reduce the number of nighttime feedings over weeks 2 and 3. Start by feeding about 0.5 mL per feeding. Increase to 1 mL per feeding by the end of the first week. The rule of thumb is to let the kit determine the amount fed. Feed amounts equal to approximately 10% of bodyweight per 24-hour period. If diarrhoea develops it is probably due to overfeeding, either in the strength of the mixture or in the quantity of total liquid intake. Kits should be weighed daily and should show a slow weight gain. There is usually a loss of weight for the first day or two until the kit's system gets used to the milk substitute and the shock of being separated from its jill. Overfeeding can also lead to bloat, so it is important not to force more feeding if the kit refuses after some nursing.

By 3 weeks of age kits generally are taking 6–8 mL of formula from the bottle every 4 hours and not during the night if they are starting to eat out of a bowl. Use a low, flat dish. Offer a bowl of formula and also a bowl filled with soaked mushy ferret food (can also be mixed with formula). Three-week-old kits can still be offered formula feedings three times a day. Be aware that they can stumble into a dish of formula and get cold and wet. They will learn to drink from the bowl very quickly. Kits cannot survive on mush alone until at least week 4. They do poorly on an adult diet before 5 weeks of age.

At each feeding or shortly afterwards the kit must be toileted because its muscles are not yet developed.

This can be done using a cotton wool ball or washcloth moistened with warm water to wipe the anogenital area very gently until urination and defaecation takes place. It is also good to lightly stroke the stomach and back legs. Kits may not defaecate after every feeding, but they must urinate. Kits start to urinate and defaecate on their own at approximately 3 weeks of age (at about the same time as they start to eat solid food).

Weaning can take place after 4 weeks of age although naturally raised kits generally wean at 6–8 weeks. The weaning solid food should be adult diet softened with a little formula and water to make a soup or mush (**Fig. 26.7**). Generally decrease the formula added after 4–5 weeks. Monitor the kit's weight. If the kit is not gaining from eating the mush, then the addition of a supplemental calorie, protein and fat to the mush can be used. Carnivore Care (Oxbow Pet Products, Murdoch, NE) or similar supplement can be mixed into the mush for

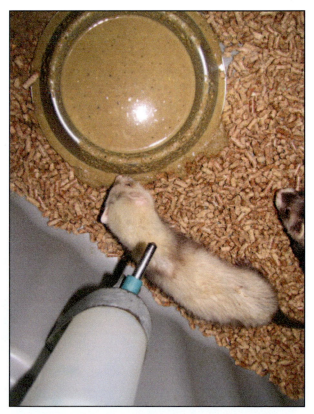

Fig. 26.7 Gruel made with formula; a water bottle is also offered. This ferret is 6 weeks old.

additional nutrition. Use approximately 1 teaspoon of Carnivore Care per cup of adult food.

PAEDIATRIC DISORDERS

Neonatal mortality and deformities

Mortality rate is greatest during the first 3–4 days of life, then drops dramatically after day 5. Common causes of death include cannibalism if the jill is stressed or primiparous. Stillbirths occur particularly if there is prolonged gestation, but also if the jill is undernourished, stressed or ill.

Severe congenital defects have been documented in ferrets including agenesis of limbs, anencephaly, hemivertebrae, scoliosis, spina bifida, gastroschisis and cranioschisis. Other congenital defects seen include cleft lip, cleft palate, corneal dermoids, missing digits, kinked tail and short tail (**Fig. 26.8**).

Entangled umbilical cords

Definition/overview

Umbilical cords can become tangled as the placenta is not separated.

Aetiology/pathophysiology

Kits in large litters are occasionally born so rapidly that the jill is unable to chew the placenta off each individual, creating a mass of kits bound together by their umbilical cords. This tangle may be exacerbated if kits are born on coarse, sharp-edged shavings. The entangled kits cannot nurse so they quickly become hypoglycaemic. The jill cannot curl around them so they become hypothermic.

Clinical presentation

Mass of kits bound together by their umbilical cords. Kits may be hypothermic and hypoglycaemic.

Differential diagnosis

None.

Diagnostic testing

None.

Diagnosis

Tangle of umbilical cords and placenta.

Management/treatment

This may be treated by careful dissection of the placentas from each kit's umbilicus with blunt scissors as far as possible from the kit's abdomen. If the placenta has become dry, soften tissue with warmed saline. Minimise the risk by closely supervising whelping. The kits can be picked up as soon as they are born to separate the placenta.

Diarrhoea

Definition/overview

Diarrhoea present (**Fig. 26.9**).

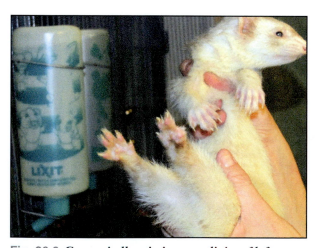

Fig. 26.8 **Congenitally missing two digits of left hind foot.**

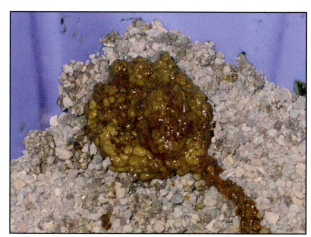

Fig. 26.9 **Diarrhoea showing poorly digested food.**

Aetiology/pathophysiology

May be caused by rotavirus alone, concurrent rota-viral and bacterial infections (i.e. *Campylobacter jejuni*, *Escherichia coli*, *Proteus* sp., *Staphylococcus aureus*, *Enterobacter cloacae*), bacterial infection alone, ferret enteric coronavirus (FRECV), coccidia or combinations of any of these. Ferret rotavirus is carried by adults and may cause diarrhoea in stressed kits or even unstressed kits if they have no passive immunity. The jill typically grooms away all evidence of diarrhoea.

Clinical presentation

Diarrhoea may be found; some evidence in the peri-rectal area and under the tail. The jill may groom the kit so it's difficult to see the actual diarrhoea. The kit may appear wet and dehydrated.

Differential diagnosis

None.

Diagnostic testing

Microscopic examination of faeces to look for coccidian. Bacterial culture and sensitivity (may take rectal culture).

Diagnosis

Presence of diarrhoea.

Management/treatment

Diarrhoea may be mild and self limiting in older kits but is potentially life threatening during the first week of life. Oral antimicrobials if bacterial component. Supportive care includes fluids and GI protectants such as famotidine, bismuth subsaliscylate. Anticoccidial medication if coccidia is present. Monitor the jill closely as kit anorexia may interrupt the normal nursing pattern and predispose the jill to mastitis and/or agalactia.

Hypothermia

Definition/overview

Decreased body temperature (below physiological 38–39°C).

Aetiology/pathophysiology

The jill is ill or a poor mother. The nest area is not sufficiently warm. Kits chill quickly and do not nurse when they are cold.

Clinical presentation

Slow-moving kits, may remain huddled with their littermates. Will not be nursing.

Differential diagnosis

Illness, diarrhoea and dehydration.

Diagnostic testing

Take body temperature. Check hydration.

Diagnosis

Hypothermia.

Management/treatment

Hold chilled kits in warm water or place on an insulated heating pad (wrapped in a towel to prevent burns, should be on low heat) or use an incubator or forced air surgical heating system (Bair Hugger, 3M Global, Brussels). Give a few drops of glucose solution orally. If dehydrated, use 0.5–2.0 mL of warmed (38–39°C) subcutaneous fluids. Correct environment so that it provides warmth to the nest. Check the jill for illness. Kits in this situation may need supplemental feeding if the jill is not able to nurse properly.

Neonatal conjunctivitis

Definition/overview

Also called ophthalmia neonatorum. Purulent discharge collecting in the conjunctival sac behind the unopened eyelids of the kit (**Fig. 26.10**).

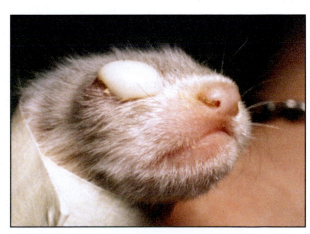

Fig. 26.10 **Neonatal conjunctivitis in a 3-week-old kit.**

Aetiology/pathophysiology

A variety of pathogens have been cultured. Route of infection is unknown although theorised to develop secondary to miniscule eyelid punctures acquired as the kit is dragged around the nest box. It may be unilateral or bilateral.

Clinical presentation

Unilateral or bilateral conjunctivitis. Kits are between a few days to 3 weeks of age. They stop nursing because of the pain associated with pressing their eyes against the dam.

Differential diagnosis

None.

Diagnostic testing

Culture and sensitivity of the purulent material.

Diagnosis

Bacterial presence, clinical signs.

Management/treatment

Administer a topical ophthalmic anaesthetic. Open the eyelids by cutting along the natural suture line with a small scalpel blade or 25 gauge needle bevel. Flush debris and apply a broad-spectrum ophthalmic ointment. Litter mates may also be affected and must be examined and treated. Repeat treatment at least twice daily until resolved. Monitor closely for nursing. If the kit does not resume nursing, hand feeding may be indicated. Prognosis is good in 3-week-old kits since the eyelids will stay open. In younger kits the eyelids may reseal and infection may recur, hence the monitoring and repeated treatments.

Rectal prolapse (see Chapters 13, 25)

Definition/overview

The rectum is prolapsed with varying lengths of tissue protruding (**Fig. 26.11**).

Aetiology/pathophysiology

This is seen following demusking that took too much tissue around the anus and/or actually damaged the rectal muscle. It can be seen with protozoal infection due to diarrhoea and tenesmus.

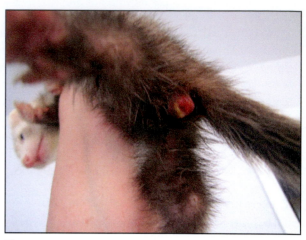

Fig. 26.11 Prolapsed rectum probably connected with the demusking surgery.

Clinical presentation

There will be prolapse of varying lengths. Depending on severity and how long the tissue has been exposed there will be oedema, erythema and ulceration with scabs. There may be faeces adherent to the tissue.

Differential diagnosis

None.

Diagnostic testing

A faecal examination for parasites should be done (rule out coccidia, cryptosporidia, giardia as causes of tenesmus, diarrhoea). Additional testing for protozoa may include ELISA, PCR.

Diagnosis

Presence of the prolapse.

Management/treatment

The exposed mucosa should be kept moist – irrigating it with 50% dextrose will also aid in reducing the prolapsed tissue. The author also uses an antibiotic ointment to lubricate the tissue. The prolapse should be reduced. Surgical correction is usually necessary to maintain the reduction. A purse-string suture rarely works. The author prefers to decrease the diameter of the anus by removing wedges of skin and thereby tightening the anus (see Chapter 25, **Figs 25.75–25.81**).

Splay-legged kits

Definition/overview
Called 'swimmers'.

Aetiology/pathophysiology
Affected kits lie on their sternum, which leads to rib compression and death secondary to anoxia by 8 weeks of age. Cause is unknown. Theorised either hereditary or husbandry related, when a rapidly growing kit is housed on smooth flooring that places excessive weight on its immature limbs.

Clinical presentation
Kit is lying on sternum with all legs splayed. Cannot place legs in normal quadruped positions for ambulation.

Differential diagnosis
None.

Diagnostic testing
Radiographs.

Diagnosis
Positioning of legs does not hold – the kit collapses.

Management/treatment
Although bracing has been tried, it has failed. Prognosis is grave.

OTHER COMPLICATIONS

Additional problems have been noted in the USA with kits shipped prior to their neutering incisions being healed. As they are usually neutered and demusked at 5 weeks of age, and shipped to a distributor at 6–7 weeks of age, they may arrive not fully healed (**Fig. 26.12**). Another complication to kit surgery are burn wounds probably due to being placed on heating pads perioperatively (**Fig. 26.13**). These problems may lead to a distributor holding back the kit from being sent to a pet shop. Unfortunately, by the time the kit is healed (1–2 weeks) it may be larger than what the pet shop wants. The distributor the author works with turns such pet shop rejects over to a local ferret shelter to be adopted.

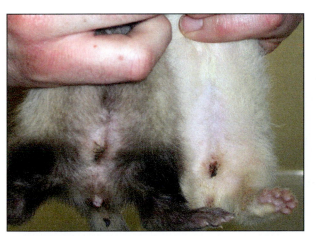

Fig. 26.12 **Non-healed ovariohysterectomy incision lines in 6-week-old kits.**

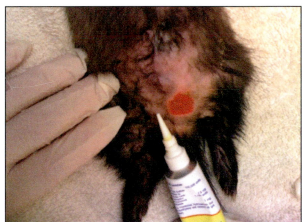

Fig. 26.13 **Burn wound in a 6-week-old kit. It took approximately 10 days to heal, and the ferret was then too large to place in a pet store. The author kept this one!**

CHAPTER 27

GERIATRICS

Cathy A. Johnson-Delaney

WHAT TO DO AND WHEN TO STOP

Ferrets live an average of 5–7 years, so can be considered geriatric at age 3. Myths about lifespan are perpetuated on the internet and by breeders and sellers, which is grossly unfair to the pet owner. It becomes the responsibility of the vet to discuss true lifespan and work with the owners when their ferret becomes geriatric even though chronologically they are 'young' in the owner's eyes. Discussing old age and death with owners, in particular children, who are truly bonded to their ferrets is difficult (**Fig. 27.1**). There are a number of issues concerning aging ferrets. This includes information about counselling and approaches that vets can use with their clients when discussing end-of-life scenarios.

It is recommended that ferrets at age 3 and above have physical examinations every 6 months. Laboratory values should be taken at age 3 to establish

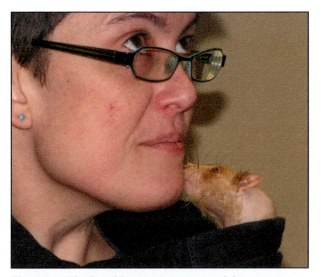

Fig. 27.1 **The bond between owner and ferret may be very strong. (Photo of Vondelle McLaughlin with Charlie, with permission.)**

a baseline, then every 12 months up to age 5, then every 6 months. Radiographs may be repeated every 6 to 12 months. Dental cleaning is usually needed every 6 months although home care regular brushing is recommended. A suggested timetable is listed in *Table 27.1*.

Comprehensive evaluation of the geriatric ferret can include:

- Full physical examination with palpation, particularly of the abdomen. Note any lumps, particularly skin lesions. Ophthalmic examination should be done, particularly to detect cataracts or lenticular sclerosis seen frequently in geriatric ferrets. Otoscopic examination, checking the integrity of the tympanic membrane and condition of the exterior canal and pinnae.
- Complete blood count (CBC), serum chemistry panel, urinalysis.
- Imaging: whole body radiographs. Ultrasonography of the abdomen should be done at least annually or more often if anomalies are found such as concurrent adrenal disease.
- A thorough oral and dental examination. Prophylaxis should be done under anaesthesia as often as necessary depending on the degree of disease seen. Radiographs of the dentition should be done at least annually or more often if disease is detected.
- Cardiac examination that includes auscultation including Doppler audio of the heart valves. Electrocardiography (ECG) may be warranted if cardiomegaly has been detected on radiographs or if the palpation of the chest seems to be less compressible than normal – heart feels enlarged. ECG is warranted especially if an arrhythmia is detected or in the cases of cardiomegaly.

Table 27.1 **Suggested geriatric ferret routine screening**	
After 3 years of age (at a minimum)	CBC, serum chemistry panel including fasting glucose (2 hours), urinalysis Thoracic radiograph Thorough physical examination with cardiac emphasis Dental cleaning Vaccinations (risk assessment for CDV; regulatory/risk assessment for rabies)
Between 3 and 6 years of age	Examination including physical, radiographs every 6 months. Additional imaging of abdomen if abnormalities detected on palpation Bloodwork at least annually Dental cleaning at least annually Risk assessment for vaccinations, administration if indicated
Older than 6 years of age: every 6 months	Examination including physical, imaging Bloodwork, urinalysis Dental cleaning Note: vaccinations still given on an annual basis based on risk assessment

Key: CBC, complete blood count; CDV; canine distemper virus.

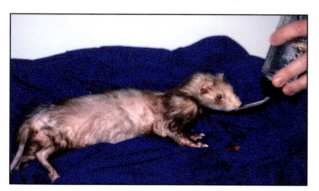

Fig. 27.2 **The geriatric ferret may be less ambulatory and need assistance with feeding and watering.**

MEDICAL CONDITIONS OF GERIATRIC FERRETS (*TABLE 27.2*)

Many of the medical issues of geriatric ferrets can be ameliorated to prolong life with a good quality. There are also many that have only palliative treatment and supportive care (**Fig. 27.2**). Often treatment is geared to allowing the longest life possible. Owners need to know that despite all efforts, it is often difficult to get the ferret beyond its projected lifespan with a good quality of life.

The ferret has one of the highest tumour rates of any mammal, and if neoplasia isn't the primary cause of death, it frequently contributes. The main geriatric problems of ferrets include neoplasia, in particular adrenal, islet cell and lymphoma, cardiomyopathy and dental disease (**Fig. 27.3**). Neurological

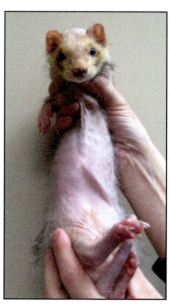

Fig. 27.3 **This 8-year-old ferret with severe adrenal disease (see Chapter 14) was surrendered to a ferret shelter as the owner could not afford medical care.**

problems frequently accompany disc disease or neoplasia. Emaciation can be due to any of the above, with pain factored in. Renal disease is also found in aging ferrets, as well as cataracts and hearing loss. Cataracts and hearing loss may not contribute to decline of quality of life though, as many ferrets have these while they are young. Renal changes include chronic interstitial nephritis and cysts. Unless the cysts are large and cause pain, they are usually incidental findings. The nephritis is not usually associated with any clinical disease.

Table 27.2 Medical conditions of geriatric ferrets

DISEASE	CLINICAL SIGNS	DIAGNOSTICS AND MONITORING	TREATMENTS
Adrenal disease (**Fig. 27.4**)	Aggression, pruritis, preputial swelling or masses, swollen vulva, alopecia, dysuria, tenesmus	Adrenal hormone panel, abdominal ultrasound, palpation, biopsy	Prevention: deslorelin implant. Tx various GnRh agonists; surgery, other antisex steroid drugs
Arrhythmias, heart block, pacemaker problems	Collapse, exercise intolerance, loss of muscle mass, hindquarters weakness	Auscultation, Doppler audio, ECG, echocardiography, blood pressure, radiographs	Terbutaline, enalapril, benazepril, pimobendan
Cataracts	White eyes	Ophthalmoscopic examination, tonometry	Usually none unless secondary glaucoma. Can have cataracts removed, although this is usually not necessary as ferret has adapted to blindness
Deafness	Doesn't respond to sounds	Audio testing, otoscopic examination, radiographs	Usually none unless secondary ear infection that is treatable with otic formulations
Dental disease	Anorexia, bruxism, hypersalivation, halitosis	Visual/endoscopic examination, radiographs	Prophylaxis, scaling, as with other carnivores. Extractions may be necessary. It may be possible to do a root canal in canine teeth if fractured and pulp is exposed (see Chapter 19)
Dilated cardiomyopathy	Collapse, exercise intolerance, loss of muscle mass, hindquarters weakness	Auscultation, Doppler audio, ECG, echocardiography, radiographs, blood pressure	Enalapril, benazepril, pimobendan, furosemide
Disc disease	Paresis hindquarters, pain, often sudden onset, reluctance to jump, climb	Radiographs, palpation, detailed neurological examination	NSAIDS, rest, acupuncture, acupressure, massage
Fibromas, fibrosarcomas	Lump	Palpation, radiographs, ultrasound, lumpectomy with histopathology	Surgery may be curative, may recur
Heart attacks: ischaemic episode	Sudden collapse, may be semi-conscious for hours, weakened	Auscultation, Doppler audio, ECG, echocardiography	IV dobutamine, atropine, lidocaine to stabilise heart; pimobendan, furosemide, low-dose aspirin
Hypertrophic cardiomyopathy	Collapse, exercise intolerance, loss of muscle mass, hindquarters weakness	Auscultation, Doppler audio, ECG, echocardiography, radiographs, blood pressure	Furosemide, diltiazem, enalapril, benazepril
Inflammatory bowel disease, malabsorption syndrome	Intermittent diarrhoea becoming continuous, weight loss, wasting	Radiographs/contrast, ultrasonography, biopsy, response to treatments	Symptomatic including loperamide, budesonide, vitamin B12, antihelicobacter treatment to start
Islet cell neoplasia	Collapse, tear at mouth, nausea, retching, hypersalivation, seizure	Episode history, fasting glucose/insulin level; surgery/biopsy or removal	Feeding programme, corticosteroids, diazoxide, doxorubicin
Lymphoma, lymphosarcoma	Lymphadenopathy generalised or local; part of inflammatory bowel syndrome	Biopsy lymph node, CBC and chemistries, radiographs, exploratory	Chemotherapeutic regimen similar to that in cats; corticosteroids

Key: BUN, blood urea nitrogen; CBC, complete blood count; ECG, electrocardiography; GnRH,; IV, intravenous; NSAID, non-steroidal anti-inflammatory drug; RBC, red blood cell; Tx, treatment.

(Continued)

Table 27.2 (continued) **Medical conditions of geriatric ferrets**

DISEASE	CLINICAL SIGNS	DIAGNOSTICS AND MONITORING	TREATMENTS
Mast cell tumours	Small, sometimes pruritic, sometimes ulcerated skin masses	Biopsy	Topical antihistamine cream, antibiotic cream. If large or bothering – surgical removal
Metabolic: renal glomerulosclerosis, glomerulonephropathy, renal hypertension; L-carnitine weakness, etc.	Less energy, general lethargy, hindquarters weakness or paresis. BUN may be elevated	CBC and chemistries, ultrasonography of kidneys (biopsy); trial with L-carnitine, blood pressure	L-carnitine and taurine supplementation, enalapril, omega 3–6–9
Metastasis	Masses	Biopsy	Remove primary tumour if possible, treat as above
Osteomas, osteosarcomas	Firm to hard masses	Radiographs, biopsy	Debulk or remove via surgery
Splenomegaly, extramedullary haematopoiesis	Large spleen	CBC, chemistries, ultrasonography, biopsy	Unless causing discomfort, no treatment. If causing problems: bone marrow must be able to make RBCs before splenectomy
Stroke	Sudden collapse, eyes partially open, dazed or semi-conscious, deficit one area of body	Physical exam, radiographs, CBC and chemistries	Nursing/supportive care. Low-dose aspirin along with omega 3–6–9 and B12 may be tried

Key: BUN, blood urea nitrogen; CBC, complete blood count; ECG, electrocardiography; GnRH,; IV, intravenous; NSAID, non-steroidal anti-inflammatory drug; RBC, red blood cell; Tx, treatment.

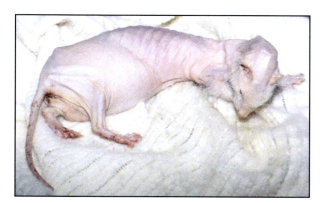

Fig. 27.4 Severe adrenal disease (see Chapter 14).

DIETARY CONSIDERATIONS

In general a diet composed of a commercial ferret food is not changed for the geriatric ferret. There has been no proof that a lower-protein commercial ferret food has any benefit as is seen in other animals with elevated BUN levels. Supplementation with omega 3–6 fatty acids may have benefits based on evidence in other species. The author uses an omega 3–6 combination along with L-carnitine, taurine, CoQ10, vitamin E, and chondroitin sulfate/glucosamine (see Appendix 10).

If the ferret has problems chewing because of tooth loss, a dook soup can be provided (see Appendix 6).

HUSBANDRY CONSIDERATIONS

If the ferret is having problems ambulating, the cage furnishings may need to be adjusted to provide sleeping areas that do not require climbing to get into them. The water bottle may need to be lowered, or a ceramic water dish may need to be added if the ferret is having problems turning its head to use a sipper tube (**Fig. 27.5**). The litter tray rim may need to be lowered for ease of getting into it. Toilet habits may deteriorate so more frequent cleaning of the cage is needed.

DOING WHAT'S BEST FOR THE FERRET

Because of emotional attachments and the effect that severe illness and/or death of the ferret may have on family members, working with the owner to alleviate guilt while providing the best for the animal becomes

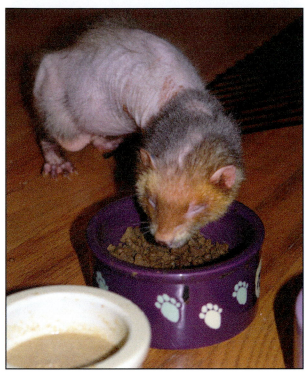

Fig. 27.5 **Food and water must be readily accessible to the geriatric ferret.**

a balancing act. The adult owner may need guidelines on breaking the news to other family members. The vet should first and foremost be realistic about prognosis and what can be offered for quality of life for the ferret. A quality-of-life scale can be used to put the management of the pet in perspective.

The issues both the owner and the vet need to address concerning the inevitable loss of the pet include accurately assessing the quality of life for the animal. Ferrets may hide a lot of symptoms and 'suffer in silence', earning the misplaced idea that they are 'stoic'. They hold off showing overt illness as long as possible. Pain can be assessed through gentle palpation and manipulation, as well as observation of demeanour, posture, alertness, eye character, inclination for eating, drinking, elimination behaviours and response to other ferrets or their owners. A ferret in pain will have a 'haunted, dull look' to their eyes. Treatment may also need to alleviate anxiety in these animals.

The owner grapples with the questions: when is the right time to euthanase? How will I know? In general, the author uses the guidelines of when the pet can no longer maintain itself and/or must be

managed on constant, opiate analgesics. The owners also must be counselled for the remaining time. Even if this is only for a few days, it may greatly aid the owner in overcoming feelings of guilt and inadequacy, and provide the family time to say goodbye. The vet can supply the needed nursing care and medications, as well as the written chart for the owner to follow. A quality-of-life scale used in dog/cat medicine can be adopted to use in ferrets. Numbers can be used to quantify the picture, and this too aids the owner in making decisions. The author uses a scale of 1 to 10, with 10 being the highest. An 'HHHHHMM' scale is used.

The HHHHHMM stands for Hurt, Hunger, Hydration, Hygiene, Happiness, Mobility, More good days than bad. Adequate pain control is ranked first. In addition to obvious types of pain, the ability to breathe properly should be assessed. In humans, dyspnoea ranked at the top of the pain scale. Along with the pain, dyspnoea can lead to anxiety and panic as well. It also takes a lot of energy to work at breathing. Appropriate pain control via oral and/ or injectable medications must alleviate the pain and distress and the owners must be capable of delivering it on a regular basis. Getting ahead of the pain curve (pre-emptive analgesia) is extremely important. Owners who have erratic daily schedules may easily let the pet lapse into pain, and dosages prescribed or types of analgesics may not be capable of reversing this. Owners must be counselled on how pain management works. The owners also must be able to recognise signs of pain. Sometimes the only way to do that is to observe the return to 'normal' activity when the pain is alleviated.

It is helpful to have a written set of symptoms to look for to send home with the owner. This list should include: dull eyes, nausea, lack of appetite and/or actively protesting hand feeding, dehydration manifested by skin tenting, sunken eyes, coolness of feet, dry mouth/anus/vulva/prepuce, reluctance to move, vocalisations upon handling or moving, black tarry stools, decreased amount of urine or faeces, inability to reach the litter tray or get away from elimination, 23.5 hours a day of sleeping with difficulty to arouse, consistently lowered body temperature and cessation of grooming. Owners often describe this terminal state as 'The ferret is no longer acting like itself and seems miserable', yet most owners want the ferret to stay for even just one more day. We tend to keep ferrets alive for our emotional and bonding needs (**Fig. 27.6**).

The general guidelines for evaluating hydration include: can the ferret drink on its own and maintain hydration? If no, then can the owner deliver subcutaneous fluids as needed? Delivering parenteral fluid therapy on an occasional basis may be acceptable, but if it is required daily, how this factors into the quality of life must be questioned. If parenteral fluids are needed, the owner must be trained to assess the hydration, and to deliver the appropriate volume safely. Written instructions should accompany the supplies and the owner should be able to demonstrate they can do this at the office. If intravenous, intraosseous or intraperitoneal fluids are needed to maintain hydration, it is doubtful that quality of life is being maintained.

Hygiene is synonymous with grooming and being able to keep itself out of its own urine and faeces: is the ferret able to keep itself groomed? If oral cancer or lesions exist and the ferret cannot clean itself, it may become depressed, and can suffer from secondary skin and infection problems due to the inability to maintain itself.

Can the ferret move around on its own or need help to satisfy its desires such as getting to a litter tray, food dish or water bottle? Is it having repeated seizures, severe weakness, ataxia? If it can still get to a litter tray, can it keep itself from stepping in or falling in its wastes? If the animal can only lie prone, is someone there to change its position or rotate the body every 2 hours or so? Owners need to realise that despite having fur, atelectasis and decubital ulcers can still form and can be extremely detrimental to the ferret (**Fig. 27.7**).

Ferrets are normally very joyous animals with a tremendous will to live. They appear to be optimistic and as Richard Bach writes in *The Ferret Chronicles*, they 'look at the best side of life and live to their highest sense of right'. When a ferret can no longer enjoy playing, petting, attention and all the things that they used to, we owe it to them to acknowledge that what made their life worth living is now gone. We tend to keep them going for us, because it is too painful to let them go. Losing a ferret is one of the hardest emotional things for us. Ferrets are the brightest of little lights, and we have to realise that it is often our wishes not the ferret's that we are following. We have to respect their right to maintain happiness (**Fig. 27.8**).

Ask the question: does the ferret experience more good days than bad? The author finds this usually is the question that really leads the owner to

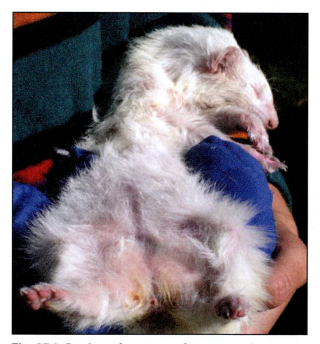

Fig. 27.6 Staying asleep or nearly comatose is common when death is near.

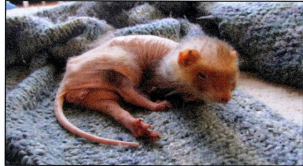

Fig. 27.7 Despite intractable adrenal disease and loss of most of the teeth, this ferret continued to be active, eating and having normal urination/defaecation.

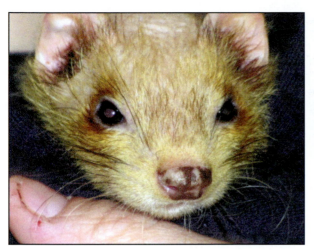

Fig. 27.8 **Geriatric ferret that still partook in normal daily activities.**

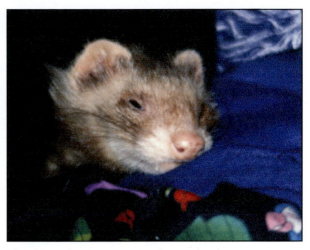

Fig. 27.9 **Sleeping excessively may be due to pain or profound weakness.**

face reality and truly assess the ferret. This can be quantified in how many days in a row the ferret is 'turned off' from its normal life. Bad days include all the signs and symptoms and undesirable experiences such as vomiting, nausea, bruxism, diarrhoea, frustration, bleeding, seizures, pain, profound weakness, ataxia, discomfort or changes in posture/mobility due to masses etc. (**Fig. 27.9**). Is the ferret resisting the medications and general handling? Does the ferret need to be hand fed constantly and puts up a struggle? Does the ferret try to hide when you approach with medications, food etc.? All of these can be used to consider the quality of life.

If the HHHHHMM scale leads owners to conclude the ferret is not ready to go but wishes to continue, and in some cases the owner is just not ready to let go yet, then the vet needs to stress the importance of maintaining close contact and evaluation to prevent suffering. The owner must agree to have the ferret re-evaluated by the vet at frequent intervals. Ask the tough question: are we keeping the ferret alive because its quality of life is adequate or are we keeping the ferret alive because we refuse to let go? The owner must be asked to consider what chronic pain feels like with no hope or understanding of it being alleviated (**Fig. 27.10**). This concept is unpleasant for all of us to address.

The vet needs to gently introduce euthanasia as an alternative to days or weeks of severe pain and complicated medical and supportive therapy when there

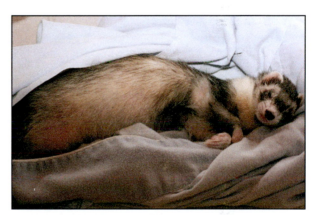

Fig. 27.10 **Reluctance to move, dull eyes usually indicates pain.**

is no hope of recovery and only increasing reliance on major pain medications and supportive care. The vet needs to discuss that it can be a painless, gentle ending to what was a wonderful life. The alternatives to 'just dying' may include seizures, uncontrolled pain, coldness/fever, bleeding, loss of control of life and dignity, all of which can be extremely traumatic – not only to the ferret but to the family members who may observe this. While the ideal of 'dying in their sleep' is hoped for, in reality, most ferrets do not 'go peacefully' (**Fig. 27.11**). Owners need to ease suffering, seek comfort from other pet owners and family members, and trust their vet to aid them in the right decision.

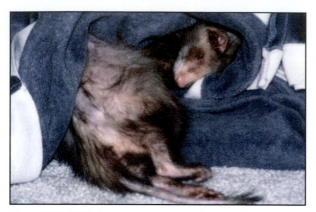

Fig. 27.11 Withdrawing from normal activity to spend all the time sleeping signals end of life.

CONCLUSIONS

With any geriatric ferret and disease process, the course of treatment depends on how severe the condition is at initial presentation: age, temperament, willingness of the owner including time and financial commitment, and evaluation of HHHHHMM. Many geriatric ferrets are presented with no alternatives but to euthanase immediately. Many neoplasias are also inoperable at the time of presentation and are severely interfering with food intake and movement, and are causing pain. If the pet is comatose, seizing or vocalising in pain, euthanasia may be the best option, but all the options including diagnostics, palliative pain treatments, etc. must be outlined for the owner. At least request that an anxiolytic and analgesic be given immediately whilst other discussions and decisions take place.

If euthanasia is the option, choices must be made about burial or cremation. Grief counselling may be available. The owner will be grappling with guilt, grief and emotional family issues. The veterinarian may have printed materials that can be of help.

CHAPTER 28

RESCUE CENTRE MEDICINE

Cathy A. Johnson-Delaney

INTRODUCTION

Working in exotic pet rescue centres is an increasing field of veterinary medicine. The vet fills a unique role in assuring that these species receive appropriate diet, husbandry and medical care. Ferrets are increasingly being relinquished to rescue centres as they age and develop serious medical conditions and owners can no longer care for them. Many young ferrets are surrendered soon after they were purchased on impulse, as the owners did not realise what they were getting into (**Fig. 28.1**). Ferrets may also be surrendered due to the human in the household developing an allergy to the ferret. Additional circumstances for surrender include behavioural problems such as biting (**Fig. 28.2**). Another source of ferrets may be from a laboratory animal facility that has finished its use of the ferrets. These ferrets are usually docile and have a complete medical history with excellent care, and are young and readily adoptable.

Many rescue centres are run by private individuals and depend on donations, adoption fees and volunteer participation in order to care for the animals. The vet can be instrumental in educating and training the volunteers about the proper care of the different species.

Rescue centre medicine is subtly different; vets have to change from primarily working with individual animals and owners to a more 'herd' health mentality as far as realistic management of space, people, budget and time is concerned. Husbandry, dietary and medical needs are different in ferret shelters than in dog/cat shelters (**Fig. 28.3**). Most vets who work with ferrets will be approached to work

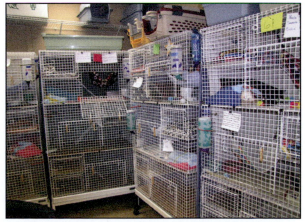

Fig. 28.2 **Eight-week-old kits, one biting the arm of the new owner.**

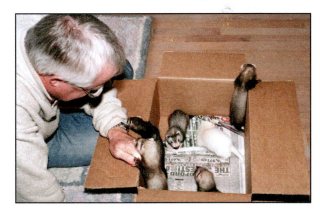

Fig. 28.3 **Caging at the Washington Ferret Rescue & Shelter (WFRS).**

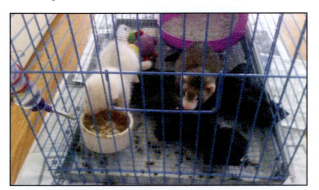

Fig. 28.1 **Eight-week-old kits.**

in one or more of these centres and need guidelines to do so.

AN EMERGING NECESSITY: FERRET RESCUE PROGRAMMES

'The needs of the many outweigh the needs of the few.' While many volunteers and animal lovers may find Mr Spock's quote contrary to their reasons for setting up or volunteering at a rescue centre, the reality is that there are always far more ferrets being abandoned and needing care than there are centres to help them. Most rescue centres would consider themselves 'no-kill' centres, i.e. the animal will be looked after until it is adopted or fostered; however, they must still have in place a policy to humanely euthanase an animal that cannot be readily treated given the funding, staffing and resources of the centre. Rescue centres must establish a policy of how much of their budget can go to treating any particular animal. This is one of the aspects of rescue centre medicine that is the most difficult for volunteer caretakers: the decision of when to euthanase an animal, who makes that decision, and the accepted humane method as well as the policy for disposal of the body. This policy needs to include not only the animals handed in in a grave condition, but those housed at the centre as well as those in foster homes. Centres should have legal documentation of surrender of a ferret to their care. **Fig. 28.4** is a sample surrender

---

I/we _____ have made the decision to surrender the following named ferret(s) and have chosen to enlist the adoption services of the Washington Ferret Rescue & Shelter, hereafter designated as WFRS, which will find new homes as appropriate.

Name of ferret: _____ Colour _____

Male/Female Age _____ Neutered: Y/N CD Vaccination date: _____

Name of ferret: _____ Colour _____

Male/Female Age _____ Neutered: Y/N CD Vaccination Date: _____

Name of ferret: _____ Colour _____

Male/Female Age _____ Neutered: Y/N CD Vaccination Date: _____

Name of ferret: _____ Colour _____

Male/Female Age _____ Neutered: Y/N CD Vaccination Date: _____

It is understood that the ferret(s) are being surrendered for their continued welfare and that the WFRS accepts said ferret(s) in an AS IS condition. It is further understood, therefore, that the WFRS assumes full legal ownership, thereby full responsibility, for any current or future illness while in the custody of the WFRS. It is also understood that items surrendered with the ferret(s) become the legal property of the WFRS, and as such will not be refunded nor returned.

Total confidentiality will be observed unless the surrendering party wishes to communicate with the *adopting* party, in which case, *this request must be put in writing* for the adopting party's acknowledgement.

The WFRS reserves the right of refusal in placing any ferret so surrendered if in their judgement certain prerequisites of ownership are not met. No ferret will be placed in any city, county, or state that restricts or bans ownership of ferrets specifically or by inclusion, nor shall any ferret be knowingly placed in a rental/condominium that excludes pet ownership, nor shall any ferret be knowingly placed in a home or institution for the purpose of ritual, rite or medical experimentation.

The WFRS guarantees to the surrendering party that their pets will receive the utmost care and consideration in the placement with a new owner and that future contact with the same will be done in the interest of continued health and welfare concerns.

The WFRS operates this Shelter as a service to ferrets and as such, is not a business. It is a non-profit 501 C corporation.

Signed _____ Date _____

Name (Printed)_____

Address_____

Phone _____ Email _____

I would like to make a donation of $ _____, to help cover the food and medical costs of the ferret(s) I am surrendering to the WFRS. Donations may be tax-deductible where applicable.

Received by WFRS staff member: _____ Date _____

Fig. 28.4 Sample surrender form.

form in current usage in the USA. Forms used by rescue centres for surrender, fostering and adoption should be reviewed by a lawyer.

Rescue frequently begins in the home of someone who takes in abandoned ferrets. While their initial reason to do so is compassion and care, without planning for increased numbers of pets within their home they are easily and quickly overwhelmed. Most people work outside the home, and additional exotic animals require extra time as well as financial commitment. Individuals soon find they need help maintaining the ferrets, hence they recruit friends or other owners of ferrets to help. Individuals also soon find out they are tied down with so many ferrets, as word usually gets out that they will take them, and more unwanted ferrets are surrendered. Those individuals who enlist the help of others to care for these ferrets usually reach the point where they realise they need to form some sort of organisation to continue, particularly if they realise they cannot keep all the ferrets themselves. They need to develop a method to adopt them to appropriate homes. Individuals who just continue to collect ferrets in the guise of 'a rescue shelter' but do not enlist the help of others and begin forming an organisation and network are hoarders. Hoarders or collectors are usually well meaning but rarely can house, feed and provide the needed medical care for these ferrets. An individual identified as a hoarder frequently comes to the attention of animal control agencies, public health agencies and even mental health agencies. Ferrets confiscated then need to be rehabilitated and placed.

Rescue centres that tend to be longer lived are those that are located in a separate facility from any one volunteer or founder's home. Location of a facility must comply with planning laws. Centres need to set a limit for the number of animals they can afford, have space for and can maintain. Volunteers frequently take home more than they can really care for too, so setting up mandatory training programmes for fosterers as well as a schedule of medical checks of the ferrets should be incorporated into the policies of the rescue centre.

THE VETERINARIAN'S ROLE

Those centres that organise will elect a board, and establish guidelines to govern acceptance of ferrets,

adoption and foster policies, and a budget. Most are staffed completely by volunteers. It is usually after individuals within the organisation have to provide medical care for the animals that a vet with a special interest in ferrets is approached. The individual vet needs to decide if her/his role will be one of volunteer *pro bono*, *per diem* surgeon, as-needed or regular consultant, and/or board member. In any role, it usually is a labour of love: working with a rescue centre will take time and commitment.

The first step is usually to negotiate reduced fees for ferrets owned by the rescue centre, although most soon realise that a knowledgeable vet can assist not only with the medical care of the animals, but help the board with many aspects including liability and insurance needs (largely due to injuries volunteers or visitors may sustain while handling the ferrets), dietary and husbandry requirements, preventive health care including parasite control, vaccinations, dental care, etc. If appointed or elected to the board of a rescue centre, the vet can also serve as a medical director and set up programmes to prevent disease outbreaks as well as training of volunteers to recognise illness.

Most centres have extremely limited funding and usually negotiate provision of at-cost or reduced-rate medications, supplies and diagnostic testing, with minimal fees for actual labour. Actual fees, costs and discounts need to be established in writing, with a clause to review the fees at least on an annual basis. Establish which centres you will work with, and set a limit. It is not unusual for word to get out that you do a service for one centre, and others try to enlist your services as well. In urban areas, a practitioner could spend all their clinical time just working with rescue animals, but economically this is not realistic. Set special appointment or visiting times for rescue ferret examinations, procedures and surgeries so that you are not taking time away from regular clinic duties. The vet's duties and services to be provided to the rescue centre in any capacity should be formalised in writing. This is extremely helpful as volunteer organisations have frequent turnover of people involved.

The vet may also assist in the development of contracts with animal control facilities and humane animal facilities that do not accept ferrets. This may include facilities inspections from the municipal animal control agency before they will transfer a ferret to the private shelter. The veterinarian also is responsible for making sure that ferrets adopted out from the shelter conform to local animal regulations: spay/neuter, vaccinations and microchipping are frequent requirements, with documentation provided to the new owner. The veterinarian is also responsible for issuing rabies vaccination certificates and other health certificates for transport as required locally.

When working with any animal rescue organisation, there will be a large turnover of volunteers and even board members. Many caregivers will experience compassion burnout, particularly if they have fostered many terminally ill and geriatric ferrets. The vet can provide assistance and training to volunteers to deal with animal death. Grief counselling should be made available.

GENERAL GUIDELINES

The vet needs to make sure the animal care is appropriate for the ferrets, including psychological needs. Animals arriving at shelters are stressed, many are in suboptimal nutritional and health status, and some may experience separation anxiety from their former owners. Volunteers accepting surrendered animals can follow an intake checklist that ensures an animal in medical need is seen by the vet. This checklist (**Fig. 28.5**) is an intake form in use by the Washington Ferret Rescue & Shelter (WFRS) in Kirkland, Washington State, USA and can be adapted for other rescue centres and species. In areas with endemic heartworm, heartworm diagnostic testing and preventive medications should be included in an intake evaluation. Some ferret facilities also require Aleutian disease titres and/or canine distemper titres as part of the admission process. The vet is instrumental in establishing the needed evaluations for a specific shelter. The vet also trains volunteers in accomplishing the checklist. Isolation and quarantine procedures and facilities should be in place for ferrets newly surrendered. Each animal admitted to the centre should have a file that includes the surrender papers, history information,

intake record and medical records. In addition to the stored paper records, computerised record keeping should be encouraged. When an animal is adopted, fostered or dies, this information is also kept in that animal's record. Storage requirements for these records should be determined by the board, and may comply with medical records retention requirements in that locality.

The vet assesses the ferret and recommends that it be either adopted, or fostered by a volunteer of the rescue centre. The centre needs to set the parameters and training programmes that qualify a volunteer to be a fosterer. Volunteering to be a fosterer should not be a way to get a free ferret. It is recommended that a contract between the centre and the trained fosterer be signed to ensure the fostered ferret returns for regular medical care and veterinary attention. Some centres that do not have permanent facilities put all animals into 'foster care', defined as housing until a permanent home and owners can be found. Other centres may have facilities to house animals deemed adoptable (good temperament, at most middle-aged, and healthy). Animals deemed needing to be fostered include those with behavioural problems, geriatric conditions or continuing medical needs. With this definition, foster care is essentially hospice care and the centre must maintain frequent contact with the foster caregivers to ensure the wellbeing of those ferrets. Fostered animals still legally belong to the centre and therefore it is necessary for the centre to track them, maintain records and ensure health and wellbeing. Samples of adoption and fostering agreements are presented in **Figs 28.6, 28.7**.

The veterinarian can also make recommendations on housing, disinfectants and cleaning methods used, protocols for sanitation, appropriate disposal of waste, appropriate storage of food and other products needed for the care of the ferrets. The facility and procedures should emphasise stress and noise reduction, no crowding, and no exposure to wildlife/vermin. Enrichment programmes should be developed including exercise pens, safe toys, care of the toys and furnishings, treats and socialisation (**Fig. 28.8**). Dietary and nutritional programmes should be developed; these may include appropriate food storage (**Fig. 28.9**).

Washington Ferret Rescue & Shelter
adopted by:
SHELTER INTAKE RECORD

date: _____

Ferret name: _____ Sex (M/F): _____ Date of arrival _____

Age: _____ Ear tattooed? Yes   No (description of tattoo) _____

Accompanying medical records or other history, papers?   (attach to this record) Yes   No

Color: lt. sable   dk. sable   silver   champagne   chocolate   albino   DEW   black(solid)

Markings: mitts   bib   hood   panda   blaze   roan   Nose: pink   speckled   black

Microchip: Yes: Number _____ ☐ Not Present

Intact (Y/N): _____ Scent Glands (Y/N): _____ Other: _____

Surrendered by:

☐ Owner   ☐ Animal Control   ☐ Humane Society   ☐ Other _____

Shelter volunteer completing intake process: _____

Condition on Arrival: ☐Excellent   ☐Good   ☐Fair   ☐Poor

Weight in grams on arrival: _____

Type of food ferret is eating if known: _____

Physical inspection:

    ☐No apparent physical problems

    ☐Hair loss _____ Fleas/dirt seen? _____

    ☐Swollen vulva _____

    ☐Scars/marks/lumps _____

    ☐Other _____

Temperament:

    ☐Biter /aggressive

    ☐Single ferret only (is not socialised)

    ☐Lap ferret

    ☐Good temperament

Intake care (check upon completion). Attach vaccination vial stickers to intake sheet

    ☐ Nails clipped   ☐ Ears cleaned, cytology: mites Y/N

    ☐ Ivermectin injection s.q. 0.2 mL   ☐ Tresaderm in ears

    ☐ Nobivac distemper (date) _____ (0.5 mL Children's oral benadryl 20 min prior)

    ☐ Imrab-3 rabies (date) _____ (0.5 mL Children's oral benadryl 20 min prior)

    ☐ Advantage or Frontline Flea Control: 2 drops between shoulder blades on skin

    ☐ Faecal flotation (date) _____ Result: _____

    ☐ Teeth (note condition) _____

Request for vet exam (Y/N) _____ Date vet exam scheduled: _____

Adoptable: (Y/N) _____ Foster (Y/N) _____

Write additional comments on back of this form.

Rev 2008

Fig. 28.5 Sample shelter intake record.

SPECIAL CONSIDERATIONS FOR HEALTH MANAGEMENT

Depending on endemic disease problems in a geographical area, and whether animals are predominantly coming from indoor or outdoor homes, backyard breeders or pet shops, the following lists of potential disease problems within a rescue centre will vary. The following are guidelines.

Anorexia with/without GI ulceration and subsequent diarrhoea or haemorrhage, just due to the stress of being surrendered, or changes in the food or habitat, is often termed 'shelter shock'. The ferret suffers severe weight loss during the first week

---

WASHINGTON FERRET RESCUE & SHELTER
CONTRACT FOR ADOPTION

I. The ferret(s) will be handled in a loving, gentle manner by all members of my household and by any guests that visit my home. The ferret(s) will be fed quality dry ferret food, have access to fresh water, will be kept indoors and will be housed in a cage or ferret-proof room when no one is at home to supervise the activities of the ferret(s).

II. If adopters are unable to spend quality time with the ferret(s), unable to keep them as pets, neglect, abuse, or mistreat the ferret(s), or must give them up for any other reason, the ferret(s) will be returned to, or reclaimed by, the Washington Ferret Rescue & Shelter (WFRS). A full refund of the adoption fee is guaranteed up to 7 days from the adoption date.

III. If the ferret's health is ever in question, the adopter will seek veterinary care. It would be appreciated if you would contact the WFRS if any health problems arise or when the ferret passes on so we may better our understanding of breeding, health, and lifespans of ferrets. Ferrets will be vaccinated yearly against Canine Distemper and it is recommended to have the ferret(s) vaccinated against Rabies with Imrab-3 once a year as required by regulations in the location of the adopter's residence. The next Canine Distemper shot due: _____ The next Rabies shot is due: _____

IV. Adopter understands that the WFRS cannot and does not make any presentations or guarantees, either expressed or implied as to the temperament, habits, or background of the named ferret(s). Therefore, in consideration of receiving the ferret(s), I hereby release the WFRS from any and all claims of liability for the actions of the ferret(s) being adopted.

This agreement applies to the following ferret(s):

_____ _____ _____
_____

Signature: _____ Date: _____
Volunteer Signature: _____ Date: _____
Questions? Call or email: _____

A copy of this contract will be kept on file at the WFRS.

Fig. 28.6 Sample contract for adoption.

WASHINGTON FERRET RESCUE & SHELTER
CONTRACT FOR FOSTERING

I. The ferret(s) will be handled in a loving, gentle manner by all members of my household and by any guests that visit my home. The ferret(s) will be fed quality dry ferret food, have access to fresh water, will be kept indoors and will be housed in a cage or ferret-proof room when no one is at home to supervise the activities of the ferret(s).

II. If adopters are unable to spend quality time with the ferret(s), unable to keep them as pets, neglect, abuse, or mistreat the ferret(s), or must give them up for any other reason, the ferret(s) will be returned to or reclaimed by the Washington Ferret Rescue & Shelter (WFRS).

III. If the ferret's health is ever in question, the fosterer will contact WFRS. The WFRS will direct the Fosterer to a WFRS-approved veterinarian or emergency facility. The WFRS may or may not authorise funds if the fostered ferret is taken for medical care without WFRS being notified for approval of costs. The Fosterer understands that the WFRS cannot and does not make any presentation or guarantees, either expressed or implied, as to the temperament, habits, or background of the named ferret(s). The Fosterer must bring the fostered ferret(s) in to the WFRS at least on an annual basis for medical examinations and vaccinations. The WFRS expects the Fosterer to attend training sessions as they are offered at the WFRS. The Fosterer understands that the ferret(s) legally belong to the WFRS that is responsible for their health and wellbeing.

Therefore, in consideration of fostering the ferret(s), I hereby release the WFRS from any and all claims of liability for the actions of the ferret(s) being fostered.

This agreement applies to the following ferret(s):

_____ _____ _____
_____

Signature: _____ Date: ____
A duplicate copy of this contract will be kept on file at the WFRS

Fig. 28.7 Sample contract for fostering.

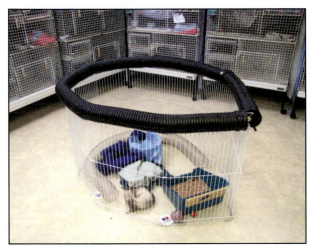

Fig. 28.8 Playpens for daily exercising at WFRS. The plastic tubing is to prevent ferrets from climbing out of the pen.

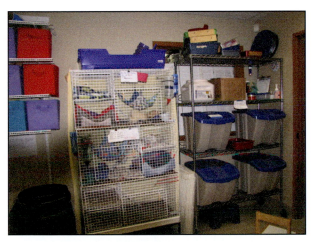

Fig. 28.9 Storage at WFRS.

of arrival, despite all other health parameters being normal. These ferrets can be placed on famotidine at 2.5 mg per ferret PO q24h and weighed daily. Hand feeding soup (Carnivore Care, Oxbow Pet Products, Murdoch, NE) (see Appendix 6) helps to nurse them through the first few days. In some cases the ferret will be taken home by one of the volunteers to nurse through this period and help it become adjusted to its new life. Stressed ferrets may also develop oral ulcers that are usually painful and contribute to anorexia. These can be treated symptomatically using sucralfate (25–125 mg/kg PO q6–8h before meals) and meloxicam (0.2 mg/kg PO q24h) along

with continuing the famotidine. Newly arrived ferrets are kept separate from the main colony until the medical issues listed below have been addressed and the ferrets seem to be adjusted to rescue centre life. The quarantine time also includes a second canine distemper virus (CDV) vaccine and a second faecal check for coccidia. Attempts at this time are made to find the ferret suitable cage mate(s) or identify potential play groups for socialisation once the ferret comes out of quarantine.

Communicable disease and parasitic problems that are of particular importance in a ferret shelter: fleas, ear mites, heartworm, coccidia, cryptosporidia, influenza, CDV, Aleutian disease and possibly enteric bacteria such as *Salmonella* sp. Occasionally fungal skin infections may be found. Ferret enteric coronavirus (see Chapter 13) may also be exhibited and these ferrets should be isolated and treated symptomatically until signs abate. Fleas and ear mites can be treated on entry, although ear mites may remain endemic in the colony despite repeated treatments. It is considered of lowered importance. Coccidia if found can be treated and these ferrets should be isolated until they are no longer shedding. Cryptosporidiosis is usually self limiting within 2–4 weeks, but ferrets should be isolated and may need supportive care including parenteral fluids. Influenza may appear similar to CDV on initial presentation. Volunteers should receive immunisation and any with influenza should stay out of the centre. During flu season it is prudent to require all visitors to wear masks and use hand sanitiser when entering the centre. Visitors are not allowed to handle the ferrets. Rabies in some localities may be considered if the ferret has been housed outdoors and has no vaccination history. This is highly unlikely, but in endemic areas it potentially is possible. Faecal parasite checks should be done upon entry into the centre, a second time during quarantine, then 2–3 times per year. In heartworm-endemic areas, a heartworm detection test should be done, then the ferret will be put on the prophylactic medication chosen to treat all those in the shelter on a regular basis. Some centres also test for Aleutian disease (see Chapter 16) and may keep any ferrets testing positive separate from their main colony even though they may not show any signs of disease.

CDV can devastate a centre (see Chapter 20). A recent outbreak occurred in a large ferret rescue centre with two sites. Initial signs were not the later stage symptoms normally associated with CDV, thus it was unrecognised in the early stages, when treatment is most effective. Signs that became associated with the disease included a red abdomen, flushed face, particularly noticeable around the base of the whiskers and around the eyes, lethargy, fever, and slight prolapse of the rectum with a dark ring around the anus, prepuce and vulva, hyperkeratosis of the foot pads, watery eyes and serous nasal discharge. There was conjunctivitis in some with eyes being stuck shut. In some there was segmenting in the hair from the throat caudally and skin sloughing. Signs and symptoms were progressive. Most of the ferrets that came down with the disease, and many that died, had received one distemper vaccination previously administered by the centre. Quarantine procedures were followed and the centre vaccinated all the ferrets again regardless of vaccination history in the face of the outbreak. What became clear was that one vaccination of an adult was not sufficient for protection. Treatment of many symptomatic ferrets was with vitamin A (50,000 IU injection SC q24h × 2 d), interferon (60–120 units SC q24h), metacam (0.2 mg/kg PO q24h), famotidine (2.5 mg/ferret SC q24h), diphenhydramine (0.5–2 mg/kg IM, IV, PO q8–12 prn), and buprenorphine (0.01–0.05 mg/kg IV, IM, SC q8–12h) if in pain. General supportive care including fluids, amoxicillin/clavulanate (12.5 mg/kg PO q12h), and hand feeding was given as needed. The outbreak lasted over 40 days, with variable incubation times. Many ferrets that were symptomatic did recover. The centre tested several symptomatic for CDV that were positive. Those that recover become negative on serology. So far there have been no signs of recurrence or neurological disease as is seen in dogs. The outbreak was very hard on the volunteers as they all have a great deal of attachment to the ferrets. Adult ferrets now receive a two-vaccination series when they are admitted to the centre, while in entry quarantine that lasts 30 days.

Aleutian disease screening is done in many ferret rescue centres using a serological test (counter-immunoelectrophoresis, CEP) (see Chapter 16).

A positive test is evidence of exposure but does not necessarily mean active disease. Many centres maintain negative premises and ferrets testing positive are euthanased. Seroprevalence has been noted at 8.5–10% in asymptomatic ferrets, although in the author's experience incidence is much lower or negative in many populations. Some shelters do not test for the disease unless there is a clinical case that may indicate transmission and incidence.

Non-communicable disease health concerns include: anorexia, GI ulceration, diarrhoea, weight loss, stress, diet and husbandry changes, geriatric conditions including heart disease, neoplasia, dental disease, trauma, and anal/rectal complications following anal sacculectomy. If unneutered, surgical neutering must be done prior to adoption or fostering. An alternative to surgical neutering is implantation of a deslorelin implant, although the adopting owner must be aware that the implant has to be replaced on a regular basis. Anal sacculectomy can be considered an elective surgery, but one that may increase the adoptability of the ferret.

Many ferrets are surrendered due to medical problems including neoplasia. This is particularly true with adrenal disease in older ferrets where the owner cannot provide medical care, usually due to financial constraints. Older ferrets surrendered may have multiple disease problems including dental and heart disease, as well as lymphoma, islet cell disease or complications from any of these. Most rescue centres have to establish a large portion, often the largest, of their budget for veterinary care and medications.

A recent problem at the WFRS has been ferrets surrendered that have been on a grain-free diet and have cysteine bladder stones requiring cystotomy. A policy at WFRS is now to radiograph every ferret with that dietary history upon surrender. Unfortunately most of them, even if asymptomatic, have urolithiasis (see Chapter 22).

Adrenal disease is addressed firstly by starting the ferret on leuprolide acetate depot 30-day injections (100 µg per female, 200 µg per male or severely affected females IM. These are repeated every 30 days). These ferrets require veterinary attention to determine if there are additional complications of the disease including preputial tumours, prostatic enlargement with subsequent urinary tract obstruction and skin lesions accompanying alopecic areas, and if the abdominal masses require surgery for the comfort of the ferret. While centres would like to have the budget to implant the ferrets with deslorelin, due to cost that may not be feasible.

Dental disease is common in surrendered older ferrets and needs to be addressed immediately. Most ferrets require some degree of dental scaling which should be done under brief anaesthesia. General dental care of rescue ferrets includes frequent tooth brushing using an enzymatic toothpaste and cotton buds. Volunteers can be trained to do this as part of the husbandry regimen. Again, older ferrets may also have more severe periodontal disease, necrotic teeth and other dental problems that should be addressed as soon as possible after the surrender.

Ferrets with chronic diseases that require continual treatment will usually be placed in the foster programme rather than put up for adoption. This allows the shelter to keep track of the health conditions and make sure care is being provided on a timely basis.

FERRET EVENTS

Many shelters conduct events that have ferrets coming together from different households. WFRS holds a 'Dooktoberfest: Ferret Frolics' as a way for owners and ferrets to get together for fun and games (**Figs 28.10, 28.11**). A veterinary clinic may be a sponsor and as such may help with insurance or fees required by facilities where the event is to be held. The veterinarian and clinic may help with publicity for the event, including contacting the media. The event may also help with fundraising by holding an auction, raffle, and/or sale of ferret items such as bedding and toys.

Ferrets that register should have some sort of a health check at registration. WFRS requires proof of current distemper and rabies vaccination, as well as cursory check by a trained shelter volunteer. This is to screen out obvious signs of disease. The ferret is also checked for fleas and if found to have them, treated with topical insecticide on the spot.

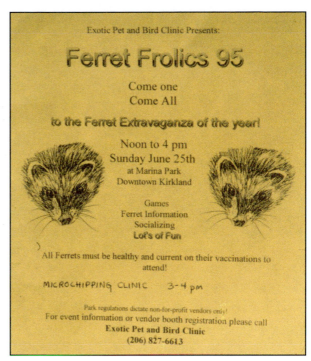

Fig. 28.10 Flyer promoting a Ferret Frolics.

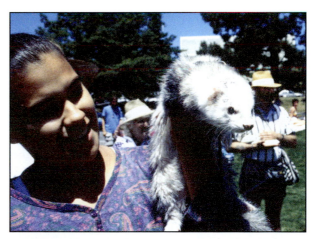

Fig. 28.11 Ferret and friend participating in the Frolics.

If a microchipping clinic is part of the Frolics, then a veterinarian and usually a veterinary technician will be on site to administer the chips. A clinic may also set up an informational table about ferret health care (**Fig. 28.12**). At this table there may be 'health kits' containing a small vial of ear cleaner, a small vial of enzymatic toothpaste and cotton buds with an

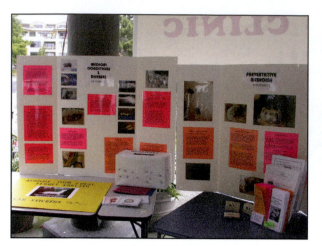

Fig. 28.12 **Health information tables.**

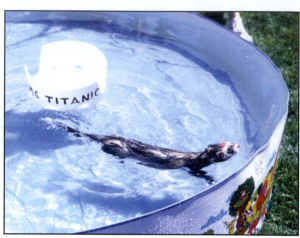

Fig. 28.13 **Sea otter game.**

instruction sheet. These are given out free of charge to attendees.

The games should be designed to be safe for owners and the ferrets. Below are listed games often run at the Frolics.

- Sea Otter – a children's wading pool, half filled with water. A 'boat' is made from a cut-down plastic water container. The ferret is put in the boat and set in the middle of the wading pool. The ferret who is fastest to swim to the edge of the pool receives an award for the worst sea otter. The slowest time, with the ferret swimming around the pool, is considered the best sea otter. Towels should be on hand for drying the ferret upon exit. This event should only be held if the ambient temperature is such that a ferret can dry off and not get cold (**Fig. 28.13**).
- Races – various types including a straight line race, a tube race or some type of obstacle course. This is a timed event. Owners can encourage their ferrets with treats or noises (**Figs 28.14, 28.15**).
- Yawning – ferrets are held by their owner and timed how many yawns in 1 minute they can do.
- Cup tipping – ferrets are presented with a number of paper cups half filled with water. They are timed as to how many they turn over in 1 minute. Towels are mandatory for drying the table between tries.

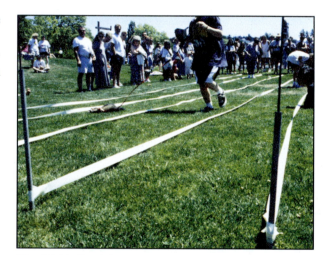

Fig. 28.14 **Straight race.**

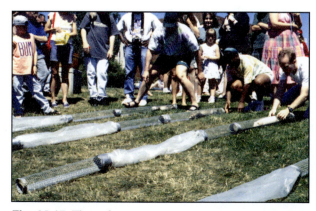

Fig. 28.15 **Tunnel race.**

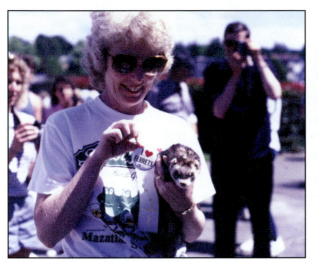

Fig. 28.16 **Awarding ribbons for winners.**

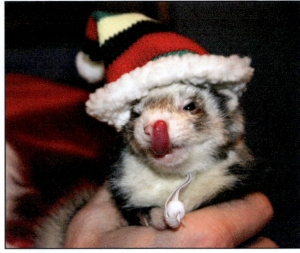

Fig. 28.17 **Costume.**

- Balloon popping – a cage is filled with inflated balloons and the ferret is placed inside. It is timed for how many the ferret pops in 1 or 2 minutes.
- Standing upright – ferrets are coaxed to stand upright and timed for how long they stand.
- Falling asleep – owners coax their ferrets to sleep deep enough that the judge can lift a hind foot without the ferret rousing. The first one to do so wins (**Fig. 28.16**).
- Costume contest (**Fig. 28.17**).

As with all events involving ferrets, sanitation must be addressed (**Fig. 28.18**). Tissue, paper towels and bottles of disinfectant should be on hand. Volunteers running the Frolics should be trained in the proper way to disinfect the spot where the ferret eliminated and to stay vigilant for mess.

FERRET VISITS

The veterinarian may also be required to provide a certificate of health for ferrets that visit schools or retirement homes (**Fig. 28.19**). The rescue centre may participate in educational booths at pet shops and fêtes with demonstration ferrets – it is a good idea to have a health certificate on site in case there is a question of safety and protection from zoonotic

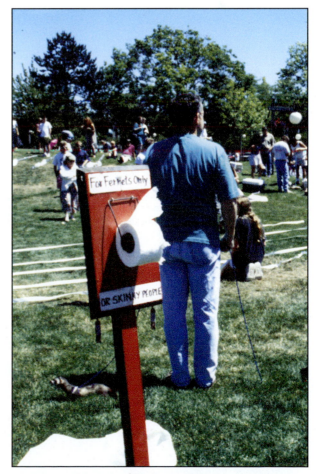

Fig. 28.18 **Tissue is provided for owners to clean up stools, urine. (Courtesy of Vondelle McLaughlin.)**

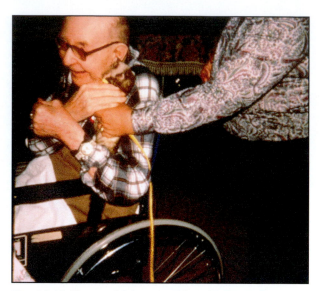

Fig. 28.19 **Ferret visiting a resident in a retirement home.**

disease. Ferrets participating in these events are ones the centre has designated as extremely docile and it also limits the public from touching or handling them. As of yet, WFRS has never had one of their ferrets on display bite anyone.

ACKNOWLEDGEMENTS

The Washington Ferret Rescue & Shelter, Kirkland, WA, USA. www.washingtonferret.org

CHAPTER 29

TOXICOLOGY

Cathy A. Johnson-Delaney

INTRODUCTION

Ferrets are susceptible to toxicosis in a similar way to dogs and cats. Because they are so curious, they are often exposed to many household toxins. A list of toxic plants is provided in Appendix 7.

More information can be obtained through the American Society for the Prevention of Cruelty to Animals (ASPCA) Animal Poison Control Center (APCC). www.aspca.org/pet-care/animal-poison-control; (888) 426-4435. A $65.00 consultation fee may be applied to your credit card. Another resource is the Pet Poison Helpline serving the USA, Canada and the Caribbean. www.petpoisonhelpline.com; (855) 764-7661. A $49.00 per incident fee applies.

In the UK, the Royal Society for the Prevention of Cruelty to Animals (RSPCA) is a resource: www.rspca.org.uk/adviceandwelfare/pets/general/poisoning and has specific information about ferrets. The Veterinary Poisons Information Service (VPIS) is available to member veterinarians, http://vpisglobal.com +44(0) 207 188 0200. There may be additional services in your area or country for small animals that will provide the basic guidelines for treating a poisoned ferret.

Always treat the patient first if symptomatic while obtaining the history and type of toxin. This includes evaluation and control arrhythmias, respiratory distress, seizures etc. Determine if a toxin is involved in the symptomatology. In cases where exposure is uncertain, a thorough work-up to determine other causes of the signs is in order. A detailed history should be taken to include questions about the environment, whether the ferret was unsupervised, what toxicants are in the environment and behavioural changes seen accompanying the onset of clinical signs.

Decontamination protocols for dogs and cats are suitable for ferrets. This includes inducing emesis if the agent is considered non-caustic. Emesis can be induced using 3% hydrogen peroxide at a dosage of 0.5 mL/kg. The ferret should be encouraged to move around after administration to help with agitation of the peroxide. Vomiting normally occurs within 10–15 minutes. If the initial dose is not successful, one additional dose may be tried. Following emesis, the mouth can be rinsed to remove any remaining hydrogen peroxide. Emesis can also be induced using apomorphine at 0.04 mg/kg IM, IV or SC. It can also be used at a dose of 0.25 mg/kg dissolved in sterile water or saline and placed in the conjunctival sac. Following emesis, the eye should be flushed to remove any remaining dug. If the patient is showing signs of excessive sedation or agitation following the apomorphine and emesis, naloxone can be used to reverse it.

Gastric lavage may be attempted, but the ferret must be anaesthetised. The water and lavage fluids (saline) should be warmed to body temperature before using. Lavage should continue until the fluid is clear. If there is a large amount of unabsorbed material in the intestines, a high enema may be done after the gastric lavage under low water pressure. The enema should be continued until the fluid runs clear.

For ingestion of caustics (emesis is contraindicated), dilution is the initial treatment of choice. Milk, yogurt or water can be given orally diluting the caustic and reducing the damage it may do. Use small volumes (1–2 mL) to avoid causing spontaneous emesis.

Following emesis or administration of a diluent (in caustic cases), activated charcoal should be administered if indicated. Caustics, petroleum distillates, metals, ethanol and ethylene glycol are poorly absorbed by activated charcoal so its use is not indicated for those. Dosage is 1–3 g/kg. For agents that undergo enterohepatic recirculation or are extended-release formulations, repeated doses of activated charcoal (use half the original dose) every 6–8 hours is indicated. Because many activated charcoal preparations contain osmotically active ingredients, there may be a shift of free water into the gut, resulting in a secondary hypernatraemia within 4 hours of administration, which may manifest as ataxia, tremors or seizures. Adjunctive fluid therapy is indicated for use with activated charcoal. Fluid therapy is often initiated anyway to treat toxicosis, so the choice of fluids should not be normal saline. Hypernatraemia may be treated with low-sodium IV fluids such as 5% dextrose in water (D5W) or half-strength saline and dextrose. Plain warm-water enemas at 5–10 mL/kg can be given to take advantage of the colon's ability to absorb water rapidly.

A cathartic may also be administered. Some activated charcoal preparations contain one. This will decrease transit time through the gut. Commonly used are sorbitol, magnesium sulphate and bulk laxatives. A cathartic should only be administered once daily even if there have been multiple doses of charcoal. With using a cathartic there is a risk of dehydration and hypernatraemia.

With topical toxicant exposure, the ferret should be thoroughly rinsed and a mild shampoo used. Many agents such as topical, spot-on flea products are oily and are not usually removed with plain water. To remove oils, bathe with a non-toxic liquid dishwashing detergent suitable for use on animals. The patient must be kept warm following the bath. If the ferret is showing neurological signs, the bath should be postponed until the ferret is controlled as the stress of bathing may exacerbate signs.

With ocular exposure, the eye should be flushed for 20–30 minutes total using saline. If saline is not available, distilled or tepid tap water can be used although this may exacerbate blepharospasm and the eyelids must be held open for the duration. After flushing, fluorescein dye should be used to check for corneal ulceration.

PARACETAMOL (ACETOMINOPHEN)

Mechanism
A pain reliever for humans for control of fever, headaches, joint or muscle pain. It causes hepatic necrosis, methaemoglobinaemia and, rarely, acute renal failure. Ferret red blood cells appear to be sensitive to oxidative stress and may be prone to the formation of methaemoglobinaemia with exposure.

Clinical presentation
Initially there may be lethargy and anorexia and the history of ingestion of the owner's pills or a children's liquid.

Treatment
Standard decontamination with emesis and/or activated charcoal performed as early as possible. A baseline blood panel should be run looking at the liver parameters (alanine aminotransferase, serum alkaline phosphatase, total bilirubin, and albumin) and repeated daily for 3–6 days. N-acetylcysteine (Mucomyst) is the treatment of choice for protecting the liver and preventing methaemoglobinaemia. It provides an alternative pathway for detoxification of the paracetamol or by conjugating the toxic metabolite N-acetyl-p-benzoquinoneimine (NAPQI). Dilute the n-acetylecysteine to a 5% solution (50 mg/mL). Use a loading dose of 70 mg/kg PO every 6 hours for 48–72 hours. Additional adjunctive medications include cimetidine (5–10 mg/kg PO, SC q6–9h). This may block the hepatic cytochrome that produces the NAPQI. Ascorbic acid at 30 mg/kg PO q6–12h may reduce any oxidised haemoglobin.

ANTICOAGULANT RODENTICIDES

Mechanism
This category contains warfarin and so-called second-generation agents such as brodifacoum, bromadiolone, chlorophacinone, diaphacinon and difethialone. These agents interfere with liver production of clotting factors II, VI, IX and X. Haemorrhage may begin usually 3–7 days after ingestion when these factors are depleted. Dosage at which decontamination and treatment should be

performed is 0.02 mg/kg. For the average ferret, this is about 0.5–1.0 g of a 0.005% bait.

Clinical presentation

Initial signs may be vague and include lethargy and anorexia. Haemorrhage may not be seen until late in the toxicosis. Bleeding may occur into the chest, abdomen, under the skin and/or in the CNS.

Treatment

For ingestions of less than 4 hours, perform emesis. Administer activated charcoal. Start vitamin K1 at 5 mg/kg divided PO q8–12h. The injectable formulation may be used orally, or an appropriate solution can be compounded. Vitamin K1 must be given with a fatty food such as peanut butter or canned cat food as bile acids are needed for proper absorption. Duration of treatment depends upon the volume of toxin ingested. It may continue for at least 2 weeks, particularly after warfarin ingestion. Second-generation anticoagulant rodenticides should be treated for at least 28 days. A coagulation panel should be taken 48 hours after stopping vitamin K1 to determine if treatment has been successful (see Appendix 2). If PT is still elevated, an additional week of vitamin K1 should be given and again the coagulation panel should be checked at the conclusion.

If the ferret is presented with haemorrhage, treatment is aimed at first stopping the haemorrhage, and correcting anaemia if present by starting with vitamin K1. There is a 24–48 hour lag period before the liver can start to produce adequate levels of clotting factors so plasma should be delivered. If plasma is not available, whole blood can be drawn from a donor ferret and the plasma separated by allowing the red blood cells to settle or by centrifuging anticoagulated blood in sterile tubes. Whole blood can be used but monitor the ferret closely for volume overload. A vitamin K1 regimen as listed above should be started.

BROMETHALIN

Mechanism

This is a rodenticide affecting the CNS. It is generally sold as a 0.01% bait. It and its metabolite demethylbromethalin uncouple oxidative phosphorylation in the CNS. This leads to loss of the Na^+-K^+ ATPase pump and retention of fluid in the brain and spinal cord, particularly within the myelin sheaths. This elevates CSF pressure. The toxic dose is not available for ferrets, but the median lethal dose varies by species. This falls between 0.25 mg/kg for pigs and up to 5.6 mg/kg for dogs. Bromethalin undergoes enterohepatic recirculation.

Clinical presentation

Signs usually develop from 24 hours to several days after ingestion. Initial signs are hindlimb weakness progressing to paresis and paralysis of the hindquarters. This ascends and eventually causes paralysis of the muscles of respiration, and death. Seizures may occur terminally.

Treatment

There is no effective treatment once the signs have begun. Treatment is aimed at aggressive decontamination. Emesis can be performed within the first 5 hours after exposure. Gastric lavage may also be an option. Activated charcoal should be administered and multiple doses (3–6 q8h) given due to the enterohepatic recirculation. Once signs have begun, treatment can only be supportive and symptomatic and may include steroids, mannitol and furosemide. The animal may deteriorate rapidly after the treatment is stopped. Mildly affected ferrets may recover but it may take days or weeks. If the ferret presents paralysed or with seizures it is a grave prognosis.

CHOCOLATE

Mechanism

Because it is sweet and fatty, chocolate is a very tempting treat for ferrets. Many owners may give them a piece because they so readily want it. Chocolate contains methylxanthines (principally theobromine and caffeine) that are cardiac and CNS stimulants.

Table 29.1 (from Dunayer, 2008) lists the relative amounts of methylxanthines found in common forms of chocolate. Total methylxanthine dosages around 10–15 mg/kg can result in gastrointestinal upset (principally vomiting and diarrhoea). At dosages above 40–50 mg/kg tachycardia may be seen.

Table 29.1 Representative theobromine and caffeine content of various chocolates

COMPOUND	THEOBROMINE, mg/30 g	CAFFEINE, mg/30 g
White chocolate	0.25	0.85
Milk chocolate	44–56	6
Semi-sweet chocolate chips	138	22
Unsweetened cooking chocolate	393	8–18
Dry cocoa powder	13–737	5–42

Dosages greater than 60 mg/kg can result in CNS stimulation with tremors and seizures. Doses over 100 mg/kg can cause acute death.

Clinical presentation

Signs depend on dosage, but most will present first with GI signs and agitation. Vomiting, diarrhoea, tachycardia, tremors, seizures and death have been reported.

Treatment

Treatment is supportive and symptomatic. Because chocolate tends to stay in the stomach for some time after ingestion, emesis may be useful up to 8 hours following ingestion. Activated charcoal should be administered and multiple doses used every 6–8 hours as long as the ferret is symptomatic. Fluid diuresis helps with the excretion of methylxanthines and should be delivered intravenously at twice the maintenance level. Caffeine can be reabsorbed through the bladder wall, so encourage the ferret to void frequently. In symptomatic ferrets, tachycardia can be controlled by beta-blockers such as propranolol. CNS stimulation and seizures respond to diazepam. Repeated vomition can be handled by an appropriate antiemetic if the vomitus is clear (initial vomiting may contain some of the chocolate).

CLEANING PRODUCTS (INCLUDING BLEACHES, SOAPS, SHAMPOOS)

Mechanism

Most cleaning products consist of anionic/nonionic surfactants. These are irritants but significant systemic toxicosis is not expected. Small ingestions may lead to nausea and vomiting, while larger ingestions may also cause diarrhoea due to a laxative effect.

Bleach and other alkaline corrosive products may cause tissue damage ranging from irritation to corrosion. The degree of injury depends on the concentration of the corrosive. Dilute solutions may be irritating, but concentrated solutions may be extremely alkaline. Those with a pH greater than 11 are corrosive. Because pain is not immediate, the ferret may continue to consume large amounts of the agent. Injury can extend beyond the oral cavity and include damage to the oesophagus and stomach. The full extent of the injury may not be evident for 24 hours.

Clinical presentation

Vomiting and diarrhoea may be seen initially. If ulceration develops there may be pain and anorexia. Secondary dehydration and electrolyte imbalances may follow.

Treatment

Immediate treatment is to dilute the agent with milk or water to reduce irritation. Vomiting of a non-caustic agent may be good in the beginning, but if it continues and the ferret is showing distress, symptomatic management may include withholding food and water for a few hours. Fluid therapy is recommended. Immediate care for alkaline corrosive ingestion is dilution with milk or water. Emesis is contraindicated. Activated charcoal does not bind these agents and may impede healing of any ulcers. Do not attempt to neutralise an alkaline substance with an acid as this may lead to the release of heat that can further damage soft tissue.

The ferret needs to be monitored for at least 24 hours. Soft food should be fed to reduce the irritation to damaged tissue. If ulcers or burns develop, liquid sucralfate should be given (75 mg/kg PO q4–6h). Nutritional support may be needed if the ferret is anorexic. A feeding tube may even be necessary. Oesophageal strictures or perforations may not show up for 2–3 weeks. Antibiotics may be part of the supportive care. Dermal and ocular exposures are treated as outlined above (bathing, flushing).

IBUPROFEN

Mechanism

It is an NSAID and is available over the counter in tablets (50, 100 and 200 mg) and a liquid formulation for children (20–40 mg/mL). Prescription-strength tablets are available in 400, 800 and 1200 mg. Ibuprofen has been used in ferrets at 1 mg/kg q12–24h. Getting into any human formulation can induce toxicosis. Ibuprofen acts by inhibiting production of prostaglandins associated with pain. In an overdose, it inhibits prostaglandins that protect gastric mucosa. This predisposes the ferret to gastric ulcers. They can also develop acute renal failure. The minimum lethal dose is 220 mg/kg.

Clinical presentation

Signs can begin as soon as 4 hours after ingestion, but it may take up to 48 hours. Most commonly seen signs are depression, ataxia, tremors or coma. Ferrets may also show GI signs including anorexia, vomiting, retching, diarrhoea and melena. Signs of renal disease include polyuria and polydipsia. Renal failure may also be seen. Serum biochemistry should be obtained for baseline BUN, creatinine and phosphorus. These should be repeated during the course of treatment to monitor kidney function.

Treatment

If the ferret is presented before signs occur, emesis and/or activated charcoal should be used. Because ibuprofen undergoes enterohepatic recirculation, repeated doses of activated charcoal should be used. If the ferret is presented comatose, oral treatments should not be attempted until the ferret is stabilised. Treatment should include IV fluids, oxygen and thermoregulation. If an endotracheal tube can be placed, then gastric lavage is possible. After lavage, activated charcoal can be placed directly in the stomach. A GI protectant should be started such as famotidine (0.25–0.5 mg/kg IV, PO, SC), cimetidine (5–10 mg/kg IM, IV, PO, SC), sucralfate (125 mg q6h PO), misoprostol (1–5 µg/kg PO q8h) and/or metoclopramide (0.2–1 mg/kg IM, PO, SC q6–8h). An acid reducer such as famotidine in combination with sucralfate should be administered

for at least 5–7 days postexposure, longer if clinical signs are still present. Misoprostal, a synthetic prostaglandin, can also be used for the first 48 hours. It has to be compounded for the ferret dose. Vomiting can be controlled with metoclopramide. Fluid diuresis at twice the maintenance rate (maintenance estimated at 25–50 mL/kg/24 h although the author has used 100 mL/kg in ill ferrets) for at least 48 hours should be done to maintain renal blood flow and reduce the risk of renal failure.

The prognosis for ibuprofen toxicosis is good with early decontamination and treatment prior to signs. Once symptoms occur, particularly if the ferret is having seizures or is comatose, the prognosis is guarded to grave.

INSECTICIDES

Mechanism

Exposure may be from sprays, granules, dusts and baits. Most products on the market contain ingredients with lower toxicity. Insecticide agents include fipronil, hydramethylnon, pyrethroids and sulfluramid. These have a wide margin of safety and generally are present in low concentrations in the products. These may cause mild to moderate GI upset if ingested. The inert ingredients in the formulation may contribute to these signs.

Clinical presentation

Mild to moderate GI upset (vomiting, diarrhoea, nausea, anorexia). Systemic signs are rarely seen.

Treatment

Symptomatic for GI distress and supportive including fluid therapy.

PAINTS

Mechanism

Ferrets may get into paint while their environment is being painted, if they are allowed free rein in the household. Exterior paints may still contain lead as pigments. Pet owners should be advised to always use paints without lead. Houses built before 1973 in the USA may still have lead-based paint indoors. Acrylic or latex (water-based) paints are still GI and dermal irritants. These paints may contain small amounts of ethylene glycol (usually less than 5%) so small ingestions are not of concern. Large ingestions may cause vomiting. Oil- and solvent-based paints and stains can cause GI upset with secondary aspiration. Inhalation of solvents can lead to CNS depression and coma.

Clinical presentation

GI signs including nausea and vomiting may be seen, primarily with water-based paint exposure. CNS depression and coma can be seen with oil-/solvent-based paint ingestion/aspiration. If the paint is on the skin/fur, local irritation may be seen.

Treatment

For ingestion, dilution should be done to reduce the risk of emesis. Emesis may be considered for large ingestions of water-based paints, although the risk of serious systemic signs with most ingestions is low. Do not induce emesis with oil-/solvent-based paints. Vomiting can be managed by giving nothing by mouth for a few hours. In dealing with oil-/solvent-based paint ingestion, the ferret should be monitored for signs of aspiration and treated appropriately using oxygen, bronchodilators and antibiotics.

For dermal exposure to acrylic/latex paints, a mild pet shampoo or liquid dishwashing detergent and warm water may aid removal of paint. If already dried on the coat, clipping it off will prevent the ferret from ingesting it during grooming. For oil-/solvent-based paints, removal can be done with vegetable or mineral oil, then the ferret is bathed in a liquid dishwashing detergent, similar to how oiled wildlife is managed.

TOPICAL FLEA PRODUCTS

These are usually of low toxicity if used according to the label. For ferrets that generally means using a fraction of a dog or cat dose. Problems arise if full dog or even cat doses are applied. At the high dose, it may cause skin irritation. It has been reported that high doses (such as an entire tube of a dose for large dogs) of pyrethrin and pyrethroid products have caused tremors or seizures in ferrets. There is also the problem that most of these products

are used off-label in ferrets. Veterinarians should counsel owners in the appropriate use of these products. Alcohol-based flea sprays may cause alcohol toxicity. The ferrets have usually been soaked with the product then confined to a small area such as a carrier. These ferrets may become ataxic or moribund. Alcohols can be absorbed dermally as well as inhaled.

Clinical presentation

Dermal irritation may be seen at the site of topical application. Tremors and seizures may be present. From alcohol-based products, ferrets may present ataxic, hypothermic, hypoglycaemic, acidotic or comatose.

Treatment

Dermal decontamination should occur using bathing in a liquid dishwashing detergent, and the ferret kept warm after the bath. Hypothermia may worsen tremors especially with pyrethroids. Regular pet shampoos are not strong enough to remove the chemical. In neurologically symptomatic ferrets, the bath should be delayed until the signs are controlled. Methocarbamol is the treatment of choice for tremors caused by pyrethroid toxicosis. Diazepam does not control tremors from permethrins. The dosage of methocarbamol is 55–220 mg/kg slowly IV. It should be given in 55 mg/kg boluses until the worst of the tremors is controlled. A 330 mg/kg/day dosage should not be exceeded. If the injectable form is not available, dissolve the dose in saline and administer rectally. Barbiturates can be used if methocarbamol is not effective, but the ferret must be closely observed for signs of respiratory depression. For seizures, diazepam may be used.

For alcohol toxicity, treatment is supportive and symptomatic. This includes rinsing the product off, IV fluid therapy (usually with dextrose added), warmth and respiratory support if the lungs have been irritated by the inhalation of fumes.

TOXIC PLANTS

Mechanism

Appendix 7 lists plants deemed potentially toxic to ferrets along with the system that may be affected.

Many common houseplants may be toxic if ingested. Ferrets allowed outside may encounter garden plants that have caused toxicity in other animals. Even ingestion of plants considered 'not toxic' can cause oral irritation, non-specific vomiting and diarrhoea. Additional plants may be listed at www.aspca.org/apcc.

Clinical presentation

Signs will depend on the system that is affected by the plant toxin. The most common signs are those of nausea, vomiting and diarrhoea, particularly if within a short time after ingestion.

Treatment

This will vary depending on what system is affected. A pet poison control database will help determine course of action. Generally treatments effective for dogs and cats can be followed for ferrets. Treatment is often symptomatic and supportive. Emesis in asymptomatic ferrets is usually advised, followed by activated charcoal to absorb plant toxins. It may take multiple activated charcoal doses. Fluid therapy should be done to maintain hydration. An anti-emetic may be needed in symptomatic ferrets.

VENLAFAXINE

Mechanism

Venlafaxine is a bicyclic antidepressant, as a serotonin, noradrenaline (norepinephrine) and weak dopamine reuptake inhibitor. For some reason its formulation seems to attract cats and ferrets and subsequent ingestion. Toxicosis has been reported in both species. In the APCC database the lowest recorded dosage causing toxicosis was 66 mg/kg. Ingestion can lead to serotonin syndrome, which is a condition caused by elevated levels of serotonin at certain CNS synapses.

Clinical presentation

The most common signs are lethargy or depression and diarrhoea. CNS signs may include hyperactivity, aggression, hyperaesthesia and fasciculations or tremors. If serotonin syndrome occurs, the ferret may exhibit GI upset, agitation, tremors, hyperthermia and tachycardia.

Treatment

Emesis is instigated in asymptomatic ferrets, followed by administration of activated charcoal. With formulations that are extended-release, multiple doses of activated charcoal should be administered. Signs may be delayed with the extended-release formulation so the ferret should be observed for at least 12 hours after ingestion. If signs are present, cyproheptadine (a serotonin antagonist) may be used to control signs at a dosage of 1.1 mg/kg PO or rectally. Seizures may be controlled with diazepam (1–2 mg/kg IV to effect). Propranolol is used for control of tachycardia (0.2–1 mg/kg PO, SC q12h).

XYLITOL

Mechanism

Xylitol is a naturally occurring sugar alcohol that is used in many foods and products as a sugar substitute. It is derived from birch trees, corn cobs, raspberries, plums and other hardwood trees and fruits. As ferrets like sweet substances there is a potential for accidental ingestion. In dogs, 100 mg/kg causes a rapid release of insulin leading to acute hypoglycaemia. In higher doses it causes liver failure. This occurs 10–60 minutes following ingestion. It has anecdotally been reported as causing death in a ferret, suggesting that it is probably toxic to ferrets similarly as to dogs.

Clinical presentation

The ferret would be likely to present with acute hypoglycaemia characterised by weakness, ataxia, lethargy, nausea and pawing at the mouth, seizures, coma and death.

Treatment

There is no antidote to xylitol. Treatment is aimed at raising the blood glucose level and protecting the liver. Decontamination may include inducing emesis and administration of activated charcoal. Fluid therapy using dextrose should be initiated as well as oral glucose. Liver protectants may include amoxicillin and milk thistle. It is advised that no products containing xylitol should be in the home.

FORMULARY

DRUG	DOSAGE	COMMENTS
Colour key: Blue: anesth/anal; Pink: anti-infective; Green: cardiopulmonary; Orange: parasiticide; Purple: gastrointestinal		
Acepromazine	0.2–0.5 mg/kg IM, SC	Sedative. May cause hypotension
Acetylsalicylic acid (aspirin)	0.5–2.2 mg/kg PO q8–24h; 10–20 mg/kg PO q24h	Analgesic; miscellaneous NSAID
Activated charcoal	1–3 g/kg PO	Antitoxicant
Alfaxan	5–15 mg/kg IM	Sedative
Alphadolone and alphaxalone	12–15 mg/kg IM initially, followed by multiple 6–8 mg/kg IV as needed to maintain	Anaesthetic
Amantadine	6 mg/kg as an aerosol q12h	Anti-infective
Amikacin	8–16 mg/kg IM, IV, SC divided q8–24h; 10–15 mg/kg IM, SC q12h	Anti-infective, potentially ototoxic, nephrotoxic
Aminophylline	4–6 mg/kg IM, IV, PO q8–12h, bronchodilator	Cardiopulmonary
Amitraz	Topical full strength to affected area q7–14d × 3–6 treatments for demodecosis; if secondary to other illness: 0.01255% solution q7d × 3 treatments then 0.0375% q7d × 3 treatments	Parasiticide
Amlodipine	0.2–0.4 mg/kg PO q12h vasodilator	Cardiopulmonary
Amoxicillin	25–35 mg/kg PO q12h; 20 mg/kg PO, SC q12h; 30 mg/kg PO q8h × 21 days; *Helicobacter*: can combine with metronidazole, bismuth subsalicylate	Anti-infective
Amoxicillin/clavulanate	12.5 mg/kg PO q12; 13–25 mg/kg PO q8–12h	Anti-infective
Amoxicillin (long-acting)	75 mg/kg SC once postsurgery	Anti-infective
Amphotericin B	0.4–0.8 mg/kg IV q7d. Total dose 7–25 mg; blastomycosis	Anti-infective; monitor for azotaemia
Ampicillin	10–30 mg/kg IM, IV, SC q8–12h	Anti-infective
Amprolium	19 mg/kg PO q24h: coccidiosis 100 mg/kg PO in food or water for 7d: isospora	Parasiticide
Anastrazole	0.1 mg/kg PO q24h	Adrenal disease agent
Apomorphine	0.1–5 mg/kg SC; (emetic, may cause excitation)	Dopamine agonist
Atenolol	3.125–6.25 mg/kg PO q24h (hypertrophic cardiomyopathy)	Cardiopulmonary

Key: ACE; angiotensin-converting enzyme; CDV, canine distemper virus; CRI, constant rate infusion; DIM, disseminated idiopathic myositis; IM, intramuscular; IP, intraperitoneal; IT, intratracheal; IV, intravenous; NSAID, non-steroidal anti-inflammatory drug; PO, per os; prn, pro re nata; SC, subcutaneous.

Continued

DRUG	DOSAGE	COMMENTS
Atipamezole	1 mg/kg IP, IV, SC	Reversal agent for dexmedetomidine, medetomidine: same volume IP, IV, SC
Atropine	0.05 mg/kg IM, SC	Miscellaneous
	0.02–0.04 mg/kg IM, SC (bradycardia); 0.1 mg/kg IT 5–10 mg/kg IM, SC (organophosphate toxicity)	Cardiopulmonary
Atropine sulphate ophthalmic solution 1%	1 drop each eye topically q24h	Ophthalmic; caution, overuse may cause toxicity
Azathioprine (Imuran)	0.9–1.0 mg/kg PO q24–72h (immunosuppressive agent, used for chronic hepatitis, inflammatory bowel disease)	Immunomodulator
Azithromycin	5 mg/kg PO q24h; mycobacteriosis: 10 mg/kg PO q12h in combination with rifampin, enrofloxacin, prednisolone	Anti-infective
Barium 20%	2–5 ml/kg PO	Gastrointestinal
Benazepril	0.25–0.5 mg/kg PO q12–24h; vasodilator for dilated cardiomyopathy	Cardiopulmonary
Bicalutamide	5 mg/kg PO q24h	Adrenal disease agent
Bismuth subcitrate colloidal	6 mg/kg PO q12h; *Helicobacter*: combine with enrofloxacin	Gastrointestinal
Bismuth subsalicylate	17.5 mg/kg PO q8–12h; *Helicobacter*: combine with either amoxicillin or enrofloxacin, add metronidazole	Gastrointestinal
Bleomycin	10 U/m^2 SC (squamous cell carcinoma)	Oncological
Budesonide	0.5 mg/kg PO q24h (compound use small enough capsule to pill directly, also treat with B12; inflammatory bowel disease, chronic diarrhoea)	Gastrointestinal
Bupivacaine	1 mg/kg epidurally; 1–1.5 mg/kg SC infiltrate	Anaesthetic
Buprenorphine	0.01–0.05 mg/kg IV, IM, SC q8–12h	Analgesic;
	12 µg/kg epidural anaesthetic	Anaesthetic (epidural)
Butorphanol	0.1–0.5mg/kg IM, SC q4–6h	Analgesic
Cabergoline	5 µg/kg q24h × 5 d	Treatment of pseudopregnancy
Calcium carbonate	53 mg/kg PO q12h for hypoparathyroidism, 100 mg/kg PO q12h pseudohypoparathyroidism	Calcium supplementation
Calcium EDTA	20–30 mg/kg SC q12h (heavy metal toxicosis)	Antitoxicant
Calcium gluconate	2.0 mg/kg/h IV starting treatment for hypoparathyroidism	Calcium supplementation
Captopril	1/8 of 12.5 mg tablet/animal PO q48h; starting dose, work up to q12–24h; (vasodilator)	Cardiopulmonary
Carbaryl powder (5%)	Topical ectoparasites q7d × 3–6 treatments	Parasiticide
Carprofen	1 mg/kg PO q12–24h	NSAID
CCNU	50 mg/m^2 q3 weeks	Oncological
Cefadroxil	15–20 mg/kg PO q12h	Anti-infective
Cephalexin	10 mg/kg SC q24h; 10–15 mg/kg PO q12h	Anti-infective
Cephaloridine	10–25 mg/kg IM, SC q24h × 5–7 d; dermatitis	Anti-infective

Key: ACE; angiotensin-converting enzyme; CDV, canine distemper virus; CRI, constant rate infusion; DIM, disseminated idiopathic myositis; IM, intramuscular; IP, intraperitoneal; IT, intratracheal; IV, intravenous; NSAID, non-steroidal anti-inflammatory drug; PO, per os; prn, pro re nata; SC, subcutaneous.

Continued

DRUG	DOSAGE	COMMENTS
Chlorambucil	1 mg/kg PO; 20 mg/m² PO	Oncological
Chloramphenicol palmitate	50 mg/kg PO q12h × 6–8 weeks (DIM)	Anti-infective
Chloramphenicol palmitate	40 mg/kg PO q8h; 25–50 mg/kg q12h; 14 d minimum for proliferative bowel disease	Anti-infective
Chloramphenicol succinate	25 mg/kg SC q24; 30–50 mg/kg IM, IV, SC q24h	Anti-infective
Chlorpheniramine	1–2 mg/kg PO q8–12h	Antihistamine
Cimetidine	5–10 mg/kg IM, IV, PO, SC q6–8h	Gastrointestinal
Ciprofloxacin	10–15 mg/kg PO q12; 10–30 mg/kg PO q24h	Anti-infective
Cisapride	0.5 mg/kg PO q8–12h	Gastrointestinal
Clarithromycin	12.5 mg/kg PO q8–12h × 14 days; *Helicobacter*: use with ranitidine bismuth citrate; 50 mg/kg PO q24h or divided q12h × 21–28 d; *Helicobacter*: use with omeprazole or ranitine, and metronidazole; 31.25 mg/kg PO q24h, combine with rifampin, clofazimine, mycobacteriosis	Anti-infective
Clindamycin	10 mg/kg PO q12h: anaerobic infections; bone, dental disease 12.5 mg/kg PO q12h: toxoplasmosis	Anti-infective
Cloxacillin	10 mg/kg IM, IV, PO q6h	Anti-infective
Cobalamin	25 μg/kg SC q7d × 6 wk, then q14d × 6 wk, then q30d (chronic diarrhoea with cobalamin malabsorption)	Gastrointestinal
Cyclophosphamide	10 mg/kg PO, SC; q24h day 1, day 14, then weekly for 3 months or until recovery has been achieved (DIM) 200 mg/m² PO, SC	Oncological, Immunosuppressive (DIM)
Cyclosporin (ciclosporin)	4–6 mg/kg PO q12h (pure red cell aplasia)	Immunomodulator
	2.5 mg/kg PO q12h (erythema multiforme)	Immunosuppressive
Cyproheptadine	1.1 mg/kg PO or rectally (venlafaxine toxicosis); serotonin antagonist; appetite stimulant at 2–4 mg/ferret PO q24–48h	Gastrointestinal, Miscellaneous or CNS usage
Decoquinate	0.5 mg/kg PO at least 2 weeks; coccidiosis	Parasiticide
Deoxycorticosterone pivalate (DOCP)	2 mg/kg IM q21d (treatment of adrenal insufficiency following bilateral adrenalectomy)	Adrenal disease agent
Deslorelin	4.7 mg implant SC q1y; 9.4 mg implant SC q1y	Adrenal disease agent
Dexamethasone	0.5–1.0 mg/kg IM, IV, SC; 2 mg/kg IM, IV (anaphylatic reaction to vaccine)	Corticosteroid
	4–8 mg/kg IM, IV once	Shock
Dexmedetomidine	5–15 μg/kg IM	Anaesthetic. Note: can reverse with atipamazole IM (same volume)
Dexdormitor and acepromazine	5–15 μg/kg plus 0.02 mg/kg IM	Sedative; anaesthetic premed
Dextrose 50%	0.25–2 mL IV (hypoglycaemia); 1.25–5% IV (infusion hypoglycaemia or anorexia)	Dextrose supplementation
Diazepam	2 mg/kg IM; 1 mg/animal IV seizure control 0.5 mg/kg IM, IV, PO q6–8h: relaxation urethral obstruction cases	Sedative
Diazoxide	5–30 mg/kg PO q12h – may be increased more if necessary 15–20 mg/kg PO q12h (insulinoma) Chapter 14	Metabolic modulator

Key: ACE; angiotensin-converting enzyme; CDV, canine distemper virus; CRI, constant rate infusion; DIM, disseminated idiopathic myositis; IM, intramuscular; IP, intraperitoneal; IT, intratracheal; IV, intravenous; NSAID, non-steroidal anti-inflammatory drug; PO, per os; prn, pro re nata; SC, subcutaneous.

Continued

DRUG	DOSAGE	COMMENTS
Digoxin	0.005–0.1 mg/kg PO q12–24h; titrate dose as needed, positive inotrope	Cardiopulmonary
Dihydrotachysterol (vit D analogue)	0.02 mg/kg PO q24h for hypoparathyroidism, 0.01 mg/kg PO twice per week pseudohypoparathyroidism	Vitamin D supplementation
Diltiazem	3.75–7.5 mg/animal PO q12; calcium channel blocker, hypertrophic cardiomyopathy	Cardiopulmonary
Diphenhydramine	0.5–2 mg/kg IM, IV, PO q8–12 prn	Antihistamine
Dithiazanine iodide	6–20 mg/kg PO (microfilaricide)	Parasiticide (heartworm)
Dobutamine	0.01 mL/ferret IV prn	Cardiopulmonary
Dorzolamide	1 drop topically q8h	Ophthalmic; carbonic anhydrase inhibitor, glaucoma
Doxapram	1–11 mg/kg IM, IV; respiratory stimulant	Cardiopulmonary
Doxorubicin	1 mg/kg IV q21d × 4 treatments; 20–30 mg/m² IV	Oncological
Doxycycline	10 mg/kg PO q12h	Anti-infective
Enalapril	0.25–0.5 mg/kg PO q12–24–48h; ACE inhibitor for dilated cardiomyopathy	Cardiopulmonary
Enflurane	2% maintenance	Anaesthetic
Enrofloxacin	10–30 mg/kg IM, PO, SC q12–24h; 8.5 mg/kg PO q12–24h; *Helicobacter*: combine with bismuth subsalicylate; 5 mg/kg q12h; *Helicobacter*: combine with bismuth subcitrate colloidal	Anti-infective; injection should only be done once, then PO
Epinephrine	0.02 mg/kg IM, IT, IV, SC	Cardiopulmonary
Epoetin alpha	50–150 U/kg IM, PO q48h	Hormone to stimulate red blood cell production
Erythromycin	10–15 mg/kg PO q6h	Anti-infective
Etomidate	1 mg/kg IV	Sedation (induction, intubation)
Famotidine	0.25–0.5 mg/kg IV, PO, SC q12h; anecdotally this is often given at 2.5 mg per ferret PO q24h as it works out to be 1/4 of a 10 mg tablet, sold over the counter for humans. Crush and mix with dab of nutrient gel	Gastrointestinal
Fentanyl citrate	10–30 µg/kg/h IV via CRI postoperative 10–30 µg/kg/h IV via CRI perioperative after loading dose of 5–10 µg/kg IV	Analgesic
Fentanyl/droperidol	0.15 ml/kg IM	Sedative, preanaesthetic dose of atropine may be necessary
	0.5 ml/kg IM	Higher-dose anaesthetic
Fentanyl/fluanisone	0.3 mg/kg IM	Sedative
Finasteride	10 mg/kg PO q12–24h (androgen inhibitor, useful to shrink prostate)	Adrenal disease agent
Fipronil	Topical: 1 pump of spray or 1/3 to 1/2 cat dose q60d 0.2–0.4 mL topical q30d	Parasiticide
Fluconazole	10 mg/kg PO q24h	Antifungal
Fludrocortisone	0.05–0.1 mg/kg PO q24h or divided q12h	Mineralocorticoid

Key: ACE; angiotensin-converting enzyme; CDV, canine distemper virus; CRI, constant rate infusion; DIM, disseminated idiopathic myositis; IM, intramuscular; IP, intraperitoneal; IT, intratracheal; IV, intravenous; NSAID, non-steroidal anti-inflammatory drug; PO, per os; prn, pro re nata; SC, subcutaneous.

Continued

DRUG	DOSAGE	COMMENTS
Flumazenil	0.01–0.2 mg/kg IM	Reversal agent for benzodiazepines (diazepam, midazolam)
Flunixin meglumine	0.03 mg/kg IM q8h prn; 0.3 mg/kg PO, SC q24h	Miscellaneous, not recommended anymore, NSAID
Flurbiprofen sodium ophthalmic	1–2 drips q12–24h	Ophthalmic NSAID
Flutamide	10 mg/kg PO q12–24h (androgen inhibitor, useful to shrink prostate)	Adrenal disease agent
Furosemide	1–4 mg/kg IM, IV, PO, SC q8–12h; diuretic	Cardiopulmonary
Gabapentin	3–5 mg/kg PO q8–12h	Analgesic (neurotropic pain) May cause sedation at higher dosages
Gentamycin	5 mg/kg IM, SC q24h for 5 days; 2 mg/kg PO q12h × 10–14d 2–4 mg/kg IM, IV, SC q12h	Anti-infective; injectable form can be used orally, not systemically absorbed from gut. IV should be diluted and given over at least 20 minutes; Potentially ototoxic, nephrotoxic
Glucagon	15–40 ng/kg/min IV via CRI for emergency treatment of hypoglycaemia, insulinoma	Hormone for use in insulinoma
Glycopyrrolate	0.01 mg/kg IM	Anticholinergic
Gonadotropin-releasing hormone (GnRH)	20 µg/ferret IM, SC repeat in 2 weeks; (oestrus termination)	Hormone
Griseofulvin	25 mg/kg PO q24 × 21–30 d	Anti-infective
Hairball laxative	1–2 mL/ferret PO q24–48h	Gastrointestinal
Heparin	100 U/ferret (0.45–1.35 kg) SC q24h × 21 d (heartworm) 200 U/kg IM, SC q12h × 5 d (decrease thromboembolism, alternate heartworm therapy regimen)	Cardiopulmonary, Miscellaneous
Human chorionic gonadotrophin (hCG)	100 IU IM, SC; repeat in 14–28 d to bring jill out of oestrus	Hormone
Hydrocortisone sodium succinate	25–40 mg/kg IV; (shock)	Corticosteroid
Hydrogen peroxide	2.2 mL/kg PO; (emetic)	Gastrointestinal
Hydromorphone	0.1–0.2 mg/kg IM, IC, SC q6–8h	Analgesic, opioid
Hydroxyzine	2 mg/kg PO q8h	Antihistamine
Ibuprofen	1 mg/kg PO q12–24h	NSAID
Imidaclopid	0.1–0.4 mL topically along dorsum q30d	Parasiticide; use small cat vial
Imdaclopid/moxidectin	1.9–3.3 µg/kg topically along dorsum q30d	Parasiticide; use small cat vial
Insulin glargine	0.5 IU SC q12h	Antidiabetic
Insulin NPH	0.1–6 U/kg or to effect SC, usually q12h	Antidiabetic
Insulin Ultralente	1 IU/ferret SC q24h	Antidiabetic
Interferon α–2a	60–120 units PO, SC q24h	Canine distemper

Key: ACE; angiotensin-converting enzyme; CDV, canine distemper virus; CRI, constant rate infusion; DIM, disseminated idiopathic myositis; IM, intramuscular; IP, intraperitoneal; IT, intratracheal; IV, intravenous; NSAID, non-steroidal anti-inflammatory drug; PO, per os; prn, pro re nata; SC, subcutaneous.

Continued

DRUG	DOSAGE	COMMENTS
Iohexal	0.25–0.5 ml/kg IV; (myelography); 10 mL/kg PO, dilute 1:1 with water for gastrointestinal constrast study	Miscellaneous
Ipecac 7%	2.2–6.6 mL/ferret PO	Gastrointestinal
Iron dextran	10 mg/ferret IM once	Iron supplementation
Isoflurane	5% induction, 2–3% maintenance	Anaesthetic
Isotretinoin	2 mg/kg PO q24h (cutaneous epitheliotropic lymphoma)	Oncological
Itraconazole	25–33 mg/kg PO q24h	Antifungal
Ivermectin	200–400 µg/kg PO, SC: 1:20 dilution with propylene glycol for topical treatment of ear mites; repeat in 14 d; 0.05–0.1 mg/kg PO, SC: heartworm microfilaricide; 3–4 weeks postadulticide treatment; 0.55 mg/ferret PO q30d: heartworm preventative (Heartgard) small cat dose; 0.05 mg/kg PO q30 d (heartworm prevention)	Parasiticide
Kaolin/pectin	1–2 mL/kg PO q2–6h prn	Gastrointestinal
Ketamine	10–30 mg/kg IM;(tranquillisation) 30–60 mg/kg IM (anaesthesia)	Anaesthetic; dependent on dosage
Ketamine plus acepromazine	20–35 mg/kg IM, SC and 0.2–0.35 mg/kg IM	Anaesthetic, depth dependent on dosage
Ketamine plus dexmedetomidine	5 mg/kg IM plus 0.03 mg/kg IM	Anaesthetic
Ketamine plus diazepam	25–35 mg/kg IM and 2–3 mg/kg IM	Anaesthetic, depth dependent on dosage
Ketamine plus medetomidine	4–8 mg/kg IM and 50–100 µg/kg IM	Anaesthetic, depth dependent on dosage. Can reverse medetomine with atepamazole
Ketamine plus midazolam	50–10 mg/kg IV and 0.25–0.5 mg/kg IV	Anaesthetic
Ketamine plus xylazine	25 mg/kg IM and 2 mg/kg IM	Anaesthetic
Ketoconazole	10–30 mg/kg PO q12–24h; 5 mg/kg SC q24–48h	Anti-infective
Ketoprofen	1–3 mg/kg PO, IM, SC q24h	NSAID
Lactulose syrup	0.15–0.75 mL/kg PO q12h	Gastrointestinal
L–asparaginase	200–400 iu/kg IM, SC q30d	Oncological
L–carnitine	Empirical. 15–50 mg/day PO	Supplement for heart, liver
Latanoprost	1 drop topically q24h	Ophthalmic; prostaglandin analogue, glaucoma
Levothyroxine	50–100 µg PO q12h	Synthetic thyroid hormone replacement
Leuprolide acetate 30 d depot	100 µg/animal <1 kg; 200 µg/animal >1 kg IM q30d	Adrenal disease agent
Lidocaine	1–2 mg/kg total SC, use as local anaesthetic infiltrate	Anaesthetic
Lime sulphur	Dip q24 × 7 d: dermatomycosis; use with griseofulvin; Dip 1:40 dilution q7d × 6 wk (demodectic mange)	Anti-infective, parasiticide
Lincomycin	11 mg/kg PO q8h	Anti-infective
Loperamide	0.2–2 mg/kg PO q12h	Gastrointestinal
Lufenuron	30–45 mg/kg PO q30d (flea larvicide)	Parasiticide
Mannitol	0.5–1 g/kg IV slowly over 20 minutes	Agent used in treatment of shock

Key: ACE; angiotensin-converting enzyme; CDV, canine distemper virus; CRI, constant rate infusion; DIM, disseminated idiopathic myositis; IM, intramuscular; IP, intraperitoneal; IT, intratracheal; IV, intravenous; NSAID, non-steroidal anti-inflammatory drug; PO, per os; prn, pro re nata; SC, subcutaneous.

Continued

DRUG	DOSAGE	COMMENTS
Mebendazole	50 mg/kg PO q12h × 2 d	Parasiticide
Medetomidine	80 µg/kg IM	Sedative. Can reverse with atepamazole
Medetomidine and butorphanol	80 µg/kg IM and 0.1–0.2 mg/kg IM	Anaesthetic
Melarsamine with prednisolone and ivermectin	2.5 mg/kg IM one injection followed by two injections 24 h apart on days 30 and 31; Pred: 1 mg/kg PO q24 to day 31; Ivermectin 50 µg/kg PO once monthly until heartworm free	Parasiticide protocol for heartworm treatment
Melatonin	0.5–1 mg/animal PO q24h prn; 5.4 mg implant SC	Adrenal disease agent
Meloxicam	0.2 mg/kg PO, IM, SC q24h	NSAID
Meperidine	5–10 mg/kg IM, SC q2–4h	Analgesic
Methotrexate	0.5 mg/kg IV	Oncological
Methocarbamol	75 mg/kg PO q8h; 55–220 mg/kg slow IV, in 55 mg/kg boluses to control tremors associated with pyrethroid toxicosis	Muscle relaxant
Metoclopramide	0.2–1 mg/kg IM, PO, SC q6–8h	Gastrointestinal
Metronidazole	35–50 mg/kg PO q24; 10–20 mg/kg q12h; *Helicobacter*: combine with amoxicillin, bismuth subsalicylate; 15–20 mg/kg PO q12h × 14 days (gastrointestinal protozoa)	Anti-infective; Parasiticide
Midazolam	0.25–0.5 mg/kg IM, SC	Sedative
Midazolam and butorphanol	0.5 mg/kg IM and 0.2 mg/kg IM	Anaesthetic (can be used as preanaesthetic combination)
Milbemycin oxime	1.15–2.33 mg/kg PO q30d; heartworm prevention	Parasiticide
Milk Thistle	Empirical. Try 10–50 mg/kg orally daily. Mix into delivery solution	Herbal. Dosage can be increased
Miconazole topical cream	Apply to lesions q8–12h until lesions resolve	Anti-infective. Wear gloves to apply cream, potentially zoonotic
Misoprostol	1–5 µg/kg PO q8h	Gastrointestinal
Morphine	0.5–5 mg/kg IM, SC q2–6h; 0.1 mg/kg epidural anaesthesia	Analgesic; Anaesthetic
Moxidectin	0.1–0.17 mg SC once; heartworm adulticide treatment or use as preventative q6 months	Parasiticide
N–acetylecysteine	5% solution (50 mg/mL); 70 mg/kg PO q6h for 48–72 h for paracetamol (acetaminophen) toxicosis	Antitoxicant
Nalbuphine	0.5–1.5 mg/kg IM, IV q2–3h	Analgesic
Naloxone	0.01–0.3 mg/kg IM, IV; 0.04 mg/kg IM, IV, SC	Miscellaneous opioid reversal. May use up to 1 mg/kg
Nandrolone decanoate	1–5 mg/kg IM q7d	Anabolic steroid
Neomycin	10–20 mg/kg PO q6h	Anti-infective; Potentially ototoxic, nephrotoxic
Neostigmine methysulphate	40 µg/kg IM or 20 µg/kg IV for myasthenia gravis diagnostic testing	Parasympathomimetic
Netilmicin	6–8 mg/kg IM, IV, SC q24h; severe staphyloccal infections	Anti-infective
Nitroglycerin 2% ointment	1/16–1/8 inch/animal q12–24h; vasodilator; apply to shaved loose thigh or pinna	Cardiopulmonary

Key: ACE; angiotensin-converting enzyme; CDV, canine distemper virus; CRI, constant rate infusion; DIM, disseminated idiopathic myositis; IM, intramuscular; IP, intraperitoneal; IT, intratracheal; IV, intravenous; NSAID, non-steroidal anti-inflammatory drug; PO, per os; prn, pro re nata; SC, subcutaneous.

Continued

DRUG	DOSAGE	COMMENTS
Nutri–cal	1–3 mL/ferret PO q6–8h	Nutritional supplement
Octreotide	1–2 μg/kg q8–12h	Hormone (synthetic somastatin) for use in insulinoma
Osaterone acetate	0.25–0.5 mg/kg q24h × 7 d	Hormone indicated for prostatomegaly
Omeprazole	0.7 mg/kg PO q24h; 4 mg/kg PO q24h × 28 d; *Helicobacter*: use with clarithromycin and metronidazole	Gastrointestinal
Oseltamivir	5 mg/kg PO q12h × 10 d	Anti-infective
Oxyglobin	6–15 mL/kg IV over 4 h	Synthetic oxygen carrier
Oxymorphone	0.05–0.2 mg/kg IM, IV, SC q8–12h	Analgesic
Oxytetracycline	20 mg/kg PO q8h	Anti-infective
Oxytocin	0.2–3 U/kg IM, SC	Hormone
Paramomycin	165 mg/kg PO q12h × 5 d (cryptosporidiosis)	Parasiticide; potentially renal toxic
Penicillamine	10 mg/kg PO q24h (copper toxicity)	Antitoxicant
Penicillin G (sodium or potassium)	20,000 IU/kg IM q14h; 40,000–44,000 IU/kg IM, SC q24h	Anti-infective
Penicillin with benzathine penicillin	40,000–44,000 IU/kg IM, SC q72h	Anti-infective
Pentamidine isethionate	3–4 mg/kg SC q48h; *Pneumocystis* pneumonia	Anti-infective
Pentazocine	5–10 mg/kg IM q4h	Analgesic
Pentobarbital sodium	36 mg/kg IP	Anaesthetic, Miscellaneous
	30 mg/kg IV, 1–2 mg/kg PO q12h (seizure control, oral elixir) 2–10 mg/kg/h IV via CRI if diazepam not effective	
Pentoxiphylline	5 mg/kg PO q12h; (disseminated idiopathic myositis) 20 mg/kg PO q12h (systemic coronavirus)	Phosphodiesterase inhibitor, multiple effects
Phenobarbital	1–2 mg/kg PO q8–12h (seizure control) 2–10 mg/kg/h IV via CRI (seizure control if diazepam ineffective)	Antiseizure
Phenoxybenzamine	3.75–7.5 mg/ferret PO q24–72h (smooth muscle relaxation for urinary obstruction)	Potential gastrointestinal or cardiovascular side-effects
Phenytoin	40 mg/kg PO q8h	Antiseizure. May cause gingival hyperplasia
Pilocarpine 2%	1 drop topically q6–12h	Ophthalmic; do not use if uveitis
Pimobendan	0.5–1.25 mg/kg PO q12h; increase cardiac contractility with dilated cardiomyopathy or mitral valve disease	Cardiopulmonary
Piperazine	50–100 mg/kg PO q14d	Parasiticide
Potassium bromide	22–30 mg/kg q24h PO if used with phenobarbitol; 70–80 mg/kg q24h PO if used alone	Antiepileptic
Polyprenyl	3 mg/kg PO 3 times week; (systemic coronavirus)	Immunostimulant
Prazosin	0.05–0.1 mg/kg PO q8h (smooth muscle relaxant for urethral obstruction)	Potential gastrointestinal or cardiovascular side-effects
Praziquantal	5–10 mg/kg PO, SC, repeat in 10–14 d (cestodes); 25 mg/kg PO × 3 d (trematodes)	Parasiticide

Key: ACE; angiotensin-converting enzyme; CDV, canine distemper virus; CRI, constant rate infusion; DIM, disseminated idiopathic myositis; IM, intramuscular; IP, intraperitoneal; IT, intratracheal; IV, intravenous; NSAID, non-steroidal anti-inflammatory drug; PO, per os; prn, pro re nata; SC, subcutaneous.

Continued

DRUG	DOSAGE	COMMENTS
Prednisolone sodium succinate	22 mg/kg IV give slowly before blood transfusion	Corticosteroid
Prednisolone/prednisone	0.25 mg/kg PO q12h × 5 d, then 0.1 mg/kg q12h × 10 d (postadrenalectomy); 0.25 mg/kg PO q12–24h (hypoadrenocortism) 0.25–1 mg/kg PO divided q12h gradually increase to 4 mg/kg/d prn, up to 2 mg/kg/day when given with diazoxide; (insulinoma) 1 mg/kg PO q24h × 7–14 d (post heartworm adulticide treatment) 1.25–2.5 mg/kg PO q24h (eosinophilic gastroenteritis, gradually decrease when signs abate to q48h) 2 mg/kg PO q24h (palliative for lymphosarcoma); 2.2 mg/kg PO q24h (chronic inflammatory bowel disease)	Corticosteroid
Prednisolone	1 mg/kg PO q12h for 3 mo, then q24h until recovery achieved. Taper off dosage. (DIM)	Corticosteroid, antiinflammatory, immunosuppressant
Proligestone	50 mg SC (induce ovulation when jill has been in oestrus 10 d); not available in USA	Hormone
Propentophylline	5 mg/kg PO q12h; (DIM)	Phosphodiesterase inhibitor
Propranolol	0.2–1 mg/kg PO, SC q12h; β–blocker hypertrophc cardiomyopathy	Cardiopulmonary
Prostaglandin F2-α	0.1–0.5 mg/ferret IM prn (metritis, expel necrotic debris) 0.5 mg/ferret IM (induce delivery, follow with oxytocin)	Hormone
Pyrantel pamoate	4.4 mg/kg PO, repeat in 14 d	Parasiticide
Pyrethrins	Topical q7d as needed (fleas)	Parasiticide; use products labeled for kittens, puppies
Pyrimethamine	0.5 mg/kg PO q12h; (toxoplasmosis, protozoa)	Parasiticide
Pyridostigmine bromide	1 mg/kg PO q8h; (megaoesophagus, myasthenia gravis); dog doses 0.5–3 mg/kg	Parasympathomimetic
Ranitidine bismuth citrate	24 mg/kg PO q8h (*Helicobacter*: use with clarithromycin); not available in USA	Gastrointestinal
Ranitidine HCl	2.5–3.5 mg/kg PO q12h	Gastrointestinal
Rifampin	30 mg/kg PO q24h; combine with clofazimine and clarithromycin; (mycobacteriosis); alternative used 10 mg/kg PO q12h along with azithromycin, enrofloxacin and prednisolone	Anti-infective
Rehmannia-6	1/2 capsule daily for renal disease	Chinese herbal used for renal protection
Selamectin	10–15 topically q30d (fleas, ear mites); 18 mg/kg topically (heartworm prevention)	Parasiticide
Sevoflurane	To effect	Anaesthetic
Stanozolol	0.5 mg/kg PO, SC q12h (anaemia)	Anabolic steroid; caution in hepatic disease
Sucralfate	25–125 mg/animal PO q6–12h; requires acidic pH; give before meals; 75 mg/kg PO q4–6h following cleaning products toxicosis	Gastrointestinal

Key: ACE; angiotensin-converting enzyme; CDV, canine distemper virus; CRI, constant rate infusion; DIM, disseminated idiopathic myositis; IM, intramuscular; IP, intraperitoneal; IT, intratracheal; IV, intravenous; NSAID, non-steroidal anti-inflammatory drug; PO, per os; prn, pro re nata; SC, subcutaneous.

Continued

DRUG	DOSAGE	COMMENTS
Sulfadiazine	60 mg/100 mL drinking water or 60 mg per 100 g of food (toxoplasmosis). May treat for 2 weeks plus extended time after cessation of signs	Anti-infective, parasiticide
Sulfadimethoxine	300 mg/kg daily in drinking water for 2 weeks; 25 mg/kg IM PO, SC, q24h; 30–50 mg/kg PO q12–24h; 50 mg/kg PO, then 25 mg/kg q24h × 9 d (coccidia)	Anti-infective; parasiticide
Sulfamethazine	1–5 mg/mL drinking water	Anti-infective
Sulfasoxazole	50 mg/kg PO q8h	Anti-infective
Taurine	30–50 mg/day PO (based on feline supplementation)	Supplement for heart, liver
Terbinafine cream	Apply to lesions q8–12h until lesions resolve	Anti-infective. Wear gloves to apply cream, potentially zoonotic
Terbutaline	2.5–5 mg/kg PO q12–24h	Miscellaneous; arrhythmias and heart block
Tetracycline	20 mg/kg PO q8h; 25 mg/kg PO q12h	Anti-infective
Theophylline	4.25–5 mg/kg PO q8–12h; bronchodilator	Cardiopulmonary
Thiabendazole, dexamethasone, neomycin (otic)	2 drops in each ear q24h × 7 d, off 7 d, on 7 d (ear mites)	Parasiticide
Thiacetarsemide	0.22 mL/kg q12h IV for 2 d	Heartworm (adulticide)
Thiopental 2%	8–12 mg/kg IV	Miscellaneous, induction for anaesthesia
Thyrogen (human recombinant TSH)	100 µg for stimulation thyroid for testing	Diagnostic agent
Thyroxine	0.2–0.4 mg/kg q12h	Hormone
Tiletamine/zolazepine	12 mg/kg IM	Sedative
	22 mg/kg IM	Anaesthetic
Tramadol	1–5 mg/kg PO q12–24h; higher dose more severe pain	Analgesic
Trilostane	5 mg PO q24h	Does not seem to work for hyperadrenalcorticism as it does in dogs
Trimethoprim/sulfadiazine	30 mg/kg PO q12h; 5 mg/kg PO q24h; pyelonephritis: 15 mg/kg IV q12h	Anti-infective
Tylosin	50 mg/kg IM, IV q12h; 10 mg/kg PO, SC q8–12h	Anti-infective
Ursodeoxycholic acid (Ursodiol)	15 mg/kg PO q12h; (chronic hepatopathies)	Bile acid, hepatic agent
Vincristine	0.12–0.2 mg/kg IV; 0.75 mg/m^2 IV	Oncological
Vitamin A	625–800 IU/kg PO q24h; 50,000 IU per ferret SC q24h × 2 d (in CDV outbreak)	Adjunctive treatment canine distemper; dermatitis various aetiologies
Vitamin B complex	1–2 mg/kg IM prn (dose based on thiamine)	Vitamin supplementation

Key: ACE; angiotensin-converting enzyme; CDV, canine distemper virus; CRI, constant rate infusion; DIM, disseminated idiopathic myositis; IM, intramuscular; IP, intraperitoneal; IT, intratracheal; IV, intravenous; NSAID, non-steroidal anti-inflammatory drug; PO, per os; prn, pro re nata; SC, subcutaneous.

Continued

DRUG	DOSAGE	COMMENTS
Vitamin C	50–100 mg/kg PO q12h; 30 mg/kg PO q6–12h for acetaminophen toxicosis	Vitamin supplementation, adjunctive treatment CDV
Vitamin E	200–400 IU q8–24h	Vitamin supplementation, dermatitis various aetiologies
Vitamin K	0.2–2.5 mg/kg IM, PO prn; 5 mg/kg divided q8–12h rodenticide toxicosis	Vitamin supplementation, antitoxicity
Xylazine	0.1–0.5 mg/kg IM, SC	Sedative; may cause hypotension, bradycardia, arrhythmias
Yohimbine	0.2 mg/kg IV 0.5–1 mg/kg IM	Miscellaneous: xylazine reversal
Zanamivir	12.5 mg/kg intranasal	Anti-infective

Key: ACE; angiotensin-converting enzyme; CDV, canine distemper virus; CRI, constant rate infusion; DIM, disseminated idiopathic myositis; IM, intramuscular; IP, intraperitoneal; IT, intratracheal; IV, intravenous; NSAID, non-steroidal anti-inflammatory drug; PO, per os; prn, pro re nata; SC, subcutaneous.

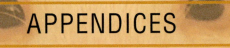

APPENDICES

APPENDIX 1 COMPOSITION OF CEREBRAL SPINAL FLUID IN CLINICALLY NORMAL ADULT FERRETS

PARAMETER	COUNT	COMMENT
Neutrophils (%)	Range 0–38 Mean ± SD 2.1 ± 8.9	
Monocytes (%)	Range 0–100 Mean ± SD 26.4 ± 33.1	
Lymphocytes (%)	Range 0–100 Mean ± SD 71.4 ± 33.2	
WBC	Range 0–8 cells/µL Mean ± SD 1.6 ± 1.8 cells/µL	Blood contamination significantly affected by blood contamination of sample
RBC	<100 RBCs/µL Mean ± SD 20.3 ± 28.8 RBCs/µL	
Protein	Range 20.0–68.0 mg/dL Mean ± SD 31.4 ± 10.6 mg/dL	

Key: RBC, red blood cell; WBC, white blood cell.
Adapted from Platt SR, Dennis PM, McSherry LJ, Chrisman CL, Bennett RA (2004) Composition of cerebrospinal fluid in clinically normal adult ferrets. *American Journal of Veterinary Research* **65(6):**758–760.

APPENDIX 2 COAGULATION VALUES

ANALYTE	MEAN ± SD	MINIMUM–MAXIMUM
PT (seconds)	10.9 ± 0.3	10.6–11.6
PTT (seconds)	20.0 ± 1.0	18.6–22.1
PTT + ellagic acid (seconds)	18.1 ± 1.1	16.5–20.5
Fibrinogen (mg/dL)	107.4 ± 19.8	90.0–163.5
Antithrombin (%)	96.0 ± 12.7	69.3–115.3

Values obtained using an ACL 3000 automated system (Instrumentation Laboratory, Bedford, MA, USA). Key: PT, prothrombin time; PTT, parathyroid hormone.
From Fox JG (2014) Normal clinical and biological parameters. In Fox JG, RP Marini RP (eds). *Biology and Diseases of the Ferret, 3rd Edition*. John Wiley & Sons, Ames, IA. pp. 157–185, with permission.

APPENDIX 3 HAEMATOLOGY AND SERUM CHEMISTRY VALUES OF NORMAL FERRETS

Haematology

PARAMETER	OBSERVED RANGE
WBC (10^3/mm^3)	1.7–13.4
RBC (10^3/mm^3)	9.7–13.2
Haematocrit (%)	47–59
Haemoglobin (g/dL)	14.5–18.5
Mean corpuscular volume (fL)	49.6–60.6
Mean corpuscular haemoglobin concentration (mmol/L)	17.8–20.9
Mean corpuscular haemoglobin (fmol/L)	1.0–1.2
Total protein (g/dL)	6.2–7.7
Neutrophils (%)	22–75
Platelets (10^9/L)	171.7–1280.6
Bands (%)	0–2
Lymphocytes (%)	20–73
Monocytes (%)	0–4
Eosinophils (%)	0–3
Basophils (%)	0–1

Key: RBC, red blood cell; WBC, white blood cell.

From Marini RP, Otto G, Erdman S, Palley L, Fox JG. (2002) Biology and diseases of ferrets. In Fox JG, Anderson LC, Loew FM, Quimby FW (eds). *Laboratory Animal Medicine, 2nd edition.* Academic Press, San Diego CA. pp. 483–517; Fox JG (2014) Normal clinical and biological parameters. In Fox JG, RP Marini RP (eds). *Biology and Diseases of the Ferret, 3rd Edition.* John Wiley & Sons, Ames, IA. pp. 157–185.

Serum chemistry

SERUM ANALYTE	SI UNIT	USA UNIT
Alkaline phosphatase	31–66 IU/L	31–66 U/L
Alanine aminotransferase	78–140 IU/L	78–140 U/L
Albumin	33–42 g/L	3.3–4.2 g/dL
α–Amylase	19.4–61.9 IU/L	19.4–61.9 U/L
Aspartate aminotransferase	78–149 IU/L	78–149 U/L
Bile acids (serum)	0.0–28.9 µmol/L	0.0–11.81 µg/mL
Bilirubin, total	0–1.71 µmol/L	0–0.1 mg/dL
Calcium	1.87–2.47 mmol/L	7.5–9.9 mg/dL
Carbon dioxide	16–28 mmol/L	16–28 mEq/L
Chloride	118–126 mmol/L	118–126 mEq/L
Cholesterol	3.08–5.41 mmol/L	119–209 mg/dL
Creatinine	26.52–70.72 µmol/L	0.3–0.8 mg/dL
Fructosamine	121.1–201.6 µmol/L	121.1–201.6 µmol/L
Gamma glutamyl transferase	0.2–14.0 IU/L	0.2–14.0 U/L
GLDH	0.0–2.5 IU/L	0.0–2.5 IU/L
Glucose	5.5–7.5 mmol/L	99–135 mg/dL
Iron	11.7–56.3 µmol/L	65.4–314.7 µg/dL
Lactate dehydrogenase	221–752 IU/L	221–752 IU/L
Lipase	262.1–1017.5 IU/L	262.1–1017.5 IU/L
Magnesium	0.9–1.6 mmol/L	2.2–3.9 mg/dL
Phosphorus	1.55–2.54 mmol/L	4.8–7.6 mg/dL
Potassium	4.1–5.2 mmol/L	4.1–5.2 mEq/L
Protein, total	50–68 g/L	5.0–6.8 g/dL
Sodium	152–164 mmol/L	152–164 mEq/L
Triglycerides	0.11–0.36 mmol/L	10–32 mg/dL
Urea nitrogen	3.93–8.93 mmol/L	11–25 mg/dL
Uric acid	41.64–101.12 µmol/L	0.7–2.7 mg/dL

Key: GLDH, glutamate dehydrogenase.
From Marini RP, Otto G, Erdman S, Palley L, Fox JG (2002) Biology and diseases of ferrets. In Fox JG, Anderson LC, Loew FM, Quimby FW (eds). *Laboratory Animal Medicine, 2nd edition*. Academic Press, San Diego CA. pp. 483–517; Fox JG (2014) Normal clinical and biological parameters. In Fox JG, RP Marini RP (eds). *Biology and Diseases of the Ferret, 3rd Edition*. John Wiley & Sons, Ames, IA. pp. 157–185.

Protein electrophoresis fractions and acute-phase proteins in clinically normal ferrets

ANALYTE	UNITS	CLINICALLY NORMAL MEAN ± SE	CLINICALLY NORMAL MINIMUM–MAXIMUM
Total protein	g/dL	6.1 ± 0.1	4.9–7.2
A/G ratio		0.95 ± 0.03	0.57–1.28
Albumin	g/dL	2.87 ± 0.05	2.13–3.37
Albumin	%	45.8 ± 1.1	36.1–56.2
Alpha 1	g/dL	0.35 ± 0.02	0.12–0.55
Alpha 1	%	5.9 ± 0.3	2.7–9.7
Alpha 2	g/dL	0.63 ± 0.02	0.42–0.82
Alpha 2	%	10.4 ± 0.2	7.6–13.5
Beta	g/dL	1.46 ± 0.05	0.85–2.16
Beta	%	24.3 ± 0.6	16.5–33.6
Gamma	g/dL	0.58 ± 0.02	0.31–0.88
Gamma	%	9.8 ± 0.4	5.6–14.6
SAA	mg/L	18.1 ± 1.3	5.5–37.0
CRP	mg/L	11.8 ± 0.7	2.0–21.5
HP	mg/mL	0.32 ± 0.03	0.03–0.75

Key: A/G, albumin/globulin; CRP, C-reactive protein; HP, haptoglobin; SAA, serum amyloid A; SE, standard error.

From Ravich M, Johnson-Delaney C, Kelleher S, Hess L, Arheart KL, Cray C (2015) Quantitation of acute-phase proteins and protein electrophoresis fractions in ferrets. *Journal of Exotic Pet Medicine* **24(2):**201–208.

APPENDIX 4 HORMONES

Cortisol

Males	0.13–2.70 µg/dL	Mean 0.9 ± 0.63 µg/dL
Females	0.55–1.84 µg/dL	Mean 0.86 ± 0.29 µg/dL

Insulin

4.6–43.4 normal range	Equivalent units 33–311 pmol/L

Tri-iodothyronine (T3)

Males	0.45–0.78 ng/mL	Mean 0.58 ± 0.9 ng/mL
Females	0.29–0.73 ng/mL	Mean 0.53 ± 0.13 ng/mL

Thyroxine (T4)

Males	1.01–8.29 µg/dL	Mean 3.24 ± 1.65 µg/dL
Females	0.71–3.43 µg/dL	Mean 1.87 ± 0.79 µg/dL

From Fox JG (2014) Normal clinical and biological parameters. In Fox JG, Marini RP (eds). *Biology and Diseases of the Ferret, 3rd edition*. Wiley Blackwell, Ames IA. pp. 157–185, with permission.

Thyroxine (T4)

Males	29.9 ± 5.8 ng/mL
Females	21.8 ± 3.3 ng/mL

From Schoemaker N, von Zealand, Y. Chapter 14 this text.

Sex hormone values are from Dr. Jack Oliver, Clinical Endocrinology Service, College of Veterinary Medicine, University of Tennessee. The neutered ferret group consists of animals castrated (13 males) or spayed (13 females) early, with a mean age of 1.5 years when the hormones were measured. The sexually intact males (40 ferrets) and females (40 ferrets) are 6–9 months old.

There is some variation in hormone levels by season. Neutered or spayed ferrets do have elevations in sex steroids corresponding to the season of the year (unpublished data, C. Johnson-Delaney).

Oestradiol (pmol/L)	
Neutered ferret	30–180
Intact male	103–238
Intact female	109–299
17–hydroxyprogesterone (nmol/L)	
Neutered ferret	<0.1–0.8
Intact male	<0.1–1.9
Intact female	<0.1–20.4
Androstenedione (nmol/L)	
Neutered ferret	<0.1–1.5
Intact male	<0.1–10.8
Intact female	<0.1–30.6

APPENDIX 5 URINALYSIS DATA FOR ADULT FERRETS

PARAMETER	MALE	FEMALE
Volume (mL/24h)*	26 (8–48) (n = 40)	28 (8–140) (n = 24)
Sodium (mmol/24h)*	1.9 (0.4–6.7) (n = 40)	1.5 (0.2–5.6) (n = 24)
Potassium (mmol/24h)*	2.9 (1.0–9.6) (n = 40)	2.1 (0.9–5.4) (n = 24)
Chloride (mmol/24h)*	2.4 (0.7–8.5) (n = 40)	1.9 (0.3–7.8) (n = 24)
Specific gravity (refractometer)**	1.059 ± 0.007	1.047 ± 0.007
Total protein (mg/dL) (refractometer)**	9.6 ± 1.4	7.6 ± 1.2
Protein by strip (mg/dL)	30–100	Trace–30
pH by pH meter**	6.2 ± 0.1	6.3 ±0.3
pH by strip	6.0–6.5	6.0–6.5
Leucocytes by strip	Negative	Negative
Nitrite by strip	Negative	Negative
Glucose by strip	Negative	Negative
Ketone by strip	Negative	Negative
Bilirubin by strip	Negative	Negative
Blood by strip	Negative	Negative – 2+ haemolysed in one case
Urobilinogen by strip	0.2	0.2

Sediment: Urine sediment from all ferrets had amorphous urates present. Most contained mucous strands and/or protein sheaths. The males were intact so urine samples had sperm cells and several samples from both sexes (intact males and females) had rare RBCs. Squamous epithelial cells, WBCs, cocci, uric acid and Ca oxalate crystals were rarely seen.

* values given as mean plus (range).

** values given as mean ± standard deviation.

Volume, sodium, potassium and chloride were collected over a 24-hour period. All other parameters were by cystocentesis from 8 males and 8 females, sexually intact, 1–2 years of age. They were sedated with ketamine/xylazine at Marshall BioResources. Samples were evaluated by the Diagnostic Laboratory of the Division of Comparative Medicine, Massachusetts Institute of Technology. Strips used were Multistix 10 SG (Siemens, Washington, DC) reagent strips provided semiquantitative results.

Key: Ca, calcium; RBC, red blood cell; WBC, white blood cell.

From Fox JG (2014) Normal clinical and biological parameters. In: Fox JG, Marini RP (eds). *Biology and Diseases of the Ferret, 3rd Edition.* John Wiley & Sons, Ames. pp. 157–186, with permission.

APPENDIX 6 DOOK SOUP RECIPE: TO MAKE APPROXIMATELY ONE MEAL

- Pulverise/grind regular ferret food into a powder. 1 tsp powder plus enough water or broth to make it fluid – may need to soak for over an hour or more until it is lumpy chowder consistency. Mix this with:
- Carnivore Care® (Oxbow Animal Health, Murdock, NE) mix with low-sodium organic chicken broth or water: approx 1 heaped tsp CC plus enough liquid to make it soupy. Emeraid-Carnivore (Emeraid LLC, Cornell, IL) can also be used instead of the Oxbow product, although it may cause loose stool.
- 1 tsp Nutrical (optional). May be needed at first to increase palatability.
- 1 heaped tsp chicken or turkey baby food, or cooked chicken purée. (Thoroughly cook a chicken including bones; process so that the bones are ground into it; purée. Portions of this can be frozen in ice cube trays, then one cube is used for each meal).
- Additional nutrients may be added such as omega 3–6 fatty acid oil (half teaspoon per day). Taurine at 25–50 mg/serving is indicated in older ferrets.
- Mix all of the above with enough additional broth or water to make it 'soupy'.
- The ferret may need encouragement to eat – often feeding off a finger or spoon may be needed to get one started. Can also do by syringe.
- Meal: usually 30 mL of CC-based food per 1 kg ferret at least 3 times a day – the requirement is to prevent weight loss. If the ferret will take it on its own from a bowl, it may need more than the 30 mL.

APPENDIX 7 BETTER SAFE THAN SORRY – A GUIDE TO 'DANGEROUS' PLANTS

No list of plants 'safe' or 'dangerous' to all pets can be complete or completely accurate. A lot of controversy surrounds the designation of plants as safe or hazardous to birds and other pets. Plants considered poisonous are on the list based on medical experiences from human, livestock, poultry or isolated pet incidents. Once a plant has been implicated in a poisoning, no matter what the circumstance, it remains so in the medical literature. Only avocado toxicity has been documented in birds in a controlled study. For most, we really don't know whether plants listed are really poisonous in all cases, including how much and what part of the plant was ingested or touched. It is best not to risk allowing any pet to get near a listed 'poisonous plant'. 'Better safe than sorry' is a good caution: replace any of your potentially dangerous plants with some of the many varieties of safe alternatives.

Whether a plant is safe, hazardous, or poisonous depends on a number of things including the species, habits and tastes, as well as the portion of the plant ingested and growth conditions. Effects will vary according to the animal species, type of digestive system, past history of chewing on plants, bodyweight, stomach contents (or lack thereof), hydration, pre-existing health conditions, age, boredom and whether ingestion is normal activity, of dietary necessity or abnormal due to stress-induced appetite or nutritional changes. Many poisonous plants are foul tasting and under normal circumstances an animal will not eat them unless forced to due to confinement, starvation, or lack of proper nutrients in the diet. Plants can vary in toxicity and then affect the animal. The plants listed here are designated by common name as well as Latin name, but discrepancies in naming are common. You may have to do some research with your local gardener to correctly identify vegetation on your property or in your home. The amount and portion of the plant eaten, as well as the time period over which it was eaten, may influence the digestion and absorption of toxic components into the animal's system. The toxic component of the plant may vary according to the plant's own water content.

Before offering any bark, branches or leaves from 'safe' trees, scrub with a non-toxic disinfectant (such as dilute bleach), rinse and dry well.

Bromegrasses, burdocks, barleys, blackberries, boysenberries, raspberries, cacti, cocklebur, sandbur, foxtail, goathead, needlesgrass, pyracantha, rose and triple awns present mechanical hazards from the awns, spines or thorns, which may directly puncture skin or mouth. If punctured and a piece of the plant remains in the animal, infection and abscess may result. Nettles have irritating hairs, and some cacti and members of the Euphorbia family produce irritating saps or latex.

Special problem plant groups

Though not necessarily toxic, some plant groups present other hazards. Trees with rough bark primarily on their trunks often have new branches with smooth bark. That part of the following trees can be used. The rough bark cannot be adequately disinfected. Trees with safe 'smooth' branches include big leaf maple, vine maple, sugar maple and firs. Pines, western hemlock, cedars, junipers and spruces are not recommended because some contain potentially toxic oils, saps or tars.

Alder is not recommended as the bark may have a laxative effect. Apple, apricot, peach, nectarine, plume and prune tree branches are safe, but the pits and seeds are toxic. The fruits themselves are safe, nutritious and enjoyed by many animals. Remove pits and seeds before feeding them to your pet. Avocado or its pit should never be offered to birds.

Inclusion or omission from either of these lists does not guarantee the safety or toxicity of a plant. The information is gleaned from the literature. It is recommended that you investigate the properties of every plant you use around you pet(s). If you cannot identify the plant and ascertain its safety, do not use it.

Dangerous plants

These plants are considered potentially toxic to pets. All or part of the listed plant may be deemed hazardous. Items starred (*) have been used in aviaries without reported problems and may be considered of questionable hazard to birds. It is extrapolated that if the plant is toxic to birds, it is probably toxic to mammals. Symptoms have been reported in various species of animals and humans, and so by extrapolation could cause the same symptoms in ferrets.

COMMON NAME	LATIN NAME	SYMPTOMS
Autumn crocus/Meadow saffron	*Colchicum autumnale*	GI
Avocado	*Persea Americana*, esp. var. *Fuerte, Nabal*	GI
Azalea	*Azalea sp., Rhododendron sp.*	GI
Baneberry	*Actaea sp.*	GI
Beans		
Castor	*Ricinus communis*	GI
Horse, Fava, Broad, Java	*Vicia faba*	BL
Glory, Scarlet runner	*Phaseolus lunatus*	CY
Mescal	*Sophora sp.*	CNS
Rosary peas, Indian licorice	*Abus precatorius*	GI
Bird of paradise, Poinciana	*Casealpiria sp., Strelitzia, Poinciana sp.*	GI
Bleeding heart or Dutchman's breeches	*Dicentra spectabilis*	CNS
Bloodroot	*Sanguinaria canadensis*	GI
Boxwood	*Buxus sp.*	GI

Key: BL, blood anomalies; CNS, central nervous system; CV, cardiovascular; CY, signs associated with cyanide poisoning; GI, gastrointestinal; IR, irritant; RE, reproductive; UR, urinary.
Excerpt from Better Safe Than Sorry, Cathy Johnson DVM, Bird Talk 1987.

Continued

COMMON NAME	LATIN NAME	SYMPTOMS
Bracken fern	Psteridium aquilirnum	BL
Buckthorn	Rhamnus sp.	GI
Bulb flowers		
Amaryllis	Amaryllis sp.	GI
Daffodil, Narcissus	Narcissus sp.	GI
Hyacinth	Hyacinthus orientalis	GI
Iris	Iris sp.	GI
Caladium	Caladium hybrids	IR
Calla lily	Zantedeschia aethiopica	IR
Cardinal flower	Lobelia sp.	CNS
Chalis or Trumpet vine	Solandra sp.	GI
Cherry tree, bark, pits	Prunus sp.	CNS
Chinaberry tree	Melia sp.	CNS
Christmas candle or rose	Helleborus niger	GI
Clematis or Virginia bower	Clematis sp.	CNS
Coral plant	Jatropha multifida	GI
Cowslip, Marsh marigold	Caltha palustris	CNS
Daphne	Daphne sp.	GI
Death camas	Zigaderius venenosus	CNS
Dieffenbachia, Dumb cane	Dieffenbachia segume, picta	IR
Elderberry	Sam bucus	CNS
Elephant's ear, Taro (not root)	Colocasia antiquorum, esculenta	IR
Eucalyptus tree* (not dyed, treated)	Eucalyptus sp.	CY
Euonymus or Spindle tree	Euonymus sp.	GI
False hellebore	Veratrum sp.	CV
Firethorn*, Pyracantha	Pyracantha sp.	IR
Four o'clock	Mirabilis jalapa	GI
Foxglove	Digitalis purpurea	CV
Golden chain	Laburnum anagyroides	CNS
Grass: Johnson, Sorghum, Sudan, Broomcorn	Sorghum sp.	CY
Ground cherry	Physalis	GI
Hemlock		
Poison	Conium maculatum	CNS
Water	Cicuta maculate	CNS
Henbane	Hysoscyamus niger	CNS
Holly	Ilex sp.	GI
Honeysuckle*	Lonicera sp.	GI

Key: BL, blood anomalies; CNS, central nervous system; CV, cardiovascular; CY, signs associated with cyanide poisoning; GI, gastrointestinal; IR, irritant; RE, reproductive; UR, urinary.
Excerpt from Better Safe Than Sorry, Cathy Johnson DVM, Bird Talk 1987.

Continued

COMMON NAME	LATIN NAME	SYMPTOMS
Horsechestnut or Buckeye	*Aesculus sp.*	GI
Horsetail	*Equisiteum arvense*	CNS
Hydrangea	*Hydrangea macrophylla*	CNS
Ivy*, English, varieties	*Hedera sp.*	GI
Jack-in-the-Pulpit or Indian turnip	*Arisaema sp.*	IR
Jasmine	*Cestrum sp.*	GI, CNS
Jimsomweek or Thornapple	*Datura sp.*	CNS
Kentucky coffee tree	*Gymocladus dioica*	CNS
Lantana	*Lantana camara*	CNS
Larkspur	*Delphinium sp.*	CV
Lily-of-the-valley	*Convallaria majalis*	CV
Locusts		
Black	*Robinia psudoacacia*	GI
Honey	*Gleditsia*	RE
Lords and ladies or Cuckoopint	*Arum sp.*	GI
Lupines or Bluebonnet	*Lupinus sp.*	CNS
Marijuana or Hemp	*Cannabis sativa*	CNS
Mayapple, Mandrake	*Podophyllum peltatum*	GI
Mistletoe	*Phoradendron sp.*	GI
Mock orange	Southern: *Prunus caroliniana, Poncirus sp., Philadelphus sp.*	GI, CNS
Monkshood, Aconite	*Acoritum sp.*	CV
Moonseed	*Menispermum canadense*	CNS
Morning glory	*Ipomeas p.*	CNS
Mushrooms – Amanita, others	*Amanita sp. Others*	GI, CNS
Nettles	*Urtica sp, Lasportea sp., Nidosculus sp.*	CNS, CV, IR
Nightshades: Deadly, Black, Garden, Woody, Bittersweet, Eggplant, Jerusalem Cherry, Potato shoots	*Solanum sp.*	GI, CNS
Oaks	*Quercus sp.*	GI
Oleander	*Nerium sp.*	CV
Oleander, yellow	*Thevetia peruviana*	CV
Periwinkle	*Vinca rosea*	CNS
Philodendrons*: var Split leaf, Swiss cheese	*Philodendrons sp., Monstera deliciosa*	IR
Pigweed	*Amaranthus sp.*	BL
Poinsettia*	*Euphorbia pulcherrima*	IR
Poison ivy	*Toxicodendron radicans, Rhus toxicodendron*	IR

Key: BL, blood anomalies; CNS, central nervous system; CV, cardiovascular; CY, signs associated with cyanide poisoning; GI, gastrointestinal; IR, irritant; RE, reproductive; UR, urinary.
Excerpt from Better Safe Than Sorry, Cathy Johnson DVM, Bird Talk 1987.

Continued

COMMON NAME	LATIN NAME	SYMPTOMS
Poison oak:		
Western	*Toxicodendron diversilobum*	IR
Eastern	*T. quercifolium*	IR
Pokeweed or Inkberry	*Phytolacca americana*	GI
Privet	*Ligustrum vulgare*	GI
Rain tree	*Samonia samon*	GI
Ranunculus, Buttercup	*Ranunculus sp.*	CNS
Red maple	*Acer rubrum*	GI
Rhubarb leaves	*Rheum rhaponticum*	UR
Rhododendrons, Azaleas, Laurels	*Rhodendron sp.*	GI
Sandbox tree	*Hara crepitans*	GI
Skunk cabbage	*Symplocarpus foetidus*	IR
Sorrel, Dock	*Rmex sp.*	CNS
Snowdrop	*Galanthus nivalis*	GI
Spurges	*Euphorbia sp.*	GI, IR
Pencil tree	*Euphorbia tirucalli*	GI, IR
Snow on the mountain	*E.marginata*	GI, IR
Candelabra tree	*E. lacteal*	GI, IR
Crown of thorns	*E.milii*	GI, IR
Sweet pea, related peas	*Lathyrus odoratus, sp.*	CNS
Tansy ragwort	*Senecio jacobei*	CNS
Tobacco, Tree tobacco	*Nicotiana sp.*	CNS
Vetch	*Vicia*	CY
Virginia creeper	*Parthenocissus quinquefolio*	GI
Wisteria	*Wisteria sp.*	GI
Yews	*Taxus sp, Podocarpus sp.*	CV, GI
Yellow jasmine	*Gelsemium sp.*	CNS

Key: BL, blood anomalies; CNS, central nervous system; CV, cardiovascular; CY, signs associated with cyanide poisoning; GI, gastrointestinal; IR, irritant; RE, reproductive; UR, urinary.
Excerpt from Better Safe Than Sorry, Cathy Johnson DVM, Bird Talk 1987.

APPENDIX 8 ECHOCARDIOGRAPHIC REFERENCE VALUES IN FERRETS ANAESTHETISED WITH ISOFLURANE OR A KETAMINE/MIDAZOLAM COMBINATION

PARAMETER (UNIT)	ISOFLURANE				KETAMINE/MIDAZOLAM			
	MEAN	SD	RANGE	MEDIAN	MEAN	SD	RANGE	MEDIAN
IVSd (mm)	3.4	0.4	2.5–4.4	3.4	3.6	0.7	2.0–5.0	3.3
IVSs (mm)	4.4	0.6	3.3–5.4	4.4	4.8	1.1	2.7–7.7	4.7
LVIDd (mm)	9.8	1.4	6.8–12.7	9.6	8.8	1.5	6.3–12.0	8.6
LVIDs (mm)	6.9	1.3	4.5–9.7	6.9	5.9	1.5	2.7–8.7	6.0
LVWd (mm)	2.7	0.5	1.8–3.7	2.7	4.2	1.1	3.0–7.0	4.0
LVWs (mm)	3.8	0.8	2.4–5.9	3.8	5.8	9.9	4.3–8.0	5.7
FS (%)	29.5	7.9	13.9–48.7	28.0	33.0	14.0	0–57.0	36.0
Ao (mm)	4.4	0.6	3.3–6.0	4.2	5.3	1.0	3.0–7.3	5.3
LA (mm)	5.8	0.9	3.2–7.3	5.7	7.1	1.8	4.7–12.0	6.7
LA:Ao	1.3	0.2	1.0–1.8	1.3	1.3	2.7	0.8–2.0	1.4
HR (bpm)	238	20	225–244	234	273	31	240–330	300

Key: Ao, aortic diameter; FS, fractional shortening; IVSd and IVSs, thickness of interventricular septum in diastole and systole; LA, left atrium diameter; LVIDd and LVIDs, left ventricular internal diameter in diastole and systole; LVWd and LVWs, thickness of left ventricular free wall in diastole and systole; SD, ± standard deviation.

From Johnson–Delaney CA (2007) Ultrasonography in ferret practice. In: Lewington JH (ed). *Ferret Husbandry, Medicine and Surgery, 2nd Edition*. Saunders Elsevier, Philadelphia PA. pp. 417–429, with permission;

Stepien RI, Benson KG, Wenholz BS (2000) M-mode and Doppler echocardiographic findings in normal ferrets sedated with ketamine hydrochloride and midazolam. *Veterinary Radiology and Ultrasound* **41(5):**452–456; Vastenberg MH, Boroffka SA, Schoemaker NJ (2004) Echocardiographic measurements in clinically healthy ferrets anesthetized with isoflurane. *Veterinary Radiology and Ultrasound* **45(3):**228–232.

APPENDIX 9 RADIOGRAPHIC KIDNEY MEASUREMENTS

Table 1 Direct kidney length measurements

VARIABLE		N	MEAN	SE	SD	95% CI
Right kidney	Total	53	30.13	0.45	3.25	29.23–31.02
	Females	20	27.95	0.57	2.53	26.77–29.14
	Males	33	31.44	0.51	2.94	30.40–32.49
Left kidney	Total	53	29.33	0.43	3.12	28.47–30.19
	Females	20	27.25	0.44	1.95	26.34–28.16
	Males	33	30.60	0.58	3.03	29.52–31.67

Table 2 Direct kidney width measurements

VARIABLE		N	MEAN	SE	SD	95% CI
Right kidney	Total	53	14.83	0.23	1.66	14.37–15.29
	Females	20	13.77	0.23	1.00	13.30–14.27
	Males	33	15.47	0.29	1.66	14.89–16.06
Left kidney	Total	53	14.63	0.21	1.52	14.22–15.05
	Females	20	13.57	0.28	1.24	12.98–14.15
	Males	33	15.28	0.23	1.3	14.82–15.74

Table 3 Ratio of kidney length to the second lumbar vertebra

VARIABLE		N	MEAN	SE	SD	95% CI
Right: L2	Total	53	2.26	0.03	0.19	2.21–2.31
	Females	20	2.19	0.04	0.16	2.11–2.26
	Males	33	2.31	0.03	0.19	2.24–2.37
Left: L2	Total	53	2.20	0.02	0.18	2.15–2.25
	Females	20	2.13	0.03	0.11	2.08–2.18
	Males	33	2.24	0.03	0.19	2.17–2.31

Key: CI, confidence interval; SD, standard deviation; SE, standard error.
Median length of L2 was 13.3 mm (slightly longer in males than females).
Kidney length to L2 ratio: right kidney 2.21–2.31; left kidney 2.15–2.25.
Kidney width to L2 ratio: right kidney 1.09–1.14; left kidney 1.07–1.12.
Significant association between kidney size and weight or sex but not age.
Measurements listed in millimetres. Taken from ventrodorsal survey radiographs. All ferrets had 6 lumbar vertebrae.
From Eshar D, Briscoe JA, Mai W (2013) Radiographic kidney measurements in North American pet ferrets (*Mustela furo*).
Journal of Small Animal Practice **54:**15–19, with permission.

APPENDIX 10 NUTRACEUTICALS AND HERBALS FORMULATIONS

All formulations were formulated by the author and used in clinical practice for many years with noticeable beneficial results. Whenever possible, nutraceuticals and herbals should read 'USP' on the label. Otherwise quality can be variable and questionable. All brands used can be checked for integrity with such organisations as www.consumerlabs.com. Unfortunately in the US, supplements are not regulated and potency or efficacy may vary considerably between brands and even between batches.

Normally these are placed in 60 mL (2 ounces) bottles so clients can shake well. Otherwise we recommend stirring with a chopstick before drawing up the dosage. Keep refrigerated.

Cardiac formula

1000 mg L-carnitine
1000 mg taurine
1000 mg CoQ10
400 IU vitamin E

In omega 3–6–9 solution to equal 30 mL (recommend Optomega from USANA*, but theoretically a blended omega 3–6 oil could be used. Care must be taken to prevent rancidity. Optomega must remain refrigerated and remains a liquid at household refrigerator temperatures).

Dosage 0.5–1 mL per ferret per day.

Liver formula

1000 mg silybins (active ingredient of milk thistle)
500 mg dandelion
1000 mg L-carnitine
1000 mg taurine
1000 iu vitamin E
400 mg CoQ10
400 mg S-adenosylmethionine (SAMe)
In omega 3–6–9 (Optomega or equivalent) to equal 30 mL.
Dosage 0.5–1 mL/kg orally once daily.
It is advised to administer lactulose and B complex separately.

Geriatric/arthritis formula

1800 mg chondroitin sulphate
600 mg glucosamine
16 mg manganese (1 scoop equine Cosequin™ powder)**
1000 mg L-carnitine
1000 mg taurine
1000 IU vitamin E
400 mg CoQ10
In omega 3–6–9 (Optomega or equivalent) to equal 30 mL.
Dosage 0.5–1 mL/kg orally once daily.

Immune formula

400 mg CoQ10
550–600 mg eleuthro
550 mg dandelion
1200 mg echinacea
10,000 IU vitamin A
1000 IU vitamin E
800 mg ginseng
In omega 3–6–9 (Optomega or equivalent) to equal 30 mL.
Dosage 1 mL/kg orally once daily.

Calming formula

800 mg L-theanine
1000 mg L-tryptophan
400 mg CoQ10
480–500 mg valerian
In omega 3–6–9 (Optomega or equivalent) to equal 30 mL.
Dosage 1 ml/kg orally 1–2 times a day.

Skin formula

1200 mg echinacea
10 mg lycopene
1000 mg L-carnitine
1000 IU vitamin E
10,000 IU vitamin A
400 mg Coq10
In omega 3–6–9 (Optomega or equivalent) to equal 30 mL.
Dosage 0.5–1 mL/kg orally once daily.

*Optomega: USANA, Salt Lake City, UT, USA. Http://usana.com
**Cosequin: Nutramax Labs, Edgewood, MD, USA. www.nutramaxlabs.com

APPENDIX 11 DIFFERENTIAL DIAGNOSIS TABLE

This chart is not all inclusive, but is a starting point for diagnosis.

CLINICAL SIGNS	DIFFERENTIAL DIAGNOSIS	DIAGNOSTIC OPTIONS	THERAPY
Abdominal enlargement, mass	Pregnant, full/blocked bladder secondary to urolithiasis/prostatic involvement, splenomegaly, neoplasia, GI foreign body, *Mycobacterium* granuloma, histoplasmosis, cystic kidneys	Hx, PE, CBC/chems, Rads, U/S. Abdominal tap & cytology. FNA of mass (U/S guided), biopsy, exploratory laparotomy, C&S, acid-fast stains. Diagnostics for adrenal disease if mass adrenal	Dependent on diagnosis
Abdominal enlargement, fluid	Ascites, cardiomyopathy, peritonitis, neoplasia	Hx, PE, Rads, U/S, abdominal tap & cytology, cardiac evaluation, CBC/chems	If cardiac, appropriate cardiac treatments including furosemide. If peritonitis, antibiotics. If neoplasia consider laparotomy, excision, chemotherapy (lymphoma)
Abortion	*Salmonella*, septicaemia, trauma, underlying metabolic disease	Nx of aborted material, C&S; Hx, PE of jill, full work-up	Appropriate antibiotics for jill. Consider OHE. Supportive care
Alopecia	Dermatomycosis	Fungal culture, KOH prep, Wood's light	Griseofulvin, topical antifungals. Discuss zoonotic potential with owner
Alopecia	Ectoparasites (such as *Sarcoptes scabei*), *Ctenocephalides* (flea allergic dermatitis)	Visual examination, skin scraping	Ivermectin, topical flea powders (feline); topical flea/tick treatments. Environmental control
Alopecia (symmetrical indicative of endocrinopathy: rat tail, comedones, swollen vulva)	Hyperadrenocorticism (adrenal disease- hyperplasia, adenoma, carcinoma), hyperoestrogenism (adrenal disease, ovarian remnant in spayed female; intact female)	Hx, PE, CBC/chems, serum hormone panel, Rads, U/S, laparotomy	Adrenal disease: surgical excision, leuprolide acetate depot, deslorelin implant. Hyperoestrogenism: remove ovarian remnant. Intact female: may use hCG to cycle out for surgery prep, OHE, blood transfusions and supportive care if concurrent anaemia
Alopecia	Mast cell tumour	Biopsy/histopath	Surgical excision, antihistamines, topical if not surgically
Alopecia	Seasonal variation (tail primarily)	Rule out adrenal disease	No Tx
Anorexia (without significant weight loss, acute, may see as part of many other disease conditions. Frequently the sole presenting symptom. If greater than 24 hours, may see some degree of depression, dehydration, tarry stool, hindquarters paresis/ataxia, seizures, generalised weakness) See weight loss	Dental disease, GI foreign body, trichobezoar, gastroenteritis, *Helicobacter*-associated ulcers, cardiomyopathy, upper respiratory disease, pneumonia, neoplasia, pain, liver disease, kidney disease, cystitis. Peracute anorexia: gastric dilatation, *Clostridium*, gorging in juveniles	Hx, PE, CBC/chems, Rads (contrast studies), U/S, echocardiography, dental examination, UA, faecal occult blood, laparotomy, enterotomy/gastrotomy if foreign body. GI endoscopy, biopsy, histopathology	Supportive care: fluids, oral supplementation such as dook soup; correct underlying problems

Vitamin B complex may help stimulate appetite |

Key: BUN, blood urea nitrogen; CBC, complete blood count; chems: serum biochemistries; CSF, cerebrospinal fluid; C&S, culture and sensitivities; DIM, disseminated idiopathic myofasciitis; ECG, electrocardiogram; FNA, fine needle aspirate; FRSCV, ferret systemic coronavirus. GI, gastrointestinal; hCG, human chorionic gonadotrophin; Hx, history; IBD, inflammatory bowel disease; IO, intraosseus; IV, intravenous; KOH, potassium hydroxide; LSA, lymphosarcoma; NSAID, non-steroidal anti-inflammatory drug; Nx, necropsy; OHE, ovariohysterectomy; PCR, polymerase chain reaction; PE, physical examination; Rads, radiographs; SC, subcutaneous; Tx, treatment; UA, urinalysis; U/S, ultrasonography.

Continued

CLINICAL SIGNS	DIFFERENTIAL DIAGNOSIS	DIAGNOSTIC OPTIONS	THERAPY
Conjunctivitis	Canine distemper	Serology, PCR conjunctival swab; rule out primary, conjunctiva/eye irritation (eye examination, staining)	Vitamin A, vitamin C, interferon, vaccination, supportive care
	Influenza	Hx, exposure to humans ill, PE, CBC/chems, Rads, eye examination, staining	Supportive, symptomatic care for comfort, control secondary bacterial infections. May need antihistamines, cough suppressants, dook soup, NSAIDs
	Foreign body/corneal lesion	Hx, eye examination including staining	Remove foreign body, keratectomy/ treatment as in other species
Constipation	GI foreign body, dehydration (may follow diarrhoea)	Hx, PE, CBC/chems, Rads (contrast studies)	Correct dehydration. Treat underlying GI problem. If foreign body, exploratory laparotomy/ enterotomy, gastrotomy. Laxatives or motility enhancers rarely needed. Supportive care
Cyanotic mucous membranes	Respiratory compromise, pneumonia, pleural effusion, cardiomyopathy, dyspnoea, heartworms	PE, auscultation, Rads, Thoracentesis or tracheal wash-cytology, analysis, C&S, Gram's stain; heartworm tests, full cardiac evaluation	Oxygen, supportive care until diagnosis. If pneumonia may need bronchodilators. If pleural effusion may need chest drainage, furosemide
Dental disease (gingivitis, periodontitis, fractured teeth, plaque, caries)	Underlying systemic disease contributions	Oral examination, oral radiographs (note: full PE, diagnostics recommended particularly if anaesthesia required for dental work)	Appropriate dental measures (as in other carnivores)
Diarrhoea	Rotavirus	Serology (3–4 wk old kits), faecal flotation & smear, rads +/- contrast, CBC/chems to assess overall condition	Fluids, symptomatic, supportive care
	Proliferative bowel disease, IBD, GI neoplasia	PE, faecal flot/smear, Rads +/- contrast, CBC/chems, endoscopy, biopsy, histopathology (done at exploratory laparotomy)	*Helicobacter* treatment regimen; chloramphenicol, enrofloxacin. If IBD, azathioprine. If neoplasia, chemotherapy can be tried. Supportive and symptomatic care
	GI foreign body	Hx, PE, Rads (contrast), CBC/ chems prior to surgery if necessary to remove. Faecal examination may show foreign material	May need laparotomy (gastro/ enterotomy) if material can't pass. Fluid therapy, supportive care including analgesics
	Salmonella	Faecal/rectal C&S, Hx particularly of raw diet	Fluids, supportive care, appropriate antibiotics. Zoonotic potential
	Aleutian disease	Serology	Supportive care
	Eosinophilic gastroenteritis, suspected food allergy	GI biopsy definitive	Diet change (such as a lamb/rice diet), prednisone, antibiotics

Continued

CLINICAL SIGNS	DIFFERENTIAL DIAGNOSIS	DIAGNOSTIC OPTIONS	THERAPY
	GI parasitism (e.g. coccidia, giardia, cryptosporidia etc.)	Faecal flotation/smear, specialised tests for protozoa	Sulfas (coccidia), metronidazole (giardia), specific antiparasitism drugs for other parasites as in other species. Cryptosporidia may not respond to medications, should be self-limiting. Symptomatic and supportive care
Dyspnoea	Acute: anaphylaxis or allergic reaction	Vaccination reaction, insect/arachnid bite or sting	Corticosteroids, antihistamines, oxygen support, epinephrine, bronchodilators, supportive. Analgesic may be needed for painful sting
	Electric shock (pleural oedema, oropharyngeal acute oedema/inflammation)	Hx (chewing on cord?), PE, may have oral lesions, Rads	Corticosteroids, diurectics, fluids, antibiotics if oral lesions or severe pulmonary oedema
	Heat stress (may be panting, open-mouth breathing)	Hx, elevated ambient temperature; elevated core temperature	Lower core body temperature: fluids, cool cloth/pack to neck/shoulders, tepid water bath
	Pleural oedema due to cardiomyopathy, heartworms, trauma	Hx, Rads, cardiac evaluation, heartworm tests, CBC/chems, thoracentesis, fluid cytology/analysis	Oxygen, supportive care for trauma including analgesics. Cardiomyopathy: diurectics, inotropics, vasocilators. Heartworm therapy
	Pleural effusion due to a space occupying mass in thorax, LSA, *Pseudomonas luteola* mediastinitis	Rads, CBC/chems, thoracentesis, fluid cytology/analysis, C&S, workup for LSA may include bone marrow biopsy	LSA: chemotherapy; antibiotics if bacterial, supportive, symptomatic
	Pneumonia (human influenza, canine distemper, *Bordetella bronchiseptica,* blastomycosis, histoplasmosis, coccidiodomycosis, *Klebsiella, E.coli, Pseudomonas, Proteus* etc.	Hx, Rads, tracheal wash, C&S, cytology	Influenza: symptomatic, antihistamines, cough suppressants; antibiotics for bacteria aetiology. Fungal: systemic antifungals. All require supportive care
	Trauma: diaphragmatic hernia. Fractures: ribs, cranium, nasal bones, jaws, dental. Direct chest trauma e.g. crush, compression, haematoma	Hx, PE, Rads, CBC/chems, thoracentesis if fluid present	Supportive. Analgesics. When stable, consider surgical correction of diaphragmatic hernia as in other species. Repair fractures as in other species.
Fever (elevated core temperature with no Hx of elevated ambient temperature)	DIM, FRSCV, canine distemper, septicaemia, systemic disease including pyelonephritis; pain/inflammation	Hx, PE. Otic/rectal temperature. CBC/chems, UA. If suspect DIM, muscle biopsy. Rads, U/S, abdominocentesis if suspect FRSCV	Appropriate therapies per aetiology. If pain, inflammation: analgesics, NSAIDs. Septicaemia: antibiotics. Supportive care. DIM may treat with ciclosporin, muscle relaxants. FRSCV supportive only

Key: BUN, blood urea nitrogen; CBC, complete blood count; chems: serum biochemistries; CSF, cerebrospinal fluid; C&S, culture and sensitivities; DIM, disseminated idiopathic myofasciitis; ECG, electrocardiogram; FNA, fine needle aspirate; FRSCV, ferret systemic coronavirus. GI, gastrointestinal; hCG, human chorionic gonadotrophin; Hx, history; IBD, inflammatory bowel disease; IO, intraosseus; IV, intravenous; KOH, potassium hydroxide; LSA, lymphosarcoma; NSAID, non-steroidal anti-inflammatory drug; Nx, necropsy; OHE, ovariohysterectomy; PCR, polymerase chain reaction; PE, physical examination; Rads, radiographs; SC, subcutaneous; Tx, treatment; UA, urinalysis; U/S, ultrasonography.

Continued

CLINICAL SIGNS	DIFFERENTIAL DIAGNOSIS	DIAGNOSTIC OPTIONS	THERAPY
Haematuria (stranguria, dysuria)	Urolithiasis, cystitis, prostate enlargement/neoplasia, pyelonephritis	Hx (grain-free diet), UA (cystocentesis), Rads including contrast, catheterisation, U/S, rule out adrenal disease component for prostate involvement	May need catheterisation if obstructed, with protocol same as cats; cystotomy, treatment for adrenal disease (prostate including treatment of cysts), analgesics, muscle relaxants, supportive care
Hypersalivation (see also neurological signs, vomiting). Most often this is a sign of nausea	Dental/oral irritation (fractured tooth, foreign body wedged in arch, reactions to bitter/toxic plant or substance)	Hx, PE including oral examination. Full work-up should be considered especially if toxin suspected	Correct dental condition. Remove foreign body. Follow appropriate antidote/remedies as in dog/cat if toxic plant, toxin involved
	Gastritis, ulcer (*Helicobacter*), gastroenteritis (parasitic, bacterial), pancreatitis (pain/nausea associated), GI foreign body	Hx, PE including oral examination. CBC/chems, abdominal palpation, Rads (contrast if suspect foreign body particularly), U/S may show ulcer	Antimicrobials, antiparasitics if indicated. Famotidine, sucralfate, GI protectants, analgesics for pain associated with conditions. Gastrotomy/enterotomy may be needed for foreign body
	Heat stress	Hx, elevated ambient temperature, elevated otic/rectal temperature	Lower core body temperature; fluids, cool cloth/pack to neck, shoulders, tepid water bath
	Insulinoma (beta/islet cell tumour)	Blood glucose (< 60 mg/dL), CBC/chems, insulin level (although that takes time), Rads, U/S, exploratory lapratomy	Supportive. Surgical excision of pancreatic nodules or lobectomy; diazoxide, prednisone, frequent meals
	Misc. conditions (electric shock, theoretically rabies)	Electric shock: see above. Rabies: post mortem, histopathology and immunoassay	Electric shock: as above. Rabies: none. Zoonotic potential, notify public health authorities if this suspected
Icteric mucous membranes (jaundice)	Liver disease including hepatitis (bacterial), cirrhosis/lipidosis, sequellae to diabetes mellitus or pancreatitis. cholecystitis, toxicosis	Hx, PE, including dietary information (ingestion of oils, fats, sugars), CBC/chems, Rads, U/S, liver biopsy	Supportive especially fluids. Antimicrobials if bacterial. Dietary – good source of calories needed (dook soup); liver supportive supplements including milk thistle. If diabetes: insulin/diet therapy, GI protectants as needed. May need analgesics. Toxins: appropriate antidotes as per dog/cat
Mastitis	Neoplasia, bacterial infection (haemolytic *E.coli*), trauma from nursing	PE, C&S exudate, biopsy if neoplastic	Remove kits, fluids, antibiotics. Surgical resection, analgesics, supportive care
Neurological signs (seizures, convulsions, ataxia) See also hypersalivation, paralysis, weakness	Seizures (any of the below): prior to diagnosis, treat the seizure	At least try to get a blood sample for glucose level before giving dextrose/glucose. Hyperglycaemia (diabetes) is rare in the ferret, but it has been documented	First aid: isotonic dextrose (IO, IV, SC), oral glucose, diazepam or phenobarb (IV) to stop seizure
	Acute seizure or convulsion: anaphylaxis or allergic reaction	Vaccination reaction, insect bite or sting	Corticosteroids, antihistamines, oxygen support, adrenaline, supportive. Analgesic may be needed for painful sting. Usually will not need diazepam

Continued

CLINICAL SIGNS	DIFFERENTIAL DIAGNOSIS	DIAGNOSTIC OPTIONS	THERAPY
	Azotaemia (renal disease, failure)	CBC/chems, BUN elevated, UA, Rads, U/S, biopsy	Fluid therapy to lower BUN, supportive care. Feline kidney diets have been tried
	Toxicosis (plants, chemicals, pesticides, materials around home)	Hx, PE, exposure to toxins. Pass materials in faeces/stomach contents. CBC/chems, UA	Appropriate antidotes per toxin. Generally follow guidelines as for dogs/cats. Supportive care
	Trauma	Hx, PE, Rads, CBC/chems	Anti-shock therapy, analgesics, corticosteroids, antimicrobials. Surgical as appropriate
Organomegaly	Spleen: idiopathic hypersplenism, splenomegaly due to anaesthesia, LSA	PE, Rads, U/S, biopsy	Dependent on aetiology
	Adrenal enlargement: hyperplasia, adenoma, adenosarcoma	PE, endocrine assays, U/S, biopsy, histopathology	See treatment for hyperadrenocorticism (adrenal disease)
	Lymph nodes: lymphadenopathy due to systemic infection, LSA, mycobacteriosis	PE, CBC/chems, FNA, cytology C&S, Grams/acid fast stain, biopsy, histopathology	Surgical removal of a node if peripheral for diagnostics. Systemic infection: appropriate antimicrobials. LSA – see LSA therapy. Mycobacteriosis: zoonotic potential, treatment regimens probably effective
	Abdominal: gastric or enteric (neoplasia or foreign body, bloat, volvulus)	Hx, PE, Rads (contrast), exploratory laparotomy	If foreign body, passage or surgical removal. Neoplasia: excision or chemo depending on aetiology. For acute volvulus, follow protocol as for dogs
	Bladder: urinary obstruction, lithiasis, neoplasia. Renal: cysts, hydronephrosis, neoplasia. Bladder obstruction may be secondary to prostatic enlargement (adrenal disease)	PE, cystocentesis, UA, Rads, contrast cystogram/excretory urogram, U/S especially prostate, exploratory laparotomy, serum endocrine panel if prostate abnormal	Urolithiasis see under haematuria, appropriate cystotomy, catheterisation. Renal, if unilateral remove affected kidney. Cyst drainage
	Cardiomegaly, dilatative or hypertrophic cardiomyopathy, rule out heartworms	PE, Rads, ECG, echocardiography. Occult heartworm tests, CBC/chems. Cardiac biopsy rarely done	Appropriate cardiac therapies per type of cardiomyopathy. If heartworms present follow protocol as in dogs/cats
Pale mucous membranes	Anaemia due to hyperstrinism (unspayed female, ovarian remnant in spayed female), advanced adrenal disease. Neoplasia including LSA (involving bone marrow or red cell depletion/consumption by spleen), pure red cell aplasia	PE, CBC including reticulocyte count, U/S, endocrine assays, bone marrow biopsy, cytology/histopathology, exploratory laparotomy to obtain spleen biopsy, other masses if found	Supportive. Blood transfusion to stabilise. Erythropoietin, adrenal disease treatment. hCG to cycle female out of oestrus prior to OVH, surgical excision of remnant ovarian tissue, adrenalectomy, splenectomy, appropriate chemotherapy per type neoplasia

Key: BUN, blood urea nitrogen; CBC, complete blood count; chems: serum biochemistries; CSF, cerebrospinal fluid; C&S, culture and sensitivities; DIM, disseminated idiopathic myofasciitis; ECG, electrocardiogram; FNA, fine needle aspirate; FRSCV, ferret systemic coronavirus. GI, gastrointestinal; hCG, human chorionic gonadotrophin; Hx, history; IBD, inflammatory bowel disease; IO, intraosseus; IV, intravenous; KOH, potassium hydroxide; LSA, lymphosarcoma; NSAID, non-steroidal anti-inflammatory drug; Nx, necropsy; OHE, ovariohysterectomy; PCR, polymerase chain reaction; PE, physical examination; Rads, radiographs; SC, subcutaneous; Tx, treatment; UA, urinalysis; U/S, ultrasonography.

Continued

CLINICAL SIGNS	DIFFERENTIAL DIAGNOSIS	DIAGNOSTIC OPTIONS	THERAPY
	Hypothermia	Core temperature, Hx	Warmth, warm fluid therapy
	Trauma, shock	Hx, PE, diagnostics appropriate for injury	Supportive, fluid therapy, possibly corticosteroids, follow guidelines for cat shock
	Cardiac compromise, failure (poor perfusion), cardiomyopathy	Hx, PE, ECG, echocardiography, CBC/chems, Rads	Appropriate cardiac therapy based on type of cardiomyopathy. Supportive care including Cardiac formula (see Appendix 10)
Paresis/paralysis (see also weakness, neurological signs)	Any debilitating systemic illness including Aleutian disease, DIM, neoplasia, renal disease	General diagnostic workup, serology for AD	Supportive, correct per disorder
	Anorexia, starvation	PE, diet Hx, CBC/chems. Assess if underlying disease condition, malabsorption, gastroenteric condition, metabolic or neoplastic condition that is preventing utilisation of food	Parenteral feeding. Assist feeding using dook soup. (see Appendix 6). Correct underlying conditions. Feed good-quality ferret food. Appetite stimulation may include fluid therapy with vitamin B complex
	Botulism (very rare)	Hx of eating rancid mink diet	Supportive including oxygen, respiratory support
	Myelitis, encephalomyelitis, DIM	PE, CBC/chems, Rads, CSF tap, cytology C&S, biopsy of muscle tissue	Supportive, appropriate antimicrobials if bacterial. Analgesics. If DIM, ciclosporin along with muscle relaxants may be tried
	Post exercise: hypoglycaemia (insulinoma), cardiomyopathy	Hx, PE, CBC/chems especially blood glucose, cardiac evaluation	As appropriate per insulinoma or cardiomyopathy
	Rabies	Hx, postmortem, histopathology, immunoassay	None, zoonotic potential. Notify public health authorities
	Mycobacterium infection	Rads, CSF tap, C&S, acid-fast stain, cytology	Zoonotic potential. Treatment involves multiple antibiotics
	Trauma (spinal injury, abdominal/limb trauma – consider crush/compression injury from dog bite, fall); intervertebral disc disease	Hx, PE, Rads, CBC/chems, CT, MRI particularly to image spinal canal, cord	Treat appropriately for shock, pain, respiratory/circulatory compromise. If abdominal organ compression/rupture signs may not appear for a few hours after injury, orthopaedic repair if fractures; analgesics
Pruritis	Bacterial dermatitis (esp. *Staph*)	C&S, biopsy/histopathology	Appropriate antibiotics, topicals, medicated bath for soothing. NSAIDs for comfort
	Ectoparasites (fleas, sarcoptes mites)	PE, skin scraping, cytology	Appropriate antiparasitics including topical flea products, environmental control; zoonotic potential
	Hyperadrenocorticism (adrenal disease)	CBC/chems, endocrine panel, U/S	Adrenal disease treatment protocol. NSAIDs, antihistamines as supportive care
	Mast cell tumour	Biopsy, histopathology	Surgical excision, antihistamines (systemic, topical)

Continued

CLINICAL SIGNS	DIFFERENTIAL DIAGNOSIS	DIAGNOSTIC OPTIONS	THERAPY
Respiratory signs (coughing, dyspnoea, sneezing, conjunctivitis, upper respiratory disease)	Cardiomyopathy, pneumonia, influenza, canine distemper, *Mycoplasma* sp., irritants, neoplasia, heat stress, corneal injury/ulcer, mechanical pressure from abdomen, diaphragmatic hernia, space-occupying masses, tooth abscess	Hx, PE, Rads, thoracentesis, tracheal wash, C&S exudates, cytology, cardiac evaluation, occult heartworm test, ophthalmic examination, sinus/lacrimal flush, oral/dental examination	Appropriate for aetiology
Respiratory signs (rhinitis, sinusitis)	Infectious, foreign bodies, particulates or irritants, tooth abscess	Hx (exposure to chemicals, dusts), oral examination, Rads, sinus flush C&S/cytology exudates or flush fluids	If possible, remove foreign bodies or materials, antimicrobials, antihistamines, decongestants, decrease exposure to chemicals, irritants. Appropriate therapy for dental abscess
Seizures (see also neurological signs)	Epilepsy, insulinoma, acute toxicity, extreme pain, renal failure, heart failure, neoplasia, starvation, heat stroke, trauma, canine distemper	Hx, PE, CBC/chems, Rads, cardiac evaluation. Other diagnostics per aetiology	Stabilise before diagnosis. Benzodiazepam IO/IV or intrarectally. Phenobarb may be needed to stop the seizure. Fluids (isotonic dextrose 5% to start then other crystalloid), additional dextrose if hypoglycaemic. Appropriate therapy per diagnosis
Stranguria, dysuria (see also haematuria)	Urolithiasis, cystitis, urethral obstruction (rule out prostate involvement, adrenal disease)	Hx (grain-free diet), PE, UA, Rads, U/S, serum endocrine panel if prostate abnormal	Appropriate antimicrobials. If stones, cystotomy, catheterisation. If prostate involvement, may need to drain cysts, surgically correct; adrenal disease protocol
Swollen vulva	Oestrus, hyperadrenocorticism (adrenal disease) in spayed female, ovarian remnant in spayed female	Hx, CBC/chems, serum endocrine panel, U/S, exploratory laparotomy	For oestrus: to stop, hCG or leuprolide acetate depot or deslorelin, OHE, surgical excision of ovarian remnant, therapy protocol for adrenal disease. If concurrent anaemia, see above
Vomiting, regurgitation (see also neurological signs, seizures, hypersalivation, trauma)	Pain (especially head pain)	Hx, PE, full work-up	Analgesics as needed, antiemetic to control
	Nausea, GI foreign body, gastric ulcer (*Helicobacter*), gastritis, gastroenteritis (any cause), heat stress, ingestion of toxic material, liver/pancreatic disease, megaoesophagus	Hx, PE, CBC/chems, Rads (contrast), endoscopy of stomach for ulceration, biopsy	Appropriate antibiotics for *Helicobacter*, general gastroenteritis, probiotics, antiemetics, GI protectants. Appropriate antidote if toxin. Other medications per aetiology. Surgery for foreign body, obstruction
	Neoplasia (insulinoma)	Blood glucose, U/S, laparotomy	Surgical excision of nodules/pancreatic resection; prednisone, frequent meals as per insulinoma protocol, GI protectants whenever on prednisone

Key: BUN, blood urea nitrogen; CBC, complete blood count; chems: serum biochemistries; CSF, cerebrospinal fluid; C&S, culture and sensitivities; DIM, disseminated idiopathic myofasciitis; ECG, electrocardiogram; FNA, fine needle aspirate; FRSCV, ferret systemic coronavirus. GI, gastrointestinal; hCG, human chorionic gonadotrophin; Hx, history; IBD, inflammatory bowel disease; IO, intraosseus; IV, intravenous; KOH, potassium hydroxide; LSA, lymphosarcoma; NSAID, non-steroidal anti-inflammatory drug; Nx, necropsy; OHE, ovariohysterectomy; PCR, polymerase chain reaction; PE, physical examination; Rads, radiographs; SC, subcutaneous; Tx, treatment; UA, urinalysis; U/S, ultrasonography.

Continued

CLINICAL SIGNS	DIFFERENTIAL DIAGNOSIS	DIAGNOSTIC OPTIONS	THERAPY
	Azotaemia, renal disease	Hx, PE, CBC/chems, electrolytes, UA	Fluid diuresis and electrolyte corrections, GI protectants, antiemetics, supportive care. Feline renal diets are unproven
	Carsickness, motion sickness	Hx	Diphenhydramine, famotidine or cimetidine prior to car ride
	Rabies (rare)	Postmortem, histopathology	None. Zoonotic potential, notify public health authorities
Weakness (see also neurological signs, other aetiologies)	Hypoglycaemia due to insulinoma; sepsis, starvation, severe GI disease preventing absorption or nutrient loss through diarrhoea, hypermotility, parasitism	Hx, PE, CBC/chems, Rads (contrast study for GI disease), microbiology, U/S, exploratory laparotomy for GI biopsy, faecal flotation and smear	Per aetiology. Insulinoma protocol if hypoglycaemic. Appropriate antimicrobials/antiparasitics, GI protectants if GI disease present
	Hyperadrenocorticism (adrenal disease)	Hx, PE, serum endocrine panel, CBC/chems, U/S, exploratory laparotomy (adrenalectomy/ biopsy, histopathology)	Adrenal disease protocols
	Anaemia due to LSA, blood loss, hyperoestrinism (intact female, ovarian remnant, advanced adrenal disease)	Hx, PE, CBC/chems, bone marrow biopsy, serum endocrine panel, exploratory laparotomy for ovarian remnant, adrenal neoplasm	Appropriate per aetiology. Blood transfusion(s), erythropoietin; LSA protocol. Surgery (OHE, ovarian remnant, adrenal neoplasm). Adrenal disease protocol
	Cardiomyopathy (dilatative, hypertrophic, heartworm)	Hx, PE, cardiac evaluation, occult heartworm, CBC/chems	Appropriate medications per type of cardiomyopathy. Heartworm protocol
Weight loss (may/may not be anorectic, progressive, subacute or chronic condition)	Aleutian disease (chronic wasting disease)	Hx, PE, serology, CBC/chems with electrophoresis	None, supportive care
	Chronic GI foreign body including trichobezoar	Hx, PE, Rads, contrast study. CBC/chems prior to surgery	Surgical removal, supportive care
	Dental disease	PE including full oral examination, dental Rads	Endodontics, extractions, periodontal surgery, antibiotics, dental cleaning and prophylaxis. Post procedure, NSAIDs, analgesics, GI protectants
	FRSCV	PE, CBC/chems, U/S (may be fluid present or masses or lymphadenopathy). Abdominocentesis with cytology. Exploratory laparotomy for biopsies. Immunohistochemistry has been done on tissue	Unfortunately this may be diagnosed at necropsy. No truly effective treatment at this time

Continued

CLINICAL SIGNS	DIFFERENTIAL DIAGNOSIS	DIAGNOSTIC OPTIONS	THERAPY
	Gastroenteritis (ulcers, may also see diarrhoea, tarry stools, intermittent vomiting or retching)	Hx, PE, CBC/chems, Rads (contrast), C&S rectal/gastric secretions, endoscopy, biopsy, faecal flotation/smear. May find pain when palpating stomach if ulcers present, general abdominal discomfort	Appropriate antibiotics, GI protectants including sucralfate
	Proliferative bowel disease, (eosinophilic enteritis/colitis, bacterial, idiopathic), IBD. May also see diarrhoea, tarry stools, intermittent anorexia	PE, faecal flotation/smear, occult blood, Rads (may do contrast), U/S to look at thickness of bowel loops, motility; endoscopy or exploratory laparotomy, biopsy, histopathology	Enrofloxacin, amoxicillin, metronidazole, bismuth subsalicylate, chloramphenicol. IBD: azathioprine. Supportive care
	Intestinal parasites (may also see diarrhoea, intermittent anorexia)	Faecal flotation/smear, specialised tests for protozoa	Anthelminitics, antiprotozoals
	Megaoesophagus (may also see vomiting, regurgitation)	Barium swallow, Rads, endoscopy, fluoroscopy	Motility enhancers, small meals (elevated). Supportive care. Has not been conclusively linked to myasthenia gravis in the ferret, but therapy may be tried
	Mycotic disease (e.g. blastomycoses	Hx, geography, CBC/chems, Rads, fungal culture, cytology	Systemic antifungals
	Neoplasia (any)	Hx, PE, CBC/chems, serum endocrine assay, U/S, exploratory laparotomy, biopsy, histopathology	Supportive, specific depending on type of neoplasia
	Lymphosarcoma (may note marked lethargy, splenomegaly, lymphadenopathy, tumours in various tissues)	Hx, PE, Rads, CBC/chems, bone marrow biopsy, FNA, cytology of lymph nodes or effusions, histopathology	Chemotherapy protocol for LSA. Rarely can true excisional surgery be fully effective
	Mycobacterium infection (*M.avium, M.bovis, M.genavense* etc.)	Acid-fast stains, molecular typing of *Mycobacterium* (may also culture but lengthy process) taken from FNA or excision of lymph nodes or granulomas, Rads, U/S	Zoonotic potential. Treatment may be effective in some cases. Notify public health authorities – usually governmental laboratories handle samples

Key: BUN, blood urea nitrogen; CBC, complete blood count; chems: serum biochemistries; CSF, cerebrospinal fluid; C&S, culture and sensitivities; DIM, disseminated idiopathic myofasciitis; ECG, electrocardiogram; FNA, fine needle aspirate; FRSCV, ferret systemic coronavirus. GI, gastrointestinal; hCG, human chorionic gonadotrophin; Hx, history; IBD, inflammatory bowel disease; IO, intraosseus; IV, intravenous; KOH, potassium hydroxide; LSA, lymphosarcoma; NSAID, non-steroidal anti-inflammatory drug; Nx, necropsy; OHE, ovariohysterectomy; PCR, polymerase chain reaction; PE, physical examination; Rads, radiographs; SC, subcutaneous; Tx, treatment; UA, urinalysis; U/S, ultrasonography.

Continued

CLINICAL SIGNS	DIFFERENTIAL DIAGNOSIS	DIAGNOSTIC OPTIONS	THERAPY
	Pyelonephritis, renal disease (may also see fever, leukocytosis, depression, lethargy, polyuria, polydipsia, pain of the kidney(s) on palpation). Acute phase may also see anorexia, dysuria/ haematuria (if ascending from cystitis). Abdominal discomfort, restlessness. Chronic renal disease with azotaemia. May also see retching, dehydration	Hx, PE, CBC/chems including electrolytes, UA (cystocentesis), urinary C&S, cytology, U/S, Rads (excretory urogram)	Antibiotics, fluids (correct any electrolyte imbalance), analgesics
	Cardiomyopathy (may also see progressive exercise intolerance, lethargy, dyspnoea, ascites)	PE (note if pulse deficit, poor perfusion limbs, mucous membranes), cardiac evaluation, Rads, U/S	Appropriate cardiac medications depending on type of cardiomyopathy. Supportive care. Diuretics if pulmonary oedema +/- ascites

Key: BUN, blood urea nitrogen; CBC, complete blood count; chems: serum biochemistries; CSF, cerebrospinal fluid; C&S, culture and sensitivities; DIM, disseminated idiopathic myofasciitis; ECG, electrocardiogram; FNA, fine needle aspirate; FRSCV, ferret systemic coronavirus. GI, gastrointestinal; hCG, human chorionic gonadotrophin; Hx, history; IBD, inflammatory bowel disease; IO, intraosseus; IV, intravenous; KOH, potassium hydroxide; LSA, lymphosarcoma; NSAID, non-steroidal anti-inflammatory drug; Nx, necropsy; OHE, ovariohysterectomy; PCR, polymerase chain reaction; PE, physical examination; Rads, radiographs; SC, subcutaneous; Tx, treatment; UA, urinalysis; U/S, ultrasonography.

CHAPTER 1: GENERAL INFORMATION

Church B (2007) Ferret–polecat domestication: genetic, taxonomic and phylogenetic relationships. In: JH Lewington (ed). *Ferret Husbandry, Medicine and Surgery 2nd Edition*. Saunders Elsevier Limited, Philadelphia, PA. pp. 122–150

Hrapkiewicz K, Medina L (2007) Ferrets. In: Hrapkiewicz K, Medina L (eds). *Clinical Laboratory Animal Medicine, an Introduction, 3rd Edition*. Blackwell Publishing Professional, Ames, IA. pp. 242–279

Lewington JH (2007) Classification, history and current status of ferrets. In: Lewington JH (ed). *Ferret Husbandry, Medicine and Surgery, 2nd Edition*. Saunders Elsevier Limited, Philadelphia, PA. pp. 3–14

Matchett CA, Marr R, Berard FM, Cawthon AG, Swing SP (2012) *The Laboratory Ferret*. CRC Press, Boca Raton, FL

Marini RP, Otto G, Erdman S, Palley L, Fox JG (2002) Biology and diseases of ferrets. In: Fox JG, Anderson LC, Loew FM, Quimby FW(eds). *Laboratory Animal Medicine, 2nd Edition*. Academic Press, San Diego, CA. pp. 483–517

CHAPTER 2: NORMATIVE DATA INCLUDING COAT COLOURS

Church B (2007) Ferret–polecat domestication: genetic, taxonomic and phylogenetic relationships. In: Lewington JH (ed). *Ferret Husbandry, Medicine and Surgery, 2nd Edition*. Saunders Elsevier Philadelphia, PA. pp. 122–150

Fox JG (2014) Taxonomy, history, and use. In: Fox JG, Marini RP (eds). *Biology and Diseases of the Ferret, 3rd Edition*. Wiley Blackwell, Ames, IA. pp. 5–22

Lewington JH (2007) Reproduction and genetics. In: Lewington JH (ed). *Ferret Husbandry, Medicine and Surgery, 2nd Edition*. Saunders Elsevier Philadelphia, PA. pp. 86–121

Marini RP, Otto G, Erdman S, Palley L, Fox JG (2002) Biology and diseases of ferrets. In: Fox JG, Anderson LC, Loew FM, Quimby FW (eds). *Laboratory Animal Medicine, 2nd Edition*. Academic Press, San Diego, CA. pp. 483–517

Piazza S, Abitbol M, Gnirs K, Huynh M, Cauzinille L (2014) Prevalence of deafness and association with coat variations in client-owned ferrets. *Journal of the American Veterinary Medical Association* **244(9)**:1047–1052

CHAPTER 3: APPLIED CLINICAL ANATOMY AND PHYSIOLOGY

Beeber NL (2015) Surgery of Pet Ferrets. In: MJ Bojrab, D Waldron, JP Toombs (eds). *Current Techniques in Small Animal Surgery, 5th Edition*. Teton New Media, Jackson, WY. pp. 686–691

Evans H, An NQ (2014) Anatomy of the ferret. In: Fox JG, Marini RP (eds). *Biology and Diseases of the Ferret, 3rd Edition*. John Wiley & Sons, Ames, IA. pp. 23–67

Kroenke CD, Mills BD, Olavarria JF, Neil JJ (2014) Neuroanatomy of the ferret brain with focus on the cerebral cortex. In: Fox JG, Marini RP (eds). *Biology and Diseases of the Ferret, 3rd Edition*. John Wiley & Sons, Ames, IA. pp. 69–80

Lawes INC, Andrews PLR (1998) Neuroanatomy of the ferret brain. In Fox JG (ed). *Biology and Diseases of the Ferret, 2nd Edition*. Williams & Wilkins, Baltimore, MD. pp. 71–102

Lewington J (2005) Ferrets. In: O'Malley B (ed). *Clinical Anatomy and Physiology of Exotic Species. Structure and Function of Mammals, Birds, Reptiles, and Amphibians*. Elsevier Saunders, London, UK. pp. 237–261

Miller PE, Pickett JP (1989) Zygomatic salivary gland mucocele in a ferret. *Journal of the American Veterinary Medical Association* **194(10):**1437–1442

Triantafyllou A, Fletcher D, Scott J (2001) Histochemical phenotypes of von Ebner's gland of ferret and the functional implications. *Histochemical Journal* **33(3):**173–181

CHAPTER 4: FERRET HUSBANDRY, HOUSING AND BEHAVIOUR

Apfelbach R, Wester U (1977) The quantitative effect of visual and tactile stimuli on the prey-catching behaviour of ferrets. *Behavioural Processes* **2(2):**187–200

Bradley Bays T (2012) Behaviour of small mammals. In: Quesenberry KE, Carpenter JW (eds). *Ferrets, Rabbits and Rodents: Clinical Medicine and Surgery.* Elsevier, St.Louis, MO. pp. 545–556

Bulloch MJ, Tynes VV (2010) Ferrets. In: Tynes VV (ed). *Behaviour of Exotic Pets.* Wiley-Blackwell, Oxford, UK. pp. 59–68

Clapperton BK (1988) An olfactory recognition system in the ferret *Mustela furo* L. (Carnivora:Mustelidae). *Animal Behaviour* **36:**541–553

Clapperton BK (1989) Scent-marking behaviour of the ferret (*Mustela furo*). *Animal Behaviour* **38:**436–446

Fisher P (2006) Ferret behaviour. In Bradley Bays T, Lightfoot T, Mayer J (eds). *Exotic Pet Behaviour: Birds, Reptiles and Small Mammals.* Elsevier, St.Louis, MO. pp. 163–206

Kaufman LW (1980) Foraging costs and meal patterns in ferrets. *Physiology and Behavior* **25(1):**139–141

Moore DR, Semple MN, Addison (1983) Some acoustic properties of the neurons in the ferret inferior colliculus. *Brain Research* **269(1):**69–82

Poole TB (1966) Aggressive play in polecats. *Symposium of the Zoological Society of London* **18:**23–44

Poole TB (1972) Some behavioural differences between the European polecat, *Mustela putorius*, the ferret, *Mustela furo*, and their hybrids. *Journal of Zoology* **166:**25–35

Staton VW, Crowell-Davis SL (2003) Factors associated with aggression between pairs of domestic ferrets. *Journal of the American Veterinary Medical Association* **222(12):**1709–1712

Vinke CM, van Deijk R, Houx BB, Shoemaker NJ (2008) The effects of surgical and chemical castration on intermale aggression, sexual behaviour and play behaviour in the male ferret (*Mustela putorius furo*). *Applied Animal Behaviour Science* **115:**104–121

Zhang JX, Soini HA, Bruce KE (2005) Putative chemosignals of the ferret (*Mustela furo*) associated with individual and gender recognition. *Chemical Senses* **30(9):**727–737

CHAPTER 5: NUTRITION

Ball RS (2006) Issues to consider for preparing ferret as research subjects in the laboratory. *ILAR Journal* **47(4):**348–357

Bell JA (1999) Ferret nutrition. *Veterinary Clinics North America Exotic Animal Practice* **2(1):**169–192

Carpenter J, Harms C, Harrenstien L (1994) Biology and medicine of the domestic ferret: an overview. *Journal of Small Exotic Animal Medicine* **2(4):**151–162

Chen S (2010) Advanced diagnostic approaches and current medical management of insulinomas and adrenocortical disease in ferrets (*Mustela putorius furo*). *Veterinary Clinics of North America Exotic Animal Practice* **13(3):**439–452

Church RR (2007) The impact of diet on the dentition of the domesticated ferret. *Exotic DVM* **9(2):**30–39

De Matos REC, Morrisey JK (2006) Common procedures in the pet ferret. *Veterinary Clinics of North America Exotic Animal Practice* **9(2):**347–365

Eroshin VV, Reiter AM, Rosenthal K, *et al.* (2011) Oral examination results in rescued ferrets: clinical findings. *Journal of Veterinary Dentistry* **48(1):**8–15

Feket S Gy, Fodor K, Prohaczik A, Andrasofszky E (2005) Comparison of feed preference and digestion of three different commercial diets for cats and ferrets. *Journal of Animal Physiology and Animal Nutrition* **89(3-6):**199–202

Fox JG, McLain DE (1998) Nutrition. In: Fox JG (ed). *Biology and Diseases of the Ferret, 2nd Edition.* Williams & Wilkins, Baltimore, MD. pp. 149–172

Hoppes SM (2010) The senile ferret (*Mustela putorius furo*). *Veterinary Clinics of North America Exotic Animal Practice* **13(1):**107–122

Johnson-Delaney CA (2014) Ferret nutrition. *Veterinary Clinics of North America Exotic Animal Practice* **17(3):**449–470

Kim Y, Chongviriyaphan N, Liu C, Russell R, Wang X-D (2006) Combined antioxidant (β-carotene, α-tocopherol and ascorbic acid) supplementation increases the levels of lung retinoic acid and inhibits the activation of mitogen-activated protein kinase in the ferret lung cancer model. *Carcinogenesis* **27(7):**1410–1419

Kim Y, Chongviriyaphan N, Liu C, Russell RM, Wang XD (2012) Combined α-tocopherol and ascorbic acid protects against smoke-induced lung squamous metaplasia in ferrets. *Lung Cancer* **75(1):**15–23

Kupersmith DS (1998) A practical overview of small mammal nutrition. *Seminars in Avian Exotic Pet Medicine* **7(3):**141–147

Lederman JD, Overton KM, Hofmann NE, *et al.* (1998) Ferrets (*Mustela putorius furo*) inefficiently convert β-carotene to vitamin A. *Journal of Nutrition* **128(2):**271–279

Lewington JH (2007) Nutrition. In: Lewington JH (ed). *Ferret Husbandry, Medicine and Surgery, 2nd Edition*. Saunders Elsevier Limited, Philadelphia, PA. pp. 57–85

Li X, Glser D, Li W, *et al.* (2009) Analyses of sweet receptor gene (Tas1r2) and preference for sweet stimuli in species of carnivore. *Journal of Heredity* **100(supplement 1):**890–100

Liu C, Russell R. Wang X-D (2006) Lycopene supplementation prevents smoke-induced changes in p53, p53 phosphorylation, cell proliferation, and apoptosis in the gastric mucosa of ferrets. *Journal of Nutrition* **136:**106–112

Matchett C, Marr R, Berard F, *et al.* (2012) *The Laboratory Ferret. A Volume in the Laboratory Animal Pocket Reference Series*. CRC Press, Boca Raton, FL. pp. 16–17

Mazuri Reference Guide (2015) Available at Mazuri®/PMI International Company LLC, Brentwood, MO. www.mazuri.cl/mazuri-diet-reference-guide.pdf; www.mazuri.com. Accessed 11 May 2015

McKimmey V (2002) Ferret kits. In: Gage LJ (ed). *Hand-rearing Wild and Domestic Mammals*. Iowa State Press, Ames, IA. pp. 203–206

Orcutt CJ (2003) Ferret urogenital diseases. *Veterinary Clinics of North America Exotic Animal Practice* **6(1):**113–138

Powers LV, Brown SA (2012) Basic anatomy, physiology, and husbandry. In: Quesenberry KE, Carpenter JW (eds). *Ferrets, Rabbits, and Rodents Clinical Medicine and Surgery, 3rd Edition*. Elsevier Saunders, St. Louis, MO. pp. 1–12

Sanchez J, Fuster A, Oliver P, Palou A, Pico C (2009) Effects of β-carotene supplementation on adipose tissue thermogenic capacity in ferrets (*Mustela putorius furo*). *British Journal of Nutrition* **102:**1686–1694

Sundaresan P, Marmillot P, Liu Q, *et al.* (2005) Effects of dietary taurocholate, fat and protein on the storage and metabolism of dietary beta-carotene and alpha-tocopherol in ferrets. *International Journal of Vitamin Nutritional Research* **75(2):**133–41

CHAPTER 6: REPRODUCTION BIOLOGY

Fox JG, Bell JA, Broome R (2014) Growth and reproduction. In: Fox JG, Marini RP (eds). *Biology and Diseases of the Ferret, 3rd Edition*. John Wiley & Sons, Ames, IA. pp. 187–209

Lewington JH (2007) Reproduction and genetics. In: Lewington JH (ed). *Ferret Husbandry, Medicine and Surgery, 2nd Edition*. Saunders Elsevier, Philadelphia, PA. pp. 86–121

CHAPTER 8: PHYSICAL EXAMINATION

Chitty JR (2009) Physical examination and emergency care of the ferret. In: Keeble E, Meredith A (eds). *BSAVA Manual of Rodents and Ferrets*. BSAVA, Gloucester, UK. pp. 205–218

Ivey E, Morrissey J (1999) Ferrets: Examination and Preventive Medicine. *Veterinary Clinics North America: Exotic Animal Practice* **2(2):**471–494

Lewington JH (2007) Ferret handling, hospitalisation and diagnostic techniques. In: Lewington JH (ed). *Ferret Husbandry Medicine and Surgery, 2nd Edition*. Elsevier, Philadelphia, PA. pp. 151–166

Quesenberry KE, Orcutt C (2011) Basic approach to veterinary care. In: Quesenberry KE, Carpenter JW (eds). *Ferrets, Rabbits, and Rodents, 3rd Edition*. Saunders, Philadelphia, PA pp. 13–26

CHAPTER 9: FERRET PREVENTIVE CARE

Chitty JR (2009) Biology and husbandry of the ferret. In: Keeble E, Meredith A (eds). *BSAVA Manual of Rodents and Ferrets*. BSAVA, Gloucester, UK. pp. 193–204

Lewington JH (2007) Endocrine diseases. In: Lewington JH (ed). *Ferret Husbandry Medicine and Surgery, 2nd Edition*. Elsevier, Philadelphia, PA. pp. 346–379

Schoemacher N (2009) Ferrets: endocrine and neoplastic diseases. In: Keeble E, Meredith A (eds). *BSAVA Manual of Rodents and Ferrets*. BSAVA, Gloucester, UK. pp. 320–329

Shoemaker NJ, Schuurmans M, Moorman H, Lumeij JST (2000) Correlation between age at neutering and age at onset of hyperadrenocorticism in ferrets. *Journal of the American Veterinary Medical Association* **216(2)**:195–197

van Zeeland YR, Pabon M, Roest J, Schoemaker NJ (2014) Use of a GnRH agonist implant as alternative for surgical neutering in pet ferrets. *The Veterinary Record* **175(3)**:66

CHAPTER 10: CLINICAL TECHNIQUES

Bexfield N, Lee K (2014) *BSAVA Guide to Procedures in Small Animal Practice, 2nd Edition*. BSAVA, Gloucester, UK

Bublot I, Randolph RW, Chalvet-Monfray K, Edwards NJ (2006) The surface electrocardiogram in domestic ferrets. *Journal of Veterinary Cardiology* **8(2)**:87–93

Capello V, Lennox A (2013) *Clinical Radiology of Exotic Companion Mammals*. Wiley-Blackwell, Ames, IA

Chitty JR (2009) Physical examination and emergency care of the ferret. In: Keeble E, Meredith A (eds). *BSAVA Manual of Rodents and Ferrets*. BSAVA, Gloucester, UK. pp. 205–218

Krautwald-Junghans M, Pees M, Reese S, Tully T (2010) *Diagnostic Imaging of Exotic Pets: Birds, Small Mammals, Reptiles*. CRC Press, Boca Raton, FL

Lewington, JH (2007) *Ferret Husbandry Medicine and Surgery, 2nd Edition*. Saunders Elsevier, Philadelphia, PA

Malakoff RL, Laste NJ, Orcutt CJ (2012) Echocardiographic and electrocardiographic findings in client-owned ferrets: 95 cases (1994–2009).

Journal of the American Veterinary Medical Association **241(11)**:1484–1489

Oglesbee BL (2011) *Blackwell's Five-Minute Veterinary Consul: Small Mammal*. Wiley-Blackwell, Ames, IA

Quesenberry KE, Carpenter JW (2012) *Ferrets, Rabbits, and Rodents; Clinical Medicine and Surgery, 3rd Edition*. Elsevier Saunders, St Louis, MO

Silverman S, Tell L (2004) *Radiology of Rodents, Rabbits, and Ferrets; an Atlas of Normal Anatomy and Positioning*. Elsevier Saunders, St Louis, MO

Stepien RL, Benson KG, Forrest LJ (1999) Radiographic measurement of cardiac size in normal ferrets. *Veterinary Radiology & Ultrasound* **40(6)**:606–610

Stepien RL, Benson KG, Wenholz LJ (2000) M-mode and Doppler echocardiographic findings in normal ferrets sedated with ketamine hydrochloride and midazolam. *Veterinary Radiology & Ultrasound* **41(5)**:452–456

Wagner RA (2009) Ferret cardiology. *Veterinary Clinics of North America Exotic Animal Practice* **12(1)**:115–134

CHAPTER 11: EMERGENCY CARE

BSAVA/VPIS (2012) *Guide to Common Canine and Feline Poisons*. BSAVA, Gloucester, UK

Carpenter JW (2013) *Exotic Animal Formulary, 4th Edition*. Elsevier Saunders, St Louis, MO

Chitty JR (2009) Physical examination and emergency care of the ferret. In: Keeble E, Meredith A (eds). *BSAVA Manual of Rodents and Ferrets*. BSAVA, Gloucester, UK. pp. 205–218

Johnson-Delaney CA (2005) Ferret cardiopulmonary resuscitation. *Seminars in Avian and Exotic Pet Medicine* **14(2)**:135–-140

Lewington JH (2007) *Ferret Husbandry Medicine and Surgery, 2nd Edition*. Saunders Elsevier, Philadelphia, PA

Longley LA (2008) *Anaesthesia of Exotic Pets*. Saunders, London, UK

Meredith A (2015) *Small Animal Formulary, 9th Edition - Part B: Exotic Pets*. BSAVA, Gloucester, UK

Quesenberry KE, Carpenter JW (2012) *Ferrets, Rabbits, and Rodents; Clinical Medicine and Surgery, 3rd Edition*. Elsevier Saunders, St Louis, MO

CHAPTER 12: DISORDERS OF THE CARDIOVASCULAR SYSTEM

Andrews PL, Bower AJ, Illman O (1979) Some aspects of the physiology and anatomy of the cardiovascular system of the ferret, *Mustela putorius furo*. *Laboratory Animals* **13(3)**:215–220

Antinoff N (2002) Clinical observations in ferrets with naturally occurring heartworm disease and preliminary evaluation of treatment with ivermectin with and without melarsomine. In: *Proceedings Symposium American*

Heartworm Society: Recent Advances in Heartworm Disease. pp. 45–47

Bone L, Battles AH, Goldfarb RD, Lombard CW, Moreland AF (1988) Electrocardiographic values from clinically normal, anesthetized ferrets (*Mustela putorius furo*). *American Journal of Veterinary Research* **49(11)**:1884–1887

Bradbury C, Saunders AB, Heatley JJ, Gregory CR, Wilcox AL, Russell KE (2010) Transvenous heartworm extraction in a ferret with caval syndrome. *Journal of the American Animal Hospital Association* **46(1):**31–35

Bublot I, Randolph W, Chalvet-Monfray K, Edwards NJ (2006) The surface electrocardiogram in domestic ferrets. *Journal of Veterinary Cardiology* **8(2):**87–93

Burns R, Williams ES, O'Toole DO, Dubey JP (2003) *Toxoplasma gondii* infections in captive black-footed ferrets (*Mustela nigripes*), 1992–1998: clinical signs, serology, pathology, and prevention. *Journal of Wildlife Disease* **39(4):**787–797

Di Girolamo N, Critelli M, Zeyen U, Selleri P (2012) Ventricular septal defect in a ferret (*Mustela putorius furo*). *Journal of Small Animal Practice* **53(9):**549–553

Dudás-Györki Z, Szabó Z, Manczur F, Vörös K (2011) Echocardiographic and electrocardiographic examination of clinically healthy, conscious ferrets. *Journal of Small Animal Practice* **52(1):**18–25

Greenlee PG, Stephens E (1984) Meningeal cryptococcosis and congestive cardiomyopathy in a ferret. *Journal of the American Veterinary Medical Association* **184(7):**840–841

Heatley JJ (2007). Ferret cardiomyopathy. *Compendium's Standards of Care: Emergency and Critical Care Medicine* **8(3):**7–11

Hoefer HL (2000). Heart disease in ferrets. In: Bonagura JD (ed). *Kirk's Current Veterinary Therapy XIII: Small Animal Practice*. WB Saunders Co, Philadelphia, PA. pp. 1144–1148

Johnson-Delaney CA (2007) Ultrasonography in ferret practice. In: Lewington JH (ed). *Ferret Husbandry, Medicine and Surgery, 2nd Edition*. Butterworth-Heinemann, Oxford, UK. pp. 417–429

Kottwitz JJ, Luis-Fuentes V, Micheal B (2006) Nonbacterial thrombotic endocarditis in a ferret (*Mustela putorius furo*). *Journal of Zoo and Wildlife Medicine* **37(2):**197–201

Laniesse D, Hébert J, Larrat S, Hélie P, Pouleur-Larrat B, Belanger MC (2014) Tetralogy of Fallot in a 6-year-old albino ferret *(Mustela putorius furo)*. *Canadian Veterinary Journal* **55(5):**456–461

Lewington JH (2007) Cardiovascular disease. In: Lewington JH (ed). *Ferret Husbandry, Medicine and Surgery, 2nd Edition*. Butterworth-Heinemann, Oxford, UK. pp. 275–284

Malakoff RL, Laste NJ, Orcutt CJ (2012) Echocardiographic and electrocardiographic findings in client-owned ferrets: 95 cases (1994–2009). *Journal of the American Veterinary Medical Association* **241(11):**1484–1489

McCall JW (1998) Dirofilariasis in the domestic ferret. *Clinical Techniques in Small Animal Practice* **13(2):**109–12

Morrisey JK, Kraus MS (2012) Ferrets: cardiovascular and other diseases. In: Quesenberry KE, Carpenter JW (eds). *Ferrets, Rabbits, and Rodents: Clinical Medicine and Surgery, 3rd Edition*. Saunders, St. Louis, MO. pp. 62–77

Orcutt C, Malakoff R (2009) Ferrets: cardiovascular and respiratory system disorders. In: Keeble E, Meredith A (eds). *BSAVA Manual of Rodents and Ferrets*. BSAVA, Quedgeley, UK. pp. 282–290

Olin JM, Smith TJ, Talcott MR (1997) Evaluation of non-invasive monitoring techniques in domestic ferrets (*Mustela putorius furo*). *American Journal of Veterinary Research* **58(10):**1065–1069

Onuma M, Kondo H, Ono S, Ueki M, Shibuya H, Sato T (2009) Radiographic measurement of cardiac size in 64 ferrets. *Journal of Veterinary Medical Science* **71(3):**355–358

Powers LV (2011) Evaluation and management of bradyarrhythmias in the domestic ferret. In: *Proceedings of the Association of Exotic Mammal Veterinarians (AEMV) Scientific Program*. pp. 115–123

Sanchez-Migallon Guzman D, Mayer J, Melidone R, McCarthy RJ, McCobb E, Kavirayani A, Rush JE (2006) Pacemaker implantation in a ferret (*Mustela putorius furo*) with third degree atrioventricular block. *Veterinary Clinics of North America: Exotic Animal Practice* **9(3):**677–687

Smith SH, Bishop SP (1985) The electrocardiogram of normal ferrets and ferrets with right ventricular hypertrophy. *Laboratory Animal Science* **35(3):**268-271

Stepien RL, Benson KG, Forrest LJ (1999) Radiographic measurement of cardiac size in normal ferrets. *Veterinary Radiology and Ultrasound* **40(6):**606–610

Van Schaik-Gerritsen KM, Schoemaker NJ, Kik MJL, Beijerink NJ (2013) Atrial septal defect in a ferret (*Mustela putorius furo*). *Journal of Exotic Pet Medicine* **22(1):**70–75

Van Zeeland YRA, Wilde AC, Bosman IH, Uilenreef JJ, Egner B, Schoemaker NJ (2015). Non-invasive blood pressure measurement in minimally sedated ferrets. In: *Proceedings of the 2nd International Conference on Avian, Herpetological and Exotic Mammal Medicine*. p. 363

Vastenburg M, Boroffka S, Schoemaker NJ (2004) Echocardiographic measurements in clinically healthy ferrets anesthetized with isoflurane. *Veterinary Radiology and Ultrasound* **45(3):**228–232

Wagner RA (2006) The treatment of third degree heart block in ferrets with subcutaneous or oral isoproterenol. *Exotic DVM* **8(2):**6–7

Wagner RA (2009) Ferret cardiology. *Veterinary Clinics of North America: Exotic Animal Practice* **12(1):**115–134

Williams JG, Graham JE, Laste NJ, Rebecca L, Malakoff RL (2011) Tetralogy of Fallot in a young ferret (*Mustela putorius furo*). *Journal of Exotic Pet Medicine* **20(3):**232–236

Zandvliet MMJM (2005) Electrocardiography in psittacine birds and ferrets. *Seminars in Avian and Exotic Pet Medicine* **14(1):**34–51

CHAPTER 13: DISORDERS OF THE DIGESTIVE SYSTEM AND LIVER

Blanco MC, Fox JG, Rosenthal K, Hillyer EV, Quesenberry KE, Murphy JC (1994) Megaesophagus in 9 ferrets. *Journal of the American Veterinary Medical Association* **205:** 444–447

Burgess ME (2007) Ferret gastrointestinal and hepatic diseases. In: JH Lewington (ed). *Ferret Husbandry, Medicine and Surgery, 2nd Edition*. Saunders, Philadelphia, PA. pp. 203–223

Caligiuri R, Bellah JR, Collins BR, Ackerman N (1989) Medical and surgical management of esophageal foreign body in a ferret. *Journal of the American Veterinary Medical Association* **195(7):**969–971

Couturier J, Huynh M, Boussarie D, Cauzinille L, Shelton GD (2009) Autoimmune myasthenia gravis in a ferret. *Journal of the American Veterinary Medical Association* **235:**1462–1466

Cross BM (1987) Hepatic vascular neoplasms in a colony of ferrets. *Veterinary Pathology* **24:**94–96

Erdman SE, Correa P, Coleman LA, *et al.* (1997) Helicobacter mustelae-associated gastric MALT lymphoma in ferrets. *American Journal of Pathology* **151(1):**273–280

Fox JG, Muthupalani S, Kiupel M, Williams B (2014) Neoplastic diseases. In: Fox JG, Marini RP (eds). *Biology and Diseases of the Ferret, 3rd Edition*. Wiley Blackwell, Oxford, UK. pp. 587–625

Garcia A, Erdman SE, Xu S, *et al.* (2002) Hepatobiliary inflammation, neoplasia, and argyrophilic bacteria in a ferret colony. *Veterinary Pathology* **39:**173–179

Gary JM, Langohr IM, Lim A, Bolin S, Bolin C, Moore I, Kiupel M (2014) Enteric colonization by *Staphylococcus delphini* in four ferret kits with diarrhoea. *Journal of Comparative Pathology* **151(4):**314–317

Geyer NE, Reichle JK (2012) What's your diagnosis: gastric dilatation–volvulus. *Journal of the American Veterinary Medical Association* **241(1):**45–47

Hall BA, Ketz-Riley CJ (2011) Cholestasis and cholelithiasis in a domestic ferret (*Mustela putorius furo*). *Journal of Veterinary Diagnostic Investigation* **23(4):**836–839

Harms CA, Andrews GA (1993) Megaesophagus in a domestic ferret. *Laboratory Animal Science* **43(5):**506–508

Hauptman K, Jekl V, Knotek Z (2011) Extrahepatic biliary tract obstruction in two ferrets (*Mustela putorius furo*). *Journal of Small Animal Practice* **52(7):**371–375

Hoefer HL, Fox JG, Bell JA (2012) Gastrointestinal diseases. In: Quesenberry KE, Carpenter JW (eds). *Ferrets, Rabbits, and Rodents, 3rd Edition*. Elsevier, St. Louis, MO. pp. 27–45

Johnson-Delaney CA (2009). Anal/rectal prolapse in ferrets. *Exotic DVM* **11(2):**13–14

Johnson-Delaney CA (2005) The ferret gastrointestinal tract and *Helicobacter mustelae* infection. *Veterinary Clinics of North America Exotic Animal Practice* **8(2):**197–212

Kaye SW, Ossiboff RJ, Noonan B, *et al.* (2015) Biliary coccidiosis associated with immunosuppressive treatment of pure red cell aplasia in an adult ferret (*Mustela putorius furo*). *Journal of Exotic Pet Medicine* **24(2):**215–222

Kiupel M, Perpiñán D (2014) Viral diseases of ferrets. In: Fox JG, Marini RP (eds). *Biology and Diseases of the Ferret, 3rd Edition*. John Wiley & Sons, Ames, IA. pp. 439–517

Krueger KL, Murphy JC, Fox JG (1989) Treatment of proliferative colitis in ferrets. *Journal of the American Veterinary Medical Association* **194(10):**1435–1446

Lennox AM (2005) Gastrointestinal diseases of the ferret. *Veterinary Clinics of North America Exotic Animal Practice* **8(2):**213–225

Lennox AM (2013) GI disease in ferrets. *Clinicians Brief* Sept. pp. 76–78

Lewington JH (2007) *Ferret Husbandry, Medicine and Surgery, 2nd Edition*. Saunders, Philadelphia, PA

Marini RP, Fox JG, Taylor NS, Yan L, McColm AA, Williamson R (1999) Ranitidine bismuth citrate and clarithromycin, alone or in cvombination, for eradication of *Helicobacter mustelae* infection in ferrets. *American Journal of Veterinary Research*. **60(10):**1280–1286

Maurer KJ, Fox JG (2014) Diseases of the gastrointestinal system. In: Fox JG, Marini RP (eds). *Biology and Diseases of the Ferret, 3rd Edition*. John Wiley & Sons, Ames, IA. pp. 363–375

Murray J, Kiupel M, Maes RK (2010) Ferret coronavirus-associated diseases. *Veterinary Clinics North America Exotic Animal Practice* **13:**543–560

Patterson MM, Fox JG, Eberhard ML (2014) Parasitic diseases. In: Fox JG , Marini RP (eds). *Biology and Diseases of the Ferret, 3rd Edition*. John Wiley & Sons, Ames, IA. pp. 553–572

Perpiñán D, López C (2008) Clinical aspects of systemic granulomatous inflammatory síndrome in ferrets (*Mustela putorius furo*). *Veterinary Record* **162(6):**180–184

Reindel JF, Evans MG (1987) Cystic mucinous hyperplasia in the gallbladder of a ferret. *Journal of Comparative Pathology* **97:**601–604

Rhody JL, Williams BH (2013) Exocrine pancreatic adenocarcinoma and associated extrahepatic biliary obstruction in a ferret. *Journal of Exotic Pet Medicine* **22(2):**206–2011

Rice LE, Stahl SJ, McLeod Jr CG (1992) Pyloric adeno-carcinoma in a ferret. *Journal of the American Veterinary Medical Association* **200(8):**1117–1118

Sledge DG, Bolin SR, Lim A, Kaloustian LL, Heller RL, Carmona FM, Kiupel M (2011) Outbreaks of severe enteric disease associated with *Eimeria furonis* infection in ferrets (*Mustela putorius furo*) of 3 densely populated groups. *Journal of the American Veterinary Medical Association* **239(12):**1584–1588

Torres-Medina A (1987) Isolation of an atypical rotavirus causing diarrhoea in neonatal ferrets. *Laboratory Animal Science* **37(2):**167–171

Williams BH, Kiupel M, West KH, Raymond JT, Grant CK, Glickman LT (2000) Coronavirus-associated epizootic catarrhal enteritis in ferrets. *Journal of the American Veterinary Medical Association* **217:**526–530

CHAPTER 14: DISORDERS OF THE ENDOCRINE SYSTEM

Bennett KR, Gaunt MC, Parker DL (2015) Constant rate infusion of glucagon as an emergency treatment for hypoglycemia in a domestic ferret (*Mustela putorius furo*). *Journal of the American Veterinary Medical Association* **246(4):**451–454

Bernard SL, Leathers CW, Brobst DF, Gorham JR (1983) Estrogen-induced bone marrow depression in ferrets. *American Journal of Veterinary Research* **44(4):**657–661

Caplan ER, Peterson ME, Mullen HS, Quesenberry KE, Rosenthal KL, Hoefer HL, Moroff SD (1996) Diagnosis and treatment of insulin-secreting pancreatic islet cell tumours in ferrets: 57 cases (1986-1994). *Journal of the American Veterinary Medical Association* **209(10):**1741–1745

Chen S (2008) Pancreatic endocrinopathies in ferrets. *Veterinary Clinics of North America: Exotic Animal Practice* **11(1):**107–123

Chen S (2010) Advanced diagnostic approaches and current medical management of insulinomas and adrenocortical disease in ferrets (*Mustela putorius furo*). *Veterinary Clinics of North America: Exotic Animal Practice* **13(3):**439–452

De Matos RE, Connolly MJ, Starkey SR, Morrisey JK (2014) Suspected primary hypoparathyroidism in a domestic ferret (*Mustela putorius furo*). *Journal of the American Veterinary Medical Association* **245(4):**419–424

Desmarchelier M, Lair S, Dunn M, Langlois I (2008) Primary hyperaldosteronism in a domestic ferret with an adrenocortical adenoma. *Journal of the American Veterinary Medical Association* **233(8):**1297–1301

Fox JG, Dangler CA, Snyder SB, Richard MJ, Thilsted JP (2000) C-Cell carcinoma (medullary thyroid carcinoma) associated with multiple endocrine neoplasms in a ferret (*Mustela putorius*). *Veterinary Pathology* **37(3):**278–282

Hess L (2012) Insulin glargine treatment of a ferret with diabetes mellitus. *Journal of the American Veterinary Medical Association* **241(11):**1490–1494

Kuijten AM, Schoemaker NJ, Voorhout G (2007) Ultrasonographic visualization of the adrenal glands of healthy and hyperadrenocorticoid ferrets. *Journal of the American Animal Hospital Association* **43(2):**78–84

Lennox AM, Wagner RA (2012) Comparison of 4.7 mg deslorelin implants and surgery for the treatment of adrenocortical disease in ferrets. *Journal of Exotic Pet Medicine* **21(4):**332–335

Miller LA, Fagerstone KA, Wagner RA, Finkler M (2013) Use of a GnRH vaccine, GonaConTM, for prevention and treatment ofadrenocortical disease (ACD) in domestic ferrets. *Vaccine* **31:**4619–4623

Miller CM, Marini RP, Fox JG (2014) Diseases of the endocrine system. In: Fox JG, Marini RP (eds). *Biology and Diseases of the Ferret, 3rd Edition*. Wiley Blackwell, Ames, IA. pp. 377–400

Neuwirth L, Collins B, Calderwood-Mays M, Tran T (1997) *Veterinary Radiology and Ultrasound* **38(1):**69–74

O'Brien RT, Paul-Murphy J, Dubielzig RR (1996) Ultrasonography of adrenal glands in normal ferrets. *Veterinary Radiology and Ultrasound* **37(6):**445

Petritz OA, Antinoff N, Chen S, Kass PH, Paul-Murphy JR (2013) Evaluation of portable blood glucose meters for measurement of blood glucose concentration in ferrets (*Mustela putorius furo*). *Journal of the American Veterinary Medical Association* **242(3):**350–354

Quesada-Canales O, Suárez-Bonnet A, Ramírez GA, Aguirre-Sanceledonio M, Andrada M, Rivero M, de Los Monteros AE (2013) Adrenohepatic fusion in domestic ferrets (*Mustela putorius furo*). *Journal of Comparative Pathology* **149(2):**314–317

Ramer JC, Benson KG, Morrisey JK, O'Brien RT, Paul-Murphy J (2006) Effects of melatonin administration on the clinical course of adrenocortical disease in domestic ferrets. *Journal of the American Veterinary Medical Association* **229(11):**1743–1748

Rand J, Behrend E, Gunn-Moore D, Campbell-Ward M (2013) *Clinical Endocrinology of Companion Animals*. Wiley Blackwell Publishing, Ames, IA

Rosenthal KL, Peterson ME, Quesenberry KE, Hillyer, EV, Beeber NL, Moroff SD, Lothrop Jr CD (1993) Hyperadrenocorticism associated with adrenocortical tumour or nodular hyperplasia of the adrenal gland in ferrets: 50 cases (1987–1991). *Journal of the American Veterinary Medical Association* **203(2):**271–275

Rosenthal KL, Peterson ME, Quesenberry KE, Lothrop CD (1993) Evaluation of plasma cortisol and corticosterone responses to synthetic adrenocorticotropic hormone administration in ferrets. *American Journal of Veterinary Research* **54(1):**29–31

Rosenthal KL (1997) Adrenal gland disease in ferrets. *Veterinary Clinics of North America, Small Animal Practice* **27(2):**401–418

Rosenthal KL, Wyre NR (2012) Endocrine diseases. In: Quesenberry KE, Carpenter JW (eds). *Ferrets, Rabbits and Rodents: Clinical Medicine and Surgery, 3rd Edition*. Elsevier, St. Louis, MO. pp. 86–102

Schoemaker NJ, Schuurmans M, Moorman H, Lumeij JT (2000) Correlation between age at neutering and age at onset of hyperadrenocorticism in ferrets. *Journal of the American Veterinary Medical Association* **216(2):**195–197

Schoemaker NJ, Teerds KJ, Mol JA, Lumeij JT, Thijssen JH, Rijnberk A (2002) The role of luteinizing hormone in the pathogenesis of hyperadrenocorticism in neutered ferrets. *Molecular and Cellular Endocrinology* **197(1):**117–125

Schoemaker NJ, van der Hage MH, Flik G, Lumeij JT, Rijnberk A (2004) Morphology of the pituitary gland in ferrets (*Mustela putorius furo*) with hyper-adrenocorticism. *Journal of Comparative Pathology* **130(4):**255–265

Schoemaker NJ, Wolfswinkel J, Mol JA, Voorhout G, Kik MJL, Lumeij JT, Rijnberk A (2004) Urinary excretion of glucocorticoids in the diagnosis of hyperadrenocorticism in ferrets. *Domestic Animal Endocrinology* **27(4):**13–24

Schoemaker NJ, Kuijten AM, Galac S (2008) Luteinizing hormone-dependent Cushing's syndrome in a pet ferret (*Mustela putorius furo*). *Domestic Animal Endocrinology* **34(3):**278–283

Van Zeeland YRA, Pabon M, Roest J, Schoemaker NJ (2014) Use of a GnRH agonist implant as alternative for surgical neutering in pet ferrets. *The Veterinary Record* **175(3):**66

Wagner RA, Bailey EM, Schneider JF, Oliver JW (2001) Leuprolide acetate treatment of adrenocortical disease in ferrets. *Journal of the American Veterinary Medical Association* **218(8):**1272–1274

Wagner RA, Piché CA, Jöchle W, Oliver JW (2005) Clinical and endocrine responses to treatment with deslorelin acetate implants in ferrets with adrenocortical disease. *American Journal of Veterinary Research* **66(5):**910–914

Wagner RA, Finkler MR, Fecteau KA, Trigg TE (2009) The treatment of adrenal cortical disease in ferrets with 4.7 mg deslorelin acetate implants. *Journal of Exotic Pet Medicine* **18(2):**146–152

Wagner RA (2012) Hypothyroidism in ferrets. In: *Proceedings of the Annual Conference of the Association of Exotic Mammal Veterinarians*. Oakland, CA. pp. 29–32

Weiss CA, Scott MV (1997) Clinical aspects and surgical treatment of hyperadrenocorticism in the domestic ferret: 94 cases (1994–1996). *Journal of the American Animal Hospital Association* **33(6):**487–493

Weiss CA, Williams BH, Scott MV (1998) Insulinoma in the ferret: clinical findings and treatment comparison of 66 cases. *Journal of the American Animal Hospital Association* **34(6):**471–475

Wilson GH, Greene CE, Greenacre CB (2003) Suspected pseudohypoparathyroidism in a domestic ferret. *Journal of the American Veterinary Medical Association* **222(8):**1093–1096

CHAPTER 15: DISORDERS OF THE EARS AND EYES

Boyd K, Smith RS, Funk AJ, Rogers TD, Dobbins RM (2007) A closer look: secondary glaucoma more likely. *Lab Animal* **36(1):**13–14

Church B (2007) Ferret–polecat domestication: genetic, taxonomic and phylogenetic relationships. In: Lewington JH (ed). *Ferret Husbandry, Medicine and Surgery*. Saunders Elsevier Ltd. Philadelphia, PA. pp. 122–150

Fujishiro T, Kawasaki H, Aihara M, *et al.* (2014) Establishment of an experimental ferret ocular hypertension model for the analysis of central visual pathway damage. *Scientific Reports* **(4):**6501–6509

Lindemann DV, Eshar D, Schumacher LL, Almes KM, Rankin AJ (2016) Pyogranulomatous panophthalmitis with systemic coronavirus disease in a domestic ferret (*Mustela putorius furo*). *Veterinary Ophthalmology* **19(2)**:167–171

Lucas J, Lucas A, Furber H, *et al.* (2000) *Mycobacterium genavense* infection in two aged ferrets with conjunctival lesions. *Australian Veterinary Journal* **78(10)**:685–689

Miller PE (1997) Ferret ophthalmology. *Seminars in Avian Exotic Pet Medicine* **6(3)**:146–51

Miller PE, Marlar AB, Dubielzig RR (1993) Cataracts in a laboratory colony of ferrets. *Laboratory Animal Science* **43(6)**:562–568

Orcutt C, Tater K (2012) Dermatologic diseases. In: Quesenberry KE, Carpenter JW (eds). *Ferrets, Rabbits, and Rodents, 3rd Edition*. Elsevier Saunders, St Louis, MO. pp. 122–131

Piazza S, Abitbol M, Gnirs K, *et al.* (2014) Prevalence of deafness and association with coat variations in client-owned ferrets. *Journal of the American Veterinary Medical Association* **244(9)**:1047–1052

Verboven CAPM, Djajadininggrat-Laanen, SC, Kitslaar W-J P, *et al.* (2014) Distichiasis in a ferret (*Mustela putorius furo*). *Veterinary Ophthalmology* **17(4)**:290–293

Williams, David L (2012) The ferret eye. *Ophthalmology of Exotic Pets*. Blackwell Publishing Ltd, London, UK. pp. 73–85

CHAPTER 16: DISORDERS OF THE HAEMIC, IMMUNOLOGICAL AND LYMPATIC SYSTEMS

Ammersbach M, Delay J, Caswell JL, *et al.* (2008) Laboratory findings, histopathology, and immunophenotype of lymphoma in domestic ferrets. *Veterinary Pathology* **45(5)**:663–673

Antinoff N, Hahn K (2004) Ferret oncology: diseases, diagnostics, and therapeutics. *Veterinary Clinics of North America: Exotic Animals* **7(3)**:579–625

Antinoff N, Williams B (2012) Neoplasia. In: Quesenberry KE, Carpenter JW (eds). *Ferrets, Rabbits, and Rodents: Clinical Medicine and Surgery, 3rd Edition*. Saunders, Philadelphia, PA. pp. 103–121

Dominguez E, Novellas R, Moya A, *et al.* (2011) Abdominal radiographic and ultrasonographic findings in ferrets with systemic coronavirus infection. *Veterinary Record* **169(9)**:231

Erdman SE, Reimann KA, Moore FM, *et al.* (1995) Transmission of chronic lymphoproliferative syndrome in ferrets. *Laboratory Investigation* **72(5)**:539–546

Erdman SE, Correa P, Coleman LA, *et al.* (1997) *Helicobacter mustelae*-associated gastric MALT lymphoma in ferrets. *American Journal of Pathology* **151(1)**:274–280

Eshar D, Mayer J, Parry NM, *et al.* (2010) Disseminated histologically confirmed *Cryptococcus spp.* infection in a domestic ferret. *Journal of the American Veterinary Medical Association* **236(7)**:770–774

Garner MM, Ramsell K, Morera N, Juan-Salles C, *et al.* (2008) Clinicopathologic features of a systemic coronavirus-associated disease resembling feline infectious peritonitis in the domestic ferret. *Veterinary Pathology* **45(2)**:236–246

Malka S, Hawkins MG, Zabolotsky SM, *et al.* (2010) Immune-mediated pure red cell aplasia in a domestic ferret. *Journal of the American Veterinary Medical Association* **237(6)**:695–700

Mayer J, Burgess K (2012) An update on ferret lymphoma: a proposal for a standardized classification of ferret lymphoma. *Journal of Exotic Pet Medicine* **21(4)**:343–346

Mayer J, Erdman SE, Fox JG (2014) Diseases of the haematopoietic system. In: Fox JG, Marini RP (eds). *Biology and Diseases of the Ferret, 3rd Edition*. Wiley-Blackwell, Hoboken, NY. pp. 311–334

Mentre V, Lafon S (2014) Detection of Aleutian disease virus in 29 healthy ferrets. *Point Veterinaire* **45(345)**:62–66

Miwa Y, Matsunaga S, Nakayama H, *et al.* (2005) Spontaneous Aleutian disease in a ferret infected with the ferret-derived Aleutian-disease virus strain. *Journal of the Japan Veterinary Association* **58(7)**:484–487

Morrisey JK, Kraus MS (2012) Cardiovascular and other diseases. In: Quesenberry KE, Carpenter JW (eds). *Ferrets, Rabbits, and Rodents: Clinical Medicine and Surgery, 3rd Edition*. Saunders, Philadelphia, PA. pp. 62–77

Peripinan D, Lopez C (2008) Clinical aspects of systemic granulomatous inflammatory syndrome in ferrets (*Mustela putorius furo*). *Veterinary Record* **162(6)**:180–184

Pedersen N (2014) An update on feline infectious peritonitis: diagnostics and therapeutics. *The Veterinary Journal* **201(2)**:133–141

Piseddu E, Trotta M, Tortoli E, *et al.* (2011) Detection and molecular characterization of *Mycobacterium celatum* as a cause of splenitis in a domestic ferret (*Mustela putorius furo*). *Journal of Comparative Pathology* **144(2)**:214–218

Shigemoto J, Muraoka Y, Wise AG, *et al.* (2014) Two cases of ferret systemic coronavirus-associated disease resembling feline infectious peritonitis in domestic ferrets in Japan. *Journal of Exotic Pet Medicine* **23(2)**:196–200

Suran JN, Wyre NR (2013) Imaging findings in 14 domestic ferrets (*Mustela putorius furo*) with lymphoma. *Veterinary Radiology and Ultrasound* **54(5)**:522–531

Welchman DB, Oxenham M, Done SH (1993) Aleutian disease in domestic ferrets: diagnostic findings and survey results. *Veterinary Record* **132(19)**:479–484

CHAPTER 17: DISORDERS OF THE MUSCULOSKELETAL SYSTEM

Anres AP (1982) Surgical repair of bilateral tibial fractures and right coxo-femoral luxation in a ferret. *Veterinary Medicine/Small Animal Clinician* **August:**1220–1221

Antinoff N, Giovanella CJ (2012) Musculoskeletal and neurologic diseases. In: Quesenberry KE, Carpenter JW (eds). *Ferrets, Rabbits, and Rodents, 3rd Edition.* Elsevier, St. Louis, MO. pp. 132–140

Camus MS, Rech, RR, Seng Choy F, Fiorello CV, Howerth EW (2009) Pathology in Practice. *Journal of the American Veterinary Medical Association.* **235(8)**:949–951

Couturer J, Huynh M, Boussarie D, Cauzinille L, Shelton GD (2009) Autoimmune myasthenia gravis in a ferret. *Journal of the American Veterinary Medical Association* **235(12)**:1462–1466

d'Ovidio, D, Melidone R, Rossi G, *et al.* (2015) Multiple congenital malformations in a ferret (*Mustela putorius furo*). *Journal of Exotic Pet Medicine* **24(1)**:92–97

Eshar D, Wyre NR, Griessmyr P, Durham A, Hoots E (2010) Diagnosis and treatment of myelo-osteolytic plasmablastic lymphoma of the femur in a domestic ferret. *Journal of the American Veterinary Medical Association* **237(4)**:407–414

Fox JG (2014) Other systemic diseases. In: Fox JG, Marini RP (eds). *Biology and Diseases of the Ferret, 3rd Edition.* John Wiley & Sons, Ames, IA. pp. 421–438

Frederick MA (1981) Intervertebral disc syndrome in a domestic ferret. *Veterinary Medicine/Small Animal Clinician* **June:**835

Garner MM, Ramsell K, Schoemaker NJ, *et al.* (2007) Myofasciitis in the domestic ferret. *Veterinary Pathology* **44(1)**:25–38

Golini L, Di Guardo G, Bonnafous L, Marruchella G (2009) Pathology in Practice. *Journal of the American Veterinary Medical Association* **234(10)**:1263–1265

Hanley CS, Gieger T, Frank P (2004) What is your diagnosis? *Journal of the American Veterinary Medical Association* **225(11)**:1665–1666

JensenWA, Myers RK, Liu CH (1985) Osteoma in a ferret. *Journal of the American Veterinary Medical Association* **187(12)**:1375–1376

Maguire R, Reavill DR, Maguire P, Jenkins JR (2014) Chondrosarcoma associated with the appendicular skeleton of 2 domestic ferrets. *Journal of Exotic Pet Medicine* **23(2)**:165–171

Marks AL, Gaschen L, Tully Jr TN, Grasperge BJ, Rich GA (2010) What is your diagnosis? *Journal of the American Veterinary Medical Association* **237(9)**:1033–1034

Pfent CM, Mansell J, Pool RR, Mitchell ME (2013) Pathology in Practice. *Journal of the American Veterinary Medical Association* **242(1)**:43–45

Pignon C, Jardel N (2009) Pelvic limb lameness in a ferret. *Lab Animal* **38(1)**:9–11

Proks P, Stehlik L, Paninarova M, Irova K, Hauptman K, Jekl V (2015) Congenital abnormalities of the vertebral column in ferrets. *Veterinary Radiology and Ultrasound* **56(2)**:117–123

Ramsell KD, Garner MM (2010) Disseminated idiopathic myofasciitis in ferret. *Veterinary Clinics of North America Exotic Animal Practice* **13(3)**:561–575

Suran JN, Wyre NR (2013) Imaging findings in 14 domestic ferrets (*Mustela putorius furo*) with lymphoma. *Veterinary Radiology and Ultrasound* **54(5)**:522–531

CHAPTER 18: DISORDERS OF THE NERVOUS SYSTEM

Cathers TE, Isaza R, Oehme F (2000) Acute ibuprofen toxicosis in a ferret. *Journal of the American Veterinary Medical Association* **216(9)**:1426–1429

Ferreira X (2015) An uncommon neurologic disorder in a ferret: intervertebral disc prolapse clinical case. *I CARE*, Paris, France. p. 317

Greenlee PG, Stephens E (1984) Meningeal cryptococcosis and congestive cardiomyopathy in a ferret. *Journal of the American Veterinary Medical Association* **184(7)**:840–841

Hamir AN, Niezgoda M, Rupprecht CE (2011) Recovery from and clearance of rabies virus in a domestic ferret. *Journal of the American Association for Laboratory Animal Science* **50(2)**:248–251

Lenhard A (1985) Blastomycosis in a ferret. *Journal of the American Veterinary Medical Association* **186(1)**:70–72

Lewington JH (2007) Viral, bacterial and mycotic diseases. In: Lewington JH (ed). *Ferret Husbandry, Medicine and Surgery, 2nd Edition.* Saunders Elsevier, Philadelpha, PA. pp. 169–202

Lewis W (2009) Ferrets: nervous and musculoskeletal disorders. In: Keeble E, Meredith A (eds). *BSAVA Manual of Rodents and Ferrets*. BSAVA, Quedgeley, UK. pp. 303–310

Piazza S, Abitbol M, Gnirs K, *et al.* (2014) Prevalence of deafness and association with coat variations in client-owned ferrets. *Journal of the American Veterinary Medical Association* **244(9):**1047–1052

Yui T, Ohmachi T, Matsuda K, *et al.* (2015) Histochemical and immunohistochemical characterization of chordoma in ferrets. *Journal of Veterinary Medical Science* **77(4):**467–473

CHAPTER 19: DISORDERS OF THE ORAL CAVITY AND TEETH

Beckman B, Legendre L (2002) Regional nerve blocks for oral surgery in companion animals. *Compendium* **24(6):**439–442

Church B (2007) Ferret dentition and pathology. In: Lewington JH (ed). *Ferret Husbandry, Medicine and Surgery, 2nd Edition*. Saunders Elsevier, Edinburgh, UK. pp. 467–485

Church RR (2007) The impact of diet on the dentition of the domesticated ferret. *Exotic DVM* **9(2):**30–39

Eroshin VV, Reiter AM, Rosenthal K, *et al.* (2011) Oral examination results in rescued ferrets: clinical findings. *Journal of Veterinary Dentistry* **28(1):**8–15

Evans HE, An NQ (1998) Anatomy of the ferret. In: Fox JH (ed). *Biology and Diseases of the Ferret, 2nd Edition*. Williams & Wilkins, Baltimore, MD. pp. 19–69

Fisher RG, Edwardsson S, Klinge B (1994) Oral microflora of the ferret at the gingival sulcus and mucosa membrane in relation to ligature-induced periodontitis. *Oral Microbiology and Immunology* **9(1):**40–49

Johnson-Delaney CA (2007) Ferret dental disorders: pictorial of common clinical presentations. *Exotic DVM* **9(1):**40–43

Johnson-Delaney CA (2012) Easy-to-use antiseptic in exotics. *Veterinary Medicine* **107(5):**214

Maurer KJ, Fox JG (2014) Diseases of the gastrointestinal system. In: Fox JG, Marini RP (eds). *Biology and Diseases of the Ferret, 3rd Edition*. John Wiley & Sons, Ames, IA. pp. 363–375

Miller PE, Pickett JP (1989) Zygomatic salivary gland mucocele in a ferret. *Journal of the American Veterinary Medical Association* **194(10):**1437–1438

CHAPTER 20: DISORDERS OF THE RESPIRATORY SYSTEM

Barron HW, Rosenthal KL (2012) Respiratory diseases. In: Quesenberry KE, Carpenter JW (eds). *Ferrets, Rabbits, and Rodents: Clinical Medicine and Surgery, 3rd Edition*. Elsevier Saunders, St. Louis, MO. pp. 78–85

Carpenter JW (2013) *Exotic Animal Formulary, 4th Edition*. Elsevier Saunders, MO. pp. 560–594

Hanley CS, MacWilliams P, Giles S, Pare J (2006) Diagnosis and successful treatment of *Cryptococcus neoformans* variety *grubii* in a domestic ferret. *The Canadian Veterinary Journal* **47(10):**1015–1017

Kendrick RE (2000) Ferret respiratory diseases. *The Veterinary Clinics of North America Exotic Animal Practice* **3(2):**453–464

Kiupel M, Desjardins DR, Lim A, Bolin C, *et al.* (2012) Mycoplasmosis in ferrets. *Emerging Infectious Diseases* **18(11):**1763–1770

Kiupel M, Perpiñán D (2014) Viral diseases. In: Fox JG, Marini RP (eds). *Biology and Diseases of the Ferret, 3rd Edition*. Wiley Blackwell, Danvers, MA. pp. 439–517

Lewington JH (2007) *Ferret Husbandry, Medicine and Surgery, 2nd Edition*. Saunders Elsevier, MO.

Martínez J, Martorell J, Abarca ML, *et al.* (2012) Pyogranulomatous pleuropneumonia and mediastinitis in ferrets (*Mustela putorius furo*) associated with *Pseudomonas luteola* infection. *Journal of Comparative Pathology* **146:**4–10

Orcutt C, Malakoff R (2009) Ferrets: cardiovascular and respiratory system disorders. In: Keeble E, Meredith A (eds). *BSAVA Manual of Rodents and Ferrets*. BSAVA, Gloucester, UK. pp. 282–290

Perpiñán D, Ramis A (2011) Endogenous lipid pneumonia in a ferret. *Journal of Exotic Pet Medicine* **20(1):**51–55

Perpiñán D, Ramis A, Tomás A, Carpintero E, Bargalló F (2008) Outbreak of natural canine distemper in domestic ferrets (*Mustela putorius furo*). *The Veterinary Record* **163:**246–250

Powers LV (2009) Bacterial and parasitic diseases of ferrets. *Veterinary Clinics of North America* **12(3):**531–561

Ropstad EO, Leiva M, Peña T, Morera N, Martorell J (2011) *Cryptococcus gattii* chorioretinitis in a ferret. *Veterinary Ophthalmology* **14(4):**262–266

CHAPTER 21: DISORDERS OF THE SKIN

Hoppman E, Baron HW (2007) Ferret and rabbit dermatology. *Journal of Exotic Pet Medicine* **16(4)**:225–237

Kanfer S, Reavill DR (2013) Cutaneous neoplasia in ferrets, rabbits, and guinea pigs. *Veterinary Clinics of North America Exotic Practice* **16(3)**:579–598

Olsen GH, Turk MAM, Foil CS (1985) Disseminated cutaneous squamous cell carcinoma in a ferret. *Journal of the American Veterinary Medical Association* **186(7)**:702–703

Orcutt C, Tater K (2012) Dermatologic diseases. In: Quesenberry KE, Carpenter JW (eds). *Ferrets, Rabbits, and Rodents, Clinical Medicine and Surgery, 3rd Edition.* Elsevier, St. Louis, MO. pp. 122–131

Palmeiro BS, Roberts H (2013) Clinical approach to dermatologic disease in exotic animals. *Veterinary Clinics of North America Exotic Practice* **16(3)**:523–577

Paterson S (2006) Skin diseases and treatment of ferrets. In: Paterson S (ed). *Skin Diseases of Exotic Pets.* Blackwell Science Ltd, Oxford, UK. pp. 204–220

Rosenbaum MF, Affolter VK, Usborne AL, Beeber NL (1996) Cutaneous epitheliotropic lyumphoma in a ferret. *Journal of the American Veterinary Medicine Association* **209(8)**:1441–1444

Stauber E, Robinette, J, Basarab R, Riggs M, Bishop C (1990) Mast cell tumors in three ferrets. *Journal of the American Veterinary Medical Association* **196(5)**:766–767

Symmers WSC, Thomson APD (1953) Multiple carcinomata and focal mast-cell accumulations in the skin of a ferret (*Mustela furo L.*) with a note on other tumours in ferrets. *Journal of Pathology and Bacteriology* **65(2)**:481–493

CHAPTER 22: DISORDERS OF THE UROGENITAL SYSTEM

Antinoff N, Wiliams BH (2012) Neoplasia. In: Quesenberry KE, Carpenter JW (eds). *Ferrets, Rabbits, and Rodents Clinical Medicine and Surgery, 3rd Edition.* Elsevier, St. Louis, MO. pp. 103–121

Bulliot C (2010) Un cas de tumeur des glandes perputiales chez un feret (*Mustela putorius furo*). www.vetup.com Juin-Juillet-aout **Vol 10.2**:1–16

Coleman GD, Chavez MA, Williams BH (1998) Cystic prostatic disease associated with adrenocortical lesions in the ferret. *Veterinary Pathology* **35(6)**:547–549

Cotchin E (1980) Smooth-muscle hyperplasia and neoplasia in the ovaries of domestic ferrets (*Mustela putorius furo*). *Journal of Pathology* **130**:169–170

d'Ovidio D, Melidone R, Rossi G, *et al.* (2015) Multiple congenital malformations in a ferret (*Mustela putorius furo*. *Journal of Exotic Pet Medicine* **24(1)**:92–97

Dillberger JE (1985) Polycystic kidneys in a ferret. *Journal of the American Veterinary Medical Association* **186(1)**:74–75

Di Girolamo M, Carnimeo A, Nicoletti A, Selleri P (2015) Retrocaval ureter in a ferret. *Journal of Small Animal Practice* **56(5)**:355

Edfors CH, Ullrey DE, Aulerich RJ (1989) Prevention of urolithiasis in the ferret (*Mustela putorius furo*) with phosphoric acid. *Journal of Zoo and Wildlife Medicine* **20(1)**:12–19

Eshar D, Briscoe JA, Mai W (2013) Radiographic kidney measurements in North American pet ferrets (*Mustela furo*). *Journal of Small Animal Practice* **54**:15–19

Inoue S, Yonemaru K, Yanai T, Sakai H (2015) Mixed germ cell-sex cord-stromal tumor with a concurrent interstitial cell tumor in a ferret. *Journal of Veterinary Medical Science* **77(2)**:225–228

Jackson CN, Rogers AB, Maurer KJ, *et al.* (2008) Cystic renal disease in the domestic ferret. *Comparative Medicine* **58(2)**:161–167

Kociba GJ, Caputo CA (1981) Aplastic anemia associated with estrus in pet ferrets. *Journal of the American Veterinary Medical Association* **178(12)**:1293–1294

Liberson AJ, Newcome CD, Ackerman JI, Murphy JC, Fox JG (1983) Mastitis caused by hemolytic *Escherichia coli* in the ferret. *Journal of the American Veterinary Medical Association* **183(11)**:1179–1181

Mor N, Qualls Jr CW, Hoover JP (1992) Concurrent mammary gland hyperplasia and adrenocortical carcinoma in a domestic ferret. *Journal of the American Veterinary Medical Association* **201(12)**:1911–1912

Nelson WB (1984) Hydronephrosis in a ferret. *Veterinary Medicine* **April:** 516–521

Nguyen HT, Moreland AF, Shields RP (1979) Urolithiasis in ferrets (*Mustela putorius*). *Laboratory Animal Science* **29(2)**:243–245

Nwaokorie EE, Osborne CA, Lulich JP, Albasan H (2013) Epidemiological evaluation of cystine urolithiasis in domestic ferrets (*Mustela putorius furo*): 70 cases (1992–2009). *Journal of the American Veterinary Medical Association* **242(8)**:1099–1103

Nwaokorie EE, Osborne CA, Lulich JP, Albasa H, Lekcharoensuk C (2011) Epidemiology of struvite uroliths in ferrets: 272 cases (1981–2007). *Journal of the American Veterinary Medical Association* **239(10):**1319–1324

Peter AT, Bell JA, Manning DD, Bosu WTK (1990) Real-time ultrasonographic determination of pregnancy and gestational age in ferrets. *Laboratory Animal Science* **40(1):**91–92

Peuro DA, Walker LM, Saunders HM (1998) Bilateral perinephric pseudocysts and polycystic kidneys in a ferret. *Veterinary Radiology and Ultrasound* **39(4):**309–12

Pollock CG (2012) Disorders of the urinary and reproductive systems. In: Quesenberry KE, Carpenter JW (eds). *Ferrets, Rabbits, and Rodents Clinical Medicine and Surgery, 3rd Edition.* Elsevier, St. Louis, MO. pp. 46–61

Rosenthal KL, Peterson ME (1996) Stranguria in a castrated male ferret. *Journal of the American Veterinary Medical Association* **209(1):**62–64

Ryland LM (1982) Remission of estrus-associated anemia following ovariohysterectomy and multiple blood transfusions in a ferret. *Journal of the American Veterinary Medical Association* **181(2):**820–822

CHAPTER 23: MISCELLANEOUS CONDITIONS

Cryptococcosis

Eshar D, Mayer J, Parry NM, Williams-Fritze MJ, Bradway DS (2010) Disseminated, histologically confirmed *Cryptococcus* spp infection in a domestic ferret. *Journal of the American Veterinary Medical Association.* **236(7):**770–774

Lester SJ, Kowalewich NJ, Bartlett KH, *et al.* (2004) Clinicopathologic features of an unusual outbreak of cryptococcosis in dogs, cats, ferrets, and a bird: 38 cases (January to July 2003). *Journal of the American Veterinary Medical Association.* **225(11):**1716–1722

Malik R, Martin P, McGill J, *et al.* (2000) Successful treatment of invasive nasal cryptococcosis in a ferret. *Australian Veterinary Journal* **78:**158–159

Wyre NR, Michels D, Chen S (2013) Selected emerging diseases in ferrets. *Veterinary Clinics of North America Exotic Animals* **16(2):**469–493

Gyrovirus

Feher E, Pazar P, Kovacs E, *et al.* (2014) Molecular detection and characterization of human gyroviruses identified in the ferret fecal virome. *Archives of Virology* **159(12):**3401–3406

Feher E, Pazar P, Lengyel G, Phan TG, Banyai K (2015) Sequence and phylogenetic analysis identifies a putative novel gyrovirus 3 genotype in ferret feces. *Virus Genes* **50(1):**137–141

Hepatitis E

Cossaboom CM, Cordoba L, Cao D, Ni Y-Y, Meng X-J (2012) Complete genome sequence of hepatitis E virus from rabbits in the United States. *Journal of Virology* **86:**13124–13125

Li T-C, Yang T, Ami Y, *et al.* (2014) Complete genome of hepatitis E virus from laboratory ferrets. *Emerging Infectious Disease* **20:**1–7. Online article: http://wwwnc.cdc.gov/eid/article/20/4/13-1815_article.htm

Li TC, Yang T, Yoshizaki S, *et al.* (2016) Ferret hepatitis E virus infection induces acute hepatitis and persistent infection in ferrets. *Veterinary Microbiology* **183:**30–36

Raj VS, Smits SL, Pas SD, *et al.* (2012) Novel hepatitis E virus in ferrets, the Netherlands. *Emerging Infectious Disease* **18:**1369–1370

Smith DB, Purdy MA, Simmonds P (2013) Genetic variability and the classification of hepatitis E virus. *Journal of Virology* **87:**4161–4169

Smits SL, Raj VS, Oduber MD, *et al.* (2013) Metagenomic analysis of the ferret fecal viral flora. *PLoS One* **8:**e71595

Yang T, Kataoka M, Ami Y, *et al.* (2013) Characterization of self-assembled virus-like particles of ferret hepatitis E virus generated by recombinant baculoviruses. *Journal of Genetic Virology* **94:**2647–2656

Histoplasmosis

Greenacre CB, Dowling M, Nobrega-Lee M (2015) Histoplasmosis in a group of domestic ferrets (*Mustela putorius furo*). *Proceedings of Exotics Conference*, San Antonio, TX. Session 169, p 363

Mycobacteriosis

Byrom AE, Caley P, Paterson BM, Nugent G (2015) Feral ferrets (*Mustela furo*) as hosts and sentinels of tuberculosis in New Zealand. *New Zealand Veterinary Journal* **63(sup 1):**42–53

Lucas J, Lucas A, Furber H, *et al.* (2000) *Mycobacterium genavense* infection in two aged ferrets with conjunctival lesions. *Australian Veterinary Journal* **78(10):**685–689

Nakata M, Miwa Y, Tsuboi M, Uchida K (2014) Mycobacteriosis in a domestic ferret (*Mustela putorius furo*). *Journal of Veterinary Medical Science* **76(5):**705–709

Pseudomonas luteola

Baum B, Richter B, Reifinger M, *et al.* (2015) Pyogranulomatous panniculitis in ferrets (*Mustela putorius furo*) with intralesional demonstration of *Pseudomonas luteola*. *Journal of Comparative Pathology* **152(2–3):**114–118

Martínez J, Martorell, J, Abarca ML, *et al.* (2012) Pyogranulomatous pleuropneumonia and mediastinitis in ferrets (*Mustela putorius furo*) associated with *Pseudomonas luteola* infection. *Journal of Comparative Pathology* **146(1):**4–10

CHAPTER 24: ANAESTHESIA AND ANALGESIA

Giral M, García-Olmo DC, Gómez-Juárez M, Gómez de Segura IA (2014) Anaesthetic effects in the ferret of alfaxalone alone and in combination with medetomidine or tramadol: a pilot study. *Lab Animal* **48(4):**313–320

Hampshire V (2015) Refining analgesia strategies using lasers. *Lab Animal* **44(8):**297–298

Johnson-Delaney CA (2009) Ferrets: anaesthesia and analgesia. In: Keeble E, Meredith A (eds). *BSAVA Manual of Rodents and Ferrets*. BSAVA, Quedgeley, UK. pp. 245–253

Johnson-Delaney CA (2005) Ferret cardiopulmonary resuscitation. *Seminars in Avian and Exotic Pet Medicine* **14(2):**135–142

CHAPTER 25: COMMON SURGICAL PROCEDURES

Antinoff N, Williams B (2012) Neoplasia. In: Quesenberry KE, Carpenter JW (eds). *Ferrets, Rabbits, and Rodents Clinical Medicine and Surgery, 3rd Edition*. Elsevier, St Louis, MO. pp. 103–121

Beeber NL (2014) Surgical techniques in small exotic animals. Surgery of the ferret. In: Bojrab MJ, Waldron DR, Toombs JP (eds). *Current Techniques In Small Animal Surgery, 5th Edition*. Teton New Media, Jackson, WY. pp. 686–691

Bennet A (2008). Collateral circulation during caval occlusion in ferrets. *Proc of the Assn of Exotic Mam Vet*. p. 105

Creed JE (2014) Surgical techniques in small exotic animals. Anal sac resection in the ferret. In: Bojrab MJ, Waldron DR, Toombs JP (eds). *Current Techniques In Small Animal Surgery, 5th Edition*. Teton New Media, Jackson, WY. pp. 691–692

Creed JE, Kainer RA (1981). Surgical extirpation and related anatomy of anal sacs of the ferret. *Journal of the American Veterinary Medical Association* **179(6):**575–577

Driggers T (2008) Novel surgical technique for right-sided adrenalectomy in the ferret. *Proc of the Assn of Exotic Mam Vet*. p. 107

Fisher PG (2002) Urethrostomy and penile amputation to treat urethral obstruction and preputial masses in male ferrets. *Exotic DVM*, 3**(6):**21–25

Keeble E, Meredith A (2009) *BSAVA Manual of Rodents and Ferrets*. BSAVA, Gloucester, UK

Lewington JH (2007) Part 3 Surgery. In: Lewington JH (ed). *Ferret Husbandry Medicine and Surgery, 2nd Edition*. Saunders Elsevier, Philadelphia, PA. pp. 391–464

Miller TA, Denman DL, Lewis Jr GC (1985) Recurrent adenocarcinoma in a ferret. *Journal of the American Veterinary Medical Association* **187(8):**839–841

Mullen HS, Beeber NL (2000) Miscellaneous surgeries in ferrets. *Veterinary Clinics of North America Exotic Animal Practice* **3(3):**663–667

Protain HJ, Kutzler MA, Valentine BA (2009) Assessment of cytologic evaluation of preputial epithelial cells as a diagnostic test for detection of adrenocortical disease in castrated ferrets. *American Journal of Veterinary Research* **70(5):**619–623

Quesenberry KE, Carpenter JW (eds) (2012) *Ferrets, Rabbits and Rodents Clinical Medicine and Surgery, 3rd Edition*. Elsevier Saunders, St Louis, MO

Reavill D, Schoemaker NJ, Lennox A (2010) Ferret preputial tumors. *Proceedings of the Association of Exotic Mammal Veterinarians*. San Diego, CA. p. 103

Reichman DE, Greenberg JA (2009) Reducing surgical site infections: A review. *Reviews in Obstetrics and Gynecology* **2(4):**212–221

van Zeeland YRA, Lennox A, Quinton JF, Schoemaker NJ (2014) Prepuce and partial penile amputation for treatment of preputial gland neoplasia in two ferrets. *Journal of Small Animal Practice* **55(11):**593–596

CHAPTER 26: PAEDIATRICS

McKimmey V (2002) Ferret kits. In: Gage LJ (ed). *Hand-Rearing Wild and Domestic Mammals*. Iowa State Press, Ames, IA. pp. 203–206

Pollock CG (2012) Disorders of the urinary and reproductive systems. In: Quesenberry KE, Carpenter JW (eds). *Ferrets, Rabbits, and Rodents, 3rd Edition*. Elsevier, St Louis, MO. pp. 46–61

CHAPTER 27: GERIATRICS

Hoppes SM (2010) The senior ferret (*Mustela putorius furo*). *Veterinary Clinics of North America Exotic Animal Practice* **13(1):**107–122

Multiple authors (2009) Ferret chapters in: Keeble E, Meredith A (eds). *BSAVA Manual of Rodents and Ferrets*. BSAVA, Quedgeley, UK. pp. 193–333

Schoemaker NJ (2010) Ferrets, skunks, otters. In: Meredith A, Johnson-Delaney C (eds). *BSAVA Manual of Exotic Pets, 5th Edition*. BSAVA, Quedgeley, UK. pp. 127–138

CHAPTER 28: RESCUE CENTRE MEDICINE

Burns K (2006) The evolution of shelter medicine. *Journal of the American Veterinary Medical Association* **229(10):**1543–45

Ellis CJ (2008) Give me shelter. *Veterinary Forum* **25:**40–48

Harms CA, Stoskopf MK (2007) Outcomes of adoption of adult laboratory ferrets after gonadectomy during a veterinary student teaching exercise. *Journal of the American Association for Laboratory Animal Science* **45(4):**50–54

Koret Shelter Medicine Program, University of California at Davis. Shelter program information available. http://www.sheltermedicine.com. Accessed 31 March 2016

Prattis SM (2004) Small mammal care. In: Miller L, Zawistowski S (eds). *Shelter medicine for veterinarians and staff*. Wiley, John & Sons, Hoboken, NJ. pp. 125–140

CHAPTER 29: TOXICOLOGY

Cathers TE, Isaza R, Oehme F (2000) Acute ibuprofen toxicosis in a ferret. *Journal of the American Veterinary Medical Association* **216(9):**1426–1428

Dunayer E (2008) Toxicology of ferrets. *Veterinary Clinics of North America Exotic Animal Practice* **11(2):**301–314

Dunmayer EK (2004) Hypoglycemia following canine ingestion of xylitol-containing gum. *Veterinary and Human Toxicology* **46(2):**87–88

Graham, J (2013) Ferrets: Ibuprofen and acetaminophen toxicity. In: Mayer J, Donnelly TM (eds). *Clinical Veterinary Advisor Birds and Exotic Pets*. Elsevier Saunders, St. Louis, MO. pp. 464–465

Richardson J, Balabuszko R (2000) Managing ferret toxicosis. *Exotic DVM* **2(4):**23–26

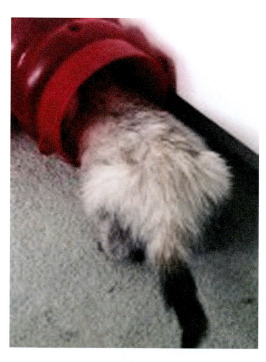